SPIRITUAL NUTRITION

Other books by Gabriel Cousens

Conscious Eating

Depression-Free for Life

Rainbow Green Live-Food Cuisine

Sevenfold Peace

Tachyon Energy:
A New Paradigm in Holistic Healing
(with David Wagner)

SPIRITUAL NUTRITION

Six Foundations for Spiritual Life and the Awakening of Kundalini

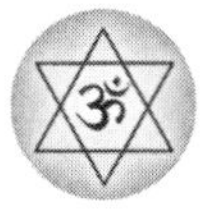

Gabriel Cousens, M.D.

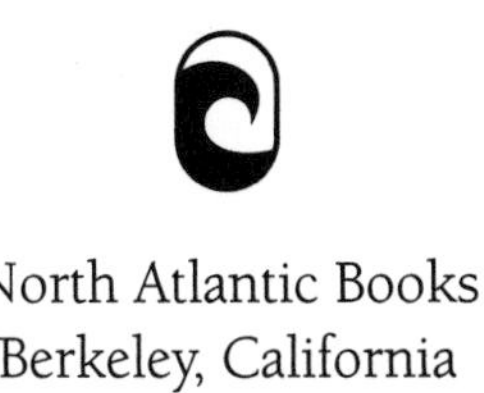

North Atlantic Books
Berkeley, California

Published by
North Atlantic Books
P.O. Box 12327
Berkeley, California 94712

and
Essene Vision Books
HC2 Box 302
Patagonia, Arizona 85624

Cover art by Jonas Hartley
Cover and book design by Maxine Ressler
Illustrations and charts by Jonas Hartley and Nan Love
Printed in the United States of America
Distributed to the book trade by Publishers Group West

Spiritual Nutrition: Six Foundations for Spiritual Life and the Awakening of Kundalini is sponsored by the Society for the Study of Native Arts and Sciences, a nonprofit educational corporation whose goals are to develop an educational and crosscultural perspective linking various scientific, social, and artistic fields; to nurture a holistic view of arts, sciences, humanities, and healing; and to publish and distribute literature on the relationship of mind, body, and nature.

Library of Congress Cataloging-in-Publication Data

Cousens, Gabriel, 1943–
Spiritual nutrition : six foundations for spiritual life and the awakening of kundalini / by Gabriel Cousens.
p. ; cm.
Originally published as: Spiritual nutrition and the rainbow diet.
Boulder, Colo. : Cassandra Press, c1986.
Includes index.
Summary: "Offers a spiritual, scientific, and intuitive blueprint for creating a diet that completely supports a person's spiritual life"—Provided by the publisher.
ISBN 1-55643-499-5 (pbk.)
1. Nutrition. 2. Kuònòdalinâi.
[DNLM: 1. Spiritual Therapies – methods. 2. Diet. 3. Medicine, Ayurvedic. 4. Yoga.]
I. Cousens, Gabriel, 1943– Spiritual nutrition and the rainbow diet. II. Title.
RA784.C6225 2005
613.2 – dc22

2004031030

2 3 4 5 6 7 8 9 MALLOY 10 09 08 07 06 05

Dedication

To Swami Muktananda Paramahansa, without whose transmission of Grace and guidance in this one's spiritual unfoldment this book would not have been able to be written.

To Swami Saraswati Prakashananda, this one's Enlightened Guru uncle whose personal guidance and Agaram Bagaram life has been a source of continual inspiration, Love, and spiritually sophisticated understanding of the post-Enlightenment maturing.

To Paavo Airola, Ph.D. and N.D., who introduced me to and personally inspired me in the field of nutrition.

To Rabbi Gershon Winkler and Kabbalist David Friedman, who helped me translate the direct apperceptions of the Truth into Kabbalistic terms and way of life.

To my soulmate and life partner, Shanti, who actively lives the Truth with me.

To my family.

To all spiritual aspirants:

> I will put my Torah in their inner parts, and write it in their hearts; and will be their God, and they shall be My people; and they shall teach no more every man his neighbor, and every man his brother, saying, 'Know the Lord;' for they shall all know Me, from the least of them to the greatest of them, sayeth the Lord . . .
>
> Jeremiah 31:32

The Torah is the living cosmic Truth of the Nothing (Ein Sof) that is already encoded in our "inner parts" (our spiritual anatomy) and heart. Spiritual Nutrition is a sacred blueprint for the awakening of our awareness to the illuminated Truth and resonance of Yah (the Divine) in our sacred spiritual anatomy (which includes the chakras, nadis, koshas, subtle bodies, and sephirotic energies). The activation of these subtle spiritual anatomies supports us in having the subjective experience of the God-radiance of who we truly are and an increase of that illumination through our ability to hold more Light. This activation helps to sustain us in the awareness of our eternal Oneness (Deveikut).

An ancient tradition says that each of the six hundred thousand people present at the communication of the Torah (Old Testament) by God to Moses on Mt. Sinai were given at least one section to interpret and share as a teaching with their brothers and sisters. In each generation these meaningful teachings of ancient wisdom are passed forward. This book is this one's sharing of Genesis 12:1 and Exodus 34:28–29.

> Get thee out of thy country, and from thy kindred, and from thy father's house, unto the land that I will show thee.
>
> GENESIS 12:1

God as the name El Shaddhai (the Nurturer) instructs Abraham: "Lech Lecha." From the viewpoint of the "culture of Liberation," (which is the focus of this book) this means *"Go to the Self"* (I AM THAT). To do this, one must let go of attachments and ego identifications with parents, culture, country, thought forms, illusion of the personality, and all identification with the body-mind-I AM complex; let go and surrender into the Divine Self. This book is a blessing to inspire and support the reader in the eternal journey of *Lech Lecha.*

> And he was there with the Lord forty days and forty nights; he did neither eat bread, nor drink water. . . . When Moses came down from Mount Sinai with the two tables of the testimony in Moses' hand, when he came down from the Mount, that Moses knew not that the skin of his face sent forth beams while He talked with him.
>
> EXODUS 43:28–29

The blessing of this book is to explain the relationship of nutrition to the Light of Communion with God so that we may journey up the mountain to partake of God's Divine sustenance.

And to the One . . . You.

Gabriel Cousens, M.D.

Please Note

Nothing in this book is intended to constitute medical advice or treatment. For development of an individualized diet or use of fasting cycles, it is advised that any person first consult his or her holistic physician. It is advised that he or she should remain under the doctor's supervision throughout any major shift in diet or while fasting.

Acknowledgments to the following for granting permission for quotes and reproductions from:

Autobiography of a Yogi, by Paramahansa Yogananda, Self-Realization Fellowship, publisher.

Tao Te Ching, by Lao Tsu, translated and copyrighted by Gia-fu Feng and Jane English, Alfred A. Knopf, Inc., publisher.

How to Get Well, Are You Confused?, Hypoglycemia: A Better Approach, and *How to Keep Slim, Healthy, and Young with Juice Fasting,* by Paavo Airola, Health Plus Publishers, publisher.

The Realms of Healing, authored and copyrighted by Stanley Krippner and Alberto Villoldo, Celestial Arts, publisher.

Live Food Longevity Recipes, by Viktoras Kulvinskas, 21st Century Publications, publisher.

Ayurveda: The Science of Self Healing, by Dr. Vas ant Lad, Lotus Press, publisher.

Kundalini: The Secret of Life, by Swami Muktananda, SYDA Foundation, publisher.

Contents

Preface

An important scientific [or spiritual] innovation rarely makes its way by gradually winning over and converting its opponents. What does happen is that its opponents gradually die out, and the next generation is familiar with it.

MAX PLANCK, THEORETICAL PHYSICIST

Self-realization is the knowing – in body, mind, and soul – that we are one with the omnipresence of God; that we do not have to pray that it come to us, that we are not merely near it at all times, but that God's omnipresence is our omnipresence; that we are just as much a part of Him now as we will ever be. All we have to do is improve our knowing.

PARAMAHANSA YOGANANDA

A generation has transitioned since the first publishing of *Spiritual Nutrition and the Rainbow Diet* (in 1986) revolutionized dietary consciousness. This new generation of readers has lived within the context of Gabriel's teachings, influenced vibrationally, as we saw ourselves changing into the at-one-ment generation within our hearts and souls. We saw the "old order" struggle through the war, politics, and "business as usual," totally in the dark of the new paradigm shift taking place in the dining room.

The Light Bearers – whether they be the cultural creatives, the wholistic camp initiates, the intuitives, those millions who have had the near death experience, the fire walkers, miracle makers, reborn Essenes, or spiritualized environmentalists – with Gabriel's redefining of spiritual frontiers, are spring boarded within a leap of faith, moving at lightning speed through the compost of a world redefined by famine, plagues, dishonesty, greed, war, terrorism, environmental toxemia, chemtrails, global warming, and mass insanity. This book helps Mother Earth detox into the world of tomorrow, which is being created in the hearts and minds of the Ones who are in "at-one-ment" with the source, "I AM THAT." More and more of the initiates are living in the eternal Now. Globally, our numbers are reaching towards the billions.

Since this transformation is so new to many, they could easily get lost within the media, swallowed in their innocence by the clouds of negativity and scholastic materialism-driven infrastructure just to end up left in despair, or even worse, in a state of numbness, munching on whole wheat tofu-burgers with organic fruit juice. Yes, Gabriel's message is timely. "Spiritual Nutrition" is the genotype with self-perpetuating inner guiding Light for our spiritualized DNA, taking quantum leaps into genetic upgrade.

This updated version, speaks to the "inner child's" current needs and creates an isle of safety, where the Light Workers can gather to be empowered, guided, and inspired to bring the Light to all those who are ready to transcend.

My story began twenty years ago. I had in the past made several attempts to meet Dr. Gabriel Cousens during my trips to California, but had to wait until we both shared the same flight to and from Yugoslavia, for the World Vegetarian Congress. Our first meeting was in total silence; I felt his special presence on the plane, without introductions. The return home was quite different. High above the clouds of confused earthly thinking, we shared experiences along the spiritual path that we had both traveled from slightly different directions. We touched upon Kundalini, kinetic mechanics of Love, God, and consciousness. I was just as excited as he was that he was creating a book on Spiritual Nutrition. Six months later, I was delighted to have the book (the first edition of *Spiritual Nutrition and the Rainbow Diet*) in my possession. The table of contents gave me an exciting menu of delicacies on which my mind was eager to feast and digest. This brother is not only Divinely inspired, but has been transformed by God in his very entrails. He tastes God as well as is one with, and dines with, yes, God.

During the last twenty years, I have witnessed an onslaught of books on nutrition that prove to be useful within a certain clinical range of individuals, but that in general create further confusion and disagreement. Finally, we have a book, *Spiritual Nutrition: Six Foundations for Spiritual Life and the Awakening of Kundalini,* that removes all contradiction.

It will become a standard for ages to come against which all other books will be measured and put into perspective of relative importance. It is truly a book on wholism that redefines the human organism on the premolecular level, and as having a relationship with all of existence.

This is not a book that any normal mortal can be expected to read in a day, but many will be enticed to go through it in a single sitting. Fasting while reading the book will help to keep the mind clear enough to understand the quantum leaps of consciousness from traditional wholistic to Divine nutrition. Reading *Spiritual Nutrition* feels like having a conversation with God over a glass of wheatgrass juice. Patiently, in the precise yet poetic language of science, spirituality, and Love, Gabriel explains the One, how we can get to know that One, and how the subtle as well as the gross universe exist and interact. We are treated to a symphony of ideas using eternal truths, well-tested theories, hypotheses, historic personalities, and spiritual phenomena as notes. Gabriel plays for us a concert of timeless, eternal wholism that oscillates our chakras with newfound happiness and outlines a natural map for activating their powers. We are shown how to bathe in an interlude of Infinite Love.

Dr. Cousens's model of Subtle Organizing Energy Fields (SOEFs), for organizing energies as they manifest in more dense forms, helps to explain the many seemingly exclusive phenomena: nutrition, breatharianism, resurrection, longevity, chakras, consciousness, and biological transmutation. We are presented with a unified theory, not only of nutrition but also of existence. He describes an energy continuum with a spectrum of laws that apply within the specific frequency range of our material plane. This theory lends itself to exploration beyond the limited precepts of nutrition into the realms of Divinity.

Dr. Cousens designs a nuclear theory of nutrition. It is of controlled fission and fusion within enzymatic cyclotrons that create new elements. These enzymatic cyclotrons control the micronuclear atomic bombs that energize our essence within the full-spectrum potential of existence. We are seduced into the experience of at-one-ment with the Source of All, our own God Presence. His poetry is divinely inspired by Love of the Divine Self and dedication to express it by Love of all. His naked personal revelation of the spiritual transformation process will leave readers eternally grateful and inspired to dedicate themselves to the inner world of adventure.

The material is subtle and abstract. With Divine kindness, Dr. Cousens keeps us from going into potential mental overload by sharing anecdotal stories for illustrating a point or personal poetry that crystallizes a moment. In each chapter, he introduces us to the intellectual terrain, then dives into the adventure of expression and play, and finally ends up summarizing, restating, unifying chapter ideas, and giving an overview from still another perspective. I never felt left behind or lost in the forest of words. Like any good teacher, he holds our hand and reassures us, for which I feel readers will be, as I was, grateful.

My first reading will certainly not be the last. *Spiritual Nutrition* has helped me a great deal to better understand my path and put more energy into correcting spots of weakness. It is a view that is taken into my everyday existence, and the SOEFs help me to understand more fully the daily phenomena of life. What I find especially exciting is that it helps to clarify the live-food concept and how the processing of food affects consciousness, energy, and spiritual aspiration. The book led me to a deeper understanding of my experiences with Kundalini energy: a reawakening that took place after a period of seven months of live food and many years of celibacy, revealing itself through physical actions in the spine, the delicacies of taste, smell of ecstatic fragrances, sounds of creation, and light of crystalline evolution as well as gifts of healing, parapsychology phenomena of ESP, astral travel, and, above all else, the meltdown of ego mass and the surrender to Love of all and desire to serve all and experience the presence of God through every manifestation. It explained my childhood communions. My experience in a seven-week coma has helped me, in retrospect, to reconfirm the experience and presence of the reality of the SOEFs as well as the holograms and vortexes of the beautiful architecture as described by Brother Gabriel.

The book is spiritual history, scientific and humanistic phenomena in a nutshell. Great thinkers have been supported and have stood on the shoulders of other great thinkers in order to see further and deeper. Dr. Cousens has built an intellectual pyramid of ideas, creating a unified field of thought.

This book is much more inclusive than the title implies. Its concepts, when applied in everyday life, ashrams, and monasteries, will lead to the highest manifestation of what some folks might call "saintly" people. It is a blueprint for creating the critical mass of conscious people necessary for the planetary transformation into a peaceful, loving, humanistic world. This book is for all God's children. For many, it will take years to read; for others, it will be understood without reading. For this book is one whose time has come to reveal the Truth to all.

As the final appreciation, I want to highlight the excellent pragmatic approach of the book. It presents an approach and information for designing our own personal Spiritual Nutrition program. It helps to clarify spiritual nutrition for the novice or even one who is old as the hills. We are inspired with the potential of total rejuvenation and filled with enthusiasm to use the given tools offered for participating in the adventure of our total fulfillment and unfoldment of our unified, individual, co-created evolutionary vision.

We are One.
All is Love,
All Ways.
Love in Service.

Enzymatically Yours,
Brother Viktoras Kulvinskas, M.S.
Live-food educator and author of *Survival into the 21st Century*
www.viktoras.org

Author's Introduction

Most of us live in the world thinking and acting as if we are the child of a barren woman – as if we were born. At some point in our evolution, we wake up and realize we are not the illusion of the body-mind complex, but THAT which exists as prior to consciousness, time, space, and Being – we were never born and will never die.

Kundalini and Liberation

The inspiration for this book came in a profound meditation in 1975 when this one received *Kundalini Shaktipat* initiation from the Enlightened spiritual teacher Swami Muktananda Paramahamsa. As consciousness emerged out of the Nothing *(B'lee mah),* a still, small voice *(chashmal)* whispered, "You should learn how to eat and live in a way that enhances the Kundalini" (the inherent spiritualizing force within each of us). Since that time, *Spiritual Nutrition and the Rainbow Diet* (the forerunner of this book), *Conscious Eating,* first and second editions, *Depression-Free for Life, Sevenfold Peace,* and *Tachyon Energy: A New Paradigm in Holistic Healing* have been published. *Spiritual Nutrition* is the second to last in this nutritional series that emerged out of that meditation. The last in this series will be on Spiritual Fasting.

This book talks about Spiritual Nutrition from the point of view of the Six Foundations for Spiritual Life. It is based on this one's spiritual, holistic medical, professional, and nutritional experience since 1975. It is being shared to support all spiritual aspirants. Its power lies in its emergence out of this one's direct personal experience with spiritual aspirants from over seventy nations, as a Liberated spiritual teacher who has been empowered to awaken *Shakti Kundalini (S'micha l'shefa/Haniha),* with thirty years practical experience with the unfolding of the Kundalini process in thousands of people, as well as the completion of the full Kundalini into the Oneness of I AM THAT in this one. This book is primarily written in the third person – using the terms "this one," "Gabriel," or "the author." This is to emphasize the shift in consciousness in which one no longer identifies with the body-mind-I AM complex.

When the vessel of the body-mind complex is strengthened and the body turns into a luminescent vehicle of Light, it serves as a doorway to open up the six *koshas* (layers of body-mind-I AM complex) to the witness consciousness of the presence and eventually the Divine Presence. This then leads to *sankalpa* and *nirvakalpa samadhi* (I AM THAT awareness), known in the Kabbalah as *Deveikut*. Eventually, we stabilize these experiences of I AM THAT into a consistent state of awareness. This is called Self-realization, or Liberation – I AM THAT awareness.

This awakening into I AM THAT is made easier and accelerated when the life force of the body-mind-I AM complex is purified and expanded until it becomes a body of Light, and the Light of the Divine shines forth. Spiritual Nutrition and the Six Foundations for Spiritual Life are designed to purify and build up the life force, or *prana*. When the life force is sufficiently purified, it merges with the I AM consciousness (of Beingness) and we are then able to spontaneously transcend time, space, and Being – to the source of awareness prior to consciousness as the I AM THAT awareness. This does not mean you can "technique" or purify your way to Liberation, however. The Six Foundations for Spiritual Life create pre-conditions that quiet the mind and draw Grace that allows us to spontaneously transcend the mind into the Nothing (I AM THAT awareness). This awakening is an act of Grace. In extremely rare cases as with Ramana Maharshi, and in our times, with Eckhart Tolle, the Grace came spontaneously prior to spiritual practice in this lifetime, but in both cases this Grace was followed by years of meditation and integration.

Spiritual Nutrition is about how to live in a way that purifies and builds the prana until ultimately the prana spontaneously merges into the I AM. It is after this point that one, through Grace, transcends the mind and merges with the Divine Self – I AM THAT.

Some of the language presented here may be new for the reader. It isn't important that the mind understand all that is written. The purpose is to surrender to the inner process of going to the Self.

The Six Foundations for Spiritual Life

Kabbalah teaches that in the beginning the finite vessels of the world were filled with Infinite Light, and they shattered because they could not hold the power of Light. *Spiritual Nutrition* is about how to repair the vessels of the body-mind complex so we can become a superconductor of the Light, and hold the Light, eternally.

The Six Foundations for Spiritual Life help us to understand the process of preparing our vessels for Whole Person Enlightenment. A key step in this process begins with a summary of the importance of veganism, live foods, spiritual fasting, and full body awakening, and how they transform us into Whole Person Enlightenment. The Six Foundations for Spiritual Life, as developed by Gabriel, are offered in Chapter 1.

Kabbalah and Yoga – Complete Paths of Liberation

This book also represents an honoring of Eastern and Western traditions. It is greatly influenced by the Torah, Kabbalah, and the mystical Essene fellowships (in which Jesus was most likely raised), and reveals some of this one's direct experiences and extensive training in a Yoga tradition. Each tradition, when deeply understood, is based in the same One God. The focus is on the merging with God – *jivanmukti* and *moksha* in the Yogic tradition, or Deveikut in the Kabbalistic tradition – as the ultimate purpose of human life.

This book offers a rare weave of the Yogic and Kabbalistic terms and teachings that are part of Gabriel's life experience. In the esoteric systems of both the Yogic path of the Kundalini and the mystical Jewish path of Kabbalah, there are many parallels that directly illustrate and help us to realize that the purpose of the spiritual path is Liberation and God-merging. This weave is an important teaching: That which we seek not only dwells within us as THAT, but exists as a living expression within the spiritual foundation of our Western culture going back more than 5,764 years. This book highlights that the Jewish tradition, especially as practiced in the esoteric Kabbalistic tradition and Living Essene Way (as taught by Gabriel), is a complete path of Liberation and God-merging. Although the full path of Liberation is not overtly recognized and practiced by many in the Jewish tradition, it clearly exists. Citing the parallel terms between the Sanskrit and Hebrew for the different states such as the void, Liberation, mantra, God-merging, meditation, and transmission of Grace clearly shows the completeness of both paths. This weave, along with the sharing of science and metaphysical science, in the service of spirit, creates an underlying integrated wonderment and sense of Oneness with all of creation. It represents this one's sense of awe as he "walks" in the mysterious paradox of the what *(Mah)* and the without what *(B'lee mah)*. *Spiritual Nutrition* shares this "sacred walk" with the reader.

A New Paradigm in Nutrition

Writing this book has been an adventure. To explore fully the relationship of nutrition to spiritual life, this one had to evolve beyond the present materialistic-mechanistic paradigm of nutrition to an expanded definition of nutrition that includes subtle energetic principles. The word *nutrient* is discussed in terms of its material, emotional, energetic, and spiritual qualities. The pillars of the materialistic-mechanistic paradigm of the last 200 years are shaken, but not discarded. The new paradigm that has evolved – the Spiritual Nutrition paradigm – more completely answers the questions: What is the purpose of nutrition? What is it we call nutrition? What is assimilated? What is that which is assimilating? What is the relationship between the nutrient assimilated and spiritual unfolding?

A new conceptual dimension of the meaning of nutrient assimilation according to these subtle energy principles is formulated. To do this adequately, a more refined model of the key energy-assimilating systems of the body is shared. This includes a detailed discussion of the body as a "human crystal" and, as such, how it functions to absorb plant material and energy into our energetic and biomolecular structures.

For proper nutrition to be of maximum benefit, it needs to be integrated into a harmonious balance of the Six Foundations practiced with Love. Please remember that the information and concepts shared in this book are given to inspire and empower the reader. Let these be as guidelines and tools, not rules. This one prays that the reader not lose sight of the right spiritual perspective for applying these concepts. Proper nutrition is best understood as a support for spiritual evolution. This book is a blueprint of how to prepare our bodies to handle the increased energy released in the quantum evolutionary leap in consciousness the world is taking. It is this one's prayer that all who read this book are benefited, and that there be an increase of peace in the world as a result of the inner peace and harmony with Nature gained from applying the understanding of Spiritual Nutrition to our lives.

When we eat in a healthy, harmonious way, our ability to attune and commune with the Divine is enhanced. With this perspective, the author suggests that rather than "living to eat," or "eating to live," *we eat to intensify our Communion with the Divine.* Our hunger for the Divine then becomes the overwhelming appetite. In this way, it is okay to become a glutton ... for the Divine.

Summary

In *Spiritual Nutrition,* the emphasis is on the live-food diet, Spiritual Fasting, the intricacies of the Kundalini/Shekhinah energies spiritualizing the body-mind-I AM complex, and the process of Liberation. New chapters are added on the role of diet in spiritual life as well as on the importance of minerals (frequencies of Light), living water, and optimal nutrition, including the issue of B_{12} for vegetarians and vegans, as well as the concept of eating to optimize phenotypic expression (genetic expression). All of the chapters have been revised and updated as necessary.

The focus is understanding how and why to turn the body-mind-I AM complex into a superconductor of the Divine. *Spiritual Nutrition* is about how to eat and live in a way to enhance our Communion (Deveikut) with the Divine. There is much more personal sharing in this new edition than was shared in the 1986 edition. It is now time to offer these insights, experiences, and poems as they were given to support the Liberation of all who are ready. It is meant to activate and support the awakening and Liberation of all Beings. This is the *dharma.* Having realized there is nothing but the One *(eyn zu-lo-to),* it is only to be shared.

Acknowledgments

Many people have put their Love and energy into the creation of this book.

The author is grateful for the patience and loving support of Shanti GoldsCousens, his life partner, who has shared, supported, and given valuable feedback at every step of the rebirthing of this book, and who helped with the three simple breathing exercises.

Love and grateful appreciation also go to Ivri Krzyz from the Tree of Life, who lovingly served as the developmental editor, copyeditor, and project manager for this book. To Yoav Agmon from Israel, who spent hours going over Hebrew and key chapters. To Rabbi David Friedman, a Safed Israel Kabbalist and artist, and Rabbi Gershon Winkler, who consulted on some of the Hebrew meanings and terms over the years. To Dr. Tru Ott, for his insights and for reviewing the mineral and water chapters.

This one wants to thank a dear brother, Kevin Ryerson, whose Love and support encouraged this one in the writing of this book, first in 1986, and for this new book. Kevin is an expert intuitive who possesses the ability to obtain highly refined bodies of information. Some of the elements of the theory in this book arose out of the seeds of the dynamic interaction of our mutual intuitive processes. Kevin and his work have also been helpful in this one's development of an understanding of the Essene way of life.

The author also thanks Davis Batson, who helped edit several key chapters and supplied the information concerning the vrittis illustration; Kiana Rose, who reviewed and gave valuable feedback on several chapters; Jonas Hartley, who created the cover artwork and all of the color illustrations; and Susan Miller Madely, who formatted a few of the charts.

The author also thanks Jane English, a Ph.D. in physics and published author and photographer, who served as science editor in the first edition of this book. The late Marcel Vogel, who had a background of 29 years as an IBM scientist and was a world-famous crystal expert, for the advice on crystals and structured water. Raffi Dillian, who shared insights on water technologies. Viktoras Kulvinskas, M.S., a world expert in live-food nutrition with a rare understanding of diet and fasting as a spiritual path, who graciously wrote the preface. Viktoras, himself, and his work have been an inspiration.

This one also wants to give loving thanks to Lisa Lissant, in whose kitchen the concept of the subtle organizing energy fields took final shape. To Adam Trombley, an astrophysicist, who helped the author understand some of the concepts of zero point physics. To Norm Mikesell, M.S., an expert in structured water, who shared his work and reviewed the sections on it. To Stephen Levine, author of *Antioxidant Adaption: Its Role in Free Radical Pathology* and avant-garde Ph.D. in biochemistry, who shared his anoxia hypothesis and reviewed the book for its biochemical accuracy. To Lee Sannella, M.D., author of *Kundalini: Psychosis or Transcendence?*, with whom he discussed the issues of the physio-Kundalini. To Father Dunstan Morissey, a forty-year Benedictine monk with whom the author enjoyed discussing biblical issues. To Bruce Lipton, Ph.D. and professor of anatomy at St. George's University School of Medicine, who checked several chapters for accuracy.

This one gives thanks and Love to all who have helped. He is grateful for God's Grace, which has allowed him to serve through the offering of this book. It has been inspiring to be part of this collective process.

Shalom-Om Shanti
Gabriel

PART I

ENERGETICS, EVOLUTION, AND SPIRITUAL ANATOMY

Introduction

Part I of this book answers the *why* questions about Spiritual Nutrition. It inspires the reader with an in-depth view of the mystical *Kundalini* – defining terms, exploring evolutionary processes, and discussing some of the intricacies of its unfolding. The Six Foundations of Spiritual Life, as developed by Gabriel, form the basis for understanding how we can nourish the Kundalini as it awakens and takes us toward the next step in the evolutionary process – *Liberation* – the purpose of life, and the purpose of this book. Unlike reporting the teachings in ancient texts, *Spiritual Nutrition* uniquely shares with the reader Gabriel's direct personal meditation and life experiences of the transformation of consciousness since the awakening of Kundalini in 1975. It is as if the Divine gave Gabriel step-by-step experiences of the unfolding of the spiritual energetics and spiritual anatomies so that he could personally explain it in detail to the contemporary spiritual aspirant. Some of the experiences are explained in prose, and some in poetry. Much of it is supported by references to highly regarded spiritual texts and masters.

A variety of spiritual anatomies and energetics are involved in the holographic spiritual unfolding. The author describes the interrelationship between the flow of the Kundalini and the *chakras, nadis, vrittis, koshas,* and *granthis.* This gives the reader greater insight into the awakening of the Kundalini. It also leads to a discussion of the reasons for and how to heal imbalanced Kundalini – information in modern and experiential cases not accessible in any other book at this time.

Once we understand the subtle systems of Kundalini – chakras, nadis, vrittis, koshas, and granthis – we can enter the next layer of subtle energetics, the subtle bodies and subtle organizing energy fields. We arrive at a deeper understanding of "aberrant" biological phenomena that cannot be explained by the current materialistic-mechanistic model of life. To answer the questions posed by the aberrant biological phenomena and to include the subtle energetics of Kundalini, we begin to realize the need for a fuller, more holistic model for life and nutrition.

As we probe deeper, we understand that we are a human crystal functioning as a series of synchronous vibrations between the solid crystals and the liquid crystals of the human body. This takes us to the understanding of bioenergetic assimilation. It ultimately helps us develop an insight into the chemistry of stress, alchemy, and meditation. When all these systems are put together in an evolutionary framework, we begin to understand the relationship of nutrition to Kundalini and transcendence. This prepares us for Part II, in which the Spiritual Nutrition paradigm helps us understand the role of nutrition in spiritual evolution and offers specific nutritional practices that support the awakening of consciousness.

Chapter 1

The Mystical Kundalini and the Six Foundations for Spiritual Life

Kundalini

Kundalini (*Shekhinah* in Hebrew) is the inner spiritualizing energy that takes us to the experiences of non-causal ecstasy, joy, peace, Love, and God awareness. These are our natural emotions in Liberation. The power of Kundalini's unfoldment activates the pre-conditions for Self-realization (Liberation). Kundalini is the Grace of God, which has the potential to transform us into the non-dualistic, holographic, living awareness of the Truth of God, of *I AM THAT.* A major purpose in understanding Spiritual Nutrition is to eat and live in a way that enhances the spiritualizing force of Kundalini. Once the Kundalini is awakened, it moves through the physical and subtle bodies, removing blocks and spiritualizing the consciousness of the aspirant. In Enlightenment, one loses the identity of aspirant and knows I AM THAT. This process of unfoldment awakens our consciousness to the higher awareness and energy of each chakra. This is the most important subtle energy system in terms of the spiritual evolution of the human species. As part of the completion process, Shakti Kundalini stored below the base of the spine merges with *Shiva* or Cosmic Awareness (the spiritual Kundalini) in the crown chakra as we disappear and enter into Self-realization (I AM THAT). This is the view from outside of the process.

Carl Jung, in *Psychological Commentary on Kundalini,* said, "When you succeed in awakening the Kundalini, so that it starts to move out of its mere potentiality, you necessarily start a world which is totally different from our world. It is the world of eternity."[1] Gopi Krishna, inspired by his own experience of Kundalini awakening, has written much to describe its meaning. He says of Kundalini, "A new center presently dormant in the average man and woman has to be activated and a more powerful stream of psychic energy must rise into the head from the base of the spine to enable human consciousness to transcend the normal limits. This is the final phase of the present evolutionary impulse in man. . . . Here reason yields to intuition and revelation appears to guide the steps of humankind. . . . This mechanism, known as Kundalini, is the real cause of all genuine spiritual and psychic phenomena, the biological basis of evolution and development of personality, the secret origin of all esoteric and occult doctrines, the master key to the unsolved mystery of creation."[2] Ramakrishna, considered by many to be one of the greatest Indian saints of the last century, taught that an individual's spiritual consciousness is not awakened unless the Kundalini is aroused. Swami Muktananda, a recent spiritual master who awakened the Kundalini energy in thousands of spiritual hopefuls, said, "It is only when the Kundalini is awakened that we become aware of our true nature, of our greatness."[3] He points out that "as long as the inner Kundalini is sleeping, it does not matter how many austerities we follow, how much Yoga we practice . . . we will never realize our identity with our inner Self. . . . The awakening of the inner Kundalini is the true beginning of the spiritual journey."[4]

Although the various Yoga traditions have been the main source of our detailed knowledge of Kundalini in the West, a spiritualizing energy that seems to be the same as Kundalini is acknowledged in many cultures. Katz, in the *Journal of Transpersonal Psychology,* describes how the Kung people of the Kalahari Desert in northwest Botswana, Africa, danced for hours to awaken the *n/um* (Kundalini) to attain the *!kia* state. He feels that the n/um is analogous to the Kundalini and the !kia is a state of transcendence.[5] He describes how about half of the Kung people were able to heat up the n/um. In the Chinese Taoist tradition, Luk, in his book *The Secrets of Chinese Meditation,* describes an awakening process that is directly parallel to Kundalini awakening.[6] In the Christian tradition, Saint Thérèse of Lisieux, when she enrolled in a Carmelite convent at the age of ten, was reported to have had several months of spontaneous spells with a "strange mélange of hallucination, comas, and convulsions."[7] Sometimes she had spontaneous movements like springing from her knees and standing on her head without using her hands. Her history is compatible with descriptions of classical Kundalini awakenings and with those reported by Lee Sannella, M.D., in *Kundalini: Psychosis or Transcendence?*[8] The ecstatic visions of the prophet Ezekiel and the psycho-physical states he describes are obvious Kundalini *kriyas*. In the Jewish-Kabbalistic system the analogous description of the *Shekhinah* in the form of *Nukba* is comparable to the Kundalini stored at the base chakra and emanates from the grandmother *Atik Yomin*. She is the crown of glory that channels the Eternal Light on all creation. In Kabbalah it is the feminine principle of the Shekhinah that descends to do the work of repairing the world. The Shekhinah descends into the realms of time, space, and Being to be the Presence in all Beings. This is an accurate description of the spiritual (cosmic) and Shakti Kundalini.

The Language of Kundalini and Liberation

As we weave the esoteric systems of both the Yogic path of the Kundalini and the mystical Jewish path of Kabbalah, it is first helpful to have a brief description of the differences in language that point to the universality of Truth. The parallel in Kabbalah to Kundalini is Shekhinah. The Shakti Kundalini initiation is *S'micha l'shefa* or *Haniha:* The void is *teheru* in Hebrew. *Par'gawd* in Hebrew is the veil between the worlds, and *eyn zu-lo-to* in Hebrew means there is Nothing but the One or I AM THAT. Transcending time, space, and Being (I AM consciousness) brings I AM THAT awareness called Self-realization or Liberation – *jivanmukti* in Yoga, or *Chaya-Yehida* consciousness in Kabbalah. In the Yogic tradition, the merging of the life force *(prana)* with the I AM consciousness is referred to as Shakti merging with Shiva in the crown chakra. In Kabbalistic tradition it is Nukba merging with *Zeir Anpin*. This integration is a pre-condition for and part of the Liberation process. When we go, prior to consciousness, into non-dual awareness (I AM THAT) we more permanently reside in the upper *sephirot* of *Binah* (Divine understanding), *Chochma* (direct knowing), and *Keter* (Divine will) – or Chaya-Yehida awareness. In Yoga, it is termed jivanmukti, which means Liberated while in the body. This merging takes us beyond the subtle existence of the I AM to the I AM THAT – *Paramatman* or *Ein Sof* – which is beyond understanding, comprehension, and description. Complete merging into Paramatman is called *moksha* – God merging or complete *Deveikut* in the Kabbalah. For simplicity in this chapter, this one has chosen to primarily stay with one system of description: the Kundalini terminology.

Kundalini, a Scientifically Acknowledged Force

In Dr. Sannella's book and through the Kundalini Crisis Clinic, of which the author was an original co-director with Dr. Sannella, we have become aware of the growing number of documented Kundalini awakenings occurring in our own Western society. A model called the physio-Kundalini cycle, so named by Izak Bentov, a physicist and meditator, has begun to evolve from observing and recording these ever-increasing Western awakenings. This cycle is a beginning scientific effort to describe the initial Kundalini awakening process from a physiological and clinical basis. The details of this process are described in Dr. Sannella's book.[9] They present a plausible physiological explanation for the initial awakening process. This model seems basically compatible with the initial stages of the classical Yoga description, except for some variance in the exact path of the energy flow after it reaches the crown chakra. The exact path is of minor significance compared with the overall shift in awareness that comes from the full awakening. As with the details of the other subtle systems, it is hard to achieve full agreement among all researchers. It is more important that this physio-Kundalini cycle obtains scientific validity and becomes a guide for helping clinicians understand that this process might be going on.

In his book, Dr. Sannella describes the physio-Kundalini cycle as a "dynamic, self-directed, self-limited process of mental and physiological purification, leading to a healthier and more developed state than what we usually consider normal."[10] The physio-Kundalini model is limited, however, in its lack of description of the subtle transformation and awakening of the human consciousness that occurs over time. Dr. Sannella alludes to this unresolved issue when he says "all the characteristic elements of the physio-Kundalini complex are included in the classic description. And yet we find quite 'ordinary' people who complete the physio-Kundalini cycle in a matter of months, whereas Yogic scriptures assign a minimum of three years for the culmination of full Kundalini awakening even in the most advanced initiates. Here we have the suggestion that full Kundalini awakening includes a larger complex, of which the physio-Kundalini process is only a part."[11] In the author's personal and clinical experience, the physio-Kundalini process is primarily a description of the initial Kundalini awakening step, which may take place almost immediately or over several months to two or more years.

There are many people who have experienced a Kundalini awakening, but because of lack of effort, discipline, interest, or awareness of the great potential, or even because of their fear of the unfolding, do not undergo a permanent transformation. They might experience profound moments of awareness in the beginning of the physio-Kundalini cycle, but without the continued and spiritually disciplined effort to nurture the unfolding power of this spiritualizing energy, profound moments of awareness become memories. The process seems to fade out.

Poetry and Power of Kundalini

The unfolding of Kundalini is the most important process in our spiritual evolution. To describe it within the limited confines of scientific terminology deprives the reader of its poetry and significance. This book represents the merging of traditional left-brained scientific hypotheses with right-brained intuitive, direct, and experiential input. At this point it seems appropriate to switch from a technical dialogue to a poetic style to communicate more multi-dimensionally.

Kundalini is the power of consciousness. As Muktananda poetically describes it, "She is the supreme creative power of the Absolute Being.... Dwelling in the center of the universe, she holds it together and maintains it. Similarly ... she dwells at the center of the human body, in the Muladhara chakra (first chakra) and controls and maintains our whole physiological system through its network of 72,000 nadis ... she makes everything work in our bodies ... our mind, senses, power of motion."[12]

Another term for Kundalini energy is prana. In Yoga, the term prana is used to describe three different manifestations of the same basic universal energy. One is the prana that is intelligent, aware of itself, and that permeates all creation as the supreme creative power of the Absolute Being. This is known as *cosmic* prana, or all-pervading or *universal* prana. The Yogic scriptures teach that Universal Consciousness evolves into prana and that the entire universe arises from prana. A scientific term we will use, analogous to universal prana, is the *virtual energy state*. It is the all-pervading, cosmic energy state from which energy condenses at a rate faster than the speed of light, to tachyon field-particles, and ultimately condenses to particles of matter moving at the speed of light (see Chapter 6). Another way the term prana is used is as the life force within the body, called *mundane* Kundalini (discussed later in this chapter). It is the form that Muktananda referred to as maintaining and controlling our whole physiological system. It is on this level, as the energizer of the human body, that the Kundalini is considered already awake. Although the vital force prana of the body is only one, there are five active forms of it at work in the body: *apana,* which expels waste; *samana,* which governs digestion on all levels and distributes nourishment in the body; *vyana,* which pervades the power of movement and governs circulation on all levels, moving from center to periphery; *udana,* which brings the energy upward in the body; and *prana,* which is breath. Prana as breath is the most common association people have with the word.

The aspect of Kundalini we refer to when we use the term Kundalini awakening is the Shakti Kundalini. This spiritual, potential energy is said to be stored in the etheric body below the base chakra. When it becomes sufficiently energized, it emerges out of its potential state and begins to move throughout the subtle nervous system, which consists of 72,000 nadis. It moves upward through the central nadi, or *sushumna.* Once activated, it begins a process of cleansing (this process is described in detail in Chapter 2).

Feeding the Kundalini

This awakening was so profound for this one, that it has been a powerful motivation for discovering all means possible for increasing the flow of spiritualizing energy in one's body. It inspired the basic theme of Spiritual Nutrition: *How do we eat and live in a way that will stimulate the awakening of, nurture, and intensify the spiritualizing energy flow of the Kundalini?*

This awakened Kundalini literally transforms the body and makes it able to withstand and conduct the more intense and subtler energies involved in spiritual evolution. Muktananda pointed out that it is only after the body has been purified that the Kundalini spiritualizing energy can act with full force. He says that "the basis of all disease and pain is the impurities which block the flow of prana in the nadis. These blockages are caused by imbalances and disorders in the three bodily humors . . . due to undisciplined habits of eating and immoderate living."[13] The main point of quoting this Yogic and Ayurvedic medical system language is not to describe the cause of all disease, but to make an important connection between Spiritual Nutrition and the unfolding, purifying, and transforming action of Kundalini. With an appropriate diet and lifestyle, the transforming and purifying action of the Kundalini takes place faster and more easily. In the following chapters this will be discussed in more detail.

When the subtle energy channels (nadis) are cleaned, the mind also becomes purified of negative thought patterns. Then a subtle process of transformation of consciousness occurs. The first stage of purification seems to correlate most closely with Dr. Sannella's physio-Kundalini process. In the author's observation of hundreds of people, after the Kundalini is awakened it usually takes from one to two years for this physio-Kundalini process to unfold. This applies to an aspirant who follows a regular spiritual discipline of meditation, devotion to God, keeping good company, living a balanced and harmonious life, and of course, following a diet supportive of the Kundalini. The second stage of permanently transforming consciousness and reaching the highest awareness seems to require not only the Grace of having the Kundalini awakened but a more heroic and dedicated personal effort. This is why Dr. Sannella reports that so many people are able to experience the physio-Kundalini cycle and yet none were reported by him to have completed the full classical cycle.

During the process of the full Kundalini spiritual transformation of consciousness, the Kundalini works to purify and awaken each chakra so that our mind merges with the highest awareness. The Kundalini energy continues to work as a spiritualizing force in the physical anatomy and in all the subtle anatomies, until it merges with the I AM consciousness of the aspirant in the Divine Oneness and awareness of the crown chakra. At this grand time, the spiritualizing process of the Kundalini is completed. One of the main purposes of Spiritual Nutrition is to share how to eat and live in a way that will enhance this Kundalini unfolding.

Shakti Kundalini, Mundane Kundalini, and Spiritual Kundalini

A model for the inner Kundalini energy flow needs to be clarified so that we can better understand the Kundalini awakening and unfolding process. Kundalini is often referred to as the "two-headed serpent" in that there are two aspects to Kundalini. One is the *spiritual* Kundalini, the all-pervading cosmic energy, the cosmic prana, or Shakti energy. The whole universe is nothing but the vibration of this cosmic prana. It is this energy that condenses to create the physical form. After the creation of the form, there is a residual cosmic energy left in the body, which is classically called Shakti Kundalini. It is said to be "coiled like a serpent" below the first chakra in the subtle body near the base of the spine. It awaits in a potential energy state ready to "spring upward." In this potential state, this Shakti Kundalini (Divine power) also supplies the vital force energy that runs all the mundane functions of the body. For clarity's sake, Gabriel has termed this partly active Shakti Kundalini as *mundane* Kundalini, and the cosmic prana as *spiritual* Kundalini. The spiritual Kundalini continually "descends" (involution) in its pure form through the crown chakra to energize directly the pineal and pituitary glands associated with it. These glands are located so close together that they create a strong electromagnetic field that oscillates within the brain tissues. The spiritual Kundalini tends particularly to move into the right or intuitive brain. From there it moves down the body energizing the different chakras and their associated organs, nerve plexuses, and glands. In this process it energetically interfaces with the force of the Shakti Kundalini arising from its source just below the base of the spine. In most cases, by the time the spiritual Kundalini reaches the stored energetic center of the Shakti Kundalini just below the base chakra, there is not enough combined energy to ignite the stored Shakti Kundalini. A certain amount of energy of the mundane Kundalini is always moving up the spinal cord area in its function as the prime life force energy of the body. As it reaches the brain, the mundane Kundalini primarily energizes the left brain, or the rational ego mind, maintaining its dualistic relationship with the spiritual Kundalini energizing the right brain. The awakening of the Shakti Kundalini requires that the combination of the spiritual and mundane Kundalini energies reach a combustion point that then sparks the awakening.

The Six Foundations for Spiritual Life

To prepare for the sparking of the purifying and spiritualizing fire of Shakti Kundalini, the integrated approach of the Six Foundations is an invaluable context in which to live. These spiritual practices prepare and maintain the physical body as a superconductor, quieting the emotions and anxieties of the mind, which helps to align the subtle bodies and allow more energy into the system. The practices also help to balance and stabilize the first three chakras as a foundation for sustaining the awakening of the superconscious upper chakras. Meditation guides us in right life and more completely aligns all seven subtle bodies so that the full organism becomes a better superconductor of the spiritual Kundalini. This is an integration of body, mind, and spirit. The Six Foundations for Spiritual Life formulated by Gabriel are:

1. **Nutrition:** *sattvic/kedusha* (holy), vegan, organic, live-food, high-mineralized, low-sugar, individualized, moderate food intake diet, well-hydrated with pure living water, and including Spiritual Fasting.
2. **Building prana (life force):** Yoga *asanas* (postures), *pranayama* (breathing practices), *Ophanim* (the energetics of the Hebrew letters), T'ai Chi, Reiki, Tachyon Energy, other energy practices, and sacred dance. These all enhance and expand the consciousness of the body-mind complex, filling it with increased life force energy or prana.
3. **Service (*seva/sheirut*) and charity (*tzedaka*):** In the process of service and charity, we are able to face our attachments to things, as well as to feel our connection to all of the family of humanity. This helps to expand consciousness through direct experience.
4. **Spiritual guidance and inspiration:** *Satsang* or *yechidut,* being in the energy of Truth in the presence of a Liberated or awakened spiritual teacher. *Satsang* gives meaning, value, heart, and energy to spiritual wisdom teachings and spiritual life energetics. *Sangha* or *chavurah (kehila)* is spending time with spiritual people or community. Expanding and refining the mind with spiritual wisdom teachings, the great scriptures such as the Zohar, the Torah, the Tao Te Ching, or the Vedas, and great mystical poetry such as that of Hafitz, Rumi, or Blake is also part of this Foundation. Wisdom literature helps formulate and focus our consciousness and expand it. Zero Point Process (Western *jnana* Yoga) as taught by Gabriel, sacred music, and spending time in Nature are also part of this Foundation.
5. **Silence:** Meditation *(hitbodedut),* prayer *(tefila),* repetition of mantra *(hagiya),* and chanting *(mizmor)* the names of God. Silence is the doorway to the Heart of God. The source of all spiritual wisdom emanates from the silence of the Divine.
6. **Kundalini Awakening:** Shaktipat initiation (S'micha l'shefa/Haniha), which is the awakening of the Divine force that is resting in potential within us. This is known as the descent of Grace. It usually occurs through a living Enlightened spiritual

> teacher, but may occur spontaneously. Once the Shakti Kundalini is activated, it begins to spontaneously move through our body, spiritualizing every cell, every aspect of the DNA, every chakra, every nadi (the channels of the subtle nervous system), every organ, and every tissue, so that consciousness becomes activated into the next evolutionary stage.

The paradox is that it is a pathless path. One cannot eat, do Yoga asanas, pray, selflessly serve, philosophize, have satsang, or even meditate to Enlightenment. The Six Foundations of Spiritual Life are not goal-oriented practices, but ways of Being that remove the *vrittis, vasanas,* or *klipot* from the mind and body. In the deep silence of the body and mind, a starting point is created that enables us to know beyond time, space, and Being the Divine Mystery of our True Self. The Six Foundations prepare us to awaken from the dream illusion of separation. The paradox is that the Six Foundations have no goal, but are ways of living that support shattering the delusion of the mind and create the pre-conditions to awaken to the Cosmic Awareness beyond all thought and experience. The spiritual experiences that come out of living the Six Foundations enhance our appetite for the Divine, but may become obstacles if we become attached to them or practice them in a goal-oriented way. It is from this perspective that the Six Foundations can best serve us. One simply needs to remember:

- We are not the body-mind-I AM complex.
- We were never born and will never die.
- One cannot lose what one never had (that is, the body-mind-I AM complex).
- One cannot attain what was never lost (Paramatman, Absolute, Enlightenment, or Infinite Light of Ein Sof).

The Six Foundations are the basic general practices in our Western culture for enhancement of the mass Enlightenment that is beginning on this planet. The Love of God is an intrinsic part of this approach. The Love of God, Divine Love, devotion to God, desire to commune with God, and surrender to God are inherent in the Six Foundations and are evolutionary impulses. They are the driving motivation behind the Six Foundations. Without Divine Love, without the burning desire to commune fully with God, the Six Foundations can become empty mechanical disciplines that have a limited impact on our spiritual evolution.

Devotion to God is the major driving force in the Kabbalistic-Jewish and Yogic traditions. It is why people seek a spiritual path. In the Eastern tradition, this Love of God is called *bhakti* Yoga. The practices of all religions and spiritual paths may also help to prepare us. Among the many, they include: Buddhism, Advaita Vedanta, Hinduism *(Sanatana Dharma)*, Zoroastrianism, Yoga, Islam, Sufism, Taoism, Christianity, Judaism, Ecstatic Kabbalah, and the Living Essene Way as taught by Gabriel.

Experiencing the Divine

One need not have the awakening of the Kundalini to experience Divine Communion. It may occur when watching the setting of the sun, when the mind becomes completely still and all time stops and one is right there in that Oneness. One of the author's first divine experiences came in the middle of a college football game. It was the last game of the season, a tie game with two minutes left to play. The author went into a state of bliss in which he experienced all on the field as One. He played perfect football for those two minutes as his team marched 80 yards to win the game in the last ten seconds. In a book titled *The Psychic Side of Sports,*[14] experiences like this are cited as common. The mind becomes so focused that we move into a meditative state.

We have the total Truth inside us all the time. Spiritual practices and the awakening of the Kundalini help us maintain contact with the awareness of our Inner Selves, rather than waiting for perfect experiences to arise spontaneously from our interaction with our environment.

Summary, Chapter 1

1. Kundalini is the Grace of God, which transforms consciousness into the non-dualistic holographic awareness of the Truth of God (I AM THAT awareness).
2. In this Kundalini process, we experience non-causal ecstasy, non-causal contentment, non-causal Love, non-causal peace, and Communion with God (Deveikut), which is our natural state.
3. There are two Kundalini energies. The mundane Kundalini emanates out of the dormant Shakti Kundalini/Shekhinah as Nukba resting below the base of the spine. It powers the physiologic functions of the body. It is a dormant remnant of the spiritual Kundalini. The spiritual Kundalini is the pure prana,

which enters through the crown chakra. The downward flow of the spiritual Kundalini into creation can be thought of as the process of involution which reaches its terminus as a dormant remnant of this cosmic Kundalini stored below the base of the spine which we call Shakti Kundalini. The Shakti Kundalini is awakened when there is a critical energetic level of intensity between the dormant Shakti Kundalini and the spiritual Kundalini to initiate the awakening. This awakening is the beginning of the next step in evolution toward Liberation.

Chapter 2

Evolution and Fruition of Kundalini into Liberation

Awakening happens as a descent of Grace. It occurs when there is enough spiritual Kundalini descending through the crown chakra to reach the energy center of the Shakti Kundalini, resting in its potential state below the base chakra, thus sparking the awakening.

An Experience of Kundalini Awakening

From this one's own direct experience witnessing the Kundalini awakening within, this one has begun to think fondly of the Kundalini as the power of God that leads us to God. It is such an incredible occurrence, such a profound ecstatic spiritual birth, that the best way this one can communicate it is to share the joy and mystery of this one's awakening. It took place during the second meeting with Swami Muktananda at a two-day meditation retreat designed to awaken the Kundalini. Muktananda activated this through a spiritual transmission called Shaktipat, a process by which a Liberated spiritual teacher with an already awakened Kundalini acts as a vehicle for the transmission of Grace of the cosmic spiritual Kundalini energy into the spiritual aspirant. This powerful energy activates the "sleeping" Shakti Kundalini energy, which is stored just below the first chakra. This is not the only way that Kundalini can be awakened, but it is powerful, effective, and considered by many to be the most direct method. It is also, historically, a traditional way. Kundalini Shaktipat transmission is referred to in the Torah's Old Testament in Deuteronomy 34:9 in the passage, "And Joshua the son of Nun was full of the spirit of wisdom, for Moses had laid his hand upon him." In Kabbalah, an accurate term for Shaktipat is S'micha l'shefa or Haniha. In the

New Testament, Shakti Kundalinipat transmission is referred to in John 20:22, which says that Jesus "blew upon them and said to them: 'Receive Holy Spirit.'" In the Yogic traditions, Shaktipat is a well recognized approach for awakening the Kundalini.

Muktananda gave Gabriel Shaktipat by hitting him with his peacock feather wand. He followed this by putting his hand over this one's mouth in a funnel and blowing directly into this one's mouth. After this he squeezed this one at the bridge of the nose and pushed his head back. After what seemed a few minutes, this one went into a deep meditation. In the midst of this, Gabriel's mouth spontaneously opened and the tongue stuck out as far as it could go. These sorts of unusual physical movements are known as kriyas, and they may also occur on emotional, mental, and spiritual levels. They may be gentle pulsations or swirling feelings over a chakra area, very vigorous physical movements, sudden changes in emotional states, spontaneous crying, rapid thought production, or spiritual visions. They are evidence of the purifying movement of the Kundalini as it travels through the nadis (subtle energy channels), spontaneously working through blocked areas of energy. Often the Kundalini puts the body into a particular physical posture to remove a specific energy block. Later it was discovered that the pose with this one's tongue sticking out is a Yoga asana (position) called the lion pose. While the lion pose was happening, there was a peaceful, wavy bliss. At some point after this, this one began to have a vision of Muktananda in which he guided this one into a fusion and awareness of the Inner Divine Self. Following this, the experience of Oneness between this one's inner world and the universe began to emerge into awareness.

A little later in the meditation, Gabriel had the inner vision of the third, fourth, and fifth chakras in their anatomical locations, all bathed in a full, golden Light. As the energy moved upward in this one's body, the eyes turned upward to the brow chakra to see Nityananda (Muktananda's guru) sitting in a lotus posture looking down at this one. As Gabriel's inner vision continued to turn upward, he experienced and saw the crown chakra blazing in what looked like thousands of lights. Sometime during this meditation, Gabriel began to experience intense pains in the sacral and lumbar areas. This back pain, in many people, is associated with the awakening of the Kundalini.

Following this awakening, Gabriel's meditation experience at home became very intense. Certain emotional issues seemed to come up intensely and then quickly pass. Gabriel continued to have more physical kriyas, including spontaneous forms of rapid and slow breathing, sequences he later found were called pranayama, Yogic breathing exercises often used to activate the Kundalini energy. About ten days after this awakening, a red rash developed on Gabriel's back, starting in the lower back, curving back and forth across the spine twice before it veered off to the left shoulder. It disappeared about a week later. Dr. Sannella and Gabriel thought it might be a stigmata representing the spiral path of the Kundalini up the spine. Gabriel also began to hear high-pitched sounds during meditation, which he later learned are called *nada*. These sounds represent the opening of higher centers.

A few weeks after the first intense session, Gabriel took another meditation retreat with Muktananda, feeling it would enhance the energy of the newly awakened Kundalini. During the retreat, Muktananda again directly channeled his activating Kundalini energy into this one. The result of this was an even more intense movement of the Kundalini energy in Gabriel's body and up the spine. Hot-cold shooting pains occurred in the upper back and neck, and there were burning pains in the thyroid area and throat region. Gabriel's head and neck spontaneously went through many different movements. Although this all seemed strange, throughout it all this one experienced a background of deep peace and a feeling of Love. As the retreat proceeded, Gabriel began to see colors and flashes of light around people, especially Muktananda. The brow chakra began to spin and pulsate. So many things seemed to be happening that it all became rather humorous. In the final meditation of the retreat, the energy began to move up Gabriel's spine with great heat and culminated in a great explosion of white Light in the head. It seemed as though this one was exploding with energy. With inner vision, this one could see his crown chakra as a golden Light, sometimes like an inverted saucer of gold and other times like thousands of golden lights. Following this explosion, this one moved into an experience of deep inner peace and knowledge. After this, as consciousness emerged out of the Nothing, a small, silent voice said, "You should learn to eat and live in a way that feeds the Kundalini." (This occurred in 1975 and is the core experience motivating the writing of this book.) In the brow chakra region, this one directly experienced a golden, brilliantly shining two-petaled lotus flower. It gave off a pure and beautiful Light. Pure ecstasy and Love became this one's total Being. While this was happening, a deep feeling of belonging and total freedom pervaded the awareness. It came with a sense of knowing that whatever the situation in life, this one could merge in this awareness and be forever content. Gabriel's consciousness and body pulsed in total ecstasy: "I AM free!" It was at this point this one realized that death did not exist for the Self. The physical body might die, but the Truth, the I AM of existence, was immortal.

This experiential report shares Gabriel's respect and feeling for the power and awesomeness of the awakened Kundalini. It has irrevocably altered this one's life. It represents only the first step of the unfolding. A little later in this initial unfolding, some of the phenomena associated with the activated Kundalini appeared to move over the top of the head and down to the stomach area. It seemed quite secondary compared to the focus of energy toward the crown chakra.

The Awakening of Shakti Kundalini

In the 1930s, when Jung wrote about the mystery of Kundalini, very few people had experienced the awakening of Kundalini or had even heard of the word Kundalini. Now Kundalini awakening is happening in mass numbers. The first Kundalini Crisis Clinic, established by Dr. Lee Sannella and Gabriel in 1976, started to supply a frame of reference and direct aid to people experiencing these awakenings. It was particularly important healing support for those in whom Kundalini awakening happened unexpectedly and spontaneously as a result of individualized practices, as compared to those in groups that acknowledged the existence of the Kundalini awakening and had some framework for integrating it.

One possible explanation for the increase in awakenings today is because of the process of *sangha* (right fellowship) plus the power of this 2000-year cycle (200 A.D.–2200 A.D.) of *prophesy,* as described by the seventeenth-century Kabbalist Moshe Haim Luzzatto. Prophesy is described as God merging (Deveikut) and delighting in this ecstatic experience of God. It is the awakening that precedes the completion of the Messianic era. As spoken in God's name by the prophet Joel (3:1–2): "I will pour out my spirit upon all flesh, and your sons and daughters will *prophesy,* your old men shall dream dreams, and your young men shall see visions, and also upon the servants and upon the handmaids in those days, will I pour out my spirit." As the time of mass awakening comes, ignorance will cease to exist in the world, and all hearts will be filled with wisdom. All humanity will become Enlightened without difficulty. In Isaiah (11:19) it says in that day "They will not do evil nor cause harm on all my holy mountain." In other words, people will be drawn to spiritual pursuits beyond material desires and evil tendencies will be transformed to good. The prophet Jeremiah (31:31–34) shared the message of *Yah* (a name of God connecting the spirit of God as breath) about this time: "I will put my Torah in their inner parts, and write it in their hearts . . . for they shall all know Me, from the least of them to the greatest of them." Zechariah (14:9) also prophesied of the awareness at the final time: "In that day shall the Lord be One and His name One." All of creation will be experienced as the scintillating Oneness of Yah as all things. It is in this Prophetic Kabbalistic context that *Spiritual Nutrition* has been written. The universe was created so we could experience the Oneness of Yah, so that we have the direct non-dual apperception of God as One – as Isaiah communicates God's message, "I AM the first and the last" (Isaiah 44:6). The spiritual technology of Spiritual Nutrition is clarified in Moshe Chaim Luzzato's *The Way of God:*

> Those who learn to become prophets do so through a number of specific techniques, which allow them to draw down to themselves Influence from Above. They remove blocks which come from the physicality of their bodies, and bring upon themselves a revelation of God's Light, which they become profoundly aware of.

We are blessed to be living in and inspired by these times. Meditation groups, spiritually oriented workshops, or even large spiritual gatherings such as peace meditations can stimulate the awakening. The increased spiritual Kundalini energy developed by the group creates enough descent of Grace that, combined with the aspirant's own inner energy and preparation, the spark may be ignited. The safest and most consistent way that a Kundalini awakening happens is through the tradition of Kundalini Shaktipat initiation (S'micha l'shefa or Haniha). This occurs when an awakened spiritual teacher with a great amount of the spiritual Kundalini flowing shares the Grace of this energy with the aspirant. When the combination of this energy with the Kundalini energy of the aspirant is enough to reach the critical ignition point, the Shakti Kundalini awakens. The sharing of this spiritual Kundalini energy through the spiritual teacher may be by look, mantra, thought, or direct touch. Such a Kundalini awakening happened to this one when Swami Muktananda actually blew his cosmic prana into this one's mouth. The awakening may often be a combination of all these ways of increasing the descending power of the spiritual Kundalini: individual preparation and build-up of the aspirant's mundane and spiritual Kundalini, group spiritual energy, and Shaktipat.

The awakening may be the intense classical variety, or it may be moderate or mild. It occurs according to the Kundalini energy build-up in each person and what his or her internal spiritual circuitry can handle. It is important to acknowledge the mild and moderate awakening, as well as the classically described awakening, as the criteria for an awakened Kundalini. For the vast majority of people, the awakening is very safe. In Gabriel's experience at the Kundalini Crisis Clinic, with Muktananda, through which tens of thousands of people were awakened, and with thousands of people over time in Gabriel's meditation groups, workshops, and at the Tree of Life, it is rare for anyone to have serious trouble with the awakening of the Kundalini. It helps to remember it is our own Divine energy that is awakened, not some foreign drug. It is, of course, comforting and helpful to have the awakening in the context of right fellowship with someone who is experienced with the workings of Kundalini.

Psychosis and Kundalini

Some claim that many patients in mental hospitals are there because of an undiagnosed Kundalini awakening. This has not been the author's experience, neither as a psychiatrist having worked in mental hospitals, nor as a spiritual teacher involved with the subtleties of Kundalini. Manic episodes, spaced-out and disorganized thinking, or intense personal and even spiritual crises are not the same as a Kundalini awakening. Labeling them as such may make people feel good, but adds confusion to the process of getting proper help. It is, however, useful to redefine and appropriately turn the crisis, whatever it is, into an opportunity for psycho-spiritual growth. It has been the author's experience, from the Kundalini Crisis Clinic and in Muktananda's main ashrams in Ganeshpuri, India and South Fallsburg, N.Y., where he often performed in the role of a psychiatrist evaluating and supporting people having serious psychological difficulties, that many of the people who had difficulties with their Kundalini awakening had a previous history of psychotic episodes or a very brittle nervous system. These people would usually be carefully stabilized and compassionately sent back home to continue their spiritual work in a less intense, Kundalini-charged situation. It is important to understand that people with this sort of background do not need to stop their spiritual work, but should be very careful about practices that artificially force the awakening of Kundalini, intensify the energy after the awakening, or that in general amplify the nervous system energy before it is ready, whether or not there has been an awakening.

A Tale of Two Siddhis (Powers)

With the awakening, a merging of the two Kundalini energies begins to take place. A dynamic polarity still exists between awakened Shakti Kundalini and spiritual Kundalini, but they begin to act synchronistically. It may be analogous to the image of two north-pole magnets facing each other as they spiral up the spine. The energy generated by this synchronistic interaction purifies and spiritualizes the body and helps to charge and awaken the chakras. The energy not only begins to move through the subtle nervous system of the whole body, but also begins to open up the sushumna, or central channel, the major path for Kundalini flow in the body. This subtle path runs vertically in the etheric body along the spine.

The more we become a superconductor for the flow of this awakened Kundalini and for the influx of the spiritual Kundalini into the system, the more actively and powerfully this partially merged dual Kundalini force works in us. Because of the energy that is generated and the centers that are awakened, we often have temporary experiences of bliss, ecstasy, Love, tremendous well-being, Divine intoxication, peace, profound inner contentment, Divine awareness of the non-dualistic Truth of God, Oneness awareness, and direct experiences of our own Inner Self. It is as if the Divine influence of God has descended to the physical plane of our body-mind-I AM complex. We begin to feel this Divine influence permeating every aspect of our life and Being. It is poetic to think of the awakened Kundalini as the Hand of God. At this point, we stop thinking of God in terms of belief. *To have the direct experience of God's Presence takes us to the place of the direct knowledge of God and our own True Nature as the Transcendent Reality. God is no longer an abstract idea but a positive reality.* The experience of the energy of God is a tremendous motivation for continuing the spiritual practices that heighten this communion. It is much easier to meditate and fast, and to follow right diet and all Six Foundations when our desire for the Communion with God and experience of the ecstatic Love of God is being fulfilled. We do not need the Kundalini awakened to experience this communion, but when it is awakened, these experiences usually come more frequently, intensely, and easily.

Once we are aware of the Kundalini energy, it is easier to know what to do to enhance its intensity. One of the subtle traps of the spiritual path, however, is to become addicted to the bliss of these experiences and begin to think of them as the goal of spiritual life rather than simply part of the wonderful, awesome process. The goalless goal is to become stabilized in the non-dualistic continual awareness of the Truth. As this happens, we lose the dualistic concept that spiritual life has a goal and there is something to attain. We begin to understand we always have been THAT . . . which we have the illusion of seeking. When the overall purpose of spiritual life is consciously in mind and these experiences of the Truth are repeated enough, temporary awareness of these experiences begins to build into a more stabilized, continuous awareness of the Truth. When the awareness of the Transcendent Reality of our existence as Divine Love, as the dual/non-dual, holographic Truth of the Self becomes our predominant awareness, a major shift in the Enlightenment process has taken place. At the point of Liberation, all seeking stops and we rest in the Nothing as the True Self we always were, are, and will be. There is nowhere to go and nothing to be. We are free. There is no direction, but we are free to move in any direction as a spontaneous happening. All actions come from a place of emptiness. Actions happen without causation. This emptiness is beyond the duality of form and formlessness. It is indescribable and mysterious. One simply becomes a body-mind-I AM complex for the unending Light of the Ein Sof to emanate through. All motivation has disappeared and one becomes what is known in ancient Kabbalistic teachings as a *merkaba* vehicle, the expression of the Divine, mysterious Will. One does not even know what action may arise next. It is very humorous.

The Evolution of the Kundalini and the Three "Knots"

The process of the Kundalini evolution may take only a short time, or it may not complete itself in this lifetime. An important factor affecting this is the intensity of our desire for the complete unbroken Love Communion with the Divine.[1] The Kundalini awakening is the first step of the opening of the sushumna pathway, which takes us to this permanent awareness of Communion. In this pathway there are three "knots" *(granthis)*, which are rarely written about, spoken about, or understood. In the Yogic literature there are vague references to the three knots and their meaning, and few references in Western literature. This one has been drawn to develop an understanding of their significance because of his own experiences of them. Some Yogis talk of them as blockages in the sushumna channel, but we will get a clearer functional understanding if we think of them as evolutionary nodal points.

Classically speaking, these knots are located at the base chakra (Brahmagranthi), the heart chakra (Vishnugranthi), and the brow chakra (Rudragranthi). These points represent the different stages in which there is an intensification of the total Kundalini energy in the system. Each stage or knot opening reflects a progressively more integrated synchronization and merging of the two polarized Kundalini energies. With each level of merging, there is an amplification and intensification of the Kundalini energy. In an indirect way, the knots regulate the flow of Kundalini in the sushumna (central channel), so that excessive energy does not flow through and "burn out" the system. Thus, the merged Kundalini energies do not move to the next level until the consciousness and conductivity of the individual have reached the capacity to hold the more intense energy and awareness. This does not mean that people do not experience higher states of awareness; it only means that these states do not become stabilized until the channels are sufficiently strengthened to hold the increased energy of the awareness. It is said that the Kundalini is very intelligent. For this reason, *it is better to allow the Kundalini to unfold spontaneously than to attempt to force it artificially with specific meditations or techniques.* In some of the Yogic teachings, three intensities of Kundalini energy are reported, which correlate with the opening of each knot.[2] The first level of energy intensity is called prana Kundalini. It corresponds to the energy released with initial awakening and the beginning synchronization and partial merging of the two polar Kundalini energies associated with the awakening. Chit Kundalini is the name of the next major increase in Kundalini intensity, which corresponds to the Kundalini power that is active after the awakening of the second knot. Para Kundalini, associated with the opening of the third knot, is the name for the most refined, most intense, and purest level of Kundalini that the body is able to conduct.

The first knot release of energy happens when the individual's awakened awareness of the first three chakras merge into one unified state of awakened awareness. The second knot represents the merging of the already unified first three chakras with the awakened Love of the heart chakra. Parallel to this is a new level of synchronicity and fusing of the two Kundalini energies spiraling up the sushumna. With each increased level of Kundalini merging, the sushumna channel itself becomes more and more open and conductive of the Kundalini.

The final knot in the sixth chakra is released when the awakened awareness of all the chakras are merged into the one non-dual awareness of the Truth. It is at this point that the Shakti Kundalini and spiritual Kundalini completely merge into one single Kundalini energy. All polarity of the Kundalini and corresponding duality in our consciousness vanish. The energy of each chakra merges into this one energy, although a remnant of each remains for body maintenance. The subtle bodies are perfectly aligned and merged in a way that the pure cosmic prana is no longer filtered and can directly enter any chakra. The primary center for energy intake becomes the pure prana taken in through the crown chakra. The very sushumna structure itself essentially dissolves into this one energy, our Union in God Consciousness. With this complete fusing of the two Kundalini energies, the evolutionary activity of the Kundalini in the spiritualization of body, mind, and spirit is essentially complete. We operate from a sense of pure knowingness, and become absorbed in the pure apperception of God Awareness. This is a quality associated with Enlightenment.

At this level of the greatly increased non-dual Kundalini energy, there is a shift in the very energy balance of our atoms. It is the hypothesis of the author that the increased energy is translated into an increased spin in the rotation of the axis of the atom and in the electron spin. With this increased energy and axis spin of the nucleus and electron, the mass of both the electron and the nucleus expands, but the orbit does not increase. The nucleus and electron are more closely bound and vibrate faster. The person can hold more energy at the atomic level, and it is harder to pull electrons away from the atom. Therefore the system is healthier, because it is harder for the more tightly held electrons to be pulled off by free radical oxidation.

Experiences of the Three Knots Opening

Much of this one's interest, understanding, and sharing about the three knots and the movement of the Kundalini is based on the teaching received from working out the meaning of his own experiences. The merging of the first three chakras occurred about eleven months after the awakening of the Kundalini. It occurred at Muktananda's Ganeshpuri ashram in India. From the time of the awakening, having tasted of the Divine Communion, the Kundalini pulled this one into deeper and deeper Communion, like a bull in heat, as some people joked. This one's role was simply to surrender to the power of the Kundalini and keep "showing up." It pained Gabriel not to be in Union. His Love for God was so intense he could barely stand it.

In one stanza of a poem from Gabriel's journal at that time (October 5, 1976), he wrote:

> How can I desire anything but You,
> Once having joined You for even a moment in the bliss of I AM free,
> There is nothing higher or more sacred than to be in total Union with You.

The Shakti of this intense desire for Communion did not allow much space to identify as a seeker. It propelled this one into meditation. Meditation time was increased to the maximum that the physical structure could tolerate. Having received Muktananda's permission to meditate more than the customary one hour a day, meditation time increased to four and a half hours per day. This was in addition to the hours of chanting songs to God, in which the entire spiritual community participated. At this intensity, most of the three one-and-a-half hour meditations per day were filled with the ecstatic bliss of Love Communion with God. Frequently merging into the blue Light of Consciousness within the Self, continual experiences of the non-dualistic reality were imprinted on the awareness, bringing this one into a peaceful and contented state, except for a flaming desire for THAT. The God-merging, Deveikut, program had been activated beyond any idea of control. It was simply a happening, with this one simply witnessing while trying to keep up with the Flame of God burning up any illusion of being other than the Flame of God. The body-mind-I AM complex felt like a plane reaching speeds and energies at which the wings were about to come off. The whole body, ego-mind, and spirit integration was undergoing intense transformation. With very little formal training or knowledge in any sort of Yoga, this mind-body complex had embarked, with much trust in God, on a voyage into the unknown. Muktananda's subtle guidance was this one's only safety line. "Going for it" describes the situation, except that this one did not know what he was going for. The unfolding was a force much greater than the mind could comprehend. The following journal entries can best illustrate the intensity of this.

Journal entry of October 31, 1976:

> Well today is another turn of *sadhana* [spiritual practice]. It started last night when going to bed. I was lying there repeating my mantra when I began to feel some increased energy. What I perceived as my vas deferens began to twitch and spasm, then I got a partial erection and a feeling of a thin column of energy going directly inside of me vertically from the perineal knot [this is a physical body knot joining the muscles at the base of the perineum]. It was painful, but not terribly painful. The night was spent in more of a meditation half sleep.
>
> In my morning meditation I felt calm, peaceful, and enjoyed the play of *chitti* [conscious]. Baba [Muktananda] came in a blue pearl and took me off somewhere. Much blue Light. Much energy. I seemed to be all Light inside. Kundalini rising. Then the pain at the base of the *Muladhara* [base chakra] began, twitching and spasming of the vas deferens-sushumna energy stream, which is usually narrow, begins to broaden and increases the intensity of the flow of upward energy. All this alternated with visions of Baba – and much celestial feeling. I am feeling very gentle and mellow, but I know a process is beginning that is very unusual and beyond my body concepts. I urge myself to let go of any illusion of control of the body and let the Kundalini be in complete control. I am determined to go all the way. Shakti is purifying me.
>
> In my afternoon meditation, it started again with lots of energy. Nice visions of Baba alternating with different energy forms. I was feeling joy and Light. Then a brief sense of a negative energy feeling-vision came and quickly passed. Obviously the play of consciousness – it almost seemed psychedelic. Then the vas deferens spasm began; much pain, hot, painful erection. My whole pelvic area to lower solar area on the inside became flaming red hot. My body began to undulate in orgasmic movements. Self-consciously I am relieved that I am the only one sitting in the meditation hall at that time of the day. But I had tinges of self-consciousness sitting in half-lotus having spontaneous pre-orgasmic undulations. Then I realized that it was not going to stop. I was going to have an orgasm right in the

> middle of the meditation hall! I could not believe that this was happening. I was not even having any sexual thoughts or feelings. I then began vigorous dry ejaculation spasms with my whole lower pelvis involved. No semen was coming out. What a surprise! With each orgasmic spasm, I could feel and see [in meditation vision] the semen shooting directly up the sushumna, broadening it and extending the sushumna channel opening all the way to my *Ajna* [brow chakra]. It filled me with intense energy. It went on for what might have been 15 to 30 minutes. It took another 15 minutes for the erection to go down. It was another one and a half hours before the perineal pain subsided.
>
> The next day, the nails of both my little toes spontaneously came off. It was as if the energy was so intense that my system could barely contain the energy. This whole process was very sobering. I felt a quiet joy in surrendering to a process that was more powerful than I and which was beyond my comprehension. But it is one thing to revel in the bliss of the Divine Communion, and another to surrender to having my internal anatomy reorganized.

Following this night- and day-long experience, whenever this one even had the glimmerings of a sexual thought, that painful ten- to twelve-inch rod of energy would begin to activate. It seemed like a shish kebab skewer piercing through the round discs of the first three innocent chakras. After returning to the United States, it did not take long to discover that this one had undergone a process of spontaneous celibacy because of this shish kebab effect. My then wife was distinctly unhappy about this. With some help from my friend Dr. Lee Sannella and the strength of our own Love, we began to take our relationship to new levels of Love and compassion. At the time we were living in a rural setting in Mendocino, California, and this one was immersed in organizing his life according to the principles of what is called *kedusha* (holiness). Working as a holistic physician was limited to half-time, which was enough to cover expenses, and the rest of the time was spent working on the land, being with family, meditating, and performing other spiritual practices. Life had never been so attuned and in balance. It was a special time for our whole family. Analyzing it now, all three basic chakras were being awakened to their higher awareness and integrated into this one's life practice. It was also a time in which the spontaneous celibacy served as a protective space for the Kundalini to complete its work on the awakening and merging of the first three chakras. After about six months, a note from Muktananda arrived, suggesting that this period of spontaneous and complete celibacy was nearing completion. When we finally felt it was the time to make Love, we both spontaneously and simultaneously merged into the wonderment of the blue Light of total Communion in the Oneness of God. It was clear that we had both been transformed by the spiritualizing power of the Kundalini.

Gabriel is neither for nor against celibacy as a spiritual practice. As in this case, there may be times when the Kundalini requires one to be celibate as part of the subtle structure reorganizing, and not as a spiritual concept. This is an important point because this one has witnessed many people causing themselves undue angst because of a superimposed practice of motivated celibacy from concept rather than as a natural flow of Kundalini. The ancient Yoga teachings include a need to balance *dharma* (right living), *artha* (wealth), *kama* (pleasure), and *moksha* (God merging). When kama is disrupted because of unnecessary pleasure deprivation, a certain unbalancing angst may arise that may disrupt and unbalance sadhana (spiritual practice). In order to maximize the unfolding, it is best to let the flow of Kundalini decide and not be stuck in spiritual concepts. The reverse of this celibacy approach is found in Kabbalah. A spiritual couple is to make Love on the Shabbat (Sabbath). However, if the Kundalini says "no," she needs to be listened to. The path is too mysterious to get caught in concepts.

Awakening of the Second Knot

The merging of the first three chakras with the heart chakra was not as dramatic or painful. It began about six months after the sequence of time associated with the first knot opening and the following integration. The second opening was marked by a vision experience of the detailed anatomy of the heart chakra, an increase in the total energy of the Kundalini spiritualizing the system, and the sudden cessation of most of Gabriel's daily meditation visions. Instead, there was the continuous experience of white Light and merging into this Formlessness. Sometimes it would be so bright in the early morning meditations that this one would think he had meditated into the daytime. This one's whole essence would be vitalized by this Light. Gabriel became aware of a broad, white Light energy emanating from the heart chakra. It was a broad vortex that connected this one with an impersonal Love and empathy with everything and everyone in the universe. Whether meditating or not, on the in or out breath, it was easy to dissolve into the white Light. This would happen even while jogging. During this time this one would often experience a blue flame in what the left-brained medical mind identified as the bottom of the right auricle of the heart. It was slightly to the right side of the heart. Sometimes this blue Light would transform itself into an image of Muktananda or Nityananda. Less frequently, there would be a similar blue flaming Light in the brow chakra that seemed aligned with the blue Light in the heart area. These were not considered visions, since their presence was felt whether or not a vision appeared. This second knot state expanded in awareness over a period of five years before the final merging of the chakras began. During this time, the heart chakra appeared as an eight-petal lotus, in the center of the heart, rather than as the customary twelve-petal lotus. During this time the daily repeated meditation experiences of the True Self as the formless white Light of consciousness slowly began to etch itself into a more permanent, awakened awareness. I AM THAT awareness was becoming more and more a part of the ground of being.

In later research it was noted that within the heart chakra there are eight petals within the twelve-petal outer *yantra*. This eight-petal form represents the spiritual heart, known as the *anandakanda* (space of bliss). Within the twelve is a circle with eight petals that is like molten gold, which is the way it appeared, and was situated in the right side of the physical body heart, which in essence is the very straight center of the physical body. It is connected with the *chittrini* nadi, which is a subtle part of the sushumna. This eight-petal form represents the spiritual or etheric heart, or *hrit pundarik* (heart lotus). It is stainless and untouched by physical impurities. It is the seat of the Self in the waking consciousness and in the dream state. It is described as the Temple of God, and it can only be reached when the sushumna is opened. It is said that within it, there are eight deities, including Indra. Inside the sushumna nadi, represented by the color red, is the *vajrini* nadi (the thunderbolt nadi) represented by fire or the sun; inside that is the chittrini nadi, which is the moon represented by water. The Divine nectar *(amrita)* drips out of the chittrini nadi. Inside the water nadi is the radiance of the *Brahma* nadi, where a throne ornamented with jewels is located. This was Gabriel's vision. This was a good lesson because only eight petals were seen, leading this one to think at first he was not seeing the whole heart chakra. It is a good lesson to simply witness what is going on and not judge, because the vision was one of the core essence and transformational experience of the heart chakra. These meditation experiences were daily teaching this one that the whole universe dwells within this one as THAT. The experience of I AM THAT was more and more becoming the ground of awakened existence.

Awakening of the Third Knot

The cycle for this awakening began to build in late October of 1981, about ten months before its culmination. After four years of gently stabilizing and expanding the awareness of the second awakening, the spiritual desire began to get very hot again. This one kept thinking of a teaching Muktananda once gave in a lecture, that when God offers you the kingdom, why settle for a handful of dust? Sadhana increased in intensity – getting up at 2:30 A.M. to gain an extra hour of meditation time, which now was closer to two hours three times per day. In early December, the first two experiences of *Nirvakalpa samadhi* occurred, in which even the I AM consciousness, or witness consciousness, dissolved into the void (teheru). All duality disappeared – beyond time, space, and Being. Everything was gone. These lasted for about an hour each. Gabriel's then wife came in during one of them and thought the body-mind-I AM complex had died. Apparently breathing had stopped for about forty-five minutes. The Kundalini does kill off the illusion of the body-mind-I AM complex. More propelled than seeking, willing to keep showing up and willing to die, this one kept showing up. There was no sense of choice or fear as the Shakti Kundalini gave one message: *Meditate until all you think is "you" disappears forever.* This was beyond any spiritual philosophy or insight – it was a spontaneous non-intellectual happening. Somewhere during this time, another chakra opened, which was above the sixth chakra. Later, this one discovered it was known as the *soma* chakra, or the *amrita* chakra, which means "nectar of the moon" or "nectar of immortality." It is actually within the *Sahasrara* or crown chakra. The Soma chakra is associated with Rahu, one of the moon's nodes. This chakra was experienced as a crescent moon, although the literature says that it often has twelve petals. It was a white moon, very luminescent. Surrounding this moon was a triangle. This chakra is the source of nectar (soma) and as the soma dripped down, this one could taste it on the palate. It just seemed to be dripping down into the palate from the brain, as if the brain were leaking nectar. The experience of the soma nectar was of a sweetness. The taste didn't seem to change with this one's state, with what he had tasted, and with what was in his mouth. This nectar just came down as a sweetness that was beyond sweetness. As this phenomenon was happening, it seemed that the subtle organism of the nadis were opening up to take the final step.

Later, these phenomena were researched in the Yogic texts. The triangle around the moon is called the *Ah Cah Tah triangle,* and has figures in it, which were not seen by this one – *Kmeshdara* and *Kmeshdari.* For this one, it was enough to taste the nectar. It is interesting to note that Kmeshdara is also known as *urdhdareta* or upward streaming or flowing, which is the ability to draw the essence in seminal fluid upward into the sushumna nadi, which is an earlier experience occurring in the first year of the seven-year cycle with Swami Muktananda. So, the connections became a little bit clearer.

Excert from journal poem entry, December 27, 1981:

> Ah – the bliss of my life, of the world, of my children, of my wife. If I die of a broken heart, it will not be out of sorrow, but because it is so full of Love, that I could not say no to more . . . and it just burst out of Love.

Journal entry, February 12, 1982:

> The bliss of the Self, the pulsating oneness, the inner joy has simply grown greater than the contraction of my ego. The critical point has past. . . . The power of the Bliss of God is greater than the safe contraction of the ego. It dies as my Liberation grows. The last stage is beginning.

Journal entry, May 29, 1982:

> Somewhere in this last year I have recognized. . . . I AM THAT! I AM THAT is more a part of my awareness than not. Destiny unfolds on the empty field of my Being. I AM the spectator watching it in the quiet ecstasy of the play; knowing I AM THAT. Just to Be is enough.

By late August of 1982, meditation had reached a steady six hours per day for about one year. The family had returned to the United States three weeks earlier. The children had to get ready to start school and someone had to find a home in which to live. This one was feeling much gratitude to his then wife, Nora, for being so understanding at that time. It is this awareness, Love, and compassionate understanding by a mate that makes it possible for a complete spiritual unfolding to happen for a family person. To completely surrender to the unfolding of the Kundalini requires the right life consent of our social context, so Nora's consent was very important. Spiritual life for family people is made easier when both partners are evolving spiritually.

This one was unable to leave India with the family because there was a strong sense that something very important was going to happen. As a wise person once said, "You cannot cross a chasm in two small jumps." At this time, the energy of the Kundalini was centered in the I AM consciousness of the sixth chakra. Although the gentle throbbing of the Kundalini in the sixth chakra had gone on for years, it now became particularly intense during meditation, feeling as if it were going to explode. After a few weeks of this intensity, it began to occur that the third knot was about to be expanded and the Kundalini was going to merge in the crown chakra. The traditional teachings often said that one needed the guru's permission for this final step of Kundalini to take place. How was this going to happen? Gabriel's relationship to Muktananda did not involve a lot of personal verbal contact. Other teachings said that the permission of the *Inner Guru,* the Self of All, was sufficient. So this one waited for inner guidance.

During one evening meditation, the energy became so intense that the mind-body complex spontaneously got up and wobbled over to the meditation hall outside Swami Muktananda's room. Sometimes in the evening he would come out and walk around this hall. About 30 seconds after this one sat down, Swami Muktananda, dressed in his long johns, opened the door and came out. He walked directly over to Gabriel. He immediately began to work his fingers over the short path from the sixth to the seventh chakra on the brow, forehead, and crown area. As he worked, the streams of the totally merged Kundalini energy began to flow upward in a V-shaped pattern to the crown chakra. His other hand was gently placed over the head. It seemed to be pulling the Kundalini energy up through the crown. With the flow firmly established, Swami Muktananda calmly turned and walked back into his room. His cosmic function of Grace for over seven years with this one was now completed. The crown chakra had clearly been initiated by Swami Muktananda and the final step of Shakti merging with Shiva in the Sahasrara chakra had been activated. This one actually saw and experienced a thin stream of energy move upward through what he later identified as the Brahma nadi, located in the center of the larger sushumna nadi.

Shattering the Glass Ceiling of Consciousness

Sometime shortly after this final initiation of the Kundalini, there was a direct shattering of what this one metaphorically calls "the glass ceiling of consciousness" – the veil. In the final stages, one is immersed in the experience of the *hiranyamaya kosha* (bliss body). One experiences being surrounded in this golden Light continuously. One is in and out of samadhi and there is a tremendous internal urging to merge with the One. There is just a thin veil (par'gawd) keeping one from that final merging. At some point, that veil, which Gabriel metaphorically calls the glass ceiling, shatters. The subtle veil of the hiranyamaya kosha that stands between one and the awareness of jivanmukti – Self-realization while in the body – just spontaneously dissolves.

This metaphor came to Gabriel one day years later at the Tree of Life Café, when the wind blew over a glass table and the whole glass top shattered. This level of shattering is what it feels like. The table became Enlightened. The thin glass ceiling, which had separated and so very slightly warped the Divine Light coming through, was no longer there and it was experiencing the direct unbroken Communication with the Divine. One literally loses "their" mind and the I AM consciousness prior to the mind becomes absorbed into the I AM THAT – the Absolute as the Absolute Eternal Nothing. It is a tremendous sense of freedom when the glass ceiling shatters. It is an explosive discontinuity with past, present, and future.

Shattered Glass Table

One day the windy Grace of Yah
Blew so hard
The glass table of the mind
Turned over and shattered
Into thousands of useless fragments.
It happened so suddenly
So effortlessly
After so many years and lifetimes
Of thinning this glass ceiling of illusion
So suddenly
The mind just shattered
Just exploded into the eternal motionless, timeless presence.

The scintillating sublime Absolute
Burst through
Uninterrupted
Alone
Disconnected from past, present, and future
And the illusion of "I" was not even there to claim it as mine.
There was no place to stand
And no one to be standing.
The Great Way
Which has no gate
Opened
And there was no "me" there to walk through.

The work of the Kundalini unfolding takes you to the place where the shattering of the glass ceiling of consciousness can potentially actually happen. The rest is Grace. For this one, the I AM shattering occurred while simply meditating, as always at the noon meditation, and on the balcony of our little apartment in India overlooking a field where the farmers were plowing with ox. A little railing prevented this one from seeing the whole landscape. One day, this one just stood up and saw the whole thing, but in reality, "the mind" and I AM shattered at that moment. Everything became totally clear and luminescent. It was just a simple moment of seemingly totally inconsequential action that marked the altering of this one forever. The process of Self-realization does not rest with the unfolding of the Kundalini or the subtleties of knowing all the intellectual ins and outs of the I AM. The I AM consciousness exists as the source of primordial *Maya* (the illusion of dualistic reality). It represents the last step before Self-realization – before moving into the timeless, spaceless, non-Being awareness of I AM THAT. It is an internal experience of consciousness shattering, and all that is left is the eternal, permanent Divine Presence permeating all of the Being, and there isn't even a Being left. The I AM disappeared and only existence remained. Concepts such as Yoga *chitta vritti nirodha* (stilling the mental activity of the mind) or the goal of Yoga as Union no longer made sense. There was never anything to come into Union with. *There was always Union from prior to Eternity.* You can't unite with that which was never separated. The point was to be in the awareness of the eternal shining Truth that Was, Is, and Will Be. *At the highest level of understanding, Yoga or Kabbalah has no goal. They are systems to help one wake up to what has always existed. There is no growth or change – only waking to the Eternal Truth.* Once the angle of the mind changes away from goals or working toward Union, life becomes easier and the Six Foundations are simply living in a way that draws the Grace that shatters the glass ceiling of the mind so one wakes to the non-dual experience of the Divine. This is the essence of Ecstatic Kabbalah and of Yoga.

It is important to understand that we will not all have the same experiences in this evolutionary process. A danger in sharing is that we tend to compare experiences. A key thing to remember is to learn, listen, and be inspired by each other's experiences, but to be content with the particular Grace that God gives us and to know that our experiences are specifically appropriate for our own spiritual expression. It is not necessary to have such an intense awakening and expansion of the three knots in order to evolve spiritually. It is more important that we be willing to experience all of God's Grace in whatever form it comes to us. The lightning flash of God's Grace needs an attracting focus on Earth, which is our full intention and devotion to be fully open to this Grace. This willingness draws the Grace. Without our desire for and ability to receive God's Grace, its effect on us is minimal. Grace comes through silence.

Silence – The Song of Yah

The spirit must know silence
Before it can sing and dance
Its own song –
The ecstatic song of Yah.

Illuminated Maya

Ah!

A sublime luminescent silence
Emanating as all of existence
Complete peace as the DNA of existence
The illusory "I" had ceased
All effort, however subtle ceased
The overwhelming aching, flaming desire to merge with God stopped
Kundalini laughed
And there was no one left to hear the laughter.

All that exists is the great silent cosmic laugh
An extraordinary glowing aliveness of the Absolute
So real that everything else became unreal
In the reality of this awakening
All previous reality seemed unreal.
In contrast this nameless Absolute illuminated reality
The meaning of Maya
The illusion of the three-dimensional world
Had a new understanding.
All of existence now glowed as the radiance of THAT.
The indescribable glory of God is the world.
Only the illuminating radiance of God IS.

This awakening opened the magical illumination of the Third Torah, which is the silent Torah (the first two are the written and oral Torah). The awakening illuminated Enoch's teaching – "Be still and know I AM THAT." This is the essence of the Living Essene Way, Ecstatic Kabbalah, and Yoga. It revealed the non-existential existence as the Ultimate Truth of all the great traditions. Maya does not mean the world is illusion or unreal. That is the unawakened view. The experience of "illuminated Maya" is the world of duality revealed in a new way – as the scintillating radiance of the Divine in different forms. At this level it is no longer traditional Maya, but the play of God Gracing our lives. One experiences all of creation as the luscious play of THAT. From that Deep Silence and complete peace spontaneously emanates the pulse of non-causal Love, contentment, and joy as a natural, unbroken background. The whole world appears in a new luminescence. Maya is the unreal black-and-white world of our projections. In illuminated Maya, all projected truths are holy lies. A flower is not unreal, but the way we experience a flower in the world of deluded, unawakened Maya is. In the real world of illuminated Maya of God's Grace, a flower is the fragrance of Yah laughing in unbroken Love and Peace, as Divine beauty. Enlightenment emanates as cosmic, undifferentiated individuality.

Awakening Continues

In this post-Kundalini state one becomes intensely human. There is another stage of heart awareness that opens in which one is subject to the heart pain of the world and of each individual. No matter how people project their pain and alienation on you, you have no choice but to keep the heart open.

Journal entry, March 7, 1985:

> As the process of increased prana intensifies in the body . . . its main effect seems to be a subtle accumulation of Love in the heart that is radiating within me most of the time. Not necessarily ecstatic Love, but a solid awareness of the Love that connects us all. . . . It is not the Love of any one thing, even God. . . . It is just Love for Love's sake . . . as the ground of my existence.

This Love is an unrelenting Love. This sensitivity does not mean one is attached to emotions; it means that the emotions go through, one experiences them, and they pass. One is not the Yogic idealized rock that emotions bounce off of, but rather is more like the Taoist water that absorbs all. In the oneness of a compassionate world connection, even the rock is eventually absorbed by the water. A poem from the Tao Te Ching, verse 49, makes this point nicely:

> The sage has no mind of his own. He is aware of the needs of others. . . . The sage is shy and humble – to the world he seems confusing. Men look to him and listen. He behaves like a little child."[3]

Since that awakening time of the third knot opening, the awareness of the Kundalini energy has rarely left the crown chakra. A steady pulse of increasing energy continued to flow in the crown chakra, yet the experience of the sushumna channel seemed to have faded. About two weeks later in meditation, while visiting Swami Prakashananda, Sai Baba of Shirdi, a very well known Indian saint who died in 1918 and with whom this one has a special connection, appeared. From the palm of his right hand a thunderbolt of energy shot into this now opened pathway. From this there was a great widening of the Kundalini path to the crown and the dissolution of the sushumna entirely. It all seemed to dissolve into the merged Kundalini energy in the crown chakra. From this time on, a vortex of energy pulsating at the top of the head was almost continuous. A continuous experience of this vortex pulsation did not occur, however, until the end of a forty-day fast seven months later. At that time the top of the crown chakra seemed to disappear, leaving an open, swirling vortex of pure prana. It is through this open vortex that the pulsation of the cosmic energy was entering the system. It is in a circle in the shape of a *kippah* (Jewish skullcap) covering the crown to the forehead and back of the head. The energy felt in the other chakras seems almost non-existent compared to this channel.

Sahaja samadhi is when, both awake and asleep, one is aware of being in the awareness of I AM THAT. As this has unfolded, it has begun to pervade more heavily even in the sleep state, in the sense that all is filled with Light. Even though the mind-body complex seems to be asleep at night, the witness is experiencing pure Light. It manifests very strongly, particularly on going to sleep and awakening, and the consciousness proceeds during sleep into the awareness of THAT being Light. This does not necessarily happen all night long, every night, but during a significant amount of time, and it seems to be increasing over time.

Like everything else on the spiritual path, the non-dualistic awareness does not become 100 percent immediately. In our dualistic thinking, many would like it one way or another to fit it in a neat box. During this one's experience of the merging of all the chakra energy and the Kundalini energy into one Divine energy, there was a profound shift to an essential identity as I AM THAT, as Non-Being. This one began to live in the dual/non-dual awareness of the Truth as a synergistic paradox. It is this one's predominant and overwhelming inherent awareness. Yet it is not the 100 percent unbroken awareness of the Truth – moksha. It appears to be an ever-increasing awareness of the non-dualistic state moving from a predominant awareness toward a constant awareness of the state.

Shriman Tapasviji Maharaj, the 185-year-old saint, once wept for three days when a close disciple of his died. When his amazed disciples asked him what was going on, he said that no matter how great a saint may be and that people call him Enlightened, his mind may sometimes become deluded by the idea that one is separate from the world or that there is duality and that someone actually dies or is lost. Although this state is temporary in such a one, Maharaj pointed out, the grief is felt for the time that it lasts.[4] He taught that no human, even if Liberated, is truly and continuously free from all attachments, grief, desire, and every trace of dualistic, I-ness or my-ness, thinking. Maharaj gives a beautiful analogy by comparing the situation to that of a large tree hit by a strong wind. The trunk moves a little and then regains its immobile state. The branches shake longer and are affected by lesser winds. The trunk is analogous to one who is Liberated from the basic false identities and dualistic thinking of the mind. The easily movable branches are like the workings of the normal dualistic mind.

The unfoldment is endless! Self-realization fructifies into full moksha. Never look back or ahead. All there is is the endless scintillating Now, rippling in the Nothing beyond comprehension.

The Process of Awakening

Reflecting on the process, it seems that the very first step is the purification of the prana, or vital life force. As the prana begins to purify and expand, there is more and more clarity about the I AM consciousness becoming the predominant consciousness, which is what we see in *hiranyamaya kosha* (bliss body). The prana eventually becomes pure enough to be absorbed into the I AM consciousness. The analogy is Shiva absorbing Shakti and becoming One, or Nukba, the feminine aspect as the Shekhinah energy merging into *Zeir Anpin*. As Oneness happens, we disappear beyond time, space and Being – I AM THAT. This book is primarily about purification of the prana via the Six Foundations so that we may merge into Shiva or Zeir Anpin. So, the first step is I AM consciousness, which is not the state of Self-realization, but just prior to it. There is still a thin veil between it and jivanmukti – Liberation while in the body. When the glass ceiling shatters, we realize I AM THAT, prior to consciousness. This is the awareness of Self-realization, Liberation, jivanmukti, or Chaya-Yehida. Then the Absolute becomes "more Absolute." In Kabbalah, there are levels of non-dual existence: Chochma, then Keter, and then the unknowable Ein Sof.

Merging the prana with I AM consciousness allows us to go beyond the I AM in an act of Grace. Building prana and awareness of the I AM is the purpose of the spiritual practices of the Six Foundations. They are designed, in the paradoxical goalless goal and pathless path, to help one shift to prior to I AM consciousness. These practices, these Six Foundations, require some effort in building, expanding, and purifying the prana, so that we can move to the first step in spiritual knowledge, which is the I AM consciousness. The second step, moving to pure awareness (I AM THAT) is without effort and can happen in an instant through Grace. With this experiential understanding, the debate of the effortless versus effort becomes resolved. The first part of moving to the I AM consciousness is one that takes effort – purification of the prana with the Six Foundations. The second step is spontaneous through Grace – moving prior to consciousness is the ultimate and final Truth. It is a state of awareness in which we are not only not identified with the body-mind-

I AM complex, but we have let go of our identification with the I AM consciousness. It is the Absolute. At that point, there is no birth, there is no death; in other words, there is no time, space, or Being.

In the Kabbalistic system, this awareness starts with the world of *Atz'ilut*. It exists at the sephirot level of Chochma and Keter. There is the constant oscillation between Binah (I AM consciousness), and Chochma (I AM THAT), and Keter (deeper I AM THAT awareness). This state in the Yogic system is called sahaja samadhi. In sahaja samadhi, we exist prior to time, space, and Being, and yet we live in the world of time and space, and let our efforts unfold in the world of time and space. The work is a manifestation of Divine Will coming through us, except there is no us; there is only the work manifesting, as one witnesses from prior to consciousness. This state of prior to the I AM, is also known as paramatman. It is the core of the Self. It is prior to consciousness. It is the sense of the Absolute, or I AM THAT. There is no sense of separation. I AM THAT awareness is the highest knowledge in which no knowledge exists. The practice of this one was primarily meditation, which amplifies the Light of the atman shining forth. *When the prana and I AM consciousness become one in meditation, this merging celebrates Liberation. When it is fully merged, irreversibly merged, 100 percent merged, it is called moksha. Before that point, it is called Self-realization or Liberation.* In the Yogic system, Liberation begins with the merging of Shiva and Shakti. In the Kabbalistic system, it is Zeir Anpin and Nukba merging.

When the glass ceiling shatters (Liberation), there are no paths; we realize we are the destination Itself. One simply abides in the Truth. Not even Love of the Self exists. All is simply the unfolding of the Eternal Consciousness and we are simply witnessing that unfolding of the Absolute through the I AM consciousness.

Subtle Kiss

The subtle kiss of Liberation
Has no lips
But you taste it
In every cell
An ecstatic wild pulsing in every DNA oscillation
Dancing freely in every chakra
Coursing through the shusumna, *ida, pingali* – all 72,000 nadis
In all four worlds.
Once kissed

You become alive
And there is nothing else worth living for
Except to be the ecstatic, naked, wild dance of Yah.
Yah's kiss is the cosmic death
And the cosmic rebirth into Immortality.
Once kissed
You become the breath of Yah as the play of the world.
Be careful who you yearn to kiss
Because there may be no return.

Wild Tao

The "I" that existed
Burst into the flame of Kundalini.
Continually flamed by meditation
In a cycle of seven incendiary years
All was destroyed
Burnt by the Divine raging fire.
There was no choice
But to cooperate with the burning.
It demanded total innocent surrender
Beyond the ignorance of the body-mind-I AM complex
And out of the flames
Danced the most sublime, passionate, non-causal contentment
Peace and joy
More powerful that any worldly attachment.
Like a coyote
It laughed
At all the illusory I
Thought to be real,
Biting through attachments.
It challenged:
"Fool, can you lose what was never yours?"
Biting deep into the illusory brain of consciousness
Killing the illusion of body-mind-I AM consciousness
That had been me.
Nothing was left
Except the untamed, wild Tao
Expressing.

Expressions

After all of the illusory "I" is gone
What remains is an ecstatic
Non-causal Love, peace, joy, and contentment.
Emanating out of the Emptiness
As the subtle tangible ground of existence
Playing as the world
Expressing through the body-mind-I AM complex
As *Tikkun Olam*
The healing and transformation of the world.
Like with the urge for Self-awakening
The passionate burning corpse
Has no choice.
The idea of any choice, spiritual or otherwise
Is coyote humor.
All this emanates in the non-causal Love
Which manifests as service to all Life
In all forms
And in all ways
Existing only to serve
Awakening of human awareness.

The I AM is the primordial Maya. Prior to this there are no desires because there is not anything or any entity to want anything. Another way to understand the shift is that *the ego can't exist without the creation of striving. The ego exists in the realm of time and space as a process that must recreate itself in every moment in order to exist. In Enlightenment, nothing needs to be created because the Absolute always Was, Is, and Will Be. God is not a verb or a process.* It is the ego that is a verb. All striving stops because the ego illusion that there is an us and something outside of us to strive for dissolves and all that is left is the eternal peace of THAT. Paradoxically, this doesn't mean that in the process of fulfilling the dharma of Beingness, one acts as if one has no desires. To experience no connection to the body may still allow one to move around in the body with I AM consciousness and beyond. This one had the occasion to test that play in both the mid-eighties and also in 2003, during the course of two repeat hernia operations performed without any anesthetic. By residing in I AM THAT, the awareness of the pain of the body-mind complex disappeared. The body-mind complex also had jaw surgery for cavitations and this one stayed in the awareness beyond the body and therefore was able to have it without anesthetic. (The author does not recommend this unless one is firmly established in I AM THAT.) This is part of the power of this state of awareness prior to consciousness. Yah provides these tests so we know that we are not just playing with spiritual words.

When consciousness gets involved with the body-mind complex, it becomes personality and we have the illusion of a separate individual. This is why, in the Zero Point Process course (a Western jnana Yoga) facilitated by Gabriel, the teaching is that "the personality is a case of mistaken identity." *Personality is consciousness conditioned by the body and mind concepts.* As we go beyond our identification with personality as the body-mind complex, we become the I AM consciousness, and then spontaneously take the final step when we go prior to the I AM consciousness to I AM THAT. In I AM consciousness, we are able to observe the play of the mind, as a witness. *In I AM consciousness, time and space have dissolved, but Being still exists.* When we begin to observe consciousness itself (the witness of the witness), this is the final phase. This is "the Awareness State." In the Awareness State, we do not carry out our activities; they are just simply going on. When the witnessing stops, all that is left is the Eternal, Chochma, Keter, and a vague sense of the Ein Sof.

Back to basics: Without the prana, we cannot attain any of this, so our first focus and the purpose of this book, *Spiritual Nutrition,* is to build, purify, and expand prana. That's our work. In that process of building the Six Foundations, we move deeper into the I AM consciousness. Although the Six Foundations have been recommended, one must understand that it is not possible to "technique" one's way to *Liberation.* There is an act of Grace in it. However, we can actively work to expand and purify the prana and all thought forms or vasanas within consciousness. That is basically the purpose of the Six Foundations. *The shift is to no longer identify with the life principle or prana, with the body, the mind, or continue to let the body-mind complex dominate. The prana becomes merged into the I AM consciousness and the I AM begins to dominate as the primary awareness. The Grace comes when we spontaneously move to the awareness prior to the I AM, the I AM THAT awareness. This is the effortless, spontaneous part of the unfolding.*

The work of this book is simply to build and purify the vital life force with the Six Foundations. These include: (1) nutrition, with vegan live foods and Spiritual Fasting; (2) building prana by means of Yoga asanas;

pranayama, ophanim; Tachyon, sacred dance, and other energetic practices; (3) service and charity; (4) satsang, Zero Point Process, and sangha (spiritual group support of consciousness), the reading of the wisdom scriptures, sattva/kedusha (holiness), sacred music, and walking in nature; (5) silence, through meditation, prayer, mantras, and chanting; (6) Shaktipat initiation, S'micha l'shefa/Haniha.

Through these processes, we transform ourselves into the sattvic/kedusha (holy) state. Then, spontaneously, the next step happens. The glass ceiling shatters. At that point, time, space, and Being disappear. This is the ultimate realization, the experience of non-dual existence prior to time, space, and Being. This state is known as *Svarupa,* which means one's own True State. To be sustained in this state is called *Svadharma.* This is the same as living in the world of Atz'ilut, remaining in Chochma, or, in terms of soul language of the Kabbalah, Chaya-Yehida. Liberation is arriving home and knowing one never left home. Although this one existed in three days of unbroken moksha at the end of the forty-day fast, the final moksha, which is extremely rare, is complete, unbroken existence in Nirvakalpa samadhi/God-merging.

In choosing to share these experiences, this one had to let go of old taboos and concepts of spirituality about how this sort of information and our experiences should be kept secret and therefore limited to a select few. There is a story about Ramanuja, who when he received a secret mantra from his guru was told that whoever receives this mantra will go to heaven, but if it is given to anyone else without the guru's permission, he will go to hell. Ramanuja immediately went up to a rooftop in the village and began to shout repeatedly "*Om Namah Shivaya.*" He explained to the people that whoever repeats this mantra will go to heaven. His guru heard him and shouted up to him, "What are you doing? Don't you know you will go to hell?" Ramanuja called back, "If all these people will go to heaven, I certainly do not mind going to hell." His guru, realizing his true motive, then blessed him for his act of Love.

Commentary on Evolutionary Kundalini Process

For most of us, the unfolding of Kundalini is a gradual process over years of consistent practice. At different points where the chakras merge and the two Kundalini energies become more synchronous and more fused, there is an increase of the overall Kundalini energy in the body-mind-I AM complex. The time before and after this merging is often experienced as one of more intense spiritual desire and longing accompanied by increased awareness. Between these points are times of integration and stabilization of the newly experienced awareness in our everyday life. With the understanding of the different cycles in the unfoldment of Kundalini, such practices as complete celibacy for periods of time may be appropriately followed when we are guided by the Kundalini working within. Following the inner guidance of the Kundalini seems more healthy than blindly following extreme practices according to the concepts of different teachers or spiritual paths. This does not mean we sit around and wait for the Kundalini to awaken before doing any spiritual practices. The Six Foundations and other general practices that help us lead a more sattvic, balanced, and harmonious life are clearly part of general spiritual development. Although one practices the basics of all Six Foundations, at certain times some practices may be more emphasized than others. There is a continual play according to the spiritual need of the person. A primary understanding of the spiritual process is that there is no set formula; there is no *Shulhan Arukh,* or set table. We must surrender to the spontaneous unfolding if we are to enter the gateless gate of Liberation. We cannot eat, practice asana, philosophize, or even meditate our way to Liberation. We just have to let go of any identity with the body-mind-I AM complex and in that heroic step we realize the Absolute that we always were. If it were so simple we would not need any Grace. The coyote speaks about how easy it is and laughs about expectations that are created in the mysterious paradox of simplicity.

Without the integration of our spiritual experiences into everyday life, it is difficult to maintain higher awareness. This is why it is so important that the awakened and merged awareness of the right life of the first three chakras be stabilized and integrated as the foundation of creating holiness in daily life. Without this foundation it is difficult to hold the energy of superconscious experiences or to stabilize them in a mature spiritual awareness.

The awakening and spiritualizing power of Kundalini often brings many spiritual experiences. The non-causal bliss, ecstasy, complete contentment, peace, and Love for God often associated with these experiences can be great motivators for continuing our spiritual practices. These experiences often bring us into the direct knowledge of our own Divine Self and give us profound inner teachings. The more often we experience this awareness in our meditation, the greater is the reinforcement of Truth to establish itself permanently in all states of our consciousness.

These profound spiritual experiences act as a sort of Divine behavior modification program, helping us to be constantly aware of our Transcendental Reality. These experiences encourage us to follow a purifying and elevating spiritual life practice in order to experience these states more often. The more the prana/Shekhinah energy is purified, the more these states are experienced. The subtle trap with spiritual experiences is that we begin to focus on the "hit" of the experience as an ego "feather in the cap," or even as the goal of spiritual life rather than as part of the process of the Kundalini evolution. All of it is a gift for our spiritual development. If we are able to understand this, we adopt an attitude that is neither for nor against experiences. We are simply free to relate to them appropriately for our spiritual benefit. *It is useful to remember that all experiences are phenomena and thus are dual. The permanent reality of non-dual God merging is the Truth of spiritual life.*

The intensity (kavanah), or fire of spiritual effort, is one of the most important factors in stimulating the Kundalini unfolding.[5,6] This has been true in this one's experience and general observations of people on various spiritual paths. The guidance, protection, and Grace from a spiritual teacher, guide, or guru, or even from active spiritual visions, such as Gabriel shared with Sai Baba of Shirdi and which many people experience with Jesus, are essential. Grace alone, however, is not enough. Salvation is not a one-sided gift from a teacher. It requires our intense effortless-effort as the first wing of the bird. Grace is the second wing. Without both, we do not fly very well. The issue is subtle in that this motivation for self-effort and devotion is affected by the cycles of Kundalini evolution. It is difficult to maintain an intense effort if it is not our time. It is also important to understand that although will power and self-effort help, they do not automatically guarantee a higher awareness. There is an ego trap of doership lurking when we rely solely on self-effort. Through our own will power we may have proudly mastered many Yoga asanas or developed many magical powers or learned all the Vedas, but we may have only aggrandized our egos and consequently blocked our spiritual growth. If someone tells you their path is the fastest or best, they are telling you they are still in a competitive, ego-based goal orientation, and therefore stuck in a subtle, unconscious level of understanding. Be wary of any advice they may give. The "path" is only your own joyous and spontaneous unfolding. The timing is up to Shakti Kundalini, not to your ego or someone else's plan. The unfolding in your sacred walk between *B'lee mah* and *Mah* is a path in which only you can walk. Power, intellectual knowledge, or skill is not the same as spiritual awareness. There seems to be an appointed time, which is beyond understanding, for it all to unfold. It is as if we suddenly understand our spiritual purpose and experience Love and devotion for God that we did not see or feel before. There is a Divine and sublime mystery in the timing and unfolding of the spiritual process. For us to be attuned to the subtleties of this, *we are best served by an attitude of Being rather than doing.* It is the act of surrender to the unfolding of one's own Kundalini. It is not about surrender to any outer form or guru. The work of true spiritual teacher is to help you surrender to your own Divine Self. This is the subtle work of the Six Foundations and the subtlety of this way. It is the surrendering way of the sacred feminine, rather than the conquering way of the masculine. This is a state of effortless-effort. This is part of the implication of this one's crown chakra being opened by the physical manifestation of Grace through Muktananda, through Sai Baba of Shirdi in meditation, and through the act of being inspired to fast for forty days. These are all forms of God's Grace intermixed with various manifestations of self-effort.

The idea of self-effort is paradoxical. It is not "techniquing" one's way to Enlightenment – an impossibility. In the Tao it is described as the pathless path: "The Great Way has no path. The clear water has no taste" (Tao Te Ching). *Another way of understanding self-effort is as surrender to God.* There are times in our spiritual evolution, whether or not the Kundalini is awakened, when there is a clear message from our inner teacher that it is time to take the next step. It may not be convenient or easy. Self-effort is choosing to follow that message no matter what the price. It may mean meditating long hours and eating very little and only light *biogenic* foods. It may mean a forty-day fast. It may mean working as a taxi driver for a few months. This is surrender to God's Will. It is saying "yes" when the flaming Kundalini shish kebab is painfully piercing ten inches up through the perineum and you do not know what strange thing is going to happen next. Self-effort is when God offers the Divine nectar and you choose not to reach for another bowl of ice cream. Self-effort is when God calls and you choose not to turn up the television. Self-effort is the will power required to say "yes" to Grace no matter what the circumstances. In this way self-effort and Grace become one. Another way to understand self-effort is *Netzah* – spiritual perseverance or spiritual will power.

The issue of self-effort and focusing inward is important because there is a continual desire by people to look only outward for salvation and to avoid self-effort. We search for a guru or teacher to do this for us. New people would often ask Swami Muktananda, in essence, "Are you the best?" as if this would ensure their salvation. It also would entitle us to "bragging rights" about our path or guru. Not only does the path or guru then become an extension of our pride, thus blocking our growth, but this becomes a foundation of cults of "my guru" or "my path." Today we see this cult phenomenon in both Eastern spiritual groups and our Western Christian and Jewish groups, as highlighted by the tragedy of Jonestown. Focusing only outward also confuses us about the importance of our own inner teacher and self-effort. A great spiritual teacher once said, "We create our Gods and gurus, but the only thing we cannot create is the Self." This is why we should know the Self. Shri Nisargadatta Maharaj, a Liberated seer from Bombay, taught that the physical guru is a milestone along the way, but the Inner Guru is with us for the full journey.[7] Shakti Kundalini/Shekhinah, a holographic energy pattern of universal consciousness that resides within us, is awakened within us and unfolds within us as a spiritualizing force.

After the Merging of the Kundalini

Journal entry from August of 1981:

> A quiet completeness pervades. Completeness.... Wholeness.... Non-beingness.... Timeless.... Spaceless. Knowing the Way by Being the Way. Totally regular ... a quietly ecstatic nobody. A merkaba ... an emanation of Divine Will. Just Being in the world as the world, yet not of it. Free to emanate God's Will. Free to move in any direction. The illusion of doership is gone. The personality is a mere result of mistaken identity. There is nothing to do, but to Be the sublime celebration of the unfolding of God's creation. In the Peace of Being, a gentle Love prevails. We are but one Heart, throbbing in the all-pervading harmonious energy of Love that is the basis of all existence. The Truth manifests as Love. We exist as Love, To Be as Love, Just to Be ... Love.

Journal entry of August 15, 1986:

> Kundalini rising is an arrow returning upward to the Heart of God. After the Heart of God has been pierced there is but one complete throbbing energy globe of God's Love, infinitely expanding in all directions from a completely still center. It is the awareness that there is only That One. There are no divisions into mine and thine, you and me, or this or that. It is direct knowledge that we are all fingers on the Hand of God. All is experienced as One in the ground of Being of God. It is to know completely in every fiber of our Being, the Truth of the first commandment: "Thou shalt have no other gods before Me" (Exodus 20:3) and "Hear, O Israel: The Lord our God, the Lord is One." (Deuteronomy 6:4). This is the non-dualistic Truth of God.

This awareness is beyond duality. Our binary brain simply cannot cope with it or express it on an intellectual basis. We fall into dualistic words like "perfect," which implies its dualistic opposite, "imperfect." Of course, not only is the word "perfect" dualistic, it carries within it all our dualistic conceptions of perfection. These perfectionistic conceptions limit our clarity in fulfilling God's Will and our understanding of others who are free to be God's Will. To be free to be God's Will means we are Liberated from any of our concepts or any other person's projections of perfection. It may mean expressing Love by compassionately and fiercely yelling at someone for them to wake up. It may mean allowing yourself to become caught in someone's state or problem to receive an insight in order to be of service. It may require using anger as a spiritual teaching, as Jesus did with the money exchangers in the Temple. We must allow whatever teaching that must come through and trust that we are an extension of God's Will. We realize that although we are not our personality, that as a vehicle of expression in the world our personality must be used as a tool regardless of its own peculiarities. It does not mean that no concepts are left, but instead we recognize them as such and at any time we can transcend them. The merging of Kundalini does not make us perfect; it shifts us into Being as a way of life. We become as the law rather than under the law. The merging of Shiva and Shakti or Zeir Anpin and Nukba (Shekhinah) takes one beyond the I AM consciousness to the undifferentiated wholeness of I AM THAT. In this awareness, even the Love of the Self disappears. It is very subtle. In that Oneness, we no longer experience the delusion, looking for the entrance to get in to the Heart of God while we actually are the pulsating Heart of God. All seeking stops. All everything stops.

In this state of wholeness, we do not experience ourselves as different or separate from anyone else. There is a continual communion of equality awareness. It is the foundation of humility – neither above nor below – and a heartfelt oneness. An example of this occurred after Jesus transcended: He came back and broke bread in humble communion with his disciples.

The Dharma of Liberated Ones

Each Enlightened Being is an individual Love song of the Divine that expresses differently in each moment as the Absolute plays through the individual soul, or *neshama,* as its source. Because of individual karmas we are drawn to different expressions of Liberated Ones. There is no one expression of Enlightenment or one superhighway. The Six Foundations are the roadway that help destroy the dream of one's individual existence separate from the breath of Yah. From this roadway, footpaths branch off, walked by the Liberated Ones. Yet all Enlightened Ones have one shared function: to help people wake up and stay awake – to share eyn zu-lo-to, Nothing but the One.

A Liberated One may appear completely regular in daily life. The great Chinese Master, Chuang Tzu, was said to appear as totally plain. In Hasidism, a form of ecstatic mystical Judaism, there is a tradition of the hidden *tzadik.* The original leader, the *Baal Shem Tov,* kept himself hidden for years as a poor householder. In India this is also common. My spiritual uncle and second Guru, Swami Prakashanada, who in 1961 was acknowledged by Swami Muktananda to be in a Liberated state, lived very simply in two rooms. He sat quietly, just Being in his state of Love. Spiritual seekers as well as many spiritually advanced monks came from the surrounding area to experience his Love or share his right fellowship and wisdom. There were no tours or public relations promotions so common in the West. We did not think about power when around him, only about the Love and spiritual wisdom of his simple Non-Beingness. In Zen it is taught that we simply continue our daily tasks like chopping wood and carrying water. The point is that this post-Kundalini awareness can be found in the simple, regular, ecstatic nobodies who are often not recognized because of our own projections and expectation of what we think a spiritual teacher should be or look like.

Because of the influx of charismatic gurus and teachers in the West, people mistakenly have come to judge a person's spiritual state based on how much charisma or psychic power he or she has or the number of students he or she has amassed. Power is not awareness; it is just power. Charisma is not awareness; it is charisma. The manifestation of these qualities such as power or number of students may have purpose in a person's mission, but should not be confused with the spiritual state itself. To be a highly charismatic, powerful teacher does not mean that person is in Liberated awareness, no matter how the teacher's style or act fits our expectations and projections of a Liberated Being. However, a Liberated One may be a highly public, charismatic figure. This is a subtle area to understand. These issues are brought up to help us not get caught in concepts. Either picture may fit our fantasies. The most important focus is our own inner state.

This one's Guru uncle, the Enlightened master Swami Prakashananda, proclaimed this one Liberated on three separate meetings after the glass ceiling of the mind shattered. At first it was hard to relate to because this one could not locate any being in the body-mind-I AM complex who could be identified in any way to be called Enlightened. But Swami Prakashananda was persistent and on the third time several weeks later, after one of his eloquent Love sharings through the interpreter Amrit Jyoti, his message was received. Swami Prakashananda then spent a whole day with this one personally, explaining how subtle the whole process was. Talking about the subtlety of what we call the ego of Liberation, Swami Prakashananda pointed out that in Liberation, all the common rules of the world of duality seem ridiculous. Yet at the same time, his main message was that even though they seem ridiculous, we must uphold the dharma, as lived in the world. By this he meant the *yamas* and *niyamas*, or *Ten Speakings* (Ten Commandments) that keep order in the world and maintain social harmony. He pointed out that this is the main way that people who first enter into the Beingness of Liberation may slip into a hole called "the ego of Liberation" and create imbalance in the outer planes. This is because they experience themselves as being beyond the rules of unawakened life. The fall of so many gurus makes this point very clear. Swami Prakashananda went on to emphasize that until we literally leave the body, unless we achieve the state of full moksha, which is very, very rare, dharma must be closely followed.

In Gabriel's lifetime, he has met perhaps two people who are in the stage of moksha. One is a disciple of Nityananda, Swami Jnananda, who this one met when the Swami was in his late nineties. This one had the rare opportunity to spend one hour in silence with him, thanks to Swami

Prakashananda. The other is Sri Ganapati Satchidananda Swamiji. Swami Jnananda was unusually inspiring to this one because he was not born in the *avadut moksha* state, as were Sri Ganapati Satchidananda Swamiji, Swami Nityananda, and Sai Baba of Shirdi. This state of full Enlightenment is different from the state of Self-realization and is experienced by very few people in the world.

The point that Swami Prakashananda made to this one was very clear. As long as we are in the body, we are still subject to the subtle pulls of money, sexuality, greed, and the lust of the body in different ways. By holding the dharma, we do not fall into the potential subtle delusion of Enlightenment that we are above all this and therefore can ignore it. It was a very strong teaching. The Rabbinical sages of the Sanhedrin called it the process of "putting a fence around the Torah." The experience of this one, as the awareness fructifies, is one of increasing Love and peace for the whole in which the expression is one of service in the world. In this context, living dharmically is the natural expression of THAT. Swami Prakashananda's warning has validity. The deeper one fructifies, the tests become more and more subtle. A corollary to this is the ancient prophetic teaching about Moses and other prophets. According to Kabbalah teachings, Yah communicates with the prophets through visions or dreams, but Moses was the only one in history who had clear direct communication with Yah. The eleventh-century Rabbi Shlomo Yitzchak gives a wise commentary on this: "Other prophets looked through the 'glass' [par'gawd – the veil] and believed that they had seen God while actually they had not, while Moses looked through the 'glass' and knew he had not seen God."[8] The message is that all experience, even if one is established in a steady state of one of the many stages of Enlightenment and feels and knows eyn zu-lo-to (I AM THAT), is still subtly illusory. In Kabbalah there are many stages of the Oneness, going all the way to the Ein Sof, which is prior to infinite time, space, and Being. The Ein Sof is beyond knowing. The mystery is beyond grasping, yet graspable on some level. At more mature stages of the Enlightenment process we simply dance ecstatically, quietly, humbly, and innocently in the mystery of the void, in the *B'lee mah* and *Mah,* or the something and the Nothing of *YHWH* (the name of God beyond time, form, and Being). Humbly following the dharma keeps us as the Divine Dance.

Some Enlightened souls feel one may stop spiritual practices once a particular level or state of awareness has happened. In the West there are many forces, such as fame, sex, wealth, power, and projected images of how a guru should be, which encourage us to become unconscious of the essential Truth. As our newspapers and consciousness journals have pointed out, many fine gurus, guides, and teachers have fallen to these subtle temptations. Because of this and because it has become a part of Gabriel's way, the spiritual dharma as the Six Foundations continue to manifest, as well as dharma in the world such as building his main sanghas at the Tree of Life Foundation in Patagonia, Arizona, and in Israel.

Swami Prakashananda Saraswati gave the author this feedback on his approach in a letter discussing this question in 1984:

> Baba [Muktananda] has given you everything and you've realized the innate perfection. In this perfection you know everything so what is there to say? It is true that sometimes even then, ignorance arises.

In another letter in 1983, Prakashananda supported these practices:

> You are quite right in your estimation of the fast and meditation. There is nothing like it to purify oneself in spite of your being complete as I have always mentioned to you. It is indeed very good for the soul, and you are absolutely right that when you say that as long as one is in the physical body, we need this therapy from time to time.

Because of occasional wobbling in non-dualistic awareness, the Six Foundations continue rather spontaneously. They reflect a prior-to-consciousness awareness as the expression of how to live as a family person in the world. These Six Foundations "put a fence around the Torah." The dual states that arise are not binding. They are just temporary modifications of the Transcendent Truth of I AM THAT. In a predominant non-dualistic awareness we become as the law, rather than under it. All laws and concepts, including our own, are games played in order to participate in society.

In this awareness, this I AM consciousness is entirely free to live out the Essene/kedusha archetypes as a dharma vehicle in the world, yet knowing it is just an archetype in the world of temporal reality, an illusion dissolved in the permanent reality of I AM THAT. We are all the expressions of the Enlightenment process, and this one chooses to honor the Ten Speakings (Ten Commandments) by killing neither Love nor joy with concepts. They are shared because they may help or be a guide for some people who share these archetypes. We can only live the Truth as we experience it. One can only manifest as the unique expression of the Unmanifest. This is why the Amidah, a Jewish daily prayer, repeatedly says, "The God of Abraham, the God of Isaac, and the God of Jacob." Each of these Great Ones was the individual's own unique manifestation. We are all in an Enlightenment process that will lead to the potential of total Enlightenment. The reader receives the benefit of the experience of this one at this particular stage of embodiment of awareness. Perfectionistic concepts of either/or belong to the dualists who want to judge, grade, and create separateness. God's kingdom has many mansions and this one is simply traveling through those palaces like everyone else. We are all flowers of Love, infinitely expanding step by step in the pulseless-pulse of the Infinite Universal Awareness.

An inspiration for this teaching of humility is the great Hasidic master, Rabbi Nachman. It was said that as soon as he achieved a new level of awareness he would immediately, with a humble heart, begin again, like one taking his first step into the realm of holiness.[9] He was said to be driven by an intense yearning for a deeper and deeper experience of God. Bassui Tokusho, a Rinzai Zen master born in 1327, felt so strongly about the need for awakened awareness to ripen that, although proclaimed by many as Enlightened, he continued intense practices for years as a roving monk before he reached a level of spiritual awareness that he felt was necessary to be able to teach others.[10] Another Zen master, Joshu (Chao-Chou), a ninth-century T'ang dynasty Zen Master, was Enlightened at age 18, and stayed with his teacher until the teacher left his body when Joshu was 58 years old. From 58 to 80 he traveled China involved in dharma debates. At 80 he felt it was time to take the role of active guru, which he did until he left the body at age 120.

Twenty Years After

Twenty Years After
And bliss bursts through every cell.
Sometimes the non-causal joy is so much
This body-mind-I AM complex
Explodes in natural
Love
Ecstasy
Supreme non-causal contentment.
It can't be contained any longer.
No amount of work or external difficulties
Can keep it quiet
The endless Light of Yah

Reflected
Through this funny body-mind-I AM complex
As extraordinary well-being
Sublime ecstatic energy
Dancing Yah's dance.
The many faces of Yah shine through
As the infinite smile
Yes
Enlightenment is an infinite smile.

Throughout history some of the great spiritual leaders have experienced what appear to be short breaks in their continual Communion with God. Since these Great Ones exist as a teaching for us in all their actions, it may be that these breaks in Oneness awareness are to teach that to apply concepts of perfectionist spiritual standards for those of us in the body is not appropriate. In the Judaic tradition, even the greatest spiritual leader, Moses, was chastised by God at the waters of Meribah (Numbers 20:12) for not sanctifying and remembering God in the drawing of water from the rock. For this lapse in awareness, Moses was not allowed to lead the people into the promised land. In the Eastern traditions, the great *avatar* Rama cried when he discovered that his wife had been abducted. At another time, when he saw his brother unconscious on the battlefield, he became grief stricken. Krishna, the master of Yoga, proclaimed as an avatar, was said to have experienced grief when his father died. These are important examples and teachings to suggest that the concept of totally unbroken Cosmic Unity Awareness while in the physical body may just be a play of the need of our dualistic minds for the safe, comfortable, and neat concept of perfection. Nevertheless, it is possible that a totally Enlightened, unbroken transcendental state exists for someone living in the human body.

This issue has been raised to shake up the concepts of the dualistic perfectionists who create misery for themselves and others by their states of non self-acceptance and by their critical judgment of the spiritual states of others. It is simply a Divine happening. This one is in a natural unfolding that is nurtured with the archetypal life that manifests itself. It is very ordinary, natural, regular, and essentially connected to everyone else in the ground of Being of that regularity. There is no focus on the conceptual goal of total Enlightenment (moksha) or on the process. It is enough to simply self-abide in the delight of Non-Being, to know the

Way by Being the Way, to delight in the infant innocence of *Bala Krishna* being as peace when the ignorant may judge it as the fool or trouble-maker instead of Bala Krishna, or see this one as a holistic physician, as Director of the Tree of Life Foundation, as a man, Yogi, student of Kabbalah, National Football Hall of Fame football player, sincere student, devoted, Loving, well-informed teacher, and so on. Whatever is seen is not the Truth; it is a projected lie on the screen of the ego. A Liberated One can move in any direction, from Bala Krishna (infant Krishna playing) to Rama (King of Dharma). The world becomes an endless cosmic playground for us to be as the authentic expression of Divine Will playing through the body-mind-I AM complex. In Kabbalah, the term is "merkaba vehicle." The Divine Will, or Keter, has guided this one in the way of Rama Krishna Paramahamsa, who knew God through many paths. This expression for this one is as an ecstatic Kabbalist, living in Deveikut, a Yogi in sahaja samadhi, a Native American Lakota Sundancer and Eagle Dancer merging with the cosmic Tree of Life, and as the unfolding of the Tao. Yet all the time, laughing in I AM THAT and not identifying with any of these ways. This has been a great teaching for students – how to live these ways in depth and not to identify with any of them – and is very confusing for those who need to be "something."

This practice of allowing oneself to fructify, after moving into the untamed universe of Self-realization, is one that we find in Yoga as well as the Jewish tradition. It is said that the great awakened holy man, Ramana Maharshi, spent at least twenty-one years of sadhana after he was awakened in his teens. The wisdom of various traditions mention the twenty-one-year cycle as part of the fructification as well. Perhaps the oldest recorded statement of this is from Jacob, who received the blessings from his father and then spent twenty to twenty-two years working through the subtleties of dealing with the dark side of Laban, his uncle, Master of the Dark Arts. In this process, Jacob achieved mastery in the world. Prior to this, he spent most of his time meditating in the tent of his mother.

Why is there this time for fruition? This step, in which I AM consciousness shatters, requires time to understand and integrate. Because the glass ceiling of consciousness shatters and because the Kundalini has unfolded and merged in the One does not necessarily mean that everything has been worked out. It is actually a time to go inward to the Self and become fearlessly rooted in the subtleties of the Self. Yet, paradoxically, there is no integration to be made because there is only wholeness.

In writing this revised edition of *Spiritual Nutrition*, reflecting back on the twenty-one-year cycle that has been completed post-Self-realization for this one, it has been a most amazing and challenging time. It is a time when this one was extremely sensitive to all that is happening in an entirely new way. It is far more than the Kundalini merging with Sahasrara. It is, in a sense, the ultimate rebirth into the Nothing, requiring one to be simultaneously absolutely normal, or what we at the Tree of Life Foundation call "awakened normality." It is the art of living in a paradoxical dual/non-dual awareness. The play of the Absolute through the world is the teaching.

One of the most beautiful stories about this state is a Kabbalistic teaching about the four Rabbis who went into the world of Pardes in the Garden of Eden. As they ascended in their travels into the deeper planes, Rabbi ben Azzai died from the ecstasy of the experience. Rabbi ben Zoma could not reconcile the difference between the world of Atz'ilut, which is the plane of non-dual direct knowing, and the plane of Asee'Yah, the physical world of total duality, and he went mad. Rabbi Elisha ben Abuya was not able to integrate the experience between the world of Atz'ilut, the direct knowing of total non-dual world, and the world of duality, Asee'Yah. He chose to see life from only the non-dual awareness and became what is known as an apostate, taking great joy in totally violating the precepts of the Jewish tradition. He is what we would call "crazy wisdom" in the Yogic tradition. Only Rabbi Akiba was able to rest in the peace of the knowledge of the four worlds: the world of Asee'Yah, the physical world, Yetsirah, the world of the astral plane, B'riYah, the world of the pure mind, and then Atz'ilut, the world of direct knowing of the Divine or totally non-dual world. He remained in a simultaneous dual/non-dual awareness – embracing the Absolute non-dual world of Atz'ilut, as well as the most dual world of Asee'Yah. Rabbi Akiba was able to live in peace with the different messages from the same symbols. For example, in the world of the Asee'Yah, the letters of the Ten Speakings (the Ten Commandments) could be seen only in one direction, while in the world of B'riYah, the letters could be seen in both directions in the same tablet, which is impossible in the world of duality.

It takes time to walk in the untamed mystery. We become the play of Bala Krishna. When the glass ceiling has shattered, one shifts consciousness from being dominated by the mind and I AM consciousness to aligning the mind and I AM with non-dual apperception of God. We are babes in this natural state. This is why some of the great Zen masters,

Yogis, and Jewish spiritual masters have waited many, many years before teaching, and this is why, often, it is good to wait maybe twenty-one years before going out in the world and teaching. This fructification period is a very delicate time. It is important to honor it.

Summary, Chapter 2

1. With the awakening of Kundalini, there is a partial fusing and synchronicity of the two energies. As awareness develops, there is an increase in total Kundalini energy, synchronicity, and fusing until the two Kundalini energies become fused as one holographic energy in the crown chakra. Our consciousness shifts into a predominant, non-dualistic, awake state of awareness of God. This is an awareness prior to I AM consciousness; it is the awareness of the world of Atz'ilut and soul levels of Chaya-Yehida, in the upper part of Binah, Chochma, and Keter in the Kabbalistic Sephirotic system.
2. The classical "three knots" (granthis) are nodal points of a quantum jump in increased Kundalini energy in the system. The first knot expansion of consciousness and energy occurs with the merging of the first three chakras. The second is associated with the merging of the first three with the heart chakra awareness. The third expansion comes with the merging of all the chakra awareness into one whole, non-dualistic, unity awareness of the Truth of God, I AM THAT. We realize there was never anything to attain and we were that Oneness all along.
3. In the spiritual unfolding there seem to be periods of much intense motivation and periods of less intense times, depending on the play of the Kundalini process. For this reason, general practice of the Six Foundations is always appropriate. Our emphasis on each of the Six Foundations may vary, according to spontaneous unfolding. There is no set program.
4. Depending on how we perceive them, these spiritual experiences may be an ego trap, a spiritual addiction, or may serve as Divine behavior modification for expanding consciousness and for encouraging us to follow practices that enhance the spiritualizing energy of the Kundalini.
5. A proper balance of Grace and self-effort is necessary for the overall evolution of the Kundalini to effectively take place.

6. Self-effort is not mere will power. It is a paradoxical effortless-effort. It is the ability to say "yes" when God's Grace occurs and we might not feel ready for whatever form it takes.
7. After the merging of Kundalini, we expand beyond a vertical evolution to an infinite expansion in all directions as the one Heart of God, as Love, as non-dualistic equality Unity Awareness.
8. In a state of non-Being rather than doing/Being, we are free to Be the Will of God as the non-specific expression of Love in the service of the awakening of humanity.
9. Kundalini awakening is but the start of another level of expansion in one of God's many mansions. We all share in this unending and gradual unfolding of the many stages of Enlightenment.
10. The more often we enter these states of deep Communion, the deeper they are etched into our consciousness, until they become our awareness, and finally create the pre-conditions for the glass ceiling to shatter the mind into the Liberation of I AM THAT.
11. After the glass ceiling shatters, one enters into a state of Liberation that over time establishes one more and more permanently in the non-dual awareness of I AM THAT.
12. A twenty-one-year cycle to fructify nurtures this sahaja samadhi, non-dual consciousness.
13. Although our dualistic, perfectionist thinking would like us to have an either/or possibility of a perfect, unbroken state of awareness, this represents an idealistic concept. We can stop judging ourselves and others, and know that it is enough just to Be.
14. The simple gift of Kundalini merging is to Know the Way by Being the Way. All that is required is to simply show up and be willing to die to the Self.

Chapter 3

The Chakra System

To more fully understand the process of Kundalini awakening and to understand the process of energy assimilation so we can create a diet that supports the Kundalini unfoldment, we must explore the chakra system as one of three main subtle energy systems of the human organism. The other two systems are the Kundalini, which we have already discussed in depth, and the subtle bodies, which will be discussed in Chapter 7. This lays the foundation for understanding the awakening of consciousness and relationship of nutrition to spiritual development.

The chakra system is a subtle energy system that has been described for thousands of years in spiritual traditions. In Sanskrit, the word *chakra* means wheel. It has come into common usage in the West through Yoga teachings that have diffused into our culture. The Tibetans refer to these energy centers as *khor-Io,* which also means wheel. In the Sufi tradition, some call them *latifas,* or subtle ones. In the Bible, John refers to these centers as the "seven seals on the back of the Book of Life." In early Christianity, they were often referred to as the "seven churches." The Kabbalists refer to these centers as "the seven centers in the soul of man." There is obviously a historical, cross-cultural tradition among many of the major religions that validates the existence of these subtle energy centers. For our purposes, the author chooses to use the commonly accepted term chakra for this system of subtle energy centers.

The chakras are subtle energy centers formed by the confluence of the nadis (72,000 hollow channels in the subtle body through which Kundalini flows). On the physical plane, the chakras are connected to the endocrine system and nervous system plexuses. At the confluences of the nadis, vortexes are created that pull the cosmic energy into the chakras and then into and energizing the endocrine and nervous system plexuses. It is the author's theory that their radiations create the subtle bodies (see Chapter 7) and interface energetically with the koshas (layers of the mind; see Chapter 5). When the chakras are balanced as a total system, the total cosmic energetic flow into the human system is maximized.

The chakra system has been described by Western clairvoyants and Eastern Yogis over the centuries. More recently, medical doctors and other researchers have begun to explore its existence and function. In the late '60s and early '70s, Dr. Hiroshi Motoyama, director of the Institute for Religion and Psychology, a Yoga expert and scientist who is considered by many to be one of the leading researchers in the area of chakras, did some important work documenting the physical reality of chakras.[1] He constructed a light-proof room that was shielded from outside electrical emissions. In this room he placed what he called his Chakra Instrument, designed to detect minute emissions of physical energy from the human body in the form of light, electrical, or electromagnetic energy. In his experiments, he placed the detectors 12 to 20 centimeters in front of the particular chakra area that the subject was trying to activate. The Chakra Instrument was able to detect a quantifiable difference when subjects concentrated directly on a particular chakra, but only when a chakra was chosen on which the subject had previously practiced mental activation. When a chakra was tested on which the subject had not previously practiced, no change was noted before or during the test. These results suggest the existence of a scientifically measurable chakra location.

In 1973 the physician W. Brugh Joy, M.D., discovered these energy centers spontaneously. He found that when he held his hands over certain areas of a patient's body, there were areas of increased heat energy. Mapping these areas, he realized that they were approximately the same as the Yoga descriptions of the chakra locations.[2] Another physician, Lawrence Bagley, M.D., in the 1984 issue of the *American Journal of Acupuncture*,[3] describes how by using the Nogier pulse, an auricular acupuncture pulse system developed by Paul Nogier, M.D., he was able to determine the location, size, shape, and rotational direction of the chakras. The author's own experience with being able to detect the physical existence of the chakra system began in 1976, while exploring the possible relationship between a person's mental state and the chakra system. The author discovered that when he let a crystal pendulum rotate over the chakra areas, it circled either clockwise or counterclockwise. One day when it rotated counterclockwise over a patient's head, his headache got worse and he felt energy-depleted. When the author purposefully rotated the crystal in a clockwise direction over the person's head, the headache disappeared and he felt more energized. It became clear in further experiments that subtle energies, such as those generated by a crystal, could be used in a way that would be healing and energizing to people.

Chakra Location

There is no absolute agreement on the number of major chakras, their location, and function. There does seem to be a general consensus, however, that there are seven main body chakras and an eighth transpersonal chakra above the head. Most agree that these chakras start at the base of the spine and ascend to the top of the head in a line approximately midway through the body. The first chakra is at the base of the spine in the perineal area. The second chakra is located between the pubic bone and the umbilicus. The third is located between the umbilicus and the solar plexus region. The fourth is in the midline at the heart level. The fifth is at the thyroid (throat) level. The sixth is between the eyes at the brow. The seventh is like a skullcap on the vertex of the skull.

(See the Chakra Diagram in the color plates.)

Some Western groups locate the second chakra over the spleen rather than in the midline area. It is the author's feeling that some of the variances in locations are due to cultural differences in where the spiritual traditions focus their energy. For example, the Chinese and Japanese tend to focus on the *hara,* located at the umbilicus or slightly below-between the second and third chakra locations. Theosophists tend to de-emphasize the second, or sexual, chakra and focus on the spleen region for the location of the second chakra. This differs from the Yogic tradition. Besides the cultural differences, the location and size of the different chakras may also vary with an individual's spiritual evolution. Motoyama, for example, found that the measurable chakra and associated meridian energies vary depending on which chakra a person tends to use the most. It may be that the Yogic traditions describe the chakra system of more evolved spiritual aspirants, for whom the spleen center is less important than it is for Westerners. In the author's work with

Western spiritual aspirants, he finds a more predominant midline second chakra; the spleen chakra seems to be a secondary center. What matters, beyond these details, is that from many perspectives, researchers and spiritual practitioners agree that chakras exist as an important system of subtle energy in the body.

It also seems to be generally agreed that each chakra has a specific energetic nature that relates to color, sound, and geometric shape. Each chakra is associated with certain mental states and with a specific spiritual awareness. Each chakra also seems to be associated with the physiology of a specific glandular system, organ system, and nerve plexus.

Dr. Motoyama validated the relationship of chakras to organs, glands, and nerve plexus by developing an instrument he named the AMI, or Apparatus for Measuring the Functional Conditions of Meridians and their Corresponding Internal Organs.[4] He found that in people who were judged by a panel of experts to have a particular chakra activated, there was a change in meridian energy related to the specific organs associated with that activated chakra.

Essential Function of the Chakras

There is general consensus on the essential function of the chakras. Differences exist, however, on the details. David Tansley, an English radionics practitioner and author of many books on subtle energies, feels the chakra system picks up energies originating from every level of the cosmos. This includes our physical, emotional, and mental selves, as well as the collective unconscious of our nation and our planet. Brugh Joy, M.D., is completely certain that the chakra system exists, but that nobody completely understands all its functions. In his book, he tentatively takes the position that the chakra system is an interdimensional transducing system.[5] He feels it is affected by thought and capable of converting matter into various levels of more subtle energy, transmitting them into the physical system. Its functioning transcends the limitations of time and space.

One of the first Westerners to describe the chakra system was the Reverend C. W. Leadbeater, a Theosophical leader and extremely well-known clairvoyant who had worked as a vice-rector of the Church of England and was well-practiced in Yoga. In his book *The Chakras,* written in 1927, he describes chakras as *centers of conduction in which energy flows from one subtle body of a person to another level of subtle body.*[6] These subtle bodies will be described in detail in Chapter 7; they are the subtle layers of energy and consciousness that surround the physical body, forming its aura. Leadbeater describes these chakras as perpetually rotating; the primary force from the higher world is always flowing into their open vortex. He sees the force as sevenfold, all its forms operating in each of these centers, but one center predominating over the others. He feels that without the absorption of this higher energy into the chakras, the physical body cannot exist. Dr. Motoyama also feels the chakras function as intermediaries for energy transfer and conversion between two neighboring subtle bodies. In Motoyama's system there are two subtle bodies: astral and causal. He feels the chakras convert energy from one body to another in either direction; *they can convert physical energy into psychological energy.*

It is generally agreed that the chakras rotate in a vortex that extends out from a point in the midline of the body, a sort of funnel for bringing the energy into the physical body. Lawrence Bagley, M.D., in his booklet *Chakra Chrome,* describes how these chakra vortexes can be measured using the Nogier pulse technique. The direction in which the vortexes rotate when they are healthy and balanced is not universally agreed upon, but the majority consensus, with which this author's research agrees, is that a clockwise rotation suggests a healthier chakra function.

Energy Flow in the Chakras

Our chakras, to a greater or lesser extent, are always active. It is common to describe chakras as either "open" or "closed," giving the impression that a chakra may somehow be blocked and energy not able to flow through it. But chakras are neither open nor closed. The difference is that some chakras have less energy flowing through them – they are less activated, meaning the energy charging through them is disrupted in its transduction through the subtle bodies.

There is also the implication that an "open" chakra, through which much energy is flowing, is better. This is not necessarily the case. For example, in working with people suffering from manic psychosis, the author has observed that their crown chakra is wide "open," or activated. It is so activated, in fact, that these patients' lives become imbalanced. People experiencing a manic psychosis often describe a rush of energy flowing through them from the top of their head. This sort of description correlates with what people experience with an activated chakra. For some clients in a hypomanic state, by specifically working to slow down the flow of energy through the crown chakra, it has been possible to lessen the excessive activation, rebalance their chakras, and thus decrease their hypomania.

Discarding the language "open" or "closed" does not negate a difference in the energy levels of the different chakras. Dr. Brugh Joy describes feeling these energy differences with his hands. This is relatively easy to do and the reader may want to experiment with this to get a feeling for chakra energy and location. Dr. Lawrence Bagley describes mapping out the difference in energy fields around the various chakras. Dr. Motoyama, with his Chakra Instrument and AMI device, has begun to quantify these differences. He has established that a chakra with more energy flowing through it has a wider range of dynamic balance between the sympathetic and parasympathetic nervous systems. He also discovered that in these more activated chakras, the associated organ systems have more energy running through them. Some of his preliminary research suggests that people with more activated chakras have more disease susceptibility in the organs related to that activated chakra.[7] The author's clinical impression, on the basis of observing many hundreds of people with activated chakras, is that disease susceptibility may be just a temporary phenomenon related to the time it takes to harmoniously incorporate an increased input of energy into the system. Disease susceptibility may also be connected to the mental overstimulation of one chakra in a way that knocks it out of harmony with the rest of the chakra system. Another explanation is that when one chakra is overstimulated by the mind, the organs associated with it have too much energy moving through them. Perhaps, in a way, it is analogous to a wire burning out when too much electricity passes through it and there is no protective fuse. The fuse in this case is common sense. This metaphor represents the *danger in trying to activate specific chakras by mind/will power, rather than letting them awaken spontaneously and naturally through meditation and the development of higher awareness.*

A highly activated chakra has more energy flowing into it through the transducing system of the subtle bodies. Therefore, more energy is flowing into the body in general, and specifically into the organs connected with that chakra. The first consideration in evaluating the meaning of an activated chakra is whether the individual is able to integrate this increased energy into his or her overall functioning. The second consideration is whether the total chakra system is in balance. As has already been pointed out, the chakras in an average person are not at exactly equal levels of activation. Depending on a person's life situation and how that person consciously or unconsciously uses the different chakras, they will vary in strength and activity over time. Being aware of the energetic balance of the total chakra system, rather than just focusing on a single unbalanced chakra, has given some additional clues about the energetic functioning of the chakra system. The author has observed that when one chakra became balanced through the crystal work and the remaining unbalanced chakras were retested, they became spontaneously balanced. It became clear to the author that *chakras have an energy entrainment system.* This is especially true of the linkage of the first, second, and third chakras as a unit and also seems to often be the case with the fifth, sixth, and seventh chakras. These two units seem to form a linkage at the fourth, or heart, chakra. It is like an infinity sign with the heart at the center.

An additional point in appreciating chakras as a total interconnected system is that there seems to exist a polarity within each chakra area. For the base chakra, polarity seems to exist between the feet or ground and the base of the spine. The second chakra polarizes between the two testicles or ovaries. The third is between the solar plexus and the spleen. The fourth is between the heart and the thymus (ancient heart). The fifth is between the thyroid and parathyroid. The polarity for the sixth and seventh chakras is between the pituitary gland associated with the brow chakra and the pineal gland, more associated with the seventh. There also seems to be some degree of polarity between the different chakras on a vertical basis, such as first and sixth and seventh, second and fifth, and third and fourth. Because of this, whenever working at the chakra level with a patient, the author will finish with an overall spiral balancing of the main chakras. One of the most common situations in which the chakras become disorganized in relationship to each other is severe emotional trauma. Doing a crystal spiral balancing alone is very helpful to someone in such a crisis.

Awakened Chakras

Chakras are either awake or asleep. This is not the same as the activity level of a chakra, which is primarily associated with keeping our organism supplied with vital life force for our general functioning. *The awak-*

ening of the chakras is primarily associated with the development of more evolved spiritual awareness. Dr. Brugh Joy has noted that an awakened chakra functions on a different level and that it feels and looks different to clairvoyants.[8] *When a chakra is awakened, it is part of a spiritually evolving process in which the mind merges with the higher awareness stored in that chakra.* In some cases, certain psychic abilities associated with the chakra are also activated. Psychic ability, however, is not necessarily a sign of spiritual evolvement or of a chakra's awakening. Psychic ability is not the same as spiritual awareness. It is misleading to associate it with the spiritual awareness that is stored in each chakra and released to the consciousness of the awakened mind.

There is general agreement that each chakra has a spiritual awareness associated with it, but no simplified system for understanding this awareness is either found or agreed upon. A variety of esoteric teachings and descriptions of powers may be associated with the awakening of the different chakras, but these will not be part of our discussion. With the awakening of each chakra, there occurs a key transition from mundane consciousness to a more complete spiritual awareness. Just as the general energies of the chakras are linked, the awakened chakras function as combined units of awareness. The first through the third chakras are linked as one unit, with the heart chakra the pivotal integrator. The fifth through the seventh chakras comprise the second unit, and its relationship to the heart is also important.

The first three chakras are life force energies primarily concerned with issues of survival on the physical and emotional planes. The spiritual awareness associated with their awakening manifests in mastery of all the issues of living in the world. *The awakening of the first three chakras is essential for integrating the knowledge of how to live in the world with a spiritually transformed consciousness. Without it, the more intense energies released by the spiritual awakenings of the upper chakras can throw us out of balance in our everyday lives.* It is difficult to be stabilized in the higher awareness without integrating the awakened first three chakras into our daily lives.

The fourth through the seventh chakras are primarily concerned with spiritual life. Their awakening activates spiritual energies and the transmutation of mundane consciousness into higher consciousness.

It is important to understand that development of higher awareness in the chakras is not necessarily linear; rather, it seems to be both simultaneous and spiral, yet neither. It is wholistic. Awareness of the different chakras seems to fuse at nodal points and to depend on the other chakras for a spiral, integrated, individualized, and simultaneous awakening at different levels of intensity. *Once the Kundalini is awakened, there is an ongoing awakening of all the chakras simultaneously, but at different levels of intensity in each chakra at various times.* An individual, for example, may be in the primary process of first and second chakra awakening but may also be reveling in the bliss of the Divine Communion of the seventh chakra. We often notice a new awareness or awakening when this awareness reaches a point of stabilization and integration in our conscious awareness. This is when our mind has fully merged with the total awareness of that chakra.

The first chakra is often known as the survival chakra. In its unawakened state, it is governed by the misconception that we are separate from Nature and need to conquer Nature in order to be safe and to survive. Its drive is to master the forces of matter. As a result, this limited awareness and lack of understanding allows us to become immersed in the material plane – fearing, doubting, and distrusting the environment. In this state, it is difficult to believe that there is a God. One's own ego is one's God. The awakening of the Kundalini energy that is stored in its potential state just below the first chakra often helps to shake us out of this limited awareness by giving us a taste of Communion with God. We learn that we are more than just physical bodies and that there is a higher purpose to life than simply making money and surviving on the material plane. This is the link between the first and sixth-seventh chakras, in which we become completely in tune with our higher vision and purpose. From fear, doubt, and non-belief, there is a shift to faith, trust, and belief in a higher force, or God. From disharmony with Nature, we move into a desire to be harmonious. We begin to understand the elements of Nature. Our sense of separation begins to diminish, and we seek to live in unity with Nature and the natural laws rather than to subjugate them. Trust in the illusion of one's ego power shifts to a trust in God. Primary fear and survival is transmuted to the awareness that there exists a Unity with a Higher Force.

The second chakra is characterized by the drive to procreate. When awakened, a shift in consciousness allows us to overcome the control of our lives by obsessive, instinctual sexual desires. This does not mean we deny sex. It means we experience it on a higher level of Communion, Love, harmony, and creativity. Physical sexual activity becomes a choice. Life becomes a creative Communion. The primordial energies of procreation are transformed into more refined, creative, aesthetic, and artistic energies. In the awakened state, the raw procreative energies of the second chakra transmute into more refined spiritual energies. Creativity without understanding can create havoc because it can degenerate into a lustful desire to pursue personal creativity at the expense of others. Understanding in the first chakra is necessary to give a grounding energy to the creativity of the second chakra.

The third chakra is marked by an innate awareness of what is happening on all planes of consciousness, both in the environment and within ourselves on a physical, emotional, mental, and spiritual level. It is a sensitive and perceptive ear to all forces. With its awakening, we transcend instinctual reactions to the psychic-emotional states of others. We become conscious of our reactive use of raw psychic-emotional power to attract, repel, project, magnify, and control others. We begin to operate in a balanced emotional state of reflection, discrimination, and sensitivity. We begin to develop a quality of sensitive perception of our inner and outer lives, to balance the raw forces of the first and second chakras and become interactors rather than reactors.

In the process of a full awakening, the solar plexus (third) chakra becomes harmonically linked with the heart (fourth) chakra. This linkage allows the information input of the solar plexus chakra to be interpreted through the Love of the heart chakra. The awakening leads to the fusion of the balanced emotion and power of the third chakra with the universal Love of the heart, or fourth, chakra. The fusion of the emotions with the Love-harmony of the fourth chakra gives us joy within, and we unite with one another in a moment of mutual sensitivity. It leads to a cooperative service between people. Ann Ree Colton metaphorically describes this fusion occurring when the lion initiate master of the solar plexus chakra lies down with the lamb initiate master of the heart.[9] This fusion marks a full awakening. It may be what Jeremiah describes in 31:33: "I will put my Torah in their inner parts, and write it in their hearts, and will be their God, and they shall be My people." This speaks to an attunement with an inner conscience or morality that is released into consciousness when the third chakra is awakened. As this awareness merges with the mind, judgment of self and others merges into an awareness of the spirit of the universal law. When the third chakra is harmonized with the heart, the awareness of the upper chakras manifests more easily as spirituality in everyday life. Another aspect of this awakening is the transmutation of the primordial desire/will power of the third chakra into attunement with the Will of God. It manifests as the awareness that *whatever God does is for the best.* It allows us to change the self-service of the first chakra to selfless service. It is another step in developing a trust in God. This awakened awareness helps us move from desire and attachment toward more sensitivity and less attachment to our desires. The awakened third chakra allows the life force of the first three chakras to be used as a strong healing power, the same power that *shamans* and *bruhus* use in their healing and magical work. A developed hara, which is the centering and grounding energy center focused on the martial arts and in some Chinese and Japanese religions, reflects the combined and integrated energy of the first three chakras.

The fourth, or heart, chakra awakens us to the experience of Love in any form in our lives. Eventually it awakens us to the experience of Universal Love. Its awakening helps us transform attached forms of Love associated with such emotions as lust, greed, pride, envy, infatuation, and even hate into a more peaceful, Universal Love. The raw instincts of self-preservation and survival are transmuted into full heart unity with all of humanity. It motivates us toward working for peace without oppression in the world. It is the Love that extends beyond the Love of our nuclear family to the one world family. An awakened heart acts as a balancing and integrating point for all the chakras. The conscience and virtue we develop from the awakening of the other chakras need Love as the energy to reach their full quality and power. It is with the awakening of this fourth chakra that we begin to experience ourselves and God as Love. Many people feel the Divine Self of all creation is centered in the heart. As the awareness of the heart chakra matured, this one regularly saw and experienced a blue flame of consciousness within his own heart. This occurred both during meditation and in everyday activities. The opening of the heart is very special.

The awakening of the fifth, or throat, chakra has to do with expression and communication of the more sublime meanings of existence. It has to do with the ability to translate all thoughts in the mind into form and shape. It involves all forms of communication such as aesthetics, art, language, music, and dance. Salespeople, lawyers, advertisers, and artists often have well developed throat chakras. The awakening reflects a shift from using the power of communication for our own selfish purposes to the communication of true inner feelings, spiritual teaching, and Truths. Through our own forms of expression, we become mediators and manifesters of the Truth. Our Being disperses peace and good tidings.

The awakening of the sixth, or brow, chakra brings us into a higher state of vision of the Truth. The mind becomes spiritualized. Intuition and attunement reach a spiritualized and integrated state of development. In the Christian world, this chakra is sometimes called the entry into the Christ mind. It is the "eye of the needle"; when fully awakened, it opens to the crown chakra. In the awakening of the sixth and seventh chakras, we become fully connected with the Inner Guru, or teacher. The full awakening of the sixth chakra as it oscillates with the seventh chakra seems to be associated with a state close to Self-realization in which we experience the Truth of the Universal Self within. It is at this stage that we directly begin to know ourselves as this awesome Truth. It is the stabilization of the I AM consciousness, becoming our primary identity. We are no longer deluded by the multiple material gods of ego, power, sex, or form. We enter into a state of Beingness rather than doingness as our primary identity. We feel at one with the Will of God. All concepts and ego blocks have been sufficiently purified out of the system, and we are free to follow the Will of God.

The awakening of the crown chakra is very much interconnected with awakening of the sixth chakra. As this awakening matures, we go beyond I AM consciousness into Self-realization of I AM THAT into an oscillation with merging with the Godhead. It is a sense of total Oneness with all of creation. Dualistic thinking fades, and we rest in the Beingness of non-dual awareness. We become more and more stabilized into the awareness of all as God. There is no separation. We become the purpose of life that we vaguely feel with the awakening of the first chakra. It is with this awareness that the merging of the heart and the sixth-seventh chakra complex becomes clearer. The philosophical debate between whether universal consciousness is centered in the heart or in the sixth-seventh chakra no longer has any meaning, because these chakras are linked on the planes of spiritual awareness. We spontaneously feel great, unrelenting Love with all. We never stop loving, because there is no one not to Love. Separation ends, and only Love exists. This is not so much an opening of the heart chakra as the experience of the Self as Love, of the World as God. It is another spiral deeper into the meaning and experience of Love. It exists as our totality of experience.

The awakening of the crown chakra also intensifies the link with higher levels of cosmic energy. We begin to directly experience the flow, or cosmic pulse of energy, into the system. We seem filled with this more refined cosmic energy, as though a barrier between ourselves and the cosmos has been lifted. The awakening of the sixth and seventh chakras goes beyond our linear time-space limitations and our words. It is a simple, yet totally other, awareness. Time, space, I AMness disappear and there is only THAT, resonating simultaneously in the dual and non-dual worlds.

Two Special Energy Portals

The thymus and the spleen represent a special type of energy receptor system. They take in prana, which is stepped down through the subtle bodies (but remains full-spectrum), separate it into all the specific colors, and send it individually to each chakra. On an intuitive level, the author feels that the spleen chakra becomes secondary to the thymus in this function as a person develops spiritually. This may be why Yogis who are already developed to a certain extent have not recognized the spleen as a major chakra. The reason either organ is able to take in full-spectrum cosmic energy may be because the interface between the vortexes of the heart and solar plexus chakras creates open spaces in the subtle body system, allowing cosmic energy to be stepped down while remaining in its full-spectrum state.

Vrittis

The vrittis are transpersonal bioenergetic mechanisms of the chakras through which the mind expresses itself as thoughts, tendencies, and desires. They represent the activity of the mind. This illustration of the chakra-vritti relationship was derived from the teachings of Shrii Shrii Anandamurti, as described in *Discourses on Tantra, Volume 1.*[10] Depending on our *karmas,* the vrittis may be active, overactive, underactive, or balanced in their expression. They are associated with *samskaras,* which are impressions of the mind. Samskaras may be expressed as *vasanas,* repeated impressions that create a mental groove or thought form pattern. In the Zero Point Process course, vasanas are called "thought form complexes" and described as having a root cause, emotion, thought, and sensory component.

Each chakra is made of petals that contain the subtle energies of the vrittis. There are a total of fifty petals for the first six chakras. These represent the fifty letters and *bija* sounds of the Sanskrit alphabet. They may also occur as composites. Each chakra has an element and Sanskrit

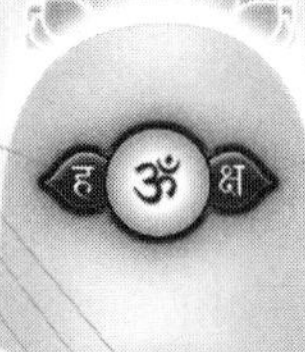

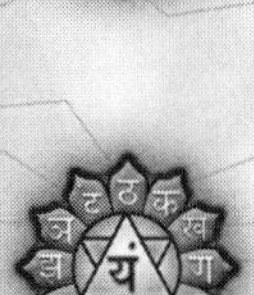
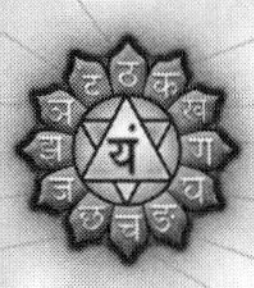

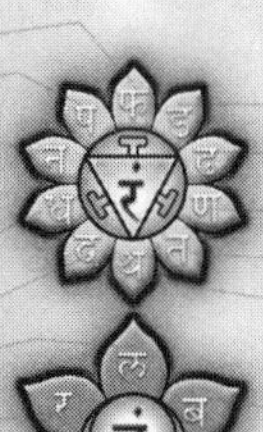

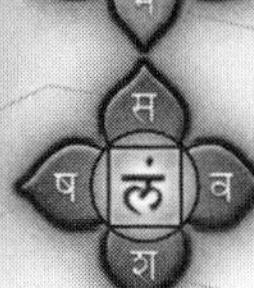

The Vrittis of the Chakras

name associated with it. Muladhara chakra is the base chakra and is associated with the Earth's four basic elements (earth, water, fire, air). Svadhishthana chakra is the second chakra and the water element – six petals. Manipura chakra is the third chakra and fire element – ten petals. Anuhata chakra is the heart and air element – twelve petals. Vishuddha chakra is the throat and Akasha (void) – sixteen petals. Ajna chakra is the sixth and the combination of the essence of two petals – all elements in purest form. Sahasrara chakra is the crown; it includes the soma chakra and transcends all the elements.

One of the purposes of Yoga asanas is to control and balance the expression of the vrittis on a daily basis. Shrii Shrii Anandamurti feels this is the most important role of Yoga asana.[11] He points out that mental expressions are brought about through the vrittis and the expression of the vrittis is affected by the different endocrine glands of the body. If there is an imbalance in a gland's hormonal secretion, the vrittis become imbalanced. Asanas, done on a daily basis, help to heal and rebalance the glands and their secretions, and therefore help to balance the expression of the vrittis in a way that optimizes expression and supports all of the Six Foundations. Dry fasting is another way. The core practices of the Six Foundations harmonize and heal expression of the vrittis so they are no longer imbalancing. Live-food diet, mantra, chanting, service, charity, meditation, Shaktipat, or awakening Kundalini all have an effect on the lives of spiritual aspirants. The Zero Point Process course taught by the author is specifically designed to balance vrittis and dissolve vasanas.

Dry fasting on *ekadashi,* which is done on the eleventh day after the full and new moons, uses the pull of the moon on the water element, which represents the *manas* (mind). Dry fasting tends to balance the *shukra,* or deep reproductive fluid that gives stability to the body on many levels and is the primary source of *ojas.* Defined as the refined product of the seven levels of *dhatus* metabolism, the ojas has as its main source the shukra, which comes from the deepest or seventh level of the *dhatus,* which is called *shukra dhatu. Ojas* is considered the purest form of all tissues. Ojas is responsible for body energy, brightness, strength, immunity, vital force, and physical and mental strength.[12] An excess in shukra, as can happen more frequently in celibates, may excite the lower vrittis, taking forms such as sexual desire, cruelty, and jealousy. The practice of ekadashi calms the shukra and brings energy toward the higher vrittis (such as Love and devotion) as food for the brain. Fasting in this way diminishes toxins and gaseous, fluid factors that rise up into the brain on and around the full and new moons. Yom Kippur (the Day of Atonement in the Jewish tradition) also uses this principle to help let go of negativities. At the Native American Sundance, the author followed the traditional way and went without food and water for the four-day dance cycle. Dry fasting is not necessary for one's physical health, but is a traditional way to affect vrittis. Although there is some theory about how it works based on our understanding of water as a carrier of impressions and therefore indirectly improves one's physical and emotional health, we only have theory. This approach to changing vrittis is more appropriate for a few people and not for the many.

Nadis

In different Yoga systems, and in the direct experience of clairvoyants, the chakras are said to have spokes, like a wheel. These spokes, called nadis, radiate out from the chakras. The word *nadi* means "stream." By definition a nadi is a hollow channel through which anything flows; examples are the blood vessels, lymph channels, and physical nerves. In the context of this book, the author refers to nadis as channels for the flow of subtle energy, or Yoga nadis. They carry the subtle prana. The 72,000 nadis intersect with the chakras and are part of their energetic structure. Nadis form a subtle energetic circuitry – a subtle nervous system of the body. It is the author's feeling that the nadis intersect with what are called the meridian lines of the Chinese acupuncture system. The place where the nadis and meridian lines intersect may be the acupuncture points. Though there is not enough research to clarify this point, the author feels the meridians and nadis are not the same. It is enough, however, to say that the nadis carry energy from the chakras into the brain, the nerves, endocrine and organ systems, the skeletal structure, and finally to the cell level.

The *Shiva Samhita*[13] describes fourteen main nadis. From the perspective of the flow of Kundalini, we will consider three of them – the main channels through which Kundalini flows: sushumna, pingala, and ida. All three originate in the *kanda* region beneath the Muladhara (base) chakra. The point where they start is called *yukta triveni* (coming together of three streams).

The pingala is considered the solar nadi. It starts on the right, beneath the base chakra, and ends in the right nostril. The ida is considered the lunar nadi. It starts on the left, beneath the base chakra, and ends in the left nostril. The sushumna is the central channel that moves straight up just behind the spinal column in the etheric body. The pingala and ida intersect with one another and the sushumna in the Ajna (brow) chakra. The place where they intersect is called mukta triveni. The ida and pingala weave around the sushumna, crossing over at each chakra. The pattern of these three nadis creates the caduceus of Hermes, the familiar winged staff with two serpents intertwined around it, known as the symbol of the Enlightened healer (hence the inspiration for the cover of this book). In Western society it has been mundanely associated with allopathic medicine.

In unusual situations, or with the use of psychedelic drugs, including ayahuasca, or putting too much effort into Yoga practices, the author has to do healing with spiritual aspirants of all traditions in which the subtle flow of Kundalini has been disrupted and inappropriately amplified or reduced in the ida or pingala rather than flowing smoothly primarily through the sushumna. This is one reason the author warns against the use of any drugs for any serious aspirant whose life focus is Liberation, or in whom the Kundalini has been awakened. The sturdy ones can do anything and get away with it, but those who are predominantly *vata,* vata imbalanced, have a low ojas, or have any previously mental imbalances run a high risk. The author has had success in rebalancing and creating healing of this disruption in the Kundalini flow through the nadis, but why take the risk?

The ida nadi or *chandra* (moon) nadi carries the feminine, cooling, yin, sattvic energy, and *kapha* qualities. In balance, it carries the energy of caring, Love, devotion, intuition, inspiration, and emotion. It also affects the function of the *manas,* or emotional and sensory mind. It strengthens bhakti Yoga qualities (devotion). When it is disrupted or out of balance, people become spacey, ungrounded, emotionally imbalanced, intuitively imbalanced, and possessive. People may become possessed by entities and suffer from insomnia, fears, nightmares, extreme emotional and psychic sensitivity, and a yin exhaustion. It is intense work to heal and rebalance these imbalances.

The pingala nadi is associated with the sun and is also known as *surya* nadi. It has masculine, yang, rajas tendencies and pitta qualities. It governs motivation, ambition, will power, and desire for deeper spiritual knowledge. It creates the tendency toward jnana Yoga (Yoga of the mind) and/or raja Yoga. An imbalanced pingala nadi creates a tendency to anger, self-righteousness, excessively critical mind, excess ambition, and egoistic, self-centered behavior.

Both of these nadis are *manovahini* nadis; they affect the energies of the mind and emotions. It is obviously important that these two nadis be balanced so that one does not become a yin, spaced-out meditator or a yang, intense, egoistic spiritual aspirant. When the prana is balanced, that is the optimal time to receive Shaktipat and activate the flow of the Kundalini. This is why the author appreciates the blessing of Shaktipat which is cosmically organized to only awaken the Kundalini when the person is ready. Kundalini awakening activated through Shaktipat as the descent of Grace, with a lineage and an awakened, empowered spiritual teacher who has received the blessings of his or her teachers to be the embodiment of Grace, is extremely safe. On the Spiritual Fasting Retreats facilitated by Gabriel and Shanti, which have been going on since 1988, and which are now at the Tree of Life in the U.S. and in retreats in Israel, more than 90 percent of the participants have a Kundalini awakening. This one-week fasting cycle combines all Six Foundations in an intense and supportive way. Since 1983 in this safe spiritual context with the author, not one person has had any problems with the Kundalini awakening. The practice of the Six Foundations and Shaktipat in this context seem to balance and maintain the ida and pingala harmony both before and after the Kundalini awakening.

The central channel, or sushumna, starts below the Muladhara chakra in the base of the spine and reaches completion in the Sahasrara chakra. It is a *chittavahini* (Beingness) nadi. In a person without the Kundalini awake, the sushumna is open at each hour with the change of ida and pingala nasal domination and at sunrise and sunset. This one experienced visions of the sushumna as three nadi tubes. On doing research, this internal vision aligned with the Yogic literature. The outer tube is called the sushumna. The middle tube is called vajra nadi and is associated with the sun. Inside this nadi is the chitrini nadi, which is associated with the cool nectar of the moon and where this one believes the nectar drips from in the soma chakra. The chitrini nadi is associated with dreams and visions. It ends in the door of Brahma. From here, in the author's experience, is a very thin nadi called the Brahma nadi, which is the final channel of Kundalini. It takes consciousness on the final step to the *Brahma Randhra* – the void between the hemispheres of the brain. It is located in the Sahasrara chakra. It is above the soma chakra, which is located in the lower part of the Sahasrara. When Muktananda personally initiated this one in this final step, the experience was that the Brahma nadi not only integrated the right and left side of the brain, but merged with Shiva (Cosmic Consciousness) in a way that exploded beyond time, space, and Being into an eternal, unbroken connection with the cosmic prana. The Brahma nadi seemed to go right through the top of the skull, creating a complete cosmic merging. This is not exactly how the scriptures describe the Brahma nadi, however, which is that it ends in the middle of the Sahasrara.

The Ten Sephirot of Nothingness

The Ten Sephirot of Nothingness which form the Kabbalistic Tree of Life represent the ten primal emanations of God. These ten represent the highest octave of the spiritual circuitry. As the Kundalini activates the nadi and chakra systems, it also begins energizing the sephirotic system. The merging of the Kundalini into the crown chakra is the next major "switch" which further opens and awakens the subtle consciousness of the sephirot. From the points of view of esoteric physics and astronomy, the sephirot are the spiritual blueprint of the macrocosm of the universe, the microcosm of the universe to its subatomic level, as well as the primal subtle anatomy of the human body. Modern string theory of physics supports this understanding. The theory of the relationship of the chakras and nadis to the sephirot is not a new understanding. The author has found confirmation of this model on a wall engraving at the Karnak Temple in Egypt which is estimated to have been built between 12,500 and 15,000 B.C. The details of the ancient sephirotic system are far too much information for this book to go into. The author teaches the primary levels of Kabbalah and the ancient spiritual technologies for illuminating the Light body through using the Holy Names of the Divine in conjunction with the sephirot in the Living Essene Way Retreats offered at the Tree of Life Rejuvenation Center.

Conclusion

The chakras, nadis, vrittis, and Kundalini energy are a completely integrated system. A change in one affects a change in the others. They all affect the expansion of consciousness.

Summary, Chapter 3

1. A subtle energy system, commonly known as the chakra system, exists. One function is transducing subtle cosmic energy into the body.
2. Each of the seven main chakras has a specific energetic nature that corresponds to a specific color, sound, and mental and spiritual awareness.
3. Each chakra is energetically associated with the physiology of a single or small group of locally associated nerve plexuses, endocrine glands, and organs.
4. Chakras are never closed; they fluctuate between more and less activation.
5. Chakra health is related to the overall synchronistic balance of the main chakras, as well as to the function of a particular chakra.
6. An awakened chakra is one in which the individual's consciousness merges with the higher awareness stored in that particular chakra.
7. There are 72,000 nadis, with fourteen basic ones and three main ones that carry the spiritualizing Kundalini. They help form the chakra system.
8. Each chakra has vrittis, which affect our psycho-emotional state.
9. The Six Foundations balance and regulate all the nadis.

Chapter 4

Healing Unbalanced Kundalini Energy

Since 1976, when the author and Dr. Lee Sanella started the first Kundalini Crisis Clinic in the world, the author has been working to understand the mystery of how Kundalini works. He has had the unique opportunity and blessing to work directly under Swami Muktananda helping people in the ashram in India and in the U.S. cope with imbalances in Kundalini. He also has had opportunities to work with people around the world in many different traditions, through the Kundalini Crisis Clinic and in his work at the Tree of Life Foundation, who have experienced some sort of difficulty with Kundalini. Fortunately, only a small percentage of people have difficulties. During this time the author has observed and treated a number of very interesting Kundalini crises (which are distinctly different from psycho-spiritual crises), which have given the author some insight. There is almost no current literature that seriously discusses the cause or correction of Kundalini imbalances with any particular insight into the situation in our modern context, so the author has been very much on his own, trying to sort this out. Based on Grace, through the author's scientific observation and the nature of people with several types of Kundalini imbalances, a theory has begun to emerge. The theory is based on several key experiences, described here as "cases," that represent the key aspects of the model.

Case #1: A man in his twenties had the Kundalini awakened. His teacher suggested that he could enhance this experience with the drug ayahuasca. Immediately after taking the ayahuasca, and for the next year until he met the author, this person suffered extreme Kundalini imbalances. These symptoms included suffering from intense nightmares, night terrors, insomnia, severe nausea, energetic depletion (he hadn't previously been depleted), spaciness, ungroundedness, severe emotional and intuitive imbalances, extreme emotional and psychic sensitivity, and what looked from the outside like extremely depleted ojas (vital life force energy). When the author met him and Graced him with Shaktipat, a rebalancing of the system occurred immediately. The energy began to flow up the sushumna, or central channel, and over the next year the person slowly regained his energy. His night terrors, insomnia, spaciness, and confusion began to recede, and over a year's period of time from receiving Shaktipat, his system came into balance. Supportive therapies included herbs to build ojas, an ojas-building diet and lifestyle with emphasis on minimizing sexual activity, and a homeopathic remedy. The person has now returned to his role as a spiritual teacher full-time and has significantly recovered from the effects of having taken the ayahuasca.

Case #2: A person who had his Kundalini awakened in another Yogic system, operated as an overachiever, was intellectually focused, and had an extreme desire for Liberation and deeper spiritual knowledge. This person had a tendency for a number of symptoms, which were amplified once the Kundalini was awakened, including: self-righteousness, anger, critical mind, egoistic and self-centered behavior, and excessive ambition for Liberation. He began to do the Yoga practices in his system extensively and intensively, which resulted in a progressive depletion of his ojas, spaciness, mental confusion, psychic sensitivity, and ungroundedness to the point that he was unable to function at all because of extreme physical weakness and exhaustion. He had to leave the ashram setting in which he was living. The person suffered symptoms from both an ida and a pingala imbalance. The treatment for him, over a period of three years, included herbs to build ojas, lifestyle, live-food diet, repeated Shaktipat to rebuild and reorganize the energy, homeopathic remedies, help to move away from pingala-driven egoistic and excessive Yogic ambitions, and support for becoming at peace with and surrendering to the unfolding of the Kundalini at a slower, more natural rate. It was necessary to repeatedly explain the principle of surrender to this person, versus the tendency of self-will and pushing with excessive practices, as a way to help this person's tendency to attempt to dominate the Kundalini. As this person began to relax and accept himself and surrender to the unfolding of the Kundalini, he slowly and steadily began to heal. Part of this was helping him accept his *pitta-vata* constitution, which is discussed in Chapter 24, and helping him accept his life-long tendency to deplete his ojas. In his acceptance and surrender, he has begun to blossom.

Case #3: This devotee of Swami Muktananda, when he would get within a block of the ashram, would begin to get agitated, violent, and out of control. Until he reached that point of physical proximity he was fairly calm. We can interpret this as an excess energetic flow in the pingala nadi. This out-of-control state could only be managed when this person did not come to the ashram because his system was not able to handle the increased energy being experienced when within a block of the ashram. The main treatment was staying away from the ashram until his system began to build and develop itself so that he could handle the increased flow of the Kundalini energy passing through.

Case #4: A woman who the author worked with in Muktananda's Ganeshpini Ashram in India would sometimes be very quiet, passive, very yin, spacey, ungrounded, emotionally imbalanced, and with insomnia and extreme emotional sensitivity. She would then quickly shift over to aggressive, violent behavior with anger, physically attacking people. This is an example of an erratic flow of the energy in the ida and pingala nadis. The treatment for her primarily was asking her to leave the ashram because she too could not handle the energy and was not open to help initially. Over time and with periodic visits, however, she appeared to get better. The other part of the treatment was to build up the ojas.

Case #5: A lady with a non-religious Christian background who had no familiarity whatsoever with Kundalini came to the Kundalini Crisis Clinic. There, she showed extreme fear, anxiety, hostility, and anger with her situation. She didn't want anything to do with the Kundalini and was very upset that this should happen to her and that it happened spontaneously. The author worked with her with general nutrition and helping her diminish the effects of the Kundalini in her life with a heavier diet. The author also was able to convince her that she shouldn't use tranquilizers as treatment for anxiety, but rather employ natural techniques to diminish her anxiety. Her relief was staying away from any kind of meditation or any kind of spiritual situation. In time the Kundalini energy began to fade out and she got the relief she wanted.

Case #6: The author worked with a woman with an excess of Kundalini-building activities experiencing fear, confusion, spaciness, ungroundedness, emotional imbalance, chronic exhaustion, out-of-control anger, critical mind, and very egoistic and self-centered behavior. This person very much wanted the Kundalini to be happening for her and wanted to continue to do her spiritual practices, pushing it very hard. The treatment was in building up the ojas and actually using a little bit of meat in the diet. This approach is exceptionally rare; in fact, this is the only person the author has ever done this with. But it worked, in that it slowed down the flow of Kundalini to a manageable level. There was a clear disregulation of her system, which could not handle the flow of Kundalini as it was. Adding meat proved miraculous, and showed how a flesh food diet does, in fact, act to slow the Kundalini. If she didn't eat meat three times per day, the Kundalini energy would overwhelm her. With a mild amount of meat in her diet three times per day, being moderate in her spiritual practices, and building ojas, she was able to progress with her spiritual work, feeling balanced and centered, and being able to continue with her life.

Case #7: Several students who were intensely meditating had a spontaneous awakening of Kundalini as a result of the meditation. They were in systems that didn't exactly acknowledge Kundalini; when they were having spontaneous, physical kriyas (uncontrolled movements of the body), they literally were getting hit by the masters with a stick or told there was something wrong with them. They thought they were going crazy. This is not exactly an imbalance in the Kundalini; however, it fits into the category of pre-conditioned religious training. Usually within an hour of discussion there was great relief in these people; they no longer thought they were going crazy. They were then clear to make choices in relation to the Kundalini unfolding versus religious rigidity in how they had been required to do their practices. This is a different type of resolution, however, and yet there is some overlap to what we have been discussing.

The theory of working with unbalanced Kundalini energy is based on the esoteric physiology that has been previously described. There are three granthis, or knots. When the Kundalini is awakened, all three are opened simultaneously, yet these three knots do act as regulators of the flow of the Kundalini. At the base of the spine is the Muladhara granthi. In the author's theory, the disregulation of the flow of Kundalini happens at the Muladhara granthi. In the physiology of the Kundalini, what is known as the kanda region, which is just below the Muladhara, or first, chakra, is where the three basic nadis, the ida, pingala and sushumna, meet and begin at the yukta triveni, just before the entrance to the Muladhara chakra. It is in this region where the disregulation is thought to occur. What happens theoretically is that there is a blockage or disregulation that occurs as the Shakti Kundalini, instead of going straight up through the middle pillar of the sushumna, is diverted through all the 72,000 nadis and chakras with their associated endocrine and nervous system components, imbalancing a variety of vrittis and physiological systems. This blockage or disregulation creates both an imbalanced and, in some cases, irregular flow primarily in the ida and pingala. As it begins to flow in the different directions it tends to significantly affect the adrenals, the base chakra, and the adrenal and kidney energies. An overstimulation of the adrenals, or weakening of the adrenals, tends to weaken the astral field. This opens people up to all sorts of psychic phenomena, creating vata imbalances, nightmares, insomnia, and astral holes. This is made much worse by the use of drugs, which also disrupt the astral field. The person in case #1 who had taken the ayahuasca and immediately began to have these kind of problems, such as vata imbalance, fears, nightmares, insomnia, extreme psychic sensitivity, and emotional and yin exhaustion is an example of this situation. It is very typical, as the energy is imbalancing and stressing the adrenals, that many people with a Kundalini imbalance have a depletion in ojas. This ojas energy is essential for holding the energy of the Kundalini. This is why Yoga practices, a proper diet, and the action of kedusha (holiness) are important for building the energies for building up the ojas as a preparation for awakening and sustaining Kundalini energy.

The author's experience is that there seem to be three types of responses to Shaktipat initiation: light, moderate, and intense. Gabriel, for example, experienced an intense Kundalini awakening and his subtle physiology was able to hold it. Many people come and receive a very mild Kundalini awakening. Because of their state of mind and their interests, that is a perfect awakening for them. Their bodies, their nadi systems, level of ojas, and basic health are best able to handle a mild awakening. Some will get a moderate awakening, which suggests that they are more ready. The exciting and important thing to be aware of, for those who want to ego-compare by wondering if they got a light, moderate, or heavy awakening, is that once the Kundalini is awakened, whether it is a small step or a leap does not matter. When the Kundalini awakens, one walks through the door into the next evolutionary level of consciousness. A mild awakening is a healthy, protective mechanism. Once a mild awakening happens, by practicing and living the Six Foundations and repeated Shaktipat, one is able to build up reserves of the ojas and the spiritual maturity that it takes to continue to enhance the continued awakening of the Kundalini. Therefore, most who have a mild awakening should be grateful that there was enough regulation in the first chakra to be able to handle it.

Another level of understanding the nature of the disregulation of Kundalini is by understanding it is associated with a concentration of contracted energy in the kanda region, which is just beneath and connected to the muladhara chakra. We can theorize that consciousness becomes concentrated in the first chakra, and in doing so it weakens the astral field. The individual's response to this can be to further contract the astral field as a way of handling the imbalance and that further concentrates the energy in the first chakra. This contraction of consciousness can cause a variety of imbalances. An example of that is the person in case #5 who had no interest and actually an overt resistance to the Kundalini. This resulted in a huge contraction of consciousness, which was displayed as insomnia, excessive fear, and anxiety.

Healing Kundalini Imbalance

The prime treatment for Kundalini imbalance from the author's experience is receiving Shaktipat from a Kundalini master (one who is Liberated and who has been initiated in a lineage). In the process of giving transmission of Shaktipat, the astral field of the person in case #1, which had been mainly disrupted and torn by drugs, and was weakened, contracted, and not able the handle the energy as it was brought into the adrenals and kidneys, begins to open to healing and the holes in the field are activated toward healing. There is an automatic linking during Shaktipat with the astral plane energy of the Kundalini master, which activates an expansion and healing of the astral plane. In this context we can think of the Shaktipat spiritual master as a model of Kundalini clarity. This process brings the other two granthis and the rest of the chakras into the total energetic and consciousness synergy. Shaktipat expands and restores the sense of the full identity and the full chakra identity to the person who had been previously contracted to a base chakra identity. In this way the astral plane can heal and expand rather than contract. When the Muladhara granthi has been activated and the adrenal and kidney energies are not strong, there is not enough energy and we have a yin deficiency. If there is an overstimulation, and the adrenals are imbalanced the other way, we get an excess of adrenaline, testosterone, and steroid production. Neither of these yin or yang responses are connected to the heart. With the receiving of Shaktipat, there is a connection and unity at the heart level with the Muladhara chakra. Once the energy begins to move up the sushumna, as in case #1 when the person received Shaktipat, the whole physiology begins to improve. The Kundalini energy moving up the central channel helps the disregulation to heal. Shaktipat opens a connection to all of the granthis. It reestablishes the appropriate flow of the energy at the central channel (sushumna) up through the crown. Esoterically people often have a vision of a blue pearl when this happens. This represents the energetic combination of the three granthis, that they have become unified in a wholeness. This is a sign of a healthy unfolding Kundalini. One of this one's teachings is that the Kundalini doesn't actually work like an elevator moving just from the first chakra to the second to the third and on up. In this one's experience since 1982, when he began operating as a Kundalini Shaktipat master/spiritual teacher, sometimes the crown chakra will appear to be activated first. Sometimes it is the heart. Sometimes, in stronger awakenings, all the chakras will be clearly experienced and activated at once. It is this integration that allows for healing the disregulation of the Kundalini. It is the integration of moving from fear in the first chakra to security, the second chakra opening up to Divine Love, and joy, and the sorrow of the heart chakra connecting to empathy and vision in the sixth chakra.

We can think of Shaktipat as the Divine Strategy of Grace. This one's experience in being a vehicle for Shaktipat is that Shaktipat initiation opens the individual to Emptiness, which allows a quiet mind, silence, and peace, which then allows the person to go to the Divine Presence as their original identity, as I AM THAT. The second thing that happens is that the three granthis are activated (and unified). The third is the state of experiencing Grace. The fourth is the activation of Divine surrender.

The second aspect of healing Kundalini imbalance is surrender. One of the issues that has clearly come up where people have had difficulty, is that the vrittis are often activated. There becomes an imbalance expressed as impatience with a deep lust, rather than a Love-desire to return to one's own original nature. The people are still involved in karmic time and form rather than peace and surrender to the unfolding of the Kundalini. Kundalini awakening is a gift of God's Love, but instead people feel impatience, pride, egoistic will power, and a lust for consciousness. This is where a lot of these imbalanced energies can originate.

Case #2 is an example where the person had such an egoistic lust for the Divine that he got impatient and began forcing Kundalini with advanced Yogic techniques. This karmic reactivation causes the congestion at the first granthi, which then converts the energy into stressing the adrenals and upsetting the flow of the kidney energies. One of the teachings, therefore, that Gabriel believes prevents people from falling into this egoistic imbalance is explaining the Divine Strategy of Grace and how one must surrender to the unfolding of one's own Kundalini energy. This does require patience, peace, and surrender rather than forcing with excessive Yogic techniques, drugs, or any other excessive techniques. The Kundalini is a feminine energy and by respecting the unfolding of the feminine energy rather than activating the karmas of past lives, of pushing, and of lust, we are able to avoid blocking or causing disregulation. This form of meditation is spontaneous and free-flowing, rather than the masculine concept of forcing and fitting into a form and a technique. This is the mystery of Kundalini – surrendering to the Kundalini and to the Grace that is being given rather than attempting to control the situation. Controlling or forcing comes from an egoistic state of past vasanas of how to deal with spiritual life. They can result in imbalance.

The issue in case #7 is excessive religious instruction that creates anxiety kriyas and blocks the first granthi. Using the Zero Point Process to eliminate these religious instructions supports the person to be free from ingrained concepts (vasanas) and to then be able to allow the Kundalini to unfold in the proper way rather than create a shutdown out of fear in the first chakra. The author must also say that the religious instruction can be from past-life activities that are activated as the Kundalini is awakened. These vasanas do need to be attended to if people are going to have a successful unfolding of the Kundalini energy. As past karmas come up, and particularly perhaps the most intense is what the author would call an egoistic lust for consciousness rather than a Love and empathy for consciousness, the vasanas of impatience, dominance, pride, and control need to be directly worked on.

This is why again this one strongly suggests the importance of surrender. It is not a surrender to the external spiritual teacher; it is a surrender to the internal flow of the Sacred Feminine within one's Self. It is surrender to magnificence of the Divine Presence within ourselves. The teachings of a Kundalini Shaktipat master and the action of Shaktipat do play a role in the successful unfolding of the Kundalini. The Liberated spiritual teacher does indeed burn up the karmas as vasanas that could potentially cause this disregulation. The master can burn up those karmas of lust for consciousness, impatience, egoistic will power, and pride, and create the spiritual space for the natural surrender to happen. A Kundalini Shaktipat master offers himself and his own life for the awakening of the students and in that act is willing to take on and burn the karmas of the students. This is part of the understanding of the Divine Strategy of Grace that is associated with the meaning of Shaktipat. Shaktipat is an awesome gift of Yah's Love that takes us into the next evolutionary stage of consciousness. The sacrifice of the Kundalini Shaktipat Master in burning the karmas of the students is part of the cycle of this gift of Grace.

The third part of the treatment is building up the ojas, which is described in Chapter 25. Emphasizing once again that drug usage depletes the ojas and disrupts the astral field, we have the example we have seen in case #1. Asana practice is specifically designed to integrate the Kundalini energies, the chakra systems, the granthis, the nadis, and the koshas (discussed in the next chapter). These definitely help to rebalance the Kundalini energy when done in moderation. Awakened Kundalini requires more glucose, but this can be achieved with a low to moderate glycemic intake as explained in the author's *Rainbow Green Live-Food Cuisine* book.[1] Eating high-glycemic foods and white sugar further depletes ojas and weakens the adrenals, as well as causes other medical problems (see the chart showing effects of a high-glycemic diet in Chapter 27).

Whether or not one experiences an imbalanced Kundalini or is simply committed to the process of spiritual Liberation, Shaktipat Initiation, surrender, and building ojas are foundational elements of an optimal and safe awakening.

Summary, Chapter 4

1. The three main aspects for healing Kundalini imbalance are Shaktipat, surrender, and building ojas.
2. Kundalini imbalance often comes from karmas of impatience, lust for consciousness, egoistic will power, and pride. These vrittis need to be healed and the vasanas need to be dissolved. The Zero Point Process and support from the spiritual teacher help with this.
3. A Kundalini Shaktipat master takes on and burns these karmas, replacing them with peace, patience, humility, and surrender to the flow.

Chapter 5

The Six Koshas

To truly understand spiritual anatomy and to continue to build the foundation for the new paradigm of Spiritual Nutrition, we must understand a basic tenet of holistic healing: the body-mind complex acts as a unit. Mind and body are not separate. The health of the body affects the health of the mind, and vice versa. While this principle is of primary importance in the Spiritual Nutrition paradigm and in holistic healing in general, it is less accepted and less emphasized in modern allopathic medicine and the materialistic-mechanistic paradigm.

The Six Foundations for Spiritual Life are an alchemical approach to purifying the layers of the body-mind complex and transforming the crude mind into the subtle mind that is ready to disappear. This is spiritual alchemy. The layers of body-mind are called *koshas*. The six-layer kosha system developed by Shrii Shrii Anandamurti, a God-realized and merged Being, best suits the teachings in this book. The koshas are intimately related to the chakras, nadis, and Six Foundations.

The first is *annamaya* kosha (food body). The second is *kamamaya* kosha (desire body), which includes desire or resistance to life. It involves our moral struggles as well as physical and psychological addictions. The third is *manomaya* kosha (emotions-mind body), which includes perceptual activities and motor-sensory, emotional, instinctual, and memory functions of the mind.

Atimanasa kosha, the fourth kosha, is what we call the first layer of the supermental mind, or higher mind. It is also known as the first of three layers of the expanded superconsciousness or causal mind. It is a natural, spontaneous, illuminated state where we first begin to transcend the bondage of time, space, and Being, allowing us to see in the past, present, and future. This layer of the mind is the layer of intuition and creative insight. It has been the author's observation that people on a highly mineralized, live-food diet have more of an opening or a tendency to open in this layer.

The clearing of the koshas is similar to what the alchemists sought. They talked about converting base metals to gold, but perhaps they were really working on how to convert a crude mind into a subtle mind. The discipline of sattva or kedusha (holiness) is the alchemist's fire. The awakening of the Self, transcending from our lower nature to the highest level of consciousness, living in "awakened normality," is the alchemical transformation. In some individuals, because of their levels of genius, a vibrational flow from this atimanasa kosha layer inspires the lower koshas to give birth to great discoveries and achievements in art and science. For example, Einstein, who received many of his ideas in dreams, made great discoveries. As Einstein put it, "There is no logical way to the discovery of these elemental laws. There is only the way of intuition." William Blake was a visionary poet who said, "The poetic genius is the true man. The body or outward form of man is derived from the poetic genius." When the lower koshas are calm and concentrated, the deep awareness of the superconscious mind can penetrate. This doesn't happen very often in everyday life, but for many people, at some time in their life, it may happen. The work is to support this opening for people so it becomes a regular experience, and part of this is connected to the quality of diet. It is through the atimanasa kosha that the desire for spiritual practice is first expressed. This kosha is also stimulated by the beauty of Nature, because Nature lifts the mind into the vibration of peace that emanates out of Nature. Wisdom literature and devotional music can also inspire one's mind to open to this level. The atimanasa kosha is the layer from which samskaras, which are the deep thought forms, get their first expression. The experience of sitting with an Awakened Being, and through entrainment with the Being's consciousness, may also stimulate the purification and opening of the atimanasa kosha.

The fifth layer is the *vijnanamaya* kosha. This is the middle layer of the causal mind. As it expands, it can grasp the total existence of the objective world. It gives the full knowledge of past, present, and future, and as this mind opens into consciousness, the qualities of mercy, gentleness, patience, serenity, success, cheerfulness, spiritual ecstasy, humility, meditation, one-pointedness, enthusiasm, imperturbability, and magnanimity are activated. The two main functions of this kosha are: (1) *viveka,* which is called discrimination, or the ability to tell the difference between the Permanent Reality and the temporal reality; and (2) *vairagya,* which is the quality of non-attachment. Viveka is the ability to know and discern the Eternal and the Absolute from the passing play of the material world of temporal reality. It involves a certain amount of discrimination. This is focused on in the Zero Point Process course (a Western form of jnana Yoga) taught at the Tree of Life by Gabriel, where people are able to experience that the "personality is a case of mistaken identity," and we are and always were the awareness prior to time, space, and Being. Vairagya, or non-attachment, which is different from detachment, tends to awaken after viveka has been awakened. It is sometimes interpreted as renunciation or avoidance of things of the world. Some people misinterpret this and try to mortify their bodies to create aversions to the mind and to the natural instincts of eating, sleeping, and sexuality. Acting in this way is a form of avoidance of life. Avoidance is not the same as vairagya. True vairagya is not a negative approach. It is an attitude of loving God, and of seeing and expanding the Universal Consciousness within all things. It is a way of seeing the finite as an expression of the Infinite, and having and being that Love of the Divine Presence in all things. Non-attachment does not mean renouncing one's family and escaping and living in a cave, but it really means embracing the whole world equally. It is equal vision. In Kabbalistic terms, it is called *hishtavut.* It means being the witness consciousness, while fully immersing oneself in the play of the world. It means living within the paradox of the dual/non-dual world. Vairagya means to be attached only to God; detachment means not even being attached to God. Vairagya is about opening your heart to the Divine, so that you are seeing the Divine in all things. This is its deep meaning: Love for the Divine. Non-attachment cannot take place until Love for the Divine is your primary way of being in the world. It is the essential, deep meaning of *tantra.* In the awakening of Enlightenment, vairagya disappears and there is only the cosmic You as I AM THAT. There is nothing left to be in non-attachment with. There is no place to stand and no-one standing.

Hiranyamaya kosha, also known as *anandamaya* kosha, is the sixth kosha, the highest level of the subtle causal mind. It is considered the bliss body. It is the beginning of the experience of the natural emotions of non-causal joy, non-causal contentment, non-causal Love, and non-causal peace. This is considered the most evolved kosha. It is the brilliant golden Light of the I AM consciousness. At this level, the consciousness of oneself as an individual unit, ego unit, has dissolved away; what remains is the intense attraction of the Supreme, and only a thin veil (par'gawd) separates the person from Self-realization-Liberation-jivanmukti (Liberation while in the body) and the process of moving into moksha, or God-merging, or Deveikut. The desire for Union, at this stage, becomes almost unbearable, relieved only when the awareness of the Divine Union takes place. When we realize the Union was there all along, the desire to go toward any goal or be or do anything disappears. In hiranyamaya kosha, one often experiences *sankalpa samadhi*. This is merging into the Light, but with a maintenance of an I AM consciousness. When one is merged long enough in this Light and the I AM disappears, it is called sahaja samadhi. This kosha bridges into the world of Liberation. In sahaja samadhi, whether awake or in the sleep state, one is in the continual experience of the Light. In this one's experience, it is a golden-white Light, as well as a golden Light. It extends slowly and steadily throughout all levels of consciousness. When it reaches a place where it is primarily awareness prior to time, space, and Being, it is called sahaja samadhi. Sahaja samadhi is a continual state in both waking and sleeping, meditating and walking around, making Love and eating. It is all there Is, Was, and Will Be.

Sahaja samadhi occurs once the hiranyamaya kosha has been transcended and the thin veil has been shattered. This is called Self-realization, or jivanmukti. In the Kabbalah, it can be defined as Chaya-Yehida. In classical Kabbalah, a person who lives at this level is called a *Kadosh* (holy person), which in ancient times was higher than the levels of *Tzadik* or *Chesed* consciousness.

Beyond the koshas and Self-realization is the total merging with God, known as moksha or complete Deveikut. This is the state of permanent nirvakalpa samadhi. Mukti is Self-realization or the state of Liberation as the overwhelming predominant awareness. In moksha, or permanent unbroken Deveikut, there is no "you" left; there is no I AM left, even as a trace intermittent oscillation. There only IS. This is a level that few Beings attain. In this lifetime, this one has met two who were in a state of moksha. There are a variety of people, however, who are in a state of Liberation or Self-realization. There is a dynamic vertical continuum between these two levels of awareness, as one fructifies from early stages of Self-realization to the unbroken awareness of complete Deveikut.

The point of describing the koshas is to get a fuller perspective on what Spiritual Nutrition is about. *Spiritual Nutrition is about purifying all of the koshas, which includes stilling the vrittis of the mind. It is about eating and living in a way that enhances one's Communion with the Divine on every level and therefore requires purifying the mind on every level.* Using the analogy of a mirror, when a mirror is dirt-free, you can see an original object very well. When it becomes dirty, the knowledge of the object becomes hazier. When the mirror of the koshas is clear, we become the Deep Stillness and the experience of the Divine Self shines through. When the koshas are clear, Grace opens us to the direct apperception that we are never anything other than the Divine Self. Grace as the final step again makes it clear we cannot "technique" our way to Self-realization. In the Kabbalah, this Grace is known as Atik Yoman – the grandmother. She is the uncertainty principle of Grace. She is the unknowable. Because of her, we are inspired to give up the idea that we were ever in control. Using another analogy makes it even clearer. Think about the koshas as layers of a magnifying glass, magnifying the Light of the Atman, which is the essential nature of who we are prior to all consciousness, prior to any aspect of the mind, prior to time, space, and any identity of self. When all of these magnifying glasses are cleansed, the Light of the Atman, which is within us, shines so brightly that we literally experience that Light within us. The first stage of really knowing this is Self-realization. The Light is so bright in sankalpa samadhi; it is the Light of a thousand suns bursting through.

Deeper than this Light is the place of nirvakalpa samadhi, where nothing exists. The work of Spiritual Nutrition, the dharma or mitzvot of Spiritual Nutrition, which includes right action and right livelihood, is simply to purify all of the koshas, so that the mind, which is the object of the Atman (soul), is so clean, and the body, which is the grossest object of the Atman, is so clean, that the mind disappears and the object and the subject become One. The dharma of Spiritual Nutrition is to purify the gross manifestations of the Atman, which includes all of the levels of the koshas. In this process, each kosha becomes fully cleansed and activated. In this process, even the body becomes a vehicle of the Atman.

The approach of Spiritual Nutrition is not to denigrate the body-mind-I AM complex, but to elevate it to the highest vehicle of consciousness. This is a major purpose of Spiritual Nutrition. It is to make the body so pure and such a vehicle of Light that, on the grossest level of physical Being, it reflects the Highest Light. As we honor the body and establish it into its original meaning, which is to be a vehicle of Light, we are opening ourselves up to experience the Divine. We open to what this one calls the presence (witness consciousness), which is a doorway to the Divine Presence. As we purify the layers of the koshas, which, in essence, are an inverted pyramid, more and more Light is magnified and shines through, so that the annamaya kosha, the kamamaya kosha, the manomaya kosha, the atimanasa kosha, the vijnanamaya kosha, and the anandamaya kosha become a huge highway of the Divine Light reverberating in us. This optimizes the pre-conditions for Liberation. The final step is a spontaneous act of Grace.

The following poem written by this one describes the subjective experience of this Light when the koshas are purified and the subject and object become One.

Incredible Light Energy of THAT

Half asleep and fully awake
The energetic body filled with indescribable, blazing Light
Explodes through the total Being
With a delectable fullness
Of Joy,
Of Peace,
Of Contentment,
Of Love,
Occurring without reason or cause,
the natural human state
Existing as the matrix of Beingness within
As phenomenon and prior,
In the silence of the night,
In the silence of meditation,
Rises like a thousand blazing suns
And settles down,
But never sets in the activity of the day.
It is always background and often foreground
To an underlying matrix
Of ecstatic, non-causal well-being, peace, Love, beauty, contentment, and joy
Emanating twenty-four and seven,
Residing as Infinite Light of Divine Presence
Uplifting this one as the One in every moment of every action

Blazing forth as the Nothing of awareness
In the silence of the Divine Presence
In the stillness of the mind and body
As the day unfolds through the night
Half asleep and fully awake
The ecstasy of the Divine Self
Is beyond cause, comprehension, and I AM.
It is Yah's permanent Grace to everyone
Incredible Light Energy of THAT
The Light of I AM THAT is all that ever Was, Is, and Will Be.

The Six Koshas and the Six Foundations

The Six Foundations serve to purify the six koshas (see chart on page 99). The first two Foundations have most effect on the annamaya kosha: eating a 100 percent organic, vegan, highly mineralized, live-food, low-sugar, sattvic-kedusha, modest food-intake diet specific to one's constitution and pure well-hydrated water intake. Spiritual Fasting is a major purification and prana-building practice for the annamaya kosha. This is the most powerful diet for activating the physical body and purifying it. A clean, vegan, live-food, organic diet, high in minerals and low in sugar will also help to create a calm mind and a mind that is open to all potentialities. These practices create a highly conscious mind, a mind that does not see limitations, and has the highest 90-mineral level of frequency able to come into it. Live-food nutrition even affects the atimanasa kosha. The annamaya kosha is also purified by the Yoga asanas. Yoga asanas that express the flow of the Kundalini and focus on activating, moving, and expanding the prana or Shekhinah energy, such as the Kali Ray Tri Yoga® system, are the most powerful Yoga asana practices. All forms of Yoga asana, however, even those that are static, will help purify the annamaya kosha to some extent. Yoga asanas balance the vrittis of the chakras, open up and activate the nadis, move and activate all the fluids in the body, integrate subtle and gross nervous systems, build flexibility, prepare one to sit comfortably for meditation, and allow a fluidity of physical gracefulness and a joyful strength of presence. The Ophanim, which is the energetics of the Hebrew letters in physical positions with the Kabbalistic breath patterns, also supports this purpose. For some people, a certain amount of physical labor or aerobic, cardiovascular exercise is also supportive. The exercise that Gabriel finds most

How Each Foundation Affects the Koshas						
Foundation	Annamaya kosha (food body)	Kamamaya kosha (pleasure body)	Manomaya kosha (emotion-mind body)	Atimanasa kosha (supermental body)	Vijnanamaya kosha (causal mind)	Hiranyamaya kosha (bliss body)
I. Nutrition						
A. Live foods	++++	+++	+++	++	+	+
B. Spiritual Fasting	++++	++++	+++	++++	+	+++
II. Building prana (life force)						
A. Yoga asanas	++++	++++	+++	++	+	+
B. Pranayama (breathing practices)	++++	+++	++++	++	+	+
C. Ophanim, T'ai Chi, Reiki, Tachyon energy, and energy practices	++++	+++	++	++	+	+
D. Sacred dance	++	+++	+++	+++	+	+++
III. Service (sheirut) and charity (tzedaka)	+	++++	+++	++	+	+
IV. Spiritual guidance and inspiration						
A.Satsang/Yechidut	+	++++	+++	++++	+++	+++
B. Zero Point Process (jnana Yoga)	+	+++	++++	++++	++++	+++
C. Sangha/Kehila (Chavurah)	+	++	+++	++++	+++	+++
D. Spiritual wisdom literature	+	+++	+++	++++	+++	+++
E. Sacred music	+	+++	++	++++	+++	++
F. Being in Nature	+	+++	++	++++	+++	++
V. Silence						
A. Meditation (hitbodedut)	+	++	+++	++++	++++	++++
B. Prayer (tefila)	+	++	++	++++	++	++++
C. Mantra (hagiya)	+	+	++	++++	++	++++
D. Chanting (mizmor)	+	++	++	++++	++	++++
VI. Kundalini awakening						
Shaktipat initiation Smicha l'shefa/ Haniha	+++	+++	+++	++++	++++	++++

potent is jumping on a rebounder, which moves the lymph. Research has shown that you need about sixteen minutes a day, and you can get great benefit in a short time period if taken in with oxygen delivered by mask, and deep breathing. Oxygen is the most important mineral in the kingdom. It is the most important mineral for supporting the immune system and mitochondrial energetic system. Pranayama is the working with the breath in a way that activates the vital energy, the five pranas of the system, as well as moves the lymph and increases oxygen in the system. Pranayama purifies the annamaya kosha, the kamamaya kosha, and especially the manomaya kosha. The manomaya kosha is strongly affected because, when the prana is steady and full, the mind becomes quiet. When the mind becomes quiet, then the Light filtering through the higher koshas can come through more easily. When the mind is active, it steals all the Light coming through to us from the Atman and we are not able to directly experience the Light that is naturally ours. A mind filled with concepts, worry, anxiety, and regrets grabs this Light to maintain its existence. Pranayama is very important, and generally increases the prana of the mind and helps expand consciousness. At the level of the annamaya kosha, pranayama is the developing of physical prana, which moves up all the way through the subtle levels to the vijnanamaya kosha.

The kamamaya kosha, the second kosha, is affected by the energy generated from the live-food diet, from Yoga asanas, and from physical activity, and gives enough clarity of mind to live according to basic moral principles. In Yoga we would call these the yamas and the niyamas, while from the biblical approach we call them the Ten Speakings (this is the literal Hebrew translation of what are commonly called the "Ten Commandments"). These are the guidelines for creating sattva/kedusha emphasized in the Fourth Foundation. In the Torah, there are actually 613 guidelines or *mitzvahs*. Each mitzvah, or practice, helps bring more Light into the system.

The Third Foundation of charity and service is the act of giving, which activates our awareness of our Oneness with all of humanity. At its highest level, it moves us from an egoistic and ethnocentric point of view to a world-centric point of view. This Foundation works on all of the levels and forces us to develop all levels of the koshas. In both the Kabbalistic and Yogic traditions, charity and service are powerful ways of altering negative karma. One of the great Kabbalistic teachings is that we mimic the Divine by the act of giving. As we receive from the Divine, we mimic Yah by giving, and in doing so we complete the cycle of life and spirit. This activates the first five koshas.

The Fourth Foundation – reading spiritual wisdom literature, sangha or kehilah, association with spiritually focused people or community, association with an awakened spiritual teacher (satsang or yechidut), sacred dance, and time in Nature – affects all six koshas.

The manomaya kosha (third kosha) is strongly affected by more sensory inputs. Increasing the prana of the mind expands consciousness on a variety of levels. Live foods, asanas, and pranayama all help to increase the prana of the mind. The Zero Point Process course, originally co-created in 1988 by the author and Steven Wolinsky, Ph.D., helps to purify the manomaya kosha. Since 1990, the author has developed his own version of Zero Point Process as a form of Western jnana Yoga to purify both the manomaya kosha and vijnanamaya kosha (fifth kosha). It is a course that Gabriel teaches at the Tree of Life, which helps people break through into a state in which consciousness controls the mind, rather than the mind controlling consciousness. It helps people to disidentify with the Being and the time-space continuum of the ego, and awake to the awareness of the Divine Presence as I AM THAT. Zero Point Process helps to free oneself of the tyranny of the mind, so that one can live in the world, as the Taoists say, "open as the sky" to all possibilities, living without expectation or hopes.

Purifying the manomaya and vijnanamaya koshas helps people to live in the moment and be in the subtle ecstasy of the Divine Presence. So, when the mind and body are quiet, through fasting, asanas, pranayama, proper diet, and Zero Point Process, it is easier to have the power to control ourselves in relationship to being able to follow the moral principles that align us with the higher functions. It is easier to calm the mind so that the higher levels can flow through, and that takes us to the atimanasa kosha (fourth kosha), the level of intuition and creativity. In classical Yoga, we talk about *pratyahara,* or withdrawal from the senses, which helps with this silence, but when one meditates, known in the Kabbalah as *hitbodedut,* the mind becomes quiet and the illusion of the outer dissolves. There is nothing to sense as separate from us. This is the spontaneous pratyahara that happens in the Deep Silence when the body-mind-I AM complex disappears in meditation. Meditation is the power of the Fifth Foundation. For this one, it was the core foundation that powered the flow of the Kundalini to destroy the dream of a separate body-mind-I AM complex. Prayer and chanting at their deepest levels dissolve into meditation and thus are part of the Fifth Foundation. The vijnanamaya kosha is influenced by the ability to understand that the personality is a case of mistaken identity. We begin to distinguish between the Ultimate Reality and the temporal reality of our myth, belief systems, concepts, and archetypes, and we awaken from the deluding dream of these.

The sixth level of the koshas, hiranyamaya kosha, is most profoundly purified and opened by meditation. There is also a greater aspect, which is Grace. Grace is something that happens spontaneously, as Atik Yomin or "*guru tattva*" in which the world is the guru. Grace is usually focalized by an awakened spiritual teacher. That Grace as the awakening of the Kundalini is also known as Shaktipat or S'micha l'shefa/Haniha. When the Kundalini is awakened and is nurtured by the Six Foundations, it is a spontaneous burning that powerfully clears, purifies, and activates the koshas. In different traditions there are different titles: the awakened spiritual teacher may be called a Kadosh in the Kabbalistic tradition, or in traditional Yoga a guru, or a Kundalini master, or a Taoist master or Zen master. They are variations of how the role of the spiritual teacher can share the spiritual vibration with the student. Each spiritual teacher has his or her own style, according to his or her particular inclination and past lives.

For this one, the Shaktipat Grace of Swami Muktananda awakened the Kundalini so that the Divine Urge or *T'shukat* Deveikut was so amplified that all that was needed was complete surrender to its spontaneous, delicious unfolding. Like a seed activated in the garden of this body-mind-I AM complex, it sprouted into the cosmic Tree of Life. All this one had to do was keep showing up each second until there was no more of this one left to show up. The predominant Foundations included hours of intense meditation each day, in which experiences occurred that dissolved the illusion of separateness. It was a sort of a Divine behavior modification. In Muktananda's ashram, not only was Gabriel meditating six hours per day, but there were also three hours of chanting each day and *Guru Darshan* (sitting in the presence of the guru) for at least one hour. A vegan diet supported all of this on the physical plane. We are the Nothing or B'lee mah expressing and experiencing the individual soul (jivan atman or neshama) through our individual body-mind-I AM complex. So, the expression of the Six Foundations will vary according to individual temperament and karmas. Not everyone has to meditate for six hours a day for years. In the same way, the expression and teaching of one who is awake will vary according to the personality and dharma of the body-mind-I AM complex.

Divine Urge

The seed of Truth
Eternally planted
Within the body-mind-I AM complex
Is awakened by Your touch.
This seed of cosmic fire
Ignites the Eternal Divine Urge
Into a roaring flame.
This one is like a bull in heat
Seeking to mate with the One
Crashing through
The illusion of all barriers
Beyond imaginary physical and mental limitation
Charging into the endless bliss of meditation
Whose experiences deprogram
The mind and body from the illusion of the world,
A form of Divine behavior modification
Slamming this one into the emptiness of Divine Stillness
A wild Love crazed moth
Irresistibly pulled toward the Divine fire.
All this one has to do is show up
And be willing to die
In the flame of the Divine Love
The I-ness is burnt to a crisp
And Yah's breath blows away the ashes.
Empty and full
As I AM THAT
Complete Peace
The urge completes its mission.
Nothing is left
No where to stand
No one standing
No seeker
And nothing to seek.
The end of all process
Nothing to Do, Be or Become

Free to move in any direction
As this one is
The wild Divine Dance of Yah.

Mantra

In addition to chanting and meditation, the use of the mantra (hagiya) is very helpful for all levels of cleaning the koshas. Depending on what tradition you come from, there are different mantras. The mantra that people are less familiar with is the Name of God "*Yod Heh Wah Heh*" (YHVH) – which is the mantra of Liberation in the prophetic-Jewish-Kabbalah tradition. It is the mantra given to Moses at the Burning Bush. It is the mantra that takes one beyond time, space, and Being – that which Was, Is and Will Be. It takes you prior to I AM consciousness. It is also the great mantra that transmutes to "I Will Be What I Will Be," which indicates our spiritual potentiality for Deveikut. This mantra is very powerful. The sacred mantras in the different traditions all work. They all represent the vibration of the Divine. Depending on your particular tradition, it is best to use a mantra that vibrates with your Inner Light. In the Yogic tradition, one powerful mantra is "*Om Namah Shivaya.*" It takes you to that Essential Oneness. The idea is about essence, because the traditional mistake in understanding the Divine Presence is somehow to relate to it as external, rather than our essential vibration. In order to become subjective, we must be subjective. These mantras, which have the vibration of the Divine, take us to that subjective awareness to help focus our concentration and then help purify all levels of the mind. This is the difference between getting a mantra from a book and an activated, empowered mantra, or what in India is known as a *chaitanya* mantra. According to our karmic tendencies, certain mantras will have particular affinities for each person. We are usually drawn to an awakened teacher who will give the activated mantra that will best serve us. Although "Yod Heh Wah Heh" has been public since Moses received it from the burning bush 3,400 years ago, it was not transmitted to this one in its awakened state until the end of a twenty-one-day water fast when it appeared visually as flaming energetic Hebrew letters that continued non-stop for six to twelve hours while this one was meditating in the temple at the Tree of Life. It taught many things and became the awakened mantra that Gabriel is to share with seekers.

We simply know the Atman, or God, by experiencing being known by God. We know God by experiencing God as the ultimate subject and source of all Being. The more we invite God into our life through clearing the koshas, the more we experience God as the living secret of life through us.

Summary, Chapter 5

1. The six koshas are the layers of the mind.
2. The koshas are intimately related to the chakras, nadis, and Six Foundations.
3. Spiritual Nutrition is about how to purify all the koshas so the Light of the Divine shines through fully.

Chapter 6

Subtle Organizing Energy Fields, a New Concept

A key in understanding the wholistic paradigm of Spiritual Nutrition and spiritual awakening lies in a new concept of what the author calls Subtle Organizing Energy Fields (SOEFs). The concept of SOEFs is a synthesis that is intuitively derived yet rooted in historical, cultural, spiritual, and scientific evidence. It incorporates an integration of nutrition with spiritual life and accounts for all the "aberrant" observations that remain unexplained by the materialistic-mechanistic paradigm. It is important to be aware that energy is not a thing but a concept that is useful for organizing and communicating phenomena and experience.

Historically and culturally, the idea that the human system is organized around an energy pattern that determines its functioning has been with us for thousands of years. The Chinese science of acupuncture is based on the subtle energy fields called *meridians* and the subtle energy called *chi*. In India, both the sciences of Yoga and Ayurvedic medicine use the word *prana* to describe the subtle energy of bodies and the life force in other living fields. In the book *The Secret Life of Plants*,[1] the concept that plants have a specific energy field and a specific energy pattern has already been popularized.

The further understanding that living systems are surrounded by subtle energy fields was greatly advanced by the discovery and use of Kirlian photography, a type of photography that demonstrates the form of SOEFs. What is critical to our understanding about SOEFs is that they exist prior to the existence of the physical form. They are not emanated from the physical form like the magnetic field lines of a bar magnet. In this hypothesis, *SOEFs are a template for physical biological forms and structures.* The

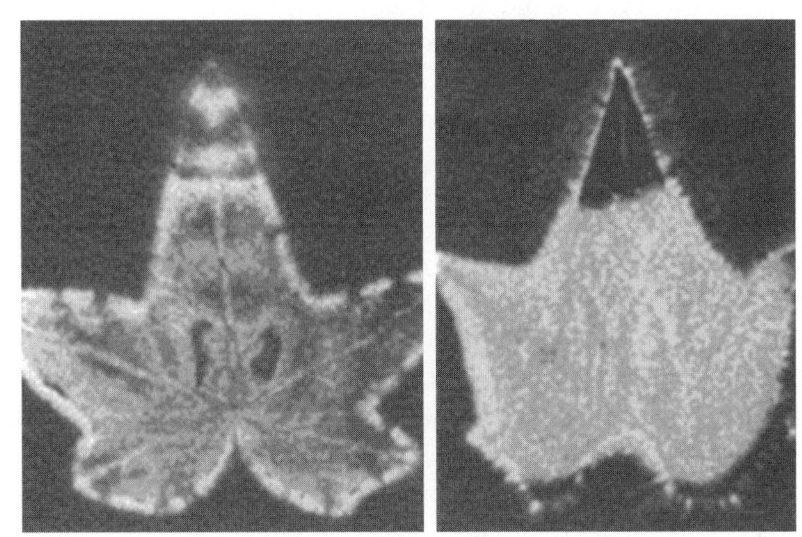

The Subtle Energy of a Leaf Shown through Kirlian Photography

photographs show an energy pattern in the shape of a complete leaf surrounding a half-missing leaf. This would not happen if the field were actually emanating from the molecular structure of the physical leaf.

More recent supportive evidence for the existence of SOEFs has been supplied by the late Marcel Vogel. In his experiments with the crystallization of cholesterol esters, Vogel was able to photograph, with a polarizing light microscope using an Ehringhouse compensator, a complete blue energy form that revealed itself a fraction of a second before the unstructured liquid cholesterol melt entered the structured crystalline phase.[2]

By accepting the concept of the pre-existence of SOEFs in both plant and human systems, this will lead us (in Part II) to an expanded view of food, which has body, life force, and SOEFs similar to the human system. *It is the dynamic interaction of these human and plant SOEFs that is important in understanding the new paradigm of Spiritual Nutrition.* The next question we might ask is, what is the source of these SOEFs?

Zero Point Physics and SOEFs

There is a theory, created by such greats as Einstein and the physicist Nikola Tesla, of how material existence comes into being. More and more, the theory is included in the "new" physics and in quantum mechanics field theory thinking. It is that our bodies exist as a precipitation out of an invisible, unbounded totality of perfect order. Several names have been applied to this invisible, unbounded totality: ether, virtual energy, anergy, or vacuum state. Gradually, some scientists are beginning to believe that matter is simply the condensation of a vibrating universal subtle energy substratum, or that it is a virtual state or a vacuum in a matrix of time and space, made of particular forms and densities of energy. In other words, matter is the manifest structure of all of Nature and the laws governing all physical phenomena. In spiritual terminology, pure consciousness, cosmic energy, and universal prana are terms analogous to this perfectly orderly, unmanifest state. SOEFs are an attempt to describe how this precipitation from subtle energy to material form takes place and how it is ordered.

What is this ether in terms of physics? Beardon, a physics philosopher, says that at the level of the ether, there is a separation of charge and mass. He calls it anergy, insisting it is not energy, but a more fundamental component of energy that exists as vacuum, virtual state, or ether. The ether, or virtual state, however, has no mass, and is not filled with this massless charge, but *is* charge.[3] It seems to be an almost limitless charge.

The potential energy that fills the cosmos is called zero point energy – energy that exists prior to the materialization of an object. Adam Trombley, an astrophysicist and expert in zero point technology, told the author in an interview that the materialization of an object in space represents one quadrillionth of the energy available in that volume of space.[4] It is from this state of zero point, or virtual, energy, that we, as a precipitation of this energy, come into existence in a physical form. The zero point energy in one cubic centimeter of space is said to equal the energy available in a million times a million tons of uranium. This is virtually limitless energy. The U.S. Department of Defense acknowledged the existence and potential importance of zero point technology when it sent out a program solicitation in 1986 that reflected an interest in esoteric energy sources for propulsion, including zero point quantum dynamic energy of vacuum space.[5]

Researchers have theorized that the first stepping down of this virtual energy is into a tachyon field space. Tachyon fields were first theorized by the outstanding German researcher Hans Nieper. *A tachyon can be thought of as a slightly contracted form of anergy, or of the virtual state trying to become a particle.* A tachyon field, sort of a quasi-state of matter, is thought to be made of quasi-particles. *It exists at the interface of energy and matter.* Philip Callahan, the entomologist who developed the first experimental evidence of tachyons by hooking a weeping fig plant up to a special electromagnetic sensing device, defines a tachyon as a particle moving faster than the speed of light.[6] He theorizes that the tachyon field energy is next stepped down as whirling, vortical forms of energy that precipitate near the speed of light as a particle of matter called a photon. The photon continues to be stepped down and patterned into material forms, and it interacts in various energetic ways with material forms. In 1990, David Wagner created physical technology to focalize and concentrate the tachyon energy in a variety of natural materials to be used as antennae for healing energization of the human system.

Energetic Continuum

The name we have coined for this process of creation and cosmic nutrition is called "energetic continuum." It is a term developed by David Wagner and this author and used in the book *Tachyon Energy: A New Paradigm in Holistic Healing.*[7] Having this framework in mind gives another perspective on the meaning of cosmic nutrition. This theory states that our body exists as a precipitation out of the invisible, unbounded, totality of perfect order. We call this unbound perfect order *zero point energy.* In the production of matter, zero point energy goes through the process of condensing into the tachyon energy, which is then converted into frequencies by the SOEFs. As the condensation of the subtle, vibrating, zero point energy moves into a more condensed, subtle energy, we get these particular forms and densities of energy known as matter. Matter, in other words, is the manifestation of Nature and the laws governing all the physical phenomena.

Zero point energy is omnipresent – it permeates the entire universe, exists in infinite quantity, and can never be exhausted. It also contains all potential. Within zero point energy is everything needed to create perfect form. That is the first characteristic. The second characteristic of zero point energy is that it is formless and unmanifest. The third is that it is omnipresent.

In summary:

- Zero point energy is omnipresent in the universe.
- It permeates everything.

- It exists in infinite quantities.
- It is completely inexhaustible.
- It contains all the potential for perfect form.

The first major step-down of this formless, unmanifested zero point energy is into tachyon energy. The German researcher Hans Nieper described tachyon as a slightly contracted form of energy trying to become a particle. It exists at the interface of energy in matter. This energy has been stepped down and patterned into material form. Simultaneously it continues to interact in energetic ways with material forms.

By increasing the amount of tachyon energy available to our system, we increase our awareness of the zero point energy because the tachyon energy is actually transmitting and concentrating the zero point energy. The result is that we improve all levels of physical, emotional, mental, and spiritual health, and enhance the process of moving into higher levels of order and therefore health in our lives. The tachyon energetic antennae (created by David Wagner) have been associated with accelerating the healing and indirectly the spiritual evolution process for those who have used this method.

The current understanding of the scientific world, as described by Ernst Wall in his book *The Physics of Tachyon,* supports some of these concepts.[8] In simplified physics terms, the lepton family of particles demonstrates the transformation of tachyon energy moving faster than the speed of light into the frequencies existing below the speed of light. The family includes the pion, the muon, and the electron. The first particle, the pion, exists just below the speed of light and has a consistent, mathematically calculable orbit that is compatible with the SOEFs. *All SOEFs exist just below the speed of light and are directly responsible for converting tachyon energy into frequencies required to evolve, organize, and create perfect form.* All forms are composed of different frequencies. The SOEFs convert tachyon energy into the particular frequency needed by the SOEF of a particular form. The SOEF holds the pion in its orbit. The pion SOEF exists just below the speed of light and interacts with the faster-than-the-speed-of-light tachyon. As the tachyon energy is converted into the pion frequency by the SOEF, the pion, in an instant, evolves into a muon. The new muon has a SOEF (orbit) that is two times larger than that of the pion. The muon SOEF still exists just below the speed of light. As the SOEF of the muon further interacts with the tachyon energy, the SOEF orbit once again expands and the muon evolves in an instant into an electron. The new electron has a SOEF orbit that is 207 times larger than that of the muon. This describes the continual process of SOEFs converting tachyon energy into whatever frequency is needed. This process then moves all the way down the energetic continuum. In this way the human being is created from the intracellular level to the macro-level of form, or any other form.

(See the Energetic Continuum illustration in the color plates.)

We can think about tachyon energy as *the binding energy of the universe, responsible for the energization of all forms on the planet.* In other words, tachyon energy is the energetic entrainment between the zero point energy and the SOEFs. The SOEFs are in direct communion with the tachyon energy at all levels. It is the SOEFs that convert the tachyon energy into all levels of frequency and form. Tachyon energy in this context is the critical factor that energizes the SOEF. The more tachyon energy we bring into our lives, the more energized and therefore more organized are our SOEFs. The energizing of the SOEFs in this theory is what creates health and rejuvenation because the subtle energy process enables us to reverse entropy. When the tachyon energy is freely flowing, we have an endless source of energy to maintain and build our SOEFs. In this context, the body-mind complex becomes a faster-than-light energy conduit, because we are linked to the unlimited zero point energy as our ultimate source of energy. Another way of understanding the energetic continuum, so that we do not become too mechanical in our thinking, is that this tachyon energy is the energy of the Shekhinah or, in a sense, the cosmic pranic energy that comes from the first emanation of the Divine. As the body-mind complex becomes more clear and balanced in our spiritual evolution, we become an increasingly better transducer and conductor of the energy. In this process the body-mind complex is able to store and transmit greater and greater amounts of this high energy. This explains some of the unusual phenomena that are described in this book.

Once the body is materialized, it becomes a focal point of the SOEFs in time and space as they emerge in their purest form. The most highly purified SOEFs resonate with the less refined SOEFs but are immersed in the bio-gravitational fields in the human body, unless we energize it and increase their degree of organization. This is distinctly different from the materialistic-mechanistic paradigm in which the physical life form is seen as the creator of the energy field, as with a magnet. Robert Toben, in his book *Space, Time, and Beyond,* points out that Einstein repeatedly stressed the view in the unified theory that the energy field creates form. The emerging particle is simply a space-time concentration of the non-linear living field.[9] In other words, the fields generate the matter, not the other way around.

Any mental and emotional tension in the system decreases the energy coming into the system by thickening and misaligning our subtle bodies. When the subtle bodies are aligned, the cosmic energy can pass through more easily. If the chakras are not getting the normal energy they need to function from direct external sources channeled through the subtle bodies, they pull more from the central Kundalini vortex. This may also result in the blockage of the transcendence process by depleting the energy of the Kundalini vortex. Tachyon energy reverses entropy and disorganization in the physical energy level and also energizes and organizes the self from the subtle body level. Clinically, we have been able to use tachyon energy to reverse stress-caused entropy at the subtle body and chakra level. Disharmony, disease, and degeneration are the result of a lifestyle that disorganizes the SOEFs and therefore creates entropy, or aging. Chronic and degenerative diseases, as well as life-threatening, self-destructive behaviors are primarily found only in humans or animals affected by human behavior. Humans at this point in history are the only life form on Earth that tries to work against the laws and wisdom of Nature. In India, this is called *prajna pratihara*, or crimes against wisdom. Because humans lack the wisdom to live a healthy lifestyle, they accelerate the entropy in the form of degenerative diseases. Only humans and domesticated animals suffer from rheumatism, diabetes, heart disease, hypertension, arteriosclerotic cardiovascular disease, multiple sclerosis, allergies, osteoporosis, and other degenerative diseases of civilization.

Pleomorphism and the Living Colloid Field

The next step in the energetic continuum takes us into the theory of pleomorphism. This is a theory that was developed in the lineage that started with Dr. Antoine Bechamp, then moved from Bechamp to Dr. Claude Bernard, and then Dr. Enderlein, who lived from 1872 to 1968. The author had the opportunity to study with one of Dr. Enderlein's German students, Dr. Maria Blecker. Dr. Enderlein proved the pleomorphic theory postulated by Bechamp through sixty years of observation of living human blood. He also proved that the cell is not the smallest unit of life and that within the cells are micro-units of life called *protids*. This is similar to Dr. Bechamp's *microzymas*. Dr. Enderlein's work also validated Bechamp's theory of pleomorphism, which states that these protid microorganisms change their form according to the conditions of the blood. Under toxic conditions, the protids undergo pleomorphic restructuring as virus, bacteria, mold, or fungus. What these researchers discovered, which can be readily seen under a microscope, is that the protids are .001 micron level, which is colloidal in size. The author has added to pleomorphism theory by suggesting that they actually form a living colloid energetic field. The living colloid field is the next step down after the energy has entered the subtle body system of chakras and the different layers of subtle bodies, which will be discussed in the next chapter. *The living colloid field represents the first receptacle of the subtle energy on the physical plane.* It is not only within the cells, but it exists in the extracellular fluid, the lymph and the blood. In other words, the living colloid field is essentially everywhere in the body. If this colloid field is healthy, it helps create and sustain health. If the living colloid field is disrupted by toxic influences, the energetic and physiological electromagnetic charges in the field change into more of a pathology and we move to progressively poorer health.

In summary, the energetic continuum goes from the formless Absolute (Ein Sof), to the zero point, to the Shekhinah, cosmic prana, or spiritual Kundalini energy, then to the tachyon level. Then it steps down from the tachyon, crossing the speed-of-light barrier to the SOEFs to the subtle body systems and chakras, the nadis, and finally into the living colloid system. This gives us a way to understand the meaning of Spiritual Nutrition and health. The SOEFs, when energized by the tachyon energy, create an energetic matrix from the protid colloid suspension in our tissues on the physical plane. This first manifests as a living colloid field in the space between and within the cells.

The living colloid field is affected by the physical environment in the body as well as by the normalizing SOEF matrix. Acid food, acid (negative) thoughts, low oxygen, environmental toxins, heavy metals, and lack of exercise all have the power to imbalance this living colloid field. These forces can shift it from a healthy, creative, energetic matrix for the development of cells and tissues into a morbid, pleomorphic expression. These negative environmental stresses create a morbid, pleomorphic change from healthy protid energies to viruses, bacteria, higher forms of yeast, mold, and fungus as the protids pleomorphically transmute and coagulate. As the morbid, pleomorphic forms – also known as yeast, mold, and fungus – begin to grow, they give off mycotoxins, or fungal poisons, which tend to break down our living tissue. They eat the sugar in our systems, the DNA, the proteins, the enzymes, and hormones. They live off our tissues and vital fluids. The mycotoxins even destroy our neurotransmitters. The pathogenic, pleomorphic forms further imbalance and acidify the system, and therefore create favorable conditions for more of these pleomorphic organisms to grow. This increases the state of mycosis (fungal infection).

In a healthy state there is a clear and full expression of vital SOEFs in the living colloid field. Here is the counterpoint to the toxic influences on the physical and mental plane. When the energetic continuum is not blocked by the toxic influences, it energizes the vital life pattern and creates a healthy, energetic living colloid field, which is the foundation for optimal health. The living colloid field is the first level of physical manifestation of life energies. The healthy living colloid field is essential for a properly functioning coagulation system and for the proper building blocks for all cellular, lymph, blood, and intracellular structures. When this living colloid field is energetically healthy, meaning there are no blocks in the energetic continuum, we have a perfect supportive field for healthy matrix and the creation, formation, and increasing life force of our cells and tissues. When the living colloid field is disrupted by degenerative influences, it acts as a sensor to the physiological imbalance. In this capacity it reacts to the environment and creates a morbid energetic field to compensate. It is this compensation, creating a morbid field, that takes us into the process of degenerative health. These protids, which seem to be independent living elements, are thought to have a critical role as a builder of health as well as a recycler of the organism. This recycling is the death and dying process. As long as the SOEF imprint on the living colloid field of the protids is not too significantly disturbed, the living colloid field acts as a builder and restorer of life. When this colloidal energetic matrix is disturbed to a significant extent, the "recycling button" or "composting button" is pushed, and the protids begin their function as recyclers/composters for whatever organism they are living in. In essence, they begin to accelerate the rate of fermentation in the system. At the turn of the nineteenth century, *candida* was seen primarily in people who were dying of cancer or other serious diseases. Candida is part of this recycling process. What was going on with these people with cancer is that the composting button had been pushed and they began to compost; they began the cycle of degeneration. This is discussed in detail in the author's book *Rainbow Green Live-Food Cuisine.*[10]

The process of chronic disease is activated in a person who is toxic enough to push the composting button. Depending on the degree of toxicity and how hard this button is being pushed, composting may lead to chronic disease, misery, and, ultimately, death. The key to restoring health is minimizing or eliminating the toxic conditions so that the composting button is turned off – eliminating the toxic conditions and increasing the amount of subtle energy coming into the system so that the degenerative process is reversed, and the composting button is turned off. On the practical level, mental peace and Love combined with a low-glycemic, high-mineralized, non-acidic, live-food, vegan diet and a healthy mind are the key factors that turn off the composting button and reestablish us in vibrant health. These create "neg-entropy," the reverse of entropy-induced aging. All of the Six Foundations help to reverse the entropy of this degeneration process. Based on the author's research, the best diet for health and Spiritual Nutrition is the Rainbow Green Live-Food Cuisine. People with moderate composting going on usually need three months on Phase I of the Rainbow Green Live-Food Cuisine, which entails no sweets and primarily raw nuts, seeds, and vegetables, to reverse this composting process (see Chapter 27 for more information on Rainbow Green Live-Food Cuisine). This is in stark contrast to food practices around the world, which generally increase the morbid influences that turn on the composting button. These morbid influences include hybrid and high-sweet fruits, radiation, intense pollution, heavy-metal toxicity, an accelerated amount of stress in the environment and within our minds, war, pestilence, plague, terrorism, use of genetically engineered food, irradiated food, processed food, fast food, junk food, refined white flour, white sugar, and canned food. All of these specifically are a morbid influence on the living colloid field as it attempts to express the pure subtle organizing energy matrix inherent in our cells and tissues.

Blockages in the Energetic Continuum

Once we understand the existence of the energetic continuum, we can concretely understand the effects of blockages in the flow of energy through the continuum. This becomes a significant insight into Spiritual

Nutrition and holistic healing. If we have a blockage in the energetic continuum, it needs to be cleared. A blockage is defined in essence as disorder or chaos in the energetic continuum, causing an energy deficiency. This may occur at the tachyon energy level or the SOEF level; it may occur with the thickening and misalignment of the subtle energy bodies that involve the emotions and mental state, or it may actually occur on the physical level with the toxicities the author has been describing. The idea of living the Six Foundations and the use of tachyonized materials and techniques is to restore the natural flow of energy through the energetic continuum. They organize that which is disorganized and create a neg-entropy, which is a youthing effect. Tachyon energy, as it is increased with the Six Foundations, restores the cells to their natural state of order and balance, thus creating health and well-being as well as enhancing spiritual awareness. To make the point clear, let's say we have a lower back pain, and this lower back pain is associated with emotional stress, which is in turn associated with a blockage in the emotional body. By upping our spiritual input and making the emotional, psycho-spiritual corrections, we are able to unblock the field, which can then eliminate the pain on the physical level. This is a short way of talking about having psychosomatic diseases. The only difference is, we are healing it from higher levels of intervention, which includes tachyon holistic healing devices, meditation, prayer, and so on.

When we have a part of the energetic continuum blocked, the aura in our system where the blockage occurs is left in a deficient energetic state and will ultimately become vulnerable to degenerative diseases as well as acute pathological invasion. When we truly understand and appreciate the importance of maintaining the energetic continuum, we have the potential of reversing entropy, creating youthing, and even the potential of such unthinkable concepts as physical immortality. This is not the goal of spiritual life; the dharma of all life is merging with God. However, the longer we stay in the body, the better chance we have of discovering that we are that which we always have been: One with God.

SOEFs and Virtual Energy

This interplay of research and theory provides the matrix for the author's hypothesis of Subtle Organizing Energy Fields. SOEFs both create and energize the template form of living systems. Emerging out of the virtual state, they are capable of organizing on any level of the human body, from tachyon to cellular structure to organ systems. These SOEFs resonate with the unlimited virtual state energy, transferring it through various step-down systems that eventually transduce it into the energy fields of the human body. The SOEFs thus resonate with and energize the body-mind complex. Virtual energy is omnipresent, thus we are always resonating to some extent with this cosmic energy. Most of the time we have only indirect or brief experiences of this, but at certain stages of spiritual evolution it is possible to experience this resonance in direct attunement, consistently and consciously. For many, this sort of experience first happens in meditation. As we become more aware of and resonant with this virtual energy state, our minds merge and identify with this awareness as the unchanging Truth and the reality of our existence. The resonance becomes part of our conscious awareness in our everyday activities. Eventually, it becomes a continual awareness and attunement with the cosmic energy. This is known as Cosmic Consciousness.

Another important ramification of zero point energy physics is relevant to the Spiritual Nutrition paradigm. Developed by Beardon, it is called the Law of Conservation of Anergy. Beardon's law states that the total equivalency of mass, energy, and massless charge is conserved.[11] If this law eventually proves to be correct, it explains how entropy can be reversed and biological transmutation (see Chapter 13) can take place in the human system without breaking any fundamental laws. It is ultimately the conversion of the essentially unlimited virtual energy into SOEFs, and the transduction of this energy into the human body, that reverses entropy and therefore aging. This explains how the body can, in effect, become a "free energy" machine, since we are linked to the unlimited virtual energy as our ultimate source of energy. If this energy is free flowing, then we have an endless source of energy to rebuild our SOEFs, and we continually reverse entropy. As a result, the body-mind complex becomes more clear and balanced in spiritual evolution, and it becomes an increasingly better transducer and conductor of anergy to energy. As this happens, the body is able to store and transmit greater and greater amounts of this higher energy. It is this process that can account for some of the many miracles said to occur in the presence of spiritual masters. For example, spontaneous healing occurred when people simply touched the robe of Jesus. We now understand that there was a flow of this pure cosmic or God energy into people, which reorganized and reenergized their SOEFs, allowing the disease processes to be reversed. People's faith allowed them to draw and be receptive to the healing energy.

Characteristics of SOEFs: Form and Energy

SOEFs have form. They can hold, gain, lose, resonate with, transduce, and transmit energy. Because of this, they are different from Rupert Sheldrake's hypothesis of morphogenic fields, described in *A New Science of Life*. His morphogenic fields are concerned only with form; they are neither a type of matter nor a type of energy.[12] Sheldrake's description of the morphogenic fields and his brilliant hypothesis of formative causation relate beautifully to the form of SOEFs. According to Sheldrake, morphogenic fields play a causal role in the development and maintenance of the forms of systems at all levels. Sheldrake uses the term "morphic unit" to describe the subunits in a system, e.g., a morphic unit for protons, another for atoms, water molecules, and muscle cells, and another for organs like kidneys. The higher morphic fields coordinate the interplay, organization, and pattern of the smaller morphic units. Like the SOEFs, these morphogenic fields correspond to the potential state of a developing system and are present before it materializes into its final form.

Once the body is manifest, it becomes a focal point for the SOEFs in time and space as they emerge in their purest form from the virtual state. These more highly purified SOEFs resonate with the less refined SOEFs that are immersed in the biogravitational fields of the human body and thus reenergize and increase their degree of organization. This is contrary to the materialist paradigm in which the physical life form is seen as the creator of the energy fields around it. To put it succinctly, these fields generate matter. The body, in this wholistic paradigm, is a form stabilized by the SOEFs.

If the energy of a SOEF is dispersed, the organizing field is disrupted, and the living system operates in a less organized way. This is one important aspect in which the form of SOEFs specifically differs from Sheldrake's theory of morphogenic fields. This dissipation, which drives the system toward disorganization, can be termed entropy. In concrete terms, the dissipation of the SOEF yields imperfect cell replication, poorer enzymatic function, decreased capacity for biological transmutation, and increased tendency toward chronic disease. This translates as aging. When the SOEFs of food are significantly depleted, to assimilate our food completely we must reenergize incoming food directly from our own life force, depleting the energy of our SOEFs. An example is eating highly refined white bread. The chromium that is necessary to aid its assimilation into the system has been depleted in the processing and must be supplied by the body. Eventually, the body becomes depleted of chromium. Analogously, when the SOEFs in food are disrupted by food processing procedures, especially with radiating our foods with over 100,000 rads (a chest X-ray is one-quarter to one-half a rad), the energetic value of the food, in terms of its ability to increase our total SOEF energy, is diminished. When we eat high-energy food, the result is just the opposite: the energy of the SOEFs is enhanced.

When SOEFs are energized, they develop a more structured and defined organization that better maintains the form and function of the human system. This energizing reverses entropy. It is this property of the SOEFs that reverses the aging process. A helpful physical model for this is shown in the figure. Brown sugar is added to water. At first, it has no defined form. It lies in a disorganized pile on the bottom of the glass. When we add vortical energy to the system by stirring with a spoon, the pile of brown sugar is pulled upward into a more defined form. When we stop the spoon and hold it in the water, it disrupts the vortical pattern, the energy in the system is diminished, the brown sugar particles begin to lose their well-defined form, and entropy takes place.

In the same way, the vortical energy patterns of the different SOEFs create different patterns of matter. As the vortical energy of the SOEFs

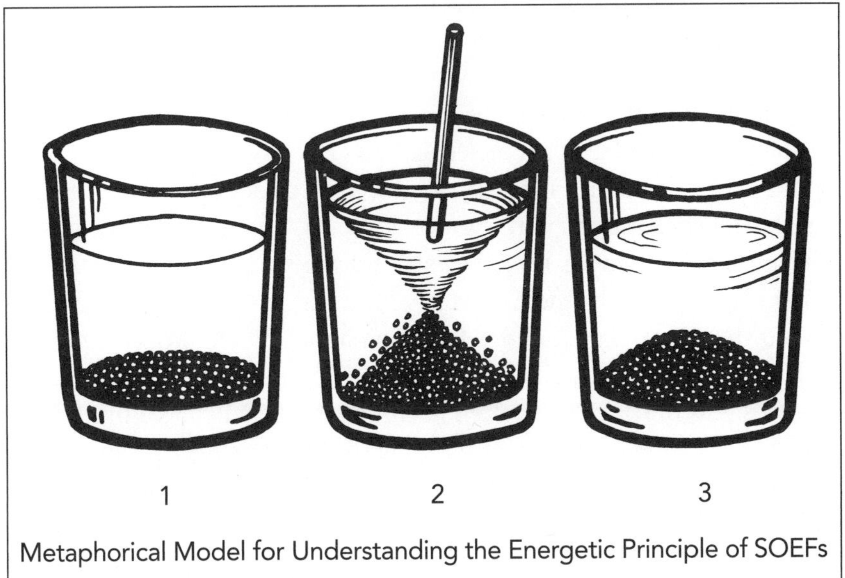

Metaphorical Model for Understanding the Energetic Principle of SOEFs

moves into the realm of time and space, they begin to organize into a physical pattern. The more energy they have, the better defined and organized are the physical structures they are organizing. The intertwined vortex structure of RNA and DNA are archetypical physical manifestations of vortex forms. They, of course, represent the key to cellular organization. From this vortex analogy and the SOEF concept, we can begin to see the connection between living an energizing, harmonious lifestyle and eating foods that are raw, organic, and living. These energized lifestyles and live foods, whose natural high energy is not dissipated by processing, can help to slow down and even reverse the aging process. Much of this book is about how an energized and organized human body supports health and spiritual evolution.

Structured Water in Biological Systems

Structured water is water that has highly organized SOEFs and therefore is a more crystalline and hydrated structure. Structured water is an excellent example of how increasing the energy in a biological system, in this case water, makes it more organized and healthier. It will help our understanding if we now take a detailed look at structured water. In structured water, both the angle of the water molecule bond and the surface tension of the water change. Structured molecules form more stable water hydration shells, and actually give more order and structure to the water.[13]

When water is exposed to moonlight, to the product Crystal Energy, or to a pyramid (these are all generators, transmitters, and/or magnifiers of subtle energy), the actual molecular configuration of the water changes. This moving from less structure to more structure represents a specific reversal of the system's entropy. Clegg reports that in a normal cell the structured water tends to gather around the surfaces of the inner and outer cell membranes and the cytoplasmic matrix of the cell.[14] It is established that the polar qualities (electromagnetic fields) of macromolecules in general and specifically of enzymes, a class of macromolecules, attract shells of structured water. Each macromolecule has a unique pattern of structured water in its shell. Biologists are shifting their view of the cell as no more than a membranous bag containing liquid water with enzymes, other macromolecules, and ions in a free solution. Cells are now regarded as containing a structured water matrix that holds enzyme systems and other macromolecules, complexed with sodium and potassium ions, in a polarized water structure.[15]

In fact, the water appears to be structured in three levels of intensity.[16] The increased intracellular structured water in these intracellular membrane locations is thought to increase the concentrations of intracellular enzymes as the structured water of the enzymes gains more affinity for the structured water in intracellular membrane sites.[17] This network of structured water, generated by the intracellular membranes and macromolecular surfaces, creates a matrix in which most intracellular metabolism takes place.[18] An increase in intracellular structured water, resulting from increased order and enzyme concentrations, is thought to improve the quality of enzymatic reactions.[19] On a practical nutritional level, there is a structuring of water around co-enzymes (vitamins) that makes it easier for them to penetrate the structured water barriers of the extracellular fluids and the intracellular system. Therefore, vitamins arrive more efficiently at the correct enzyme reaction site. The structured water around the enzymes also stabilizes the energy state of the enzyme, improving enzyme reactions.[20] An important conclusion from this research is that the more structured water there is in a system, the better the enzyme systems function, the more easily the minerals and vitamins are assimilated into the cells, and the better the enzymes metabolize.

This research is of particular significance because it correlates with the SOEF theory that the more energy in a system, the more structured it is, and the healthier and the better it functions. Nuclear magnetic resonance studies have shown that the intracellular water of cancer cells has significantly less structure than normal cells.[21] Mikesell demonstrates that when there is a decrease in structured water, there is a shift from the healthy intracellular sodium/potassium ratio.[22] This upset seems to be associated with a lower quality of health in general.[23]

Another generally accepted property of structured water is that it has a higher solubility for minerals than unstructured water. Like vitamins, minerals also become surrounded by a structured water cell because of their polarity, and are absorbed more readily for similar reasons. The implication is that people with higher SOEF energy have more structured water in their systems and are therefore better able to absorb needed minerals.

A detailed description of structured water and how to structure water is offered in Chapter 29.

Summary of Structured Water

Structured water research is of significance to us because it correlates with the SOEF theory that the more energy in a system, the more structured it is, the less entropy it experiences, and the better it functions. As an example, when there is more structured intracellular water in a system, there are more concentrated and balanced intracellular ions such as calcium, potassium, and sodium. From this new perspective we can see a positive relationship between an increased energy of our SOEFs, increased intracellular and structured water, and increased general health.

In general, there is more structured water in biological systems than in plain water. Fruits, as a biological system, have the highest percentage of water, approximately 80 to 90 percent. Their above-ground growing position exposes them to more sunlight, an established structurer of water. They are the most important source of structured water for our systems. The structured water of fruit can be said to best help cleanse the system and carry enzymes, minerals, and other nutrients most easily into the cells.

But since the focus of this book is not intracellular physiology, the author would like to shift back to the simple statement that *increased subtle energy in a living system results in more structured water in that system and therefore generally better health.* Interesting findings have been supplied by Orie Bachechi's eight-year study using Kiva lights, a balanced form of full-spectrum light. Bachechi claims that by exposing food and water to Kiva lights, the amount of structured water they contain increases.[24] He reports that many diseases, such as arteriosclerotic cardiovascular disease, high blood pressure, dry skin, kidney and gallbladder stones, ulcers, candida albicans infections, allergies, and arthritis, are ameliorated.[25] He has also found that bread made with nutrients exposed to Kiva lights contains 15 percent more protein, a result, he feels, of improved nutrient and enzyme function in the bread. It is not my interest to make health claims for Kiva lights. It would also be nice if his results from eight years of clinical research were confirmed in controlled studies by independent investigators. But his results confirm that increasing the subtle energy and therefore structured water in a system improves body function and health.

The larger theory of nutritional and holistic health is that energy flows from the zero point energy to increased subtle energy in the system, which then improves physical, emotional, mental, and spiritual well-being. This flow of cosmic energy into the biological system is what gives us the ability to reverse entropy and therefore creates a youthing process.

Summary, Chapter 6

1. Subtle Organizing Energy Fields (SOEFs) are a template for the multiple levels of organization of living systems.
2. SOEFs have both form and energy properties.
3. SOEFs resonate with the unlimited tachyon energy, and through resonance, transfer this energy to us through a series of step-down systems. As our body-mind complex becomes more spiritually transformed, it is easier for this energy to be directly transferred to us and for us to experience a direct resonance with the cosmic energy.
4. All nutrient elements have their own individual SOEFs.
5. When SOEFs are energized, they maintain and strengthen both their organization and that of the physical body. This property allows us to resist and reverse the aging process we call entropy.
6. When the energy level of SOEFs is depleted by eating low-energy foods and living energy-depleting lifestyles, the SOEFs become less organized, resulting in increased entropy and aging.
7. The existence of an energetic continuum is hypothesized.
8. The existence of a living colloid field as part of the energetic continuum is explained.

Chapter 7

Subtle Anatomies

The Subtle Body System

The subtle anatomies are another subtle energy system that needs to be explored for our complete understanding of and need for Spiritual Nutrition. As with the chakras, there is general agreement among spiritual authorities, Kabbalistic traditions, Yoga teachings, Vedantic scriptures, and Western researchers that several layers of subtle energy bodies exist. In some Western systems, two to seven subtle anatomies are reported. In most of these subtle anatomy systems, the same basic functions and levels of consciousness are generally included. In the Vedantic, and in most Yoga traditions, four bodies are reported: physical, subtle, causal, and supercausal. With each subtle body level there is an associated "mind" of functioning and awareness.

By name, the seven subtle anatomies are: etheric, emotional, mental, astral, spiritual, causal, and soul bodies. As the refined energy condenses from its cosmic or virtual state, it is stepped down via the seven subtle anatomies, which personalize it and densify it to a level at which our physical body can incorporate it. It is the author's hypothesis that these subtle anatomies work in conjunction with the chakra system in this transduction process. Each subtle anatomy has a subtle chakra system that regulates the flow of energy within it. The chakra systems also regulate the flow of energy between the different subtle anatomies. It is the author's clinical experience that the energy does not flow in just one direction from the cosmos into the body; it can also flow in the opposite direction. For example, when someone's physical energy increases, a corresponding increase in psychological energy can often be seen. By implication, some of the increased physical energy has been converted to psychological energy. In general, however, the flow is from the state of virtual energy to a more condensed form. This stepped-down energy is absorbed through the vortexes of the measurable chakra system and then into our physical anatomy. From our physical anatomy – brain, heart, organs, endocrine systems, and skeletal structures – electromagnetic fields (EMFs) are emitted and communicate with all our cells and with the external world. The chakras that are measurable with our current, limited, scientific instrumentation are those that interface between the subtle body system and the physical body. It is this level that is most commonly thought of as the chakra system.

EMFs are the final links between the etheric and physical bodies. Recent work by Jose Delgado, an internationally known Spanish neuroscientist, gives indirect evidence of the effect EMFs can have on our biological systems. Delgado uses EMFs that are one-fiftieth the strength of the Earth's own magnetic field. These fields, which the author feels are of the same nature as those transduced by the chakra system into the body, have been shown to alter the mental functioning of a variety of vertebrate nervous systems and other body system activities. For example, by exposing monkeys to different types of EMFs, Delgado could make some go to sleep and others become irritable. Researchers have also detected EMFs in the brain and around the denser area of the nervous system.

Functions of the Seven Subtle Anatomies

The seven subtle anatomies comprise what is also known as the human *aura*. The subtle bodies act in a way that is analogous to a prism, breaking cosmic energy into seven rays. Each ray tends to be the predominant energizing ray for one of the seven chakras.

The chakra system interpenetrates the seven subtle bodies and interfaces among their different levels as part of the energy transduction system. Depending on the alignment of the subtle bodies, the energy flows through with more or less resistance to the measurable chakra level. These interdimensional chakras can be thought of, metaphorically, as tubes between the subtle bodies. When all subtle bodies are aligned, then all seven interdimensional chakra "tubes" become synchronized, and cosmic energy flows through the body with the least resistance. In the figure we see the author's visualization of how the subtle bodies are an extension of the vortex energy spin of the chakras. As the vortex energy of the chakras increases, the centrifugal spin expands the subtle body. As the cosmic energy increases, our angelic wings are unfolded. Perhaps these subtle bodies are the angelic wings that are sometimes seen by people. Perhaps we are even those angels.

(See the Angel Wings: Subtle Bodies Radiating as an Extension of the Chakras illustration in the color plates.)

When the left and right hemispheres of the brain are balanced, as is commonly experienced during meditation, the subtle anatomies and chakra "tubes" are in alignment and cosmic energy flows through smoothly. Conversely, during times of mental agitation or anxiety, the subtle anatomy chakra system becomes misaligned, resulting in more resistance and less energy flowing through. At times like these, a person might describe the chakras as "closed." This decreased energy flow into the system seems to correlate to a state of constricted awareness and a feeling of disharmony.

Research by Master Charles, of MSH Associates in Virginia, seems to support the point that increased right and left brain synchronization correlates with an increased flow of spiritualizing energy into the system. MSH has developed an audiotape program called *Synchronicity, the Recognitions Experience*™ as an aid to spiritual development. In this program the brain hemispheres are progressively synchronized through sound phasing. In reviewing reports from nearly a thousand participants, the preliminary findings are that, with increased right and left brain synchronization, participants experience a more consistent, deeper meditation.[1] In post-meditation journals, participants reported an increased sense of overall harmony with themselves and their world.

The etheric, emotional, and mental bodies comprise what we would normally associate with the *conscious mind.* The seven subtle bodies as a whole comprise what can be called the *larger mind.* This larger mind is the interface between the physical body, or unconscious level of awareness, and the virtual energy level, or Cosmic Consciousness. It mediates between the body and the cosmic energy level. *We can think of the seven subtle bodies as the larger mind. The subtle body system acts as a transducing system that personalizes the energy flow from the cosmic level of virtual energy to a denser energy that our bodies can incorporate on the physical level.*

Summary, Chapter 7

1. The subtle anatomy system consists of seven subtle energy levels. It makes up what is known as the aura, or larger mind.
2. This seven-layer subtle body system mediates as a step-down transducer to conduct the flow of energy from the highly purified virtual, or cosmic, energy state to a condensed, personalized state that our bodies use as life force.
3. When all seven subtle bodies are aligned, cosmic energy flows through more intensely and with less resistance to energize and spiritualize the body-mind-spirit complex.

Chapter 8

Aberrant Biological Phenomena

There exist "aberrant" phenomena in the context of human life that, when explored more deeply, give us greater insight into the principles of spiritual anatomy, our existence as part of an energetic continuum, and the need for the new paradigm of Spiritual Nutrition. These aberrant phenomena – people who claim to have lived for many hundreds of years, biological transmutations (detailed in Chapter 13), the Divine body (non-decomposition after death), resurrection, and inedia (breatharianism) – cannot be explained by and are outside of the context of the materialistic-mechanistic paradigm that dominates Western thinking. These phenomena demand that we look beyond the old paradigm and give support to the emerging paradigm of Spiritual Nutrition.

Longevity: Approaching Physical Immortality

Let us start with evidence suggesting extended longevity that approaches physical immortality. Some Yogis presently alive in India claim they have mastered the secret of how to live for hundreds of years. The great seer Sri Nisargadatta Maharaj met such a man, who offered to teach him the secret of how he could live 1,000 years. Sri Nisargadatta, incidentally, rejected the offer because he believed that living 1,000 years was not the point of being on this planet.[1] The author agrees with Sri Nisargadatta's understanding, adding that one should court radiant health until the purpose of being on the planet – Liberation – is completed. Tapasviji Maharaj lived 185 years. He kept doing *kaya kalpa* (an Ayurvedic rejuvenation process) until he was Liberated; then he stopped. There are reports of a Trailanga Swami who, at the time Swami Yogananda wrote of him in 1946, was already reported to be 300 years old. Hotema reports that Numas De Cugna of India died in 1565 at the age of 370 years.[2] There are also reports of an ageless master called simply Babaji, who claims to have given initiation to the great saint Shankaracharya, born in 788 A.D., and to Kabir, the great Sufi saint born around 1440. In *Autobiography of a Yogi,* Swami Yogananda, a well-respected spiritual master who lived in the United States for the last 30 years of his life, describes Babaji from his interviews of those who actually spent time with him. His body was said to look like that of a 25-year-old. It was said that he did not need to eat. Yogananda's assessment of the meaning of Babaji's extraordinary physical state of maintaining his physical body for centuries is that it is to provide an example and guidance for our own fantastic possibilities.[3] The author is not asserting these anecdotes are true. They have been noted here to stimulate our imagination. As the saying goes, "Where there is smoke, there may be fire."

In Taoist teachings, immortality is described as being part of the highest state of Union with the Tao.[4] Mantak Chia, a Taoist teacher, claims that in some Taoist literature, the names of individuals who reached this state can be found. He feels the Taoist teachings talk about immortality in a concrete way rather than metaphorically.[5] The best documented Chinese man of longevity is Professor Li Chung Yun, who is reputed to have lived 256 years, from 1677 to 1933.[6] Proving his age, it is documented that at the age of 100 he was awarded a special Honor Citation for extraordinary service to his country,[7] and that he gave a series of twenty-eight lectures at the University of Sinkiang at the age of 200.

Another piece of what might be considered by some as anecdotal or symbolic evidence (and by others as hard-core proof of near immortality) are Biblical references to one person in each of the the first ten generations following Adam who lived many hundreds of years. In the Torah, Adam is reported to have lived for 930 years, Seth for 912 years, Enoch for 905 years, Methuselah for 969 years, and Noah for 950 years.

Some modern examples of longevity are cited by Hotema: Flora Thompson of North Carolina died in 1808 at the age of 152; Jose Calverto of Mexico died in 1921 at the age of 186; Thomas Garn of England died in 1795 at the age of 207. There is also Dando the Illyrian, who is said to have lived more than 500 years.[8] In the book *Maharaj,* a biography of the great holy man Shriman Tapasviji Maharaj, who lived from 1770 to 1955, to the age of 185, Maharaj meets two people, aged between 2000 and 3000 years, who were alive at the time of Krishna.[9] One man's name was Ashvatthaman; he was one of the commanders-in-chief of the Kauravas army as described in the *Mahabharata*, an epic book. He had received the boon of longevity from Drona, his father. The other man was an eight-foot-tall man who, in the course of his solitary ascetic life in the Himalayas, discovered a bush with a special herb that conveys longevity. It could be the much sought soma plant. These are fantastic anecdotes that boggle the mind with the possibility of incredible longevity.

These anecdotal, Biblical, and historically documented examples of longevity cannot be said to prove our potential absolutely, but there are enough of them to convince us to consider it a possibility. After all, a wild hog in its native state is said to live 300 years, and an eagle 500 years. Who is to say that, if we were to live according to the laws of Nature, we could not live as long as a wild hog? This one's reason for bringing up these examples is not only to demonstrate the shortcomings of the materialistic-mechanistic paradigm and give support to the existence of an energetic continuum, but also to expand our awareness to the awesome possibilities that are ours.

The Phenomenon of the Divine Body

A complete theory must also include the phenomenon of the Divine body – the finding that the bodies of certain holy people do not decompose after the spirit has left the physical shell. Examples of this discovery include the following:

- Jnaneshwar Maharaj, who had himself buried alive at the age of 21 in a cave. Three hundred years later, he was found by the great sixteenth-century saint Eknath Maharaj to have a perfectly glowing and lifelike body. Eknath Maharaj was drawn to the burial place because he was receiving messages in meditation about a tree limb that had wrapped around Jnaneshwar's neck. When he was granted permission to enter the cave, there indeed was a tree limb around the holy man's neck. He removed it and thus completed his mission.
- When the Nazis dug up the body of the Baal Shem Tov, the spiritual founder of Hasidim, not only was his body totally intact after 200 years, but a great Light streamed forth from his eyes and scared them away.
- In *A Treasury of Chassidic Tales*,[10] Rabbi Shlomo Zevin writes that

when the Nazis attempted to desecrate the grave of the great rabbi Elimelech in Lyzhansk, they found a perfectly preserved, radiant body and were thrown into a panic. Rabbi Zevin reports the same amazing discovery when the Jewish community dug up the body of Rabbi Avraham of Chechanov to protect it from Nazi desecration. They found the holy body of the tzaddik intact and whole, as though he had just been buried, though he had been buried for 68 years.[11]

- When Paramahansa Yogananda left his physical body, his body was kept out for 20 days so disciples from all over the world could come to pay their last respects. Although it is normal for a body to begin to decay within one to two days, the director of the mortuary, in a certified letter, wrote:

  The absence of any visual signs of decay in the dead body of Paramahansa Yogananda offers the most extraordinary case in our experience. No physical disintegration was visible in his body even 20 days after death. No indication of mold was visible on his skin, and no visible dessication took place in the bodily tissues. This state of perfect preservation of a body is, so far as we know, unparalleled. Yogananda's body was apparently in a phenomenal state of immutability.[12]

- It is reported that in 1859, when St. John of the Cross was exhumed 268 years after he died, his body was perfectly preserved.[13]

Resurrection

A complete theory must account for the possible phenomenon of resurrection. The most well known, of course, is that of Jesus. As pointed out in Corinthians 15:54–55, "Death is swallowed up in victory. O death, where is thy sting? O grave, where is thy victory?"

Another example of a resurrected master was Yogananda's report of the resurrection of his spiritual master Sri Yukteswar, who spent two hours with him in a Bombay hotel in 1936, four months after Yukteswar died.[14] Responding to Yogananda's amazed questions about the form Yogananda was physically hugging, Yukteswar said: "O yes, my new body is a perfect copy of the old one. I materialize or dematerialize this form any time at will, much more frequently than I did while on Earth."[15]

Yogananda also reports the phenomenon of resurrection in connection with Sri Yukteswar's guru, a householder named Lahiri Mahasaya. Just before he died he said to his devotees, "Be comforted; I shall rise again."[16] Yogananda writes that Lahiri Mahasaya resurrected himself after his physical body was cremated. He said to one devotee: "It is I. From the disintegrated atoms of my cremated body, I have resurrected a remodeled form."[17] In order to confirm the event of resurrection, Yogananda cites the testimony of three of Lahiri Mahasaya's greatest disciples that their guru appeared before them on the day after his cremation, each in a different location. One disciple claimed to have been invited to touch his physical body as proof of the physical resurrection.

Inedia

Evidence of breatharianism (inedia) actually exists in many traditions. It is unfortunate that there are occasional frauds who claim to be breatharians, but the following examples seem to be authenticated. One such person is Thérèse Neuman, a devoted Catholic woman of Konnersreuth, Germany. She abstained from food and drink, except for the ritual swallowing of one paper-thin sacramental wafer at specific times during the week and one teaspoon of water per day.[18] By ecclesiastical permission, Thérèse was allowed to be under scientific investigation for this phenomenon of inedia. The most famous investigation was by Dr. Fritz Gerlick, editor of a Protestant German newspaper, who supposedly went to expose the "Catholic fraud." Instead, he wrote her biography.

Another example of inedia is that of an 83-year-old Buddhist priest who has lived for 47 years in a cave in the Himalayan mountains. Dr. Krishnan Lal, head of a medical team of four experts who studied the monk for 43 months, reported that he lived only on sips of water. This is the closest example to inedia that we know of.

In the Taoist tradition, according to Mantak Chia, the sixth stage of spiritual evolution is marked by inedia. He claims his own teacher reached this stage in which he lived in the mountains and was able to subsist on the subtle energies of Mother Nature.[19]

There is documentation by Paramahansa Yogananda of a woman by the name of Giri Bala who stopped eating and drinking at the age of 12. At the time of his interview with her, she had not taken food or water in 56 years.[20] She affirmed that her nourishment was derived from the finer energies of the air and sunlight, as well as from the cosmic power that recharges the body through its chakras.

Most recently, a Mr. Hira Ratan Manek from India has done water fasts of 130, 211, and 411 days. He claims to derive his nutrition from the frequencies of the sun. He has conducted several world tours explaining this technique.[21]

Longevity and the New Paradigm of Nutrition

These aberrant phenomena and the existence of biological transmutation are simply not able to fit into the materialistic-mechanistic theory of nutrition based on the assumption that energy is produced by physical forms. But when we explain them with our new model of spiritual physiology, they support the wholistic paradigm of Spiritual Nutrition, which acknowledges that it is the natural course of things to have the potential for nearly immortal physical bodies and spirits. It is natural, rather than unusual, to increase the life force and degree of organization in our human system. The reason it is not experientially obvious is that our personal and world lifestyles tend to break down our system's natural organization and energy. Aging equates with the decrease in energy and organization of the pattern of the SOEFs that organize our body function. If we eat irradiated foods in which the SOEFs have been destroyed, if we eat processed, antibiotic-, and pesticide-filled foods, if we smoke, drink, take drugs, and in general lead a disharmonious, disorganized work, family, and personal life, we increase our entropy and decrease our SOEFs. By not following the universal laws of Nature, we decrease life span.

For the rationalist, who has no other framework than that of the law of entropy, these Yogic, Torah, Hasidic, and Christian stories may seem to be fantasy. But for those who understand how entropy does not completely apply to living systems as the sole governing force, the implication and explanation of these examples must be examined more closely. For example, Rabbi Moses Maimonides, a twelfth-century physician and one of the great Jewish sages in history, explained that one reason the great leaders of the first ten generations (starting with Adam) lived so long was that they were very careful of their diets.[22] It is said that they did not eat meat or any animal products, nor did they ever drink wine or any other intoxicating beverage. Their entire diet consisted only of carefully measured amounts of natural, vegetarian foods, and their only beverage was pure water. They were said to have practiced extreme moderation in sexual activity.[23] These instances in the *Torah Anthology* also point out that longevity decreased after the time of Noah because there was a change in atmospheric vitality and because meat was added to our diet.[24] I do not know the original sources of this information; some seems to have come from ancient texts and some from oral tradition or revelation. However, it is completely concordant with living a SOEF-life-affirming approach, an approach in harmony with the universal laws of Nature.

A lifetime approaching relative immortality is a possibility; healthful longevity is a practical reality. The Essenes studied and lived in harmony with Nature's laws, and they too are reported to regularly live more than 120 years.[25] The science of Ayurveda teaches that a state of immortality can be achieved if we are completely attuned to the universal laws of Nature. According to Dr. Szekeley, founder of the modern Essene movement, the Pelegasians, an ancient Greek culture, ate only nuts, seeds, vegetables, and fruits in 100-percent live form and lived to an average age of 200 years. A Greek naturopath friend has confirmed that such a culture did exist.

The book *Maharaj* contains a description of how the Mahatma Shriman Tapasviji Maharaj lived from 1770 to 1955 using the process called kaya kalpa.[26] In essence, this process is an intense adherence to and amplification of natural laws, including a total re-energizing and reorganizing of the SOEFs. He did this rejuvenation process three times: once for 90 days, then 365 days at age 150 years, and the last time for 40 days.[27] A personal witness, the book's biographer, testifies to the regrowth of new teeth, hair, and a robust young body on the last kaya kalpa rejuvenation treatment. At the age of 185, instead of repeating the process, he felt his work on Earth was complete and it was time for him to leave his body. The potentials we humans have are indeed very interesting. The essence of this treatment will be discussed in later chapters.

Today we experience imbalanced living conditions on our planet, which block the flow of cosmic energy through the energetic continuum. Our world lifestyle of radiation, pesticides, smog, strife, and other forms of pollution, hatred, violence, and war between nations makes attaining such ages in the physical body rare. However, studies of the cultures that do enjoy health and longevity show a pattern of conserving and enhancing SOEFs. In studies of cultures such as the Hunzakuts in Pakistan and the Villabamba people of Ecuador, researchers have found it is normal for people to live active lives for more than 100 years. Paavo Airola sums up the basic factors: a low-calorie, simple, primarily vegan diet accompanied by systematic undereating, exercise, fresh air, and water in the context of a contented, relaxed, and loving atmosphere, and a positive state of mind.[28] Li Chung Yun, the Chinese man documented to be 256 years old, calls it "inward calm."[29] Inner calm enhances SOEFs, while stress disrupts SOEFs and depletes the vital force. The Transcendental Meditation researchers at the annual meeting of the American Geriatrics Society in 1979 reported a study that showed that long-term Transcendental Meditators were, on the average, 12 years younger physiologically than they were chronologically.[30]

Although longevity is not the goal of Spiritual Nutrition, it is a common result in a human system with highly energized and well-organized SOEFs. Longevity is not necessarily a sign of spirituality. It is a common assumption among the holistic health and human potential movement that we are completely independent and free to create our own reality. The direct meditation experience of continual merging into Universal Consciousness and the findings of the physics of quantum mechanics over the last half century both offer a different understanding: *We are not separate and independent from the totality of the universe*. As part of the whole, we are affected by the whole. We have choice, and because of this, some responsibility, but our overall destiny is a result of our total universe. Translating this into everyday terms, just how long we live is not entirely up to us and our co-creative ability to follow Nature's laws. *To be in harmony with the universal laws of Nature maximizes the quality of our existence, but not the exact quantity.*

Divine Body, Physical Immortality, and Superconductivity

The key thing to understand about the health of the physical body in relationship with its SOEFs is that, as the energy of the system increases the SOEF, which is the matrix of the physical body, the physical body becomes stronger. The more perfectly the SOEF is aligned with the virtual energy state, the better it functions. If we damage the functioning of our system as an accumulator and superconductor of cosmic energy by destructive diet and lifestyle, the free flow of cosmic energy cannot occur. The system disorganizes, and cell replication and cellular and enzyme functions are disrupted. The results are aging and disease. The other end of the spectrum, which is our highest natural evolutionary function, is the establishment of our SOEFs to such a degree of strength, conductivity, and perfection that even on the molecular level the physical body continues to act as a stabilized SOEF superconductor after the soul has left the body. In essence, a divine or immortal body becomes a stabilized superconductor of cosmic energy.

The traditional use of the term *superconductor* refers to certain metals which, below a transition temperature near absolute zero, enter a state in which a stream of electrons can flow without encountering any resistance in the form of friction. Since friction is the cause of failure in all mechanical perpetual-motion machines, when there is no friction to impede the flow of electrical energy, the initial current is able to persist indefinitely without any further input of energy. This is a critical exception to the traditional doctrine of the impossibility of perpetual motion, or in our case, a divine or living immortal body.

The question of stability is important. A superconductor is also thought to be unperturbable. In what is called the Meissner effect, in a superconducting substance, the electron flow spontaneously rejects any external magnetic influence and thus maintains its unperturbable superconducting state. Little, in his article "Superconductivity at Room Temperature," published in *Scientific American,* speculates that if Nature wanted to protect the information contained in the genetic code of a species against all environmental influences, establishing superconducting biological systems would do it.[31] He points out that a superconductor requires a high degree of internal organization, and theorizes that a superconducting molecule could exist at room temperature. Frank Barr, M.D., in his work on the melanin hypothesis as reported in the *Brain Mind Bulletin,* suggests that melanin could be such a room-temperature superconductor.[32] Melanin is a biomolecular structure found in the brain and throughout the body that may contain the information memory necessary for directing the flow of brain chemistry molecules.

Another theoretical discussion is added by McClare who states, in his article on resonance in bioenergetics, that the classic Second Law of Thermodynamics does not exactly apply to biological systems. He feels that the energy released via resonance is exchanged so rapidly that it is not thermally available, but rather remains in a form of stored energy.[33] The implication is that the perfectly organized SOEF can resonantly transfer energy from the level of purely cosmic to the biological level without a loss of energy. He also points out that the Second Law of Thermodynamics does not state that entropy has to be created in every conceivable process, so superconductivity does not necessarily contradict the Second Law of Thermodynamics.

The existence of the physical body is then maintained, and we observe what we have called the Divine body. This explains the human potential as evidenced by the stories of St. John of the Cross, Baal Shem Tov, Rabbi Elimelech, Reb Avraham, Jnaneswar Maharaj, and Paramahansa Yogananda. Their bodies were so perfect that their SOEFs and physical bodies continued as stabilized accumulators after their souls departed.

Resurrection and SOEFs

The process of resurrection as evidenced by Jesus, Sri Yukteswar, and Lahiri Mahasaya also fits into the wholistic paradigm. The following intuitive explanation should serve as food for thought. These men had reached such a high level of spiritual perfection and their cosmic energy was so great that, by the profound awareness of their Oneness with the Source of All Creation, they could actually use their divinely attuned minds to materialize tangible physical forms from their perfected SOEFs.

Biological Transmutation and SOEFs

The knowledge of the properties of SOEFs also allows an intuitive understanding of the phenomenon of biological transmutation (described in detail in Chapter 13). In the transmutation process, the pattern for the new atoms needed is contained in the SOEF pattern, which draws component atoms into the correct relationship. Let us recall the step-down transduction of energy from virtual energy to the subtlest SOEF, then the tachyon field particles moving faster than the speed of light and finally vortexing into a particle of mass. There is a continual dynamic relationship between SOEF vortexes and physical atomic structure. As the energy from these field vortexes energizes a component atom, the axis of the atom's nucleus begins to rotate closer to the speed of light or the alchemical transmutation point. As it rotates faster, the size, but not the mass of the nucleus, appears to expand. As it expands, it interacts with the nucleus of another component atom at the same energized alchemical point within the vortical field. These two nuclei, and the enzymes involved, are all energized by the intensified energy vortexes, and the two nuclei merge to form a new atom. The enzymes Kervan[34] talks about in this process become transmitters and carriers of high levels of energy, transferring this energy at the critical alchemical point to allow the binding energy of the resulting nucleus to overcome the opposing binding energies of the two individual atoms. The enzymes, like the merging atoms, are drawn into the time and space framework of the biochemical pattern by the specific SOEF governing the interaction. A helpful way to think about this is to picture iron filings being synchronized into the pattern of a magnetic field. The filings are the atoms and the enzymes, and the magnet symbolizes the SOEF that draws them into the appropriate pattern. The availability of the specific enzymes for the transmutation process is variable. If a person is unhealthy, energy is used to fight disease and to strengthen weakened SOEFs instead of being used for enzymatic processes. As we build our health, SOEFs have more energy available for enzyme activation and transmutation.

Divine Light: The Ultimate Spiritual Nutrition

The more we transmute biologically, the less material food we need to take into our systems – we are living more and more on the cosmic prana. This process explains the phenomenon of breatharianism, or inedia, in which the nutrients we need can be completely transmuted from the molecules in air, water, and sunlight frequencies. Like longevity, inedia is not the goal of Spiritual Nutrition. But it shows the extraordinary human potential that can be explained by our new paradigm of Spiritual Nutrition.

There is another level to the meaning of inedia. It is illustrated by the more complete story of Giri Bala. At the age of 12, Giri prayed to God to send her a guru to teach her how to live without food. Much to her surprise, a guru appeared and taught her a Yoga technique, telling her: "From today you shall live by the astral Light; your bodily atoms shall be recharged by the infinite current."[35] When asked why she had been singled out to live without eating, she replied: "To prove that man is Spirit. To demonstrate that by divine advancement he can gradually learn to live by the Eternal Light and not by food."[36]

For the author, this is part of the more subtle meaning of the Torah when it says that on Mt. Sinai "Moses remained there with God for 40 days and 40 nights. He did not eat bread, nor did he drink water. As Moses descended from the mountain he did not realize that the skin of his face had become radiant. . . ." (Exodus 34:30). The implication is that Moses drew his nourishment directly from the radiance of the Divine.

Another example of subsisting on Divine Radiance is that of Enoch, who was said to have ascended alive, seen the many heavens, and then been instructed by God to return for 30 days to the Earth to share heaven's teachings with his children before he ascended again. When offered food by his children, he refused it, explaining that from the time the Ultimate One anointed him with the ointment of the glory of the Divine he had taken no food.[37] These examples are a profound expression of the deeper meaning of Spiritual Nutrition. The direct energy of God's Light is the ultimate Spiritual Nutrition. We do not have to become breatharians, but it can happen any time our awareness merges with the Divine.

Conclusion

To develop fully an understanding of spiritual anatomy and spiritual awakening, it is obvious that we must also develop an overall new paradigm of nutrition, Spiritual Nutrition, that includes the material, mental-emotional, energetic, and spiritual qualities of our Being. We have shown that the materialistic-mechanistic paradigm is far too limited to be the basis for a nutritional paradigm, because it leaves out the subtle spiritual anatomies and physiologies, and the energetic continuum itself. Findings such as biological transmutation, the existence of the Divine body phenomenon, unusual longevity, and inedia cannot be adequately explained by the materialistic-mechanistic paradigm. We have developed the SOEF concept within the wholistic paradigm of body, mind, energy, and spirit. This concept includes and accounts for these "aberrant" phenomena. The Spiritual Nutrition paradigm does not exclude the materialistic-mechanistic paradigm, but rather includes it as part of an overall totality. Much anecdotal, historical, and scientific research, along with the author's own empirical findings and intuitive insights, support this new nutritional paradigm.

There has been a subjective awareness of the energy principles and qualities in nutrition for thousands of years in traditions such as the Vedic teachings of India and spiritually advanced societies such as the Essenes of the Dead Sea scrolls. There are Biblical references to these ideas, and there are great spiritual leaders such as Enoch, Moses, and Jesus whose lives radiated these principles. Although the merging of science and spiritual knowledge has progressed to a certain level of development, it has not reached the level of refinement that will convince the minds of conservative scientists. There can be no "acceptable proof" of this material to a mind that assumes there is exclusively an objective world knowable only to the five senses. Sir Arthur Eddington, who offered the first proof of Einstein's relativity theory and who also made important contributions to the theoretical physics of the motion, evolution, and internal constitution of stellar systems, offers the following eloquent statement of the impasse:

> Verily, it is easier for a camel to pass through the eye of a needle than for a scientific man to pass through a door. And whether the door be barn door or church door it might be wiser that he should consent to be an ordinary man and walk in rather than wait till all the difficulties involved in a really scientific ingress are resolved.

The evidence is growing in support of these findings. But the author must remind readers that what is being shared is an understanding and a theory of SOEFs. This theory describes completely the dynamics of human nutrition, transmutation, and certain aberrant phenomena that do not fit into any other theory of nutrition and human life. By using the framework of this wholistic paradigm, we can develop a penetrating understanding and practical application of a system of nutrition for spiritual development. The author invites readers to consider these new concepts as tools for understanding and not necessarily as dogmatic facts. When this understanding is applied to a practical understanding of nutrition and to a relationship of nutrition to spiritual life, and the reader relates it to his or her own experience, this theory may then move into the realm of experientially known fact.

Summary, Chapter 8

1. Examples of longevity-immortality, Divine body, resurrection, and inedia have been given.
2. The SOEF theory has been used to show how these phenomena and biological transmutation are possible.
3. Liberation, or jivanmukti, is the ultimate purpose of incarnating on the planet. Longevity, inedia, and immortality of the body are secondary phenomena.
4. The Divine Light of God is the ultimate Spiritual Nutrition.

Chapter 9

The Human Crystal

Crystalline Properties of the Body

The key to understanding the assimilation of energy into our physical structure is through the awareness of our bodies as a series of synchronous, interacting, crystal structures. The human body on this level is a linkage of oscillating solid and liquid crystals that form an overall energy pattern for the total body. Each organ, gland, nerve system, cell, and protein structure, even the tissue salts in the body, shows a level of organization with some degree of crystalline function. Marcel Vogel, the world-renowned crystal expert, has pointed out that the human energy field exists as an array of oscillating energy points that have a layered structure and a definite symmetry, and that these properties fulfill the definition of a normal crystal in material form.[1]

Our bone structure has long been recognized as a solid crystal structure with piezoelectric properties. A piezoelectric effect is the creation of an electromagnetic field (EMF) pulse when a crystalline structure is physically stressed or pushed out of its normal shape. Although various esoteric traditions have implied that the pineal and pituitary glands have solid crystal structures, our skeletal bone structure is the only proven solid crystal structure in the body. As a solid crystal, it has the ability to convert vibrational energy, such as sound or light, into electromagnetic and electric energy. Crystals can absorb, store, amplify, transduce, and transmit these vibrational energies. Advanced vibrational researchers such as Glen Rein, M.D., have also shown that electromagnetic, subtle, psychic healing energies and crystal energies have similar biological effects on the body. Additional research by Dr. Rein indicates that psychic healing energies alter the measurable electromagnetic pattern of a

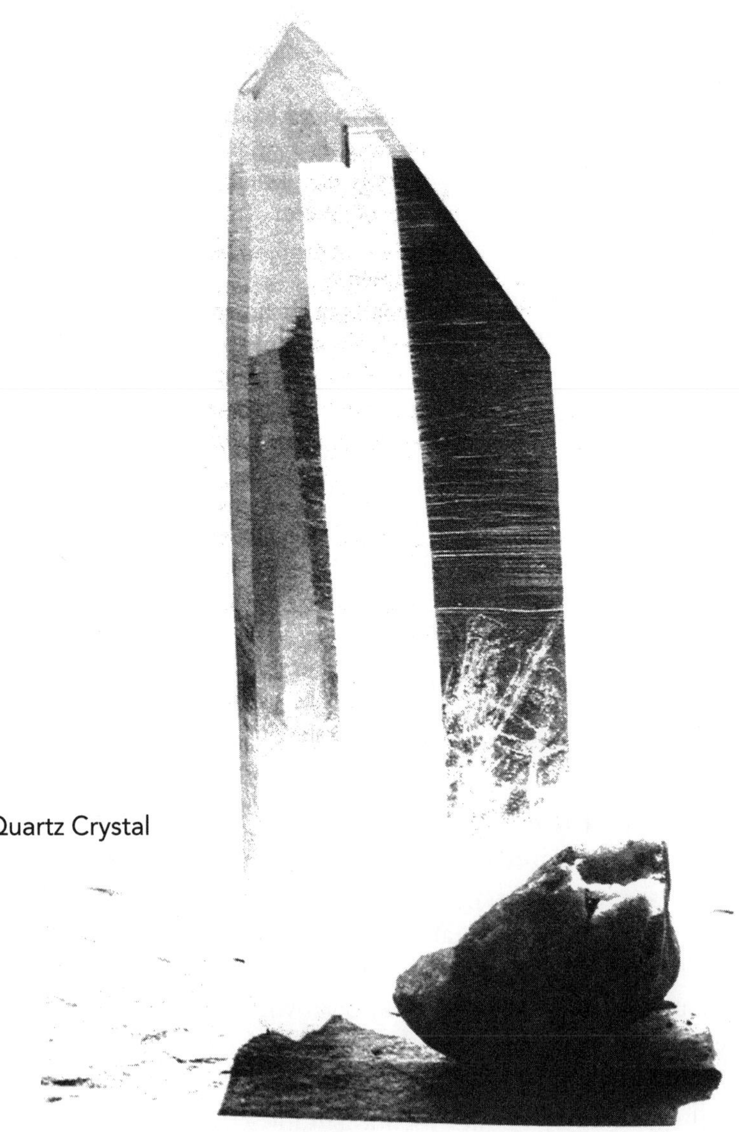

Quartz Crystal

crystal, suggesting that subtle energies can alter the physical structure of a crystal. His research suggests that subtle energies and electromagnetic energies can be converted, amplified, transduced, and transmitted by a crystal in a form of energy that has biological effects.[2] These properties of a crystal play an important role in helping us develop a model of how the body as a complex crystalline structure helps to absorb energy from the cosmos and from our food, leading us to understand the need for a new nutritional paradigm – the Spiritual Nutrition paradigm.

Our crystalline bone structure, in general, acts as an antenna for all incoming and internal body vibratory energy and information, including direct thought form energy. It resonates with all levels of nutrient energy, which it either receives directly (music, singing, and chanting) or indirectly, through the EMFs transferred from the chakras as they step down the incoming virtual energy that has entered the system through the seven subtle bodies. The brain, nervous system, and heart also give off EMFs that resonate with our bone and other crystal-like structures. The crystalline bone structure then amplifies and radiates this energy and information to the rest of the system down to the cellular and subcellular crystalline structures. This is an important way that energy and information are transferred directly to all the cells throughout the body from the chakras, as well as through the pure cosmic energy-brain-nervous system linkage.

Dr. Glen Rein has proposed an additional system of how information and energy are directly transferred to the cells.[3] This system is based on the fact that the cells are suspended in an extracellular matrix of macromolecular crystal-like connective tissue components. This matrix is filled with structured water, which also has crystal-like properties. The water in the extracellular system and the crystal-like matrix receive the resonant energy and information. In the process of receiving the incoming energy, the electrochemical formation of this matrix structure changes. This change is then transmitted as an electric current, sending energy and information throughout the whole system. This is a system that provides another pathway by which the resonating bone structure is able to send its biologically transduced, vibratory information directly to the whole cellular system. Although there are other crystal-like subsystems that resonantly take in and transmit energy, the bone structure, because it is the only solid crystal in the system, remains the main transducer. Its solid state enables it to hold memory patterns more permanently as stored EMF frequencies in the bone. Bone and spine traumas, in particular, may be stored in the bone structure, and crystal healing is often very helpful for relieving these traumas. Marcel Vogel calls the bone the storehouse of the mind.[4] Memories are also stored in the crystal-like structures of the deep connective tissue. This is the biomolecular basis for deep tissue therapies. The bones also vibrate in resonance with other vibratory sources like crystals, gems, mantras, chants, and music. We have all heard the saying "you can feel it in your bones." This helps to explain the powerful effect of religious music like Gregorian chants and Yogic *bhajans*. As human crystalline systems, we resonate in total unity, harmony, and Love with the pulse of the cosmos.

Bone-Generated Piezoelectric EMFs

When physical stress or an electromagnetic field is applied to a piezoelectric crystal, the crystal will change shape and generate an EMF.[5] Bone, quartz crystal, and tourmaline are among the few crystal forms with piezoelectric properties. Studies suggest that the crystal-like components of the extracellular matrix of bone, such as collagen and proteoglycans, possess piezoelectric qualities.[6] It has also been established that mineralized tissue such as cartilage, dentin, teeth in general, and relatively non-mineralized tissues such as keratin in skin, elastin, artery tissue, connective tissue (tendons and ligaments), and even some amino acid crystals (glycine, proline, and hydroxyproline) all have piezoelectric properties.[7]

The main forces that create pulsed piezoelectric EMFs in bone are the anti-gravity muscles, the cardiovascular system, voluntary muscles, and impact with the environment. We have also noted the ability of projected electromagnetic fields to create a piezoelectric response in bone. It is important to note that the pulsed piezoelectric EMFs that are created by bone stress have biological activity.[8] The findings suggest that the piezoelectricity created can produce an EMF of sufficient magnitude to produce a wide range of effects on living systems. Theoretically, these piezoelectric fields could affect "cell nutrition, local pH control, enzyme activation and suppression, orientation of intra- and extracellular macromolecules, migratory and proliferative activity of cells, synthetic capacity and specialized function of cells, contractility and permeability of cell membranes, and energy transfer."[9]

Research into the effects of pulsing EMFs on bone physiology has gone on for more than forty years. Much interesting research has been done on the physiological and clinical applications of pulsing EMFs on bone by prominent researchers such as Andrew Bassett, M.D., at the College of Physicians and Surgeons, Columbia University (one of the author's professors during medical school). In 1968 Dr. Bassett first introduced the author to the piezoelectric properties of bone and the effect of electrical fields on bone growth and destruction. He has put forth the hypothesis that alterations in a cell's electrical environment will create a change in the cell's physiological behavior. He has shown that pulsed EMFs diminish bone reabsorption to near normal in experimentally induced osteoporotic rat bone, and increase the rate of bone formation to be equal to those of healthy free-roaming rats. Under these pulsing fields, he found that the rate of collagen production increased.[10] Dr. Bassett also reports that, depending on the pulse pattern of the EMFs, cells receiving different EMF pulse fields were found to have different biological responses.[11] For example, a pulse burst elevates calcium content in the bone, while a single pulse lowers the calcium content. What can be deduced from this research is that pulsing EMFs affect bone function and that by varying the EMF wave, pulse, and intensity, the EMF pattern and the types of bone intracellular and extracellular response will vary. Cells of all types can be influenced by EMFs as weak as 2×10^{-10} amperes.[12]

Bone-Generated Streaming Potential EMFs

Another type of electric or electromagnetic field response is also found in bone structure. Called *streaming potentials,* this electrical field is created by the flow of ions, charged solutes, and cells such as red blood cells through the tissues, carried by extracellular fluids such as blood through the extracellular matrix. When the bone is even subtly bent from pressure by such events as walking or even by the pulse of our arteries, the extracellular fluids are pumped through the bone. An electrical potential is created as a result of the electrostatic interaction of the electrically charged fluids moving past the fixed charge in the crystalline bone structure. These electrical fluids can also interact with the piezoelectric fields of the bone.[13]

EMF fields in bone may also be produced as a result of bone's semiconductor or solid-state properties, which occur when there is a change in pressure on the bone structure. This change has been associated with an increase in electron conductivity, and hence EMF production.

Nature of Bone-Generated Energy

Depending on the generating sources, EMF intensity, pulse characteristics, and the combination of the electrical interactions within the bone structure and fluids, a particular EMF field will be generated in the bone. These properties play an important role in our theory of how vibrational energy is assimilated from food.

It is also important to understand that the energy being discussed is not simply mechanistic, heat, and electron transfer. As pointed out by McClare, there is a level of organization in biological systems – a tuned resonance between energy levels in different molecules – that enables bioenergetic systems to operate rapidly and yet efficiently.[14] He points out that energy released via resonance is exchanged so quickly that it is not thermally available, but remains a form of stored energy. This implies that 100 percent of the resonant energy is transferred and that no entropy is created in resonantly transferred energy. This is distinctly different from energy transfer in the mechanistic system, which always involves some loss of energy.

Liquid Crystal Structures in Human Systems

There are other forms of crystal-like systems in the body, and one of the most important is the liquid crystal. A liquid crystal is technically defined as having form, liquid properties, stored information, and a measurable electromagnetic field. From our perspective, it also has a SOEF, which is reflected in its stored information and EMF. A liquid crystal can act simultaneously as liquid and crystal. The larger liquid crystal systems include fatty tissue, muscle and nerve tissue, the lymphatic system, white blood cells, and the various pleural and peritoneal linings.

Muscle and nerve tissue exist as liquid crystal systems held in shape by bone and skin systems. The muscles, by the nature of their structure, have also been shown to have some piezoelectric properties. On a cellular level, all cells and cell membranes are considered liquid crystals. In *Liquid Crystals and Ordered Fluids,* edited by J. F. Johnson and R. S. Porter, it is pointed out that the various cell membranes, membrane components, and intracellular membranes function as liquid crystal structures.[15] These include the plasma membrane, mitochondrial membrane, smooth and rough endoplasmic reticulum, nuclear membranes, and chloroplast membranes.

Bodily fluids also have crystal qualities. The water molecule contains in itself the potential forms of all crystals in its primary form of a tetrahedron. Water can bring all different forms of ions into a crystalline state and hold them in solution. In addition, the more structured the water is (see Chapter 29), the higher concentration of ions it can hold. In Norm Miksell's paper on structured water, the author points out that when the body cells and tissues become diseased or cancerous, the crystalline protein structures no longer have the proper configuration to maintain the water in an optimal structured state. Ions and other solutes in the cell consequently become redistributed by the new pattern of unstructured water.[16] If the water in the cell, extracellular fluid, or blood plasma becomes structured, it will then be able to attract and hold more ions by virtue of its hydration shell patterns. When structured water is organized around a particular ion, it is able to move the ions more easily into the more structured cytoplasmic water inside the cell. Once the ionically structured water is within a cell, it helps attract the same ion into the cell.

The Body As a Series of Synchronous, Amplified Crystalline Resonant Fields

It is the author's theory that the fundamental mechanism by which the cell salt structured water and its enlarged hydration shell are able to attract additional like ions has to do with the creation of an amplified crystalline resonant field by cell salt and structured water. This amplified field is able to attract the weaker but similarly resonating crystal fields of the single ions. The single ions are drawn into and fit synchronistically into the larger resonant field pattern of the cell salt in its structured water.

This structured water and cell salt dynamic represents an important principle: *Identical crystal resonant fields emanated by micronutrients are attracted to larger resonant fields emanated by the organism's larger crystalline and liquid crystalline patterns.* This includes the total system along with individual organs, glands, cellular, subcellular, and molecular structures. The principle explains how micronutrients, through vibrating crystalline fields, are drawn to the appropriate resonating crystalline sites.

Indirect support for this idea of the overall living system as a complex of synchronistic, oscillating crystalline structures has slowly been accumulated in the scientific community. In an article by P. R. Rapp, he cites more than 450 papers that feature research aimed at cataloguing an atlas of biological and biochemical oscillators with a periodicity of one hour or less.[17] This includes oscillations in enzyme-catalyzed reactions such as photosynthesis (molecular crystalline subsystems), oscillations in protein synthesis, and oscillations in cell membranes, secretory cells, neuronal cells, skeletal cells, smooth cells, heart muscle cells, and cell movement. In a healthy state, the body's structures are a multileveled series of interacting systems and subsystems that resonate harmoniously. From this perspective, disease occurs when this synchronicity is thrown into disharmony.

The Human Organism As a Healing Vibratory Transmitter

This understanding also relates to the use of human thought's vibratory power, gems and crystals, and their elixirs in healing. Each organ system or subsystem gives off a specific measurable electromagnetic field. The EMFs are measurable, subtle vibratory fields that can have great effect on the behavior of an organism. Each crystal or gem also has a specific EMF that radiates from its piezoelectric structure. For example, ruby and emerald resonate sympathetically with the liquid crystalline structures of the heart muscle system. By amplifying the energies of these gems with light, sound, or with our own healing thoughts, we activate a stabilizing resonant EMF. In the author's work in crystal healing and meditation, it has become intuitively clear that thoughts are vibratory energy. They come from the same undifferentiated cosmic energy. "In the beginning was the Word, and the Word was with God, and the Word was God" (John 1:1). The SOEFs are also vibratory patterns coming from the same source. In this way thoughts and SOEFs are related. When one is able to tune to the SOEF pattern with the mind, it is possible to send resonant vibratory thought form energy to re-energize and reorganize the dissipated SOEF system. Crystals and gems amplify these specific resonant vibrations. This projected stabilizing EMF can help to bring a disharmonious heart muscle and its SOEF back to its normal healthy resonant vibration. The gems or crystals help to fine-tune, stabilize, and amplify the healing vibration of the thought waves required to create the specific healing, resonant EMF needed to rebalance and heal the system.

Using this same principle, we can also use specific gems or gem elixirs to energize and rebalance the individual chakras. Dark opal and tiger's eye help to rebalance the base chakra. Fire agate works on the second chakra. The solar plexus and third chakra are aided by quartz and pearl. Ruby and emerald stimulate the heart chakra. Lapis lazuli is good for the throat chakra. Quartz resonates with both the pituitary and pineal glands, or sixth and seventh chakras. Diamond is beneficial for the crown chakra.[18]

The human organism and mind can be understood as crystal transmitters. When we become a clear channel for the Divine God-force of unconditional Love, it comes through us in a way analogous to a gem or crystal being activated by our thought forms. In this enhanced state, a strong resonant field is created that is capable of reprogramming the SOEFs, chakras, and organ systems of a diseased person. By increasing the SOEF energy of a person's crystalline structure, we recreate a new and healthy field that then reorganizes the person on a spiritual, mental, emotional, and physical vibratory level. This higher Love force helps to release negative thought forms stored as dissonant vibrations within a person's system at any of these four levels. A clear example of this is the healing power of Jesus, whose mere presence or the touching of his robe brought healing. The projection of loving thought forms heals by increasing the SOEF energy, either specifically or generally. Healing groups using this principle act as amplified crystal resonators for the person being healed.

When the Kundalini is awakened, it also acts as an internal healing force by raising the energy level of the SOEFs. When the healthy SOEF pattern is raised to a more integrated and pure level, entropy-producing, negative, dissonant thought forms and emotions are forced out. They seem to come up into consciousness and are released. In one meditation group led by the author, a women in her late sixties reported seeing a vision of a particular yellow house. In sharing it, she felt a tremendous relief, because that color yellow had always been associated with the pain of her mother's death sixty years earlier. Since the yellow image came up in meditation and was released, she lost her fear and was healed of her grief. In a recent weekend seminar on meditation and nutrition, an overweight person, who for many years had been trying to control her ravenous desire for food, experienced an awakening of her Kundalini and reported one week later to have lost her intense desire for food. These two examples show how meditation and awakened Kundalini can spontaneously release dissonant patterns from different levels of our Being.

This chapter clarifies what we knew all along: People are precious gems.

Summary, Chapter 9

1. The key to understanding the assimilation of energy into our physical structure is through the awareness of our body as a series of synchronous, interacting crystal structures.
2. Our bone structure is our body's major solid crystal system. A particular EMF is generated from the crystalline bone structure. Its type depends on its generating source (piezoelectric, streaming potentials, or solid-state activity), its energy intensity, its pulse characteristic, and the combination of all these interactions within the bone structure.
3. The other major crystal-like system in the body consists of the liquid crystal structures that exist in every cell membrane, organ, gland, nerve, and muscle system.
4. Bodily fluids, because of the ions within them and the ability of water to become structured, also have crystal-like qualities.
5. An explanation of how micronutrients reach their correct sites in the body is that they are drawn by their vibrating EMFs to the appropriate resonating crystalline sites in the system.
6. Realizing the crystalline nature of the human body gives us a physical basis for understanding the efficacy of human thought vibrations, gems, crystals, flower essences, gem elixirs, and homeopathy in healing.
7. By increasing the SOEF energy of the crystalline structure of a person, we create a renewed and healthy field that reorganizes the person on a physical, emotional, mental, and spiritual vibratory level.
8. We are, indeed, precious gems.

Chapter 10

Bioenergetic Assimilation

The Questions of Assimilation

As we begin to develop the paradigm of Spiritual Nutrition, it is important to address the issue of bioenergetic assimilation. As such, we will explore the following questions:

- What is the purpose of nutrition?
- What is nutrition?
- What is the relationship between the nutrient taken in and the living system taking it in?
- What do we assimilate?
- Who is assimilating?
- What is the meaning of assimilation?
- What is the process of assimilation?
- How does our understanding of SOEFs fit into our understanding of nutrition?
- What is the relationship between the nutrient absorbed and the spiritual evolution of the person absorbing it?

To answer these questions fully, we must go beyond the materialistic-mechanistic paradigm to that of Spiritual Nutrition, which includes the material, mental, energetic, and spiritual aspects of the human organism.

Assimilating Food into the Human Body

When cosmic energy is sufficiently condensed, it arrives on our plates as food. To develop a new paradigm of the process of food assimilation into the human body requires the understanding of assimilation on both the physical and the energetic levels. We can see that the relationship of food to the human system is more than just adding up calories, vitamins, and minerals to be materially accumulated as building blocks in our bodies. On a general level, each vegetable and animal substance radiates a unique, species-specific, subtle vibration from its energy field. As solid, whole, organic, live food it maintains its SOEF. Although this is true for both plants and animals, for the rest of this discussion we will refer only to plant foods, as they exist on a more primary level in the food chain than animals.

One of the tasks of assimilation is the conversion of food as a foreign body into a likeness with our own body chemistry and vibration, especially on the levels of physical, etheric, and astral bodies. It is the relationship between the energy fields of the human system and of the substance being ingested that is important to assimilation. To assimilate food successfully, we must completely absorb the total forces of the food into our own forces. Rudolf Steiner alluded to this in 1924 when he said we should not concern ourselves with the quantity of food in metabolism, but rather with whether we can assimilate the vitality from food in the most effective way.[1] On one level, assimilation is overcoming the foreign nature or individualized SOEFs of our food. It is through the process of assimilation that we enter into a very intimate relationship with our food. Assimilating food is a major interface between ourselves and our physical environment. Assimilating food is a way of extracting energy from the environment.

Not only are we affected by the environment in which food is grown, we are also affected by the consciousness of the people who prepare our food. In Muktananda's ashrams, food was always prepared with Love so the people eating the food would receive that Love. Marcel Vogel has shown that water infused with the thought form of Love has a different taste and a different subtle vibration.[2] Live food is filled with the highest degree of structured water which best holds the vibration of our blessings. As we eat this blessed food, we eat our blessings on this subtle level. We are interacting with food on subtle energy levels as well as on the material level of assimilation. Gerhard Schmidt, M.D., points out, in *The Dynamics of Nutrition*, that nutrition is concerned with the assimilation of different levels of energy, which increase in quality the closer they are to sun or light energy.[3]

Eating allows the forces of food to penetrate us, and without proper assimilation and digestion, these foreign forces can make us ill. For example, foods injected directly into our physical bodies will typically cause an inflammation, but if taken in orally they will not, because they undergo a normal assimilation process. An old Arab proverb, that "one eats oneself sick and digests oneself back to health," illustrates this point. Digestion involves overcoming and assimilating the energetic forces in our foods, stimulating our own inner forces, and strengthening us in the overcoming of entropy. If this sounds like too much work, just think of it this way: If we are not walking around strengthening ourselves by overcoming the force of gravity, our muscles and bones begin to weaken and deteriorate, just as astronauts, in a gravity-free environment, begin to lose bone mass. To further elucidate this point, a study in Europe was done in an effort to find easier ways to feed mentally disadvantaged, institutionalized children.[4] They were fed a synthetic mixture of vitamins, minerals, calories, and proteins that was the calculated equivalent of what they had been getting on the material level from their three meals a day. After a period of time on this liquid, synthetic diet, researchers were amazed to find that the organs of taste and digestion in the children began to atrophy. One implication of this is that without the stimulating forces of the raw foods, the organs of assimilation are not energized or exercised, and therefore begin to atrophy just like bone mass in a gravity-free environment. These experiments may make us think about the long-term results caused by the consumption of high-potency synthetic vitamins, minerals, amino acids, and proteins currently practiced. This is not a statement against the use of nutritional supplements. The author suggests that synthetic supplements should be used with the awareness that assimilation involves the interaction of dynamic forces between us and the food and not just the mechanical absorption of nutrients, and that the indiscriminate use of synthetic supplements is something to be aware of.

Wholistic digestion, then, involves an intimate relationship with the nutrients we take in. It involves the liberation of the cosmic forces that are at the core of the material food. On a more subtle level, Sri Nirsargadatta, the late seer from Bombay, has pointed out that consciousness is the very essence of the food that has been assimilated.[5] Our model for nutrition and assimilation must also account for the truth of this concept.

Crystalline Bone Structure and Energy Assimilation

In the process of assimilation, the crystalline vibration of food interacts with our total oscillating crystalline system. Anyone familiar with the science of kinesiology (muscle testing) knows that when a specific food substance is brought within the body's vibratory field, it may immediately weaken, strengthen, or not appreciably affect the person.

Within the plant structure, there are different crystal-like substructures, similar to the multiple oscillating crystal-like subsystems in our own bodies. These resonate with the bone and other crystal-like structures in our bodies, amplifying and transmitting resonant energy to the body as a whole. Because bone is the only rigid crystal system in the body, it is the major "antenna" for receiving information into the body and transferring it through its crystalline properties to the rest of the body. In this process, the bone transforms the vibration of the plant into a resonant frequency that is compatible with our living system. Our crystalline bone structure acts like the crystal in a radio, which picks up radio waves and translates them into audio signals. The sound vibrations resonate with the bone structures in our ears, transmitting these vibrations as electrical vibrations or impulses to our auditory nerves. Through the bone's resonance vibration plant EMFs are transformed into specific vibrations that are similar to and hence are able to communicate information and energy to the resonating substructures in the body. In this way, specific vibrational properties of the plant energize and nurture specific organ, glandular, and cellular systems. For example, the dandelion root primarily affects the liver, while the leaf has much less effect on the liver and is best used in salads as a light cleansing tonic. At another level of awareness, it may be that only organs in a state of well-being will draw the right nutrients to themselves and reject inappropriate nutrients. When cells and organs are diseased, their resonant EMF fields are different from those of healthy cells, so they may not draw the proper nutrients to themselves to create and maintain health. It is documented that the crystal structure and EMF field generated by arthritic bone are different than in normal bone.[6]

Interplay of Our Tri-System and Crystalline Bone Structure

On another level, plant energy is also assimilated through a dynamic interplay of the crystalline bone structure with the tri-system of our circulatory, nervous, and meridian systems. The Chinese have been familiar with this tri-system relationship for thousands of years. By use of pulse diagnosis on the vascular system, they explain the condition of the various meridians, organs, glands, nerves, and bone systems. A theoretical explanation for how vibrational remedies are taken into the body – in *Gem Elixirs and Vibrational Healing,* Volume 1, by Gurudas – also discusses the interplay of this synchronous tri-system.[7] It helps us understand how energy can be transferred from the physical level to the etheric system of the chakras. In this transfer, meridians act as a bi-directional resonant transfer system between the two levels.

The meridian system also has a direct link with the nervous and circulatory systems, as it is a template for them and the whole physical body. It is the most physical templating energy system organized by the SOEFs, carrying more of the body's life force in its crystal-like structures. In Genesis 4:10 we read of Abel's blood speaking to God from the Earth. This can be understood as the crystalline life force sending out its message. The most important of these resonating forces are the hemoglobin structures in the red blood cells and the minerals in plasma. The nervous system carries more of the mental consciousness forces through the electromagnetic fields. It helps stimulate and direct cellular growth, including the direction and growth of the blood vessels in the system. Our bone structure is also penetrated by the nervous system. C-fibers and knob-like nerve receptors are found in different types of bone tissue. When the nerve tissues conduct nerve impulses, the physiological changes associated with these pulses create an external EMF.[8] These EMFs may interact with bone EMFs.

Although still theory, there is some evidence suggesting that the meridian, nervous, and circulatory systems form a stable overall system that transmits the transformed and amplified energy of the bone to the rest of the body subsystems, down to the cellular level. Vibrations from the bone also help to stabilize and energize the meridian system. It is well known that the piezoelectric energies stimulated in the bone by walking create an EMF that programs the maintenance of the bone structure. The pulsating of the heart and blood vessels creates a piezoelectric response in bone that may create a stabilizing maintenance EMF in the bone.[9] Dr. Bassett points out that the EMFs from the cardiovascular system might play a major role as some sort of stabilizing signal as they interact with locally generated piezoelectric and streaming potentials.[10] Although the evidence for this sort of relationship is not conclusive, it supports our hypothesis.

Theory of Assimilation

The first step in our assimilation theory starts with the sun activating the chlorophyll in plant cells. Energized chlorophyll, which contains a holographic vibration of the whole plant, transfers its resonant energy and information into the electromagnetic field of the iron in red blood cells. Chlorophyll and hemoglobin only differ by one atom: Chlorophyll has magnesium in its structure, while hemoglobin has iron. The red blood cells, newly energized and programmed from their interaction with the chlorophyll, circulate back through the bone system. Red blood cells transmit their new EMF energy and information to the bone via direct resonance and the streaming potential, or electrical fluidium effect. The bone amplifies and transmits it to the rest of the system (see the first figure). The red blood cell and hemoglobin systems also transfer resonant plant energy directly to cells and tissues through the resonant transfer of their own EMFs.

In addition to the red blood cell EMFs, the blood plasma, charged by plant and body cell EMFs and other input EMFs, also transmits electromagnetic fields, which are carried by mineral compounds. These plasma crystalline EMFs are transferred to bone, and at the same time charged and reprogrammed by the new bone pattern. They leave the bone structure with the information needed to be drawn by their own EMFs to the appropriate location in the system. The red blood cells and plasma help to stabilize the general patterns of the body. When their charge becomes fatigued, circulation through the bone recharges them. In essence, red blood cells and plasma are both programmers of the bone crystal and programmed by it. The programmed ionic EMFs of the plasma also help to stabilize the meridian system, which in turn helps to program and balance the neurological system (see the second figure). The bone then sends out a pattern harmonic with the whole body. The

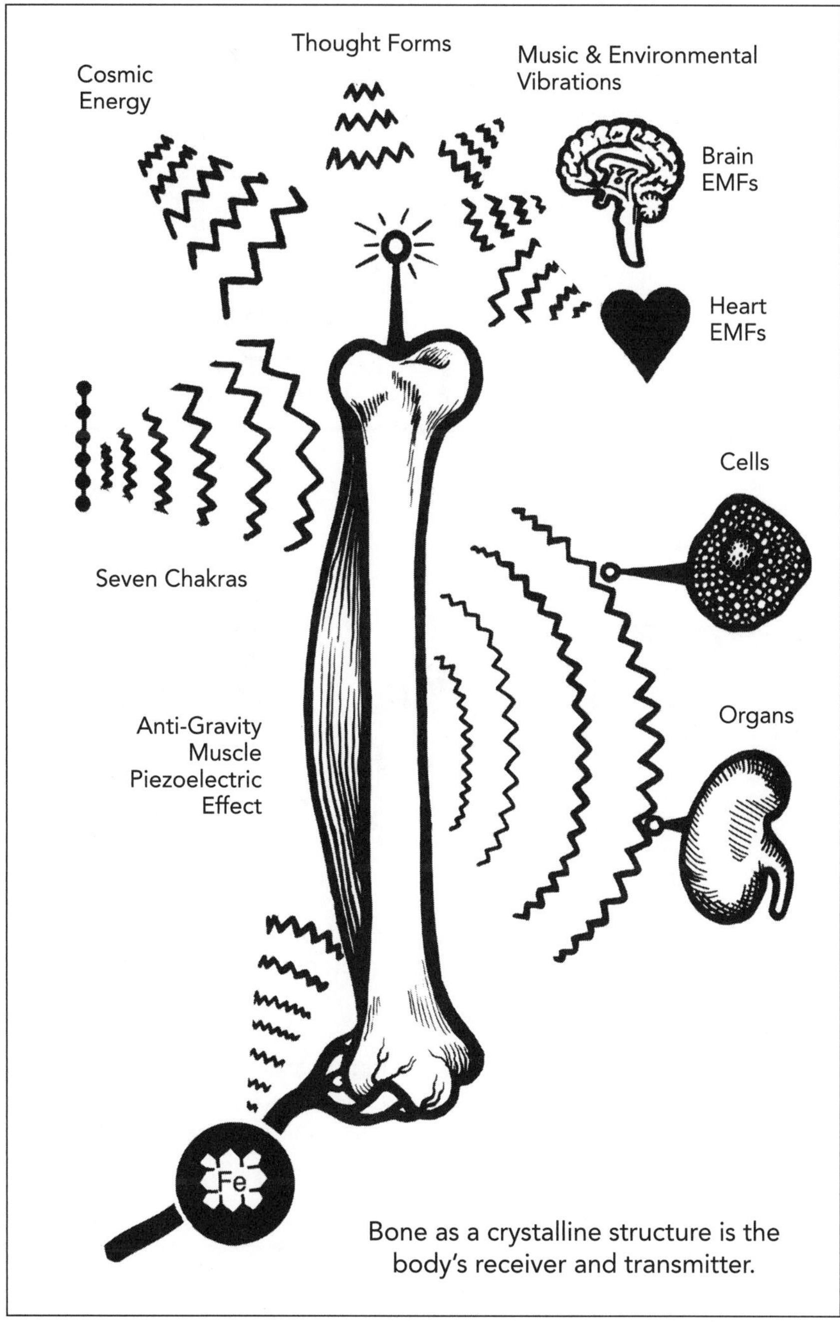

Bone as a crystalline structure is the body's receiver and transmitter.

red blood cells and plasma also leave the bone and carry specific patterns to specific locations in the body and help to stabilize the general EMFs of the body. This tri-system and the crystal energies of the bone are

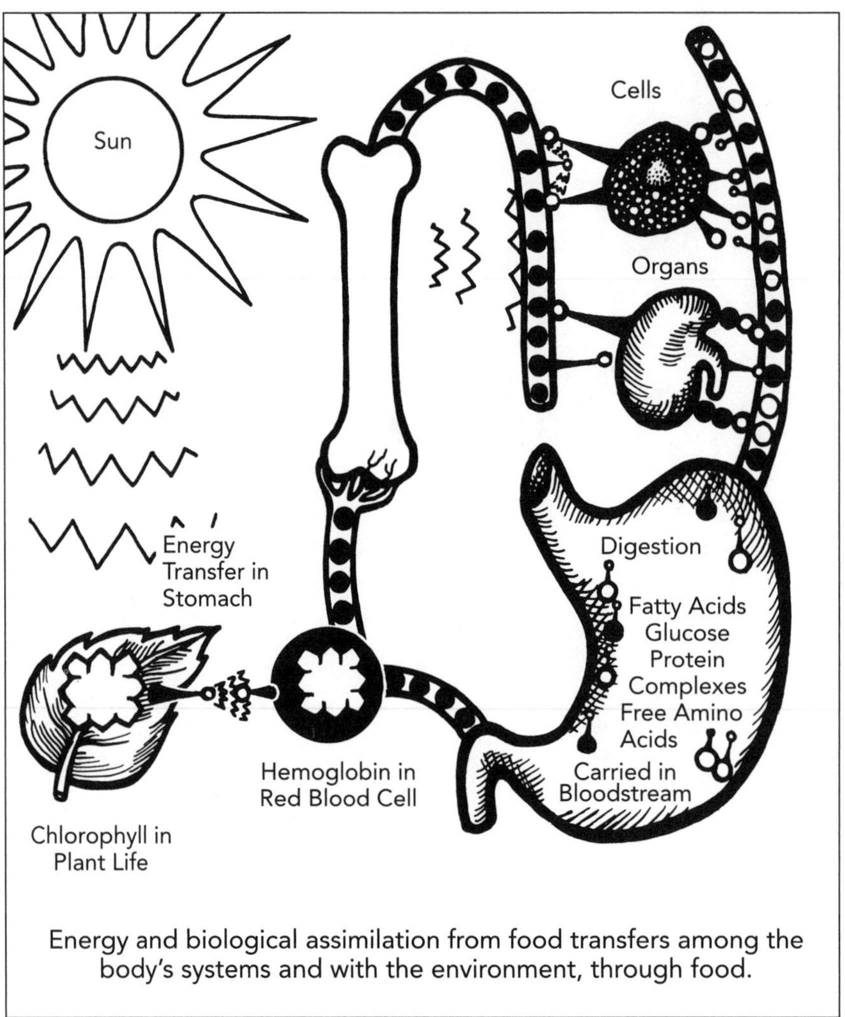

Energy and biological assimilation from food transfers among the body's systems and with the environment, through food.

a multiple-feedback, self-stabilizing, energy-conducting system. These three systems and the crystalline bone structure interact synchronistically and simultaneously.

Energy Transfer from and Absorption of Molecular Structures

Energy and material are transferred from food into our system in another way as well. This transfer is through the individual simple sugars from complex carbohydrates, crystal-like proteins, free amino acids, and negatively charged fatty acid formations. These nutrients are crystalline formations that carry specific energies and EMF patterns. They are drawn to areas like a particular gland, organ, or cell that have energy field patterns that attract the specifically programmed nutrient by like resonance. These nutrients resonantly and molecularly link into the larger resonating molecular field, releasing their energy into this larger field to re-energize it. This is how the energy of the templating SOEF is recharged. This is one way SOEFs draw nutrients into their templates to build the physical structure. It explains how nutrients get to where they are needed in the body.

Micronutrients and Cell EMFs

Bruce Lipton, Ph.D., professor of anatomy at St. George's University School of Medicine in Grenada, has developed a beautiful theory, thoroughly based on current scientific data in the field of cellular biology. It explains in more detail how specifically charged micronutrients, as carriers of energy patterns of a specific food we have ingested, are resonantly attracted to a particular cell's EMF, and actually interface with, transfer their energetic patterns to, and incorporate their material forms into the cell. His theory clarifies how nutrients, which are not specifically programmed for a particular cell but are being transported in proximity to the cell by the extracellular fluids, are drawn into the cell.[11]

Certain facts are the basis of this understanding. One is that when a protein is exposed to an energy source such as light or radio wave sound, EMFs of the same frequency, or a harmonic frequency of the crystal-like protein, the protein molecule will resonate sympathetically with it. This new resonance vibration has the power to create an electromagnetic energy shift in the protein that can change its physical shape. This change may activate a new function for the protein, or it may temporarily inhibit an ongoing function. Proteins that can change shape like this are called *allosteric* proteins. In short, proteins, as crystal-like structures, are able to take in EMF energies and transform them into a biologically active signal. One familiar example of this is rhodopsin, the crystal-like protein energy receptor for light found in pigments in the rods of the eye. It takes in the energy of light and transforms it into nerve pulses that transfer this energy to the brain's vision centers. Another common example is melanin, a crystal-like protein able to absorb light energy and transform it into sound and electromagnetic energy.

The next step that Dr. Lipton adds in his theory is based on evidence that proteins are able to integrate themselves into the cell membrane. There are several different functions for these proteins in the cell membrane. There are receptor proteins involved with reception and detection of incoming electromagnetic frequencies, including EMFs of various nutrients, hormones, ions in solution, neurotransmitters, glucose molecules, free amino acids, free fatty acids, or any other nutrients needed for cellular function that are brought to the cell via the extracellular fluids. These crystal-like proteins are sensitive to very low levels of energy such as input from single ions, electrons, photons, and protons. On receiving these incoming EMF energies, these receptor proteins convert them into specific biological signals that modulate the cell membrane functioning. These signals directly affect the three other functional protein types in the cell membrane. Receptor proteins may transfer the incoming energy to enzyme proteins, which may then become activated to perform enzymatic reactions intracellularly or extracellularly. The receptor proteins may also transfer this energy to transport proteins, which transform it into electrochemical activities that regulate some of the gates and channel systems that let in specific nutrients knocking on the outside of the cell membrane doors. The receptor proteins also act in a direct physical linkage to structural proteins within the cell walls. As the receptor proteins change shape, they create a change in the physical configuration of the structural protein to which they are linked. When the configuration of the structural protein changes, it may also open or shut a particular cell membrane door.

In summary, the receptor proteins are crystal-like energy transducers that take in the information energy of the multitudinous EMFs impinging on the cell system and convert them into energy message signals to which the cell can respond. These receptor proteins are yet another system that tunes us into the energy of nutrients, as well as the more subtle geomagnetic, Earth atmospheric vibrations such as the Schuman resonance and lunar, solar, and cosmic resonance fields that affect biological life on this planet.

The cell membrane as a total unit vibrates in sympathetic resonance with incoming EMFs. Its resonant vibration is able to induce a harmonic resonance in the intracellular crystalline membranes and protein complexes like RNA and DNA. This transfer of harmonic, resonant energy is how the cell membrane sends information to the intracellular structures, and therefore has a regulatory effect on them. It is the author's theory that the cosmic, Earth, food, and bone resonant information energy can also directly transmit energy to the core intracellular structures such as the RNA and DNA. This is particularly true as we develop spiritually through proper nutrition and meditation. We become better and better superconductors of the cosmic energy as we evolve spiritually. As we become better and better superconductors of energy, there is less and less impeded resonance between the microcosm and macrocosm, resulting in the experience of awareness.

There is another piece to this system. The intracellular crystalline vibratory structures can resonantly transmit their energy information to the cell membrane and therefore can influence the cell membrane function as well. It is a two-way system. In harmonic resonance with its intracellular structures, the cell membrane sends out EMFs into the extracellular fluids, which attract the specific nutrients they need. This completes the multiple feedback cycles in the overall system of multilevel, vibrating, crystal-like systems in the body.

Several mechanisms of information energy transfer in the system have been outlined. None are contradictory. Our complex system of energy information assimilation has many checks and balances to keep us attuned.

Living Field

An additional insight into the role of energy transfer in the health of the human body is to understand this from the perspective of the quantum physics viewpoint of the *living field.* The concept of intracellular communication via electromagnetic fields has a much larger implication. This is a microcosmic expression of how the macrocosmic living field functions. As Albert Einstein once said, "The field is the only reality." What is meant by field is that we are part of the larger zero point energy. It can be jokingly referred to as the "zero point mothership," which is a source of energy, as the author has pointed out, of a million times a million tons of the uranium, at a minimum, per one cubic centimeter of space. The living field represents a picture of an interconnected universe. *The whole theory of the living field means, in essence, that we are part of something much bigger in which we are connected to All and that we are indivisible from everything.* In this living field, the memory of whatever Was, Is, and Will Be exists.

This perceptual understanding gives us the explanation of clairvoyance, and all psychic phenomena. In essence, everything becomes transported into an electrical charge that interacts with the zero point mothership. The waves, or bio-photons, which are both particles and waves, are, in essence, energy communicators that transmit energy. The concept of non-locality, which essentially means that all subatomic particles are in contact with each other whether they are one mile apart or ten thousand miles apart, becomes the basis of intuition. Researchers have clearly shown that the subatomic particles know about each other and are indeed in constant communication with each other. In essence, when we are seeing each other, we are seeing each other as frequency composites. The essence of the non-locality "discoveries" that people are making is that the mind vibrates through the mechanism of the brain and extends out indefinitely. The real question is where do we end or begin. The fact is there is no end or beginning; there is only THAT. This is the physics explanation of the experience of Liberation or Self-realization. It is nice to know from a pure quantum physics perspective that we are only THAT.

Once we understand these basic principles, we can begin to understand Dr. Fritz Albert Popp's work, which has become a bit more popular over the last thirty years. The author discovered his research in 1984. Dr. Popp's research basically shows that humans, and the light in our cells, vibrate with quantum frequencies. The body, the cells within the body, and the DNA within the cells within the body, are all resonators working like a two-way radio. Each cell gives off a particular frequency. According to Dr. Popp, the frequencies are in an optical range between 200 and 800 nanometers. He pointed out in 2001, at a conference on the living field, that cells act as resonators for sunlight, that even the ancient one-celled organisms were evolutionarily developed by resonating with sunlight and so have gifted this basic physiology through evolution into human cells. Electromagnetic wave patterns in the cells act as a guidance or force for what happens physiologically in the cell. *When you change a field pattern, you change matter. When you change matter, you change a field pattern. What is more important is that the field pattern is much more predominant in organizing the matter than vice versa.* The point is that all living systems have a bio-photon emission and this is always changing because the field patterns are being influenced constantly by all of creation. We as human resonators, or as human oscillating crystals, are affected by these electromagnetic wave patterns. In essence, living systems are open systems. They are affected by the electromagnetic wave patterns within themselves and externally. One of the concepts of this study (from Dr. Popp's work, which he doesn't claim as his own but which comes from the field of study called bio-photonics, which has been going on for about thirty years) is that *bio-photons are coherent.* This is an important concept. What coherence means in this context is that *even small emissions can affect a greater whole because a small change can change the coherence of the greater whole.* Dr. Popp points out that there are over a hundred thousand reactions in a cell in one second. One single photon is enough to trigger ten-to-the-ninth reactions (10^9, or 10,000,000,000). *Then the photon itself is not used up but returned to the living field.* This is slightly amazing. He points out something the author agrees with, that *DNA is the most important crystalline field in the interaction with matter,* and that most bio-photon emissions come from DNA. From the author's point of view, DNA is a crystalline structure. The first research to prove the existence of the structure of DNA came from crystalline radiography. As we take this a little further, we begin to understand that consciousness is a high order of coherence of field patterns in the body. *When the consciousness is healthy, we remain healthy. When consciousness is entropic and unbalanced, we become entropic and unbalanced.*

This takes us to another understanding of disease, which is that disease in essence is a rogue frequency and is chaos in the field. Aging is an increasing level of chaos in the field. Anti-aging is the restoration of coherence in the field. The work at the Tree of Life is to bring people back into the higher spiritual frequencies of coherent consciousness. The first level of coherence rests on the idea that all subatomic particles are in communication with each other so that when you change one, you in effect change all the other subatomic particles. This is because they are in constant and instantaneous communication with each other. Dr. Popp, in a 1984 paper called "Bio-Photon Emissions: New Evidence for Coherence in DNA," points out the existence of bio-photons and the energetic phenomena of ultra-weak photon emissions from living systems. Because of the principle of coherence, these bio-photon emissions are very, very weak. With cancer cells it is just the opposite because the cancer cells are no longer in coherent communication with all the other cells – the result being that the bio-photon emission of a cancer cell is greatly enhanced, and therefore pathological. Dr. Popp was able to measure this bio-photon emission with a device he created and called a "bio-photon meter." He found that 97 percent of the DNA was associated with bio-photon transmission, and only 3 percent was associated with genetic information. These ultra-weak photon emissions from living cells are different than the phenomena of bio-illuminescence, which has to do with aura. It also fits into the model of the importance of the spiritual food, or manna (the manna given to the people in the Exodus in Genesis is linked with the monatomic element iridium [see Chapter 28]) which seems to increase the electron energy of the superconductor ability of a great deal of the "junk DNA," meaning the DNA which is not used for genetic information. What Dr. Popp found was that the healthiest people have the highest amount of bio-photon emission, while the people who are the sickest have the lowest amount. In other words, as we give off light we are in a sense communicating with each other and within and between all of our cells. When people are sick, the light fades and the amount of coherent communication diminishes. Dr. Popp and his research seem to support this finding.

The existence of bio-photon emission is an important aspect of understanding why one should eat live foods, because bio-photon emissions are given off by the DNA, RNA, and other forms of macro-molecules, including enzymes, chlorophyll, and hemoglobin. Dr. Popp found that wild, organic foods give off twice as much bio-photon energy as cultivated organic crops. He also found that cultivated organic foods give off five times as much bio-photon energy as commercially grown food. Dr. Popp's research also showed that cooked and irradiated foods gave off no bio-photon energy. The message here should be obvious.

In terms of communication, Dr. Popp's work fills in some of the theoretical pieces that were not quite available in the first edition of *Spiritual Nutrition,* where the author clearly points out the importance of the electromagnetic field and the communication between the cells. The DNA communication of bio-photons communicates with the cells and sets the electromagnetic field for the cell to communicate with the rest of the body, with all the other cells, along with the intracellular communication. This is the key to how the cells know to obtain those nutrients they need. As the author explained a little earlier, once the cells have their set electromagnetic fields, they will draw the nutrients that have the proper electromagnetic fields to them. The key is the communication from the DNA to the cell wall, which then communicates through proper electromagnetic fields. This is the exciting thing. Bio-photon emission has to do with intercellular communication. When we are unhealthy, our ability for intercellular communication diminishes, and we have increasingly less of a coherent field. This, in a sense, is the physics behind the subtle organizing energy field (SOEF) because, when our coherence diminishes, that is, when the entropy of the field increases, our ability to protect ourselves from rogue fields, therefore disease and disorganization, diminishes. Now we have a comprehensive theory of how this whole system begins to work together.

The Role of the Pineal Gland

As was established earlier, the body is a resonating crystal, giving off and receiving frequencies from all of creation. Perhaps the master gland (and the author says "perhaps" because this is still theory) is the pineal gland, also known as the third eye. But the author's feeling is that it is also connected with the crown chakra, somewhere in the interface between the sixth and seventh chakras. This pineal gland regulates our sleep cycle, affects all the glands of the body as the master regulator, and it could be the master gland as a human antenna for the electromagnetic field of the cosmos. Research has shown that the pineal gland has piezoelectric properties as well. But the bottom line is that the pineal gland could be the master antenna that picks up the fields from the entire universe and then transmits energy through its bio-photon emission ability to the rest of the body. It is, again, interesting to note that the manna thought by some to be the mineral iridium (see Chapter 28) is thought, according to ancient teaching, to stimulate the activity of the pineal gland as the master communicator, which will then enhance our communication as a superconductor to the entire universe.

Please understand that this is theory, but it is backed by an increasing amount of science of a living field we are all part of, as an interconnected One. It gives us the understanding that as we become superconductors, we can have the potential to be not only disease-free, but in a sense, immortal. We simply need to be able to maintain the free and unblocked superconductor communication with the living field. The potential of this understanding is infinite and awesome.

Importance of Living Nutrients

Another collary of Dr. Popp's work, pointed out in Chapter 9 on The Human Crystal, is that every single cell is a living crystal with an optimal cellular resonance. The only thing that can sustain or regain ideal cellular resonance and health is material at that optimal frequency.

Nutrients from a non-living source do not recreate this optimal living frequency. Synthetics, by definition from a non-living source, are therefore suboptimal entropy-producing substances. These entropic substances also include additives, pesticides, and so on. Dr. Popp points out that what accesses the DNA is critical, and especially what accesses the mitochondria, the high-energy center of the cell. Alpha-lipoic acid, Co-Q-10, and B-vitamins from a non-living source, although theoretically supplying anti-oxidant support for the mitochondria, may damage the DNA because they do not present or add a body of light, that is, the bio-photon energy. The energetic and quantum physics definition of life and nutrition by Dr. Popp is that the foods we eat must add light (as bio-photons) to our bioenergetic systems and especially to our DNA structures. In every molecule of a living substance, there is at least one atom that is pure light or bio-photon energy and that upgrades the DNA, and sustains and repairs the DNA over time. The synthetics may look good and may help in the short run, but not necessarily in the long term. Theoretically, synthetic nutrients may be creating a dissonant, entropic field and may degrade the DNA. Living materials and herb complexes are needed that restore the energetic resonance of the organs, glands, and cells. The best supplements are those that match the optimal cell resonance, and therefore are aligned with Popp's work and the message of Spiritual Nutrition. If a product has any radiation, pesticides, herbicides, organophosphates, heavy metals, talcum powder, magnesium stearate, titanium dioxide, or other synthetic materials, it may potentially disrupt the energetic field. These toxins have access to the interior of the cell and may potentially damage the mitochondrial DNA in a disproportionate amount. This concept is based on the principle of coherence, described earlier in this chapter. This means that a little disturbance of the field may cause a disproportionate entropic shift in the field because it shifts the coherence. If not 100 percent organic, living, and free of toxic "tag-a-longs" (non-live source contaminants), it has the potential to disorganize both sets of the mitochondrial and nuclear DNA. According to Robert Marshal, PhD., the mitochondrial DNA is at least four times as vulnerable as the nuclear DNA.[12] This quantum physics understanding gives an additional insight into the great importance of taking pure, organic foods and supplements on every level.

Concluding Thoughts

In this theoretical system of assimilation, food becomes not only a supplier of nutrients, but also of specific energies that re-energize all levels of our SOEFs. If we think of the development of the human organism as analogous to the development of a seed crystal, another insight is available. Once the adult form of the crystal, the human physical body, has completed its growth, we only need a minimum of nutrients to maintain the homeostasis of the system. The main purpose of nutrition at this point becomes primarily the supplying of energy to maintain the SOEFs of the overall system. If we are not able to decrease the appetites that have served us well for growth, we begin to crystallize spare tires around ourselves. The idea is to eat the minimum necessary to keep the energy and conductivity of the body at a maximum. As we shift toward absorbing less condensed energies into our organism, we need less and less material food even as a source of energy.

Summary, Chapter 10

1. Understanding nutrition involves the study of the interaction of the dynamic forces of food and the dynamic forces of our total Being.
2. This dynamic interaction strengthens our own organism.
3. It is through the process of assimilation that we enter into an intimate relationship with our food and therefore with our environment.
4. Consciousness is the essence of food.
5. To assimilate food successfully, we must completely absorb the total forces of the food into our own forces.
6. The vibrations of food resonate with our bone structure; the bone structure amplifies and transmits resonant energy to the body as a whole.
7. Our bone structure resonates with all levels of nutrient energy as they are resonantly transferred from the chakras, brain, mind, nervous system, heart, and any resonating external frequency such as music, chanting, and thought.
8. Plant energy is assimilated through a dynamic interplay of the crystalline bone structure through circulatory, nervous, and meridian systems.

9. Plant energy is also transferred directly from chlorophyll to the hemoglobin in the red blood cells and the ionic structures in the blood plasma. The red blood cells and plasma transfer the plant energy directly to the cells and to the bone structure, which transmit it to the body.
10. The tissue cell salts aid in the transfer of meridian energy for the patterning of micronutrients in tissue growth. They also help stabilize the meridian energy patterns.
11. Individual crystal-like simple sugar forms, crystal-like proteins and free amino acids, and negatively charged fatty acid formations carry specific energies and EMF patterns.
12. In this theoretical system of assimilation, food becomes a supplier of not only nutrients but also of energies that re-energize all levels of our SOEFs.

Chapter 11

The Chemistry of Stress and the Alchemy of Meditation

Chemistry of Stress

The vast majority of humanity lives in the chemistry of stress. For most, the world has become a very dangerous place: individually and nationally sponsored terrorism, chronic wars, nuclear weapons, crime-ridden streets, air and food pollution, nuclear tests and reactors exploding clouds of radioactive material, whole nations thinking about voluntarily irradiating their own food, flu-like epidemics, irresponsible dumping of radioactive and toxic wastes into the water supply, businesses and people breaking down, and the divorce rate near 50 percent as people unconsciously repeat their automatic defense patterns against giving and receiving Love. For most, these are tough times. We exist in a physiology of doing rather than Being. The doing is centered on thinking that we must accumulate food, wealth, sex, or power in order to survive.

Our first three chakras are often completely out of balance, or what we commonly call "off center." In the first chakra, we are fixated on survival and fear instead of on a healthier consciousness of trust that whatever God does is for the best. This fear blocks us from experiencing our higher purpose. In the second chakra, we are stuck in sex obsessions instead of the more evolved functions of procreativity and creativity. The third chakra, whose higher awareness is sensitivity and emotional integration, is thrown into reactive emotional imbalance, excess desires, and attachment to power. Until these first three chakras are balanced and our consciousness is merged and integrated with their higher functioning, the consciousness of the heart, or Love chakra, and the superconscious fifth, sixth, and seventh chakras cannot completely emerge or be fully integrated in a way to create the alchemy of meditation.

On all levels of our Being, stress creates degeneration and aging. Mental, emotional, and physical stress cause the subtle bodies to lose their alignment with each other and block the incoming flow of cosmic energy, or prana. As the chakra vortexes are deprived of the energizing pranic life force, their vortical vibration rate is slowed, and the expansion of subtle body energy, a function of the chakra vortex, becomes contracted. The more the subtle body contracts, the harder it is for the pranic life force to get through to energize the chakras and consequently the life functions of the body. The SOEFs, depleted of prana, are more easily disorganized, enhancing the aging process of entropy. This subtle body contraction is reflective of the body-emotion-mind contraction we experience through fear about survival, distrust, and anger with the world, in relationships, and our general state of alienation. The core of this fear is rooted in our misunderstanding and fear of death.

As a result, we live our lives in the adrenal stress syndrome of the caveman who is being stalked by the saber-toothed tiger. We live as if our lives were in immediate danger. The adrenal secretion from this lack of harmony, fear, sense of separation, and alienation from our world directly contributes to the aging process. On the physiological level, we experience it as a constant overstimulation of the sympathetic nervous system, causing excessive adrenalin secretion into the blood. We commonly know it as the "uptight" feeling in mind and body. Muscle tension, nerves on edge, digestion shut down, stomach feeling nervous, and mind racing are all physiological symptoms of this adrenal stress syndrome. In this overstimulated sympathetic state, our physiological digestive system is partially shut down. Not only is the flow of prana into our SOEFs minimized, but we cannot even absorb the food energy from our stomachs. Getting the continual false signal that it is fighting for its life, our mind and body, in continual sympathetic overstimulation, eventually fatigue. If this continues long enough, we slip into body-mind breakdown, increased rate of body aging, and the potential for illness.

The biochemistry of stress is congruent with the overall aging process. It parallels the breakdown of the SOEFs patterns and the dissipation of their energy. Adrenalin is a naturally occurring catecholamine and, when released by the body under stress, it breaks down into activated metabolite forms such as adrenochrome, a well-known free radical whose excess concentrations have been, at least loosely, associated with schizophrenia.[1] These adrenalin metabolic free radicals and other free radical-like compounds break down cell membrane structures and disrupt the basic

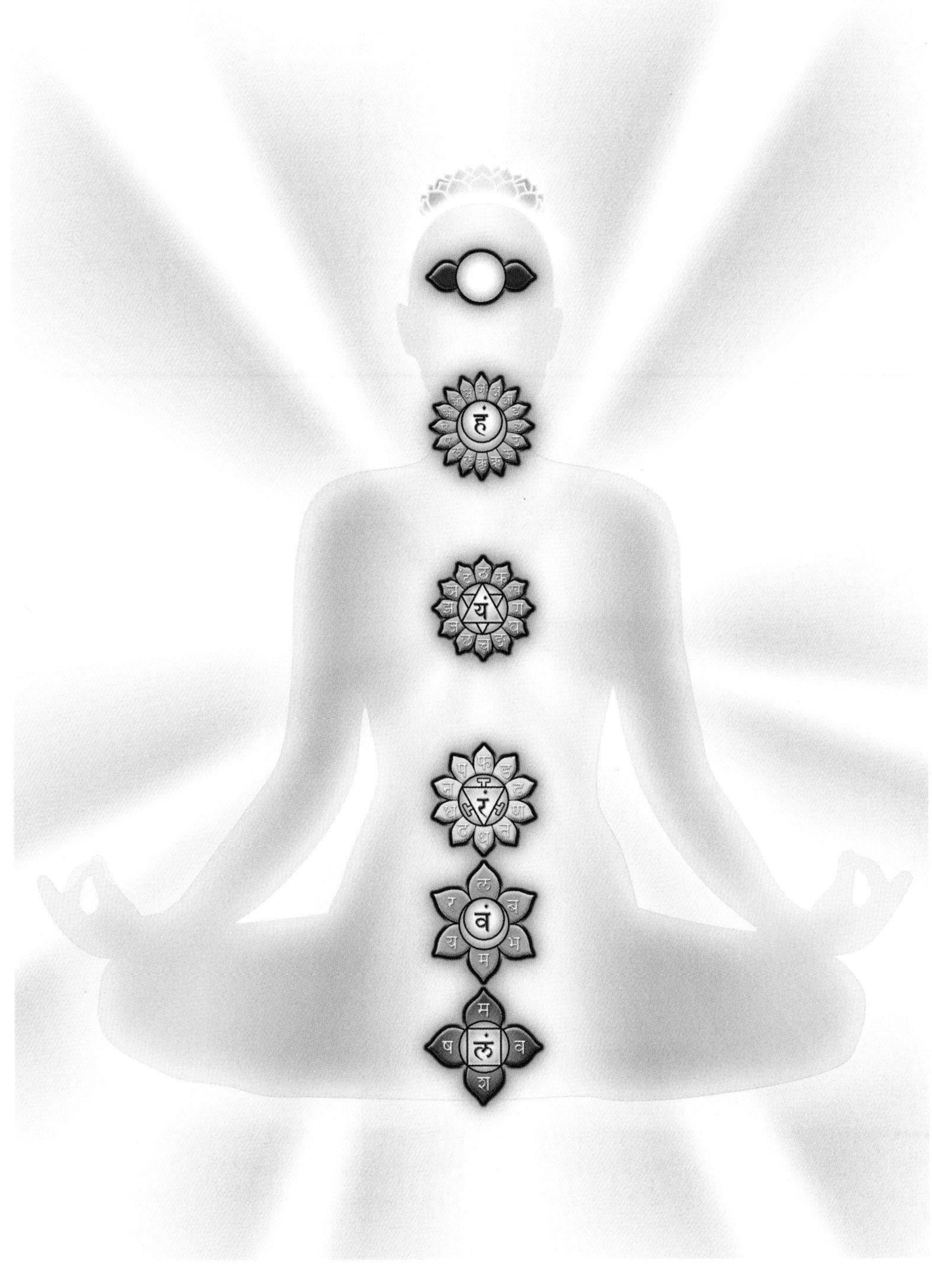

Location of Chakras in the Body

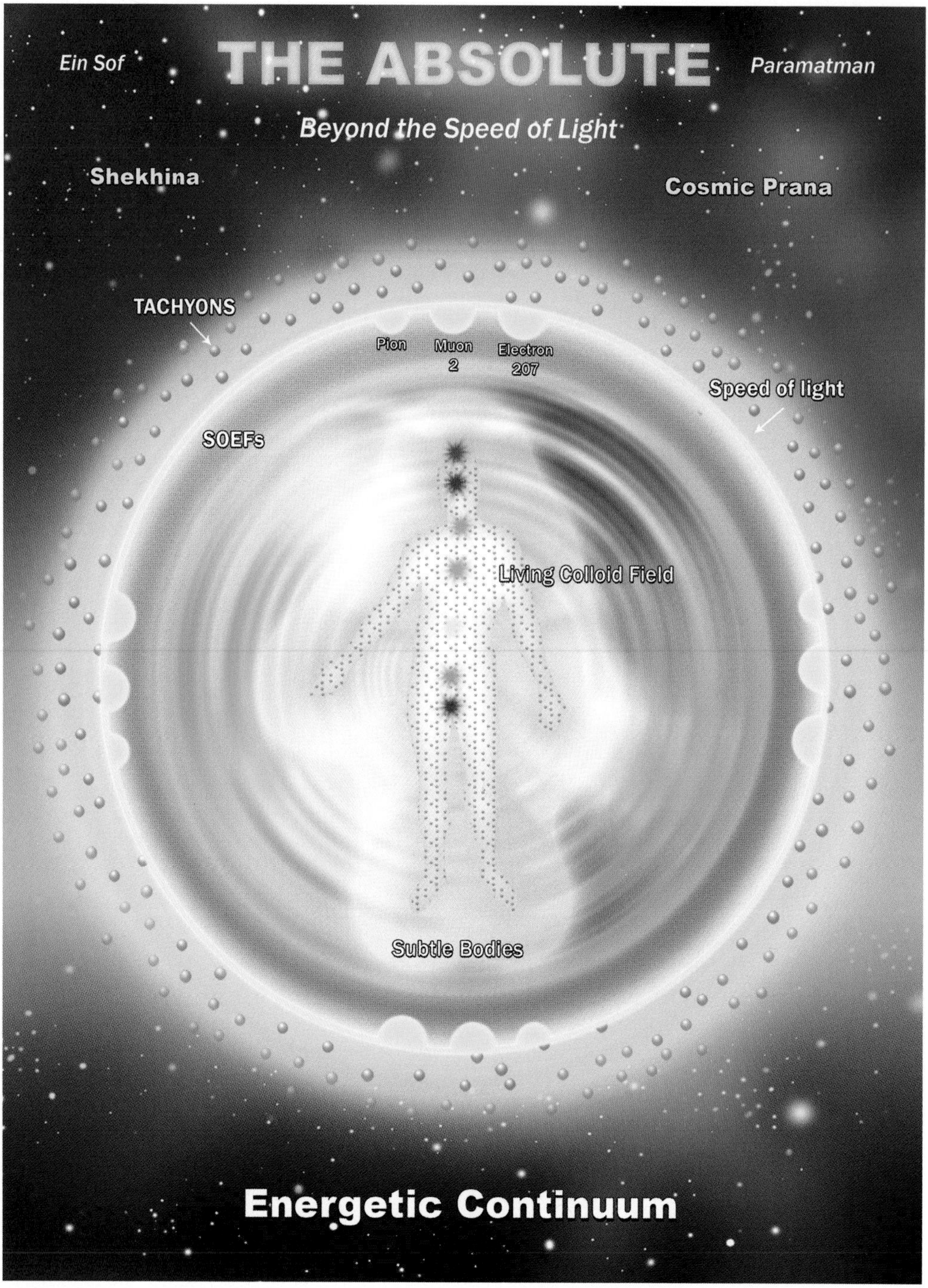

The Energetic Continuum

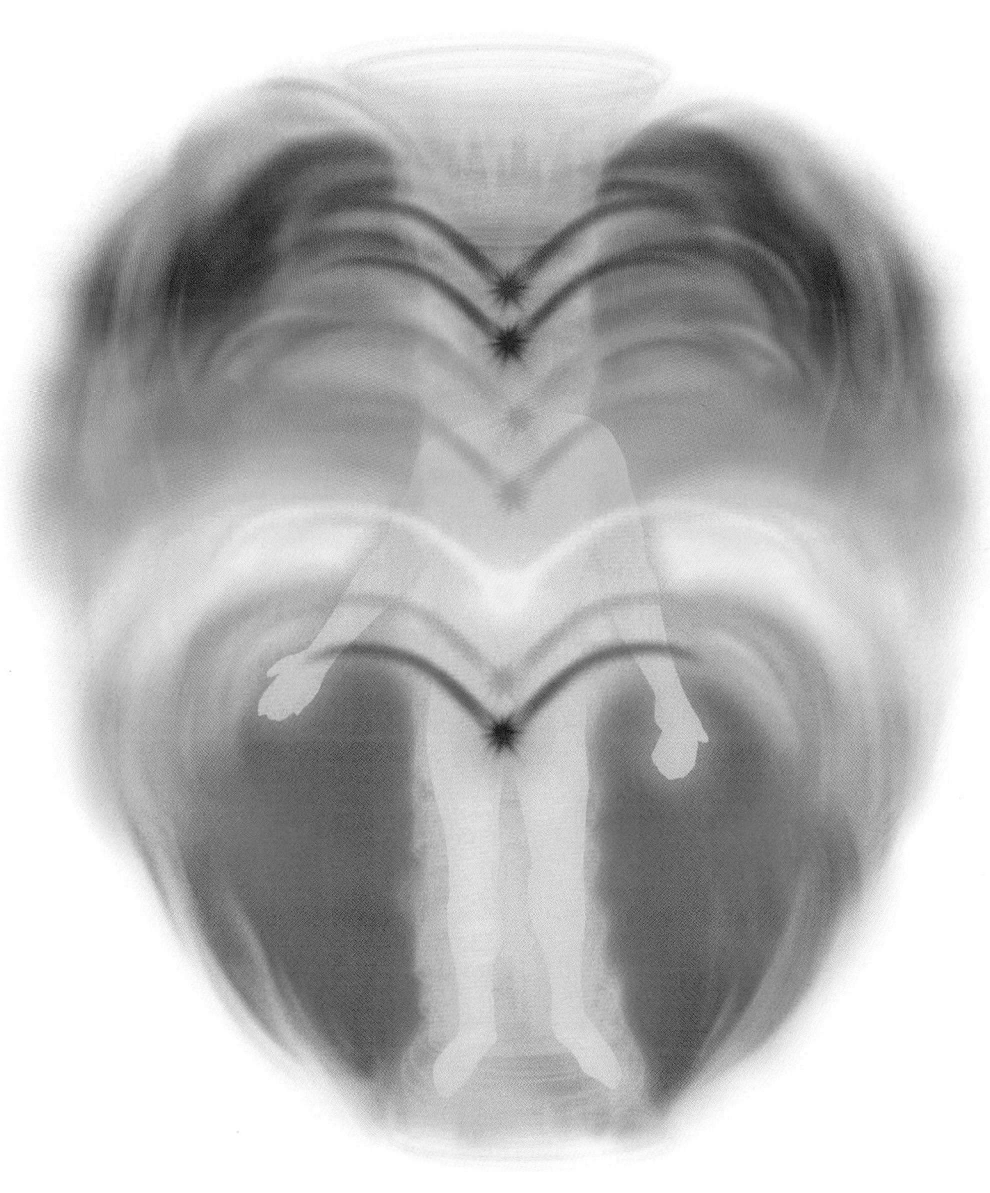

Angel Wings: Subtle Bodies Radiating as an Extension of the Chakras

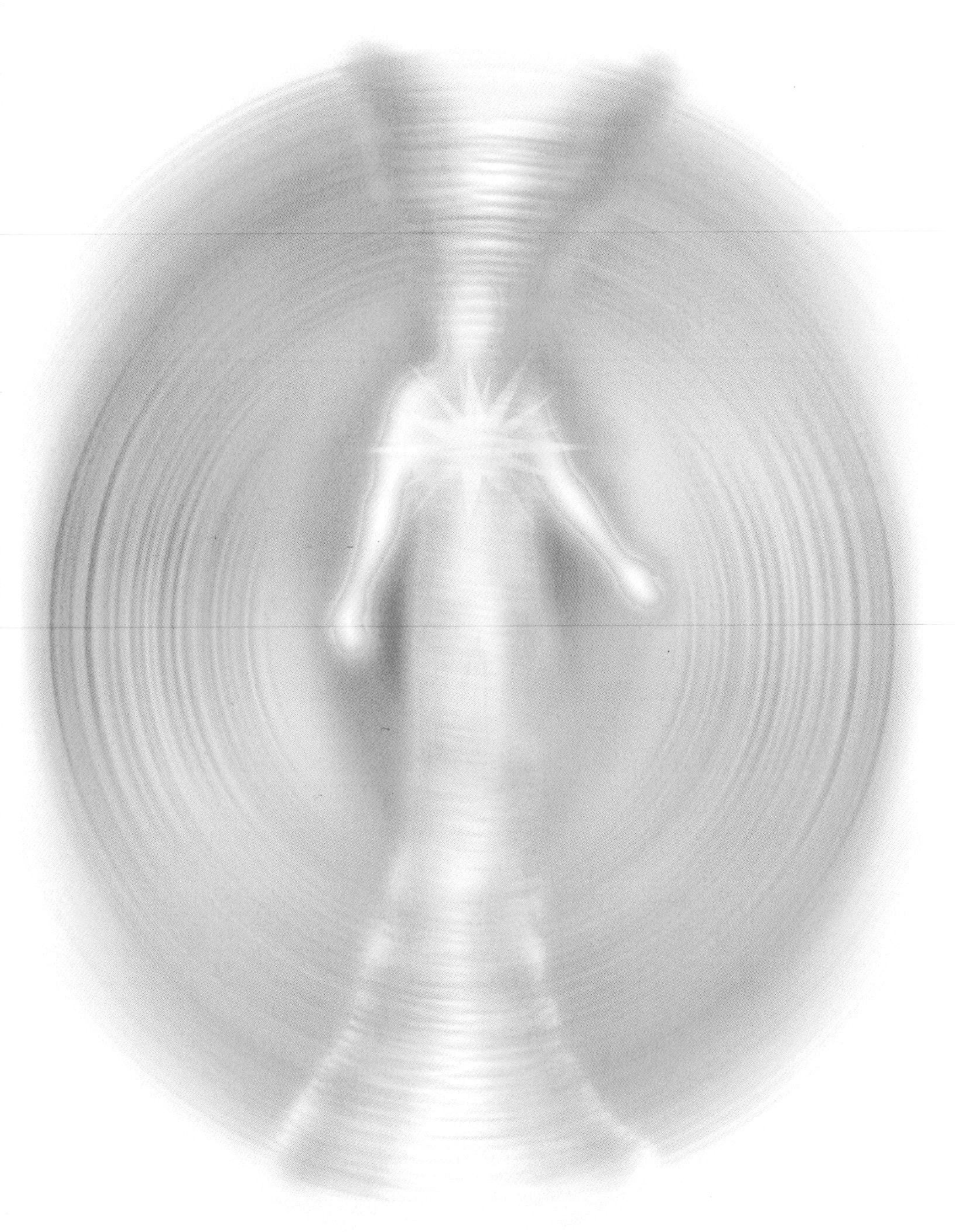

Kundalini Vortex Energy

electron transfer system of our cellular energy metabolism. The result of this is an electron leakage from the normal electron transport system, which leads to the creation of superoxide free radicals, other activated oxygen free radical-producing molecules, and additional free radicals.[2] These free radicals further oxidize in our system. The result is increased free radical damage to cell membranes, enzyme systems, and particularly artery endothelial cells (a possible precursor to atherosclerosis).[3] This free radical mediated, oxidative damage results in an accelerated aging and a chronic, degenerative disease process.[4] It represents the common biochemical endpoint for all types of stress on the system.

A simplified and useful way to understand this mechanism is that the free radicals, in essence, drain the body's molecular system of energy by stealing energy in the form of electrons. The electron energy that the free radicals "steal" is important for maintaining cell membrane structure. Dr. Levine calls these electrons the "molecular glue" that holds all levels of biological structure together, from DNA and RNA to cell membranes.[5] If one takes away the glue that holds the biological structure together, we get disorganization of cell function and cell replication, which manifests as increasing entropy and therefore aging.

It is very important to understand that sympathetic nervous system overstimulation has the same destructive endpoint effect as all other sources of stress such as physical trauma, bacterial and viral infection, and the environmental stress of pollution that is dumped on us by our society. This common effect is the destruction of oxidative cell membranes due to free radical activity. Some of these other environmental stressors that cause an excess of free radicals are ozone, sulfur dioxide and other smog components, radioactive fallout, chemical and radioactive toxins dumped into our Earth and water supplies, and foods that have undergone free radicalization.[6] Food that has been irradiated, microwaved (this is the author's hypothesis), adulterated, processed, spoiled, or undergone other "fast"-food preparations has an increased amount of free radicals and other radiolytic breakdown products. The stress of viral infections has been shown to cause increased free radicals in the system.[7] Physical trauma that results in cell membrane damage, such as swelling from bumps and bruises, causes the same free radical production resulting from the broken cell membranes.

A basic biochemical statement can be made about the meaning of stress chemistry from all causes of stress. It is that under any cause of emotional, mental, or environmental stress, the normal oxidant/antioxidant biochemical balance is thrown off. With increased free radicalization, the body's antioxidant capacity or biochemical regenerative energy is depleted. The result is that we experience decreased ability to adapt and survive free radical oxidant stresses. This results in cell membrane and other forms of biomolecular degeneration. From this we have accelerated aging and increased incidence of overt disease. This is evidenced in the epidemic increase in autoimmune disease, food allergies, and chemical hypersensitivities, now often called environmental illness. The imbalance of the oxidant/antioxidant ratio and concomitant sensitization to our own bodies and environment are the biochemical corollary of the essential disharmony and alienation from our environment, the people in it, and ourselves that stress consciousness creates. The question remains, how is this transcended?

Chemistry of Alchemy

Alchemy involves the conscious working with energy to transmute elements. For us it begins with a conscious choice to begin to reorganize our disrupted SOEFs by increasing the cosmic energy or prana coming into our system. It involves aligning ourselves with the natural laws of body, mind, and spirit in order to allow the life force to transmute us. This life force, this cosmic energy, this prana, is the God energy that is absolutely necessary for us to transcend the chemistry of stress. *This God energy is the ultimate food, and meditation is the ultimate digestive process.*

Meditation aligns and expands the subtle bodies, allowing the cosmic prana to come into our chakras and SOEFs with little resistance. As this power of God enters our system, we become rejuvenated on all levels. The reversal of entropy begins, and the physiology of stress and aging is reversed or slowed down. Hundreds of studies by Transcendental Meditation researchers since the early 1970s have validated the point that meditation reverses or slows the aging process. These researchers have shown that meditation creates a slower, more balanced metabolism with more sympathetic nervous system rest and a better sympathetic/parasympathetic nervous system balance. Unnecessary oxygen consumption, heart rate, and respiration rate have all been shown to decrease. Meditators in the studies demonstrated a decrease in high blood pressure, increased exercise tolerance in those with angina pectoris, better cardiovascular efficiency, better nervous system reaction time, improved athletic performance, better response to stress as measured by galvanic skin changes, improvement in the hearing threshold (which reflects an improved level of neurophysiological functioning), improved skills at sensory motor tasks, improved creativity testing results, higher scores on intelligence tests, increased mental speed and accuracy, improved long-term memory, increased EEG synchronicity and coherence, and decreased general anxiety.[8] On the biochemical level, researchers have found that meditators have a decrease in plasma cortisol (a major stress hormone), a decrease in adrenalin and non-adrenalin metabolites, and a decrease in blood cholesterol.[9] In the physiology of stress and aging, all these parameters have been found to move in the opposite direction to those found in meditators. This makes meditation look like the elixir of life. It is!

A most impressive study supporting this assertion was performed by R. K. Wallace on the effects of meditation on the aging process. He studied forty-seven subjects, with an average age of 52.8 years, who practiced the Transcendental Meditation technique and the TM-Siddhi techniques. He matched them to a control group and the established normal data for such a group. The testing system he used was drawn from the Morgan Adult Growth Examination, which gives reliable indicators of biological age. He found that in the subjects of the same chronological age, meditators who had been meditating less than five years had a mean biological age of 7.1 years less than that of the control group data. The mean biological age for those meditating five years or more was 15 years younger than the norms. Four of these meditators had biological ages of 27 or more years younger than expected for the normal chronological ages.[10]

How to Create the Alchemy of Spiritual Transformation

When careful gardeners plant seedling trees, they usually surround them with a wire fence to keep animals away, and they often tie the trees to a supportive stake so the wind does not blow them over. To overcome the chemistry of stress, spiritual seedlings are best aided by a spiritual protective fence or sanctuary. In ancient times and even now, the few serious spiritual aspirants retreated to caves, monasteries, and ashrams in hopes of finding such a sanctuary. There is even an ancient and incompletely understood Ayurvedic process called *kaya kalpa* in which participants lived in complete isolation for periods of forty days to a year. It was the ultimate rest. During this time, cleansing and then regenerative herbs and foods would be given. This kaya kalpa process is described in the biography of the sage Shriman Tapasviji Maharaj, a great ascetic who lived for 185 years. He used this process three times, and experienced what the biographer describes as an amazing regeneration, including the regrowth of new teeth and hair. It was said that when he did this for the first time at the age of slightly more than 100 years, he came out of it looking like a young man in his late twenties.[11] This, perhaps, represents the ultimate intensity in reversing the aging process. It also is a rare individual who can live in an isolated dark room for a year and not have the mind move into the chemistry of stress. It requires advanced spiritual development.

What is different today is that we are entering a collective age of Enlightenment on this planet. This requires an approach that is useful for large numbers of people rather than just the rare spiritual aspirant. We need to transform our own everyday life into a spiritual sanctuary, a harmonious meditative way of life that aligns our physical and all our subtle bodies, allows us to experience the full Grace of God, allows the full cosmic energy or prana to penetrate all levels of our body-mind-spirit being, filling our lives with the ecstasy of Love. This is Whole Person Enlightenment. It is our destiny – our ultimate function and purpose. It is the chemistry of meditation, which is Love. It is the wonderment of Oneness Awareness. It is knowing the Way by Being the Way.

How does one go about building a spiritual sanctuary in everyday life? For most people, a peaceful world would make the establishment of an inner experience of peace and harmony considerably easier. As one becomes more rooted in the Truth, the apparently turbulent condition of the outer world fades into the harmonious play of consciousness. Yet, for mass Enlightenment to unfold on this planet, the path to inner peace would be easier with a peaceful environment. Ultimately, we must start with experiencing the peace of our own Divine Self. This poem by Lao Tsu very beautifully describes how to create this spiritual sanctuary by starting with ourselves:

> Tao abides in non-action. Yet nothing is left undone.
> If kings and lords observed this,
> The ten thousand things would develop naturally. If they desired to act,

They would return to the simplicity of formless substance,
Without form there is no desire.
Without desire there is tranquility.
And in this way all things would be at peace.[12]

In meditation we can directly experience this completely fulfilling inner contentment. It arises from different levels of the meditation experience. It may be from the inner bliss of resonating and being filled with the Divine cosmic energy, or from the ecstasy of the at-Oneness with God as the formless and as the creation, or from the sublime Beingness of the direct awareness of the Truth. In meditation we may receive the direct experience of Love, know ourselves as Love, and experience Love for our True Inner Self and consequently the Self of All that resides in all people. These various experiences of inner bliss, sublime joy, peace, and Love fill us so wondrously that we are content beyond desire. Without desire there is peace. The practice of meditation reinforces these experiences. *Eventually the experience becomes our waking awareness and we move from the practice of doing meditation to a state of Being in life as a meditation.* This is true meditation. From this we directly experience the Torah teachings and those of Jesus that we should Love the Lord with all our heart and might and Love our neighbor as our True Self. It is from these direct meditation experiences and from the eventual stabilized direct awareness of the formless Reality of God, that we lose desire for the things and power of the world. Without desire there is tranquility. When there is tranquility based on this awareness, "all things would be at peace." From this one's own meditation experience over thirty-five years, and from observing and hearing the experiences of other meditators, this is absolutely true. A stabilized awareness in the non-dualistic Truth may not happen all at once. It may take many years to become the predominant awareness in our life, but with persistence it will happen. It is important to note that we do not become anything. What happens is that we simply become aware of the Truth of who we already are and delight in the synchronous dual/non-dual world.

Earlier we spoke of transmuting the first three chakras so we could awaken to their highest levels of awareness. In the first chakra we are confronted by fear instead of trust, rooted in the fear of death. In meditation, many people eventually have the direct experience of building an awareness that there is no death for the Self. The Self is immortal. With this awareness, the fear of death is gradually dissipated and we are free to trust. Whole books are written on this Truth, but again the author asserts from his own direct meditation experience that this fearless awareness develops and the fear of death dissolves permanently. There is no death for the Self.

Right Understanding

It is possible to meditate, to have flashy experiences, and yet never develop a right understanding. This is because people sometimes have deep patterns that resist the understanding that arises in meditation. Sometimes they become addicted to the power and energy of the experiences rather than the Truth that lies behind them. They get trapped in going for the "hit." Right understanding, which is an important part of spiritual evolvement, is the integration of our experiences with daily life; it is meditation as a practice and way of Being. It is the wisdom to distinguish the real essence of life from the illusions of life.

Right Fellowship – Sangha

Right fellowship (sangha) is extremely important in developing right understanding. It may come in the form of traditional guru-disciple relationships, through people who serve as spiritual guides or teachers, through regular meditation groups, or through spiritual group processes such as the core group process suggested by Barbara Marx Hubbard.[13] Wherever it comes from, it is a very important part of creating a spiritual sanctuary. Shivapuri Baba, an Indian holy man who practiced a live-food diet and lived for 137 years until the early 1960's, taught that the most important external aid for creating a spiritual sanctuary or right life was the fellowship of realized souls. Many, for brief periods of time, have higher awareness experiences, altered sensory states, or altered states of consciousness that do indeed take one beyond the ego, but they do not become stabilized in their daily experience.

It is rare that we reach such a stabilized awareness as our primary life orientation. It occurs more easily when the direct and sole intent of our life is to become established in the awareness of the Truth as the non-dual, holographic pure awareness of God's Light and Love. This takes spiritual discipline. This is one of the hardest parts of creating a spiritual sanctuary in regular worldly life. There are many who do well in a protected ashram situation but when they go out in the world find that they have not internalized their discipline and it slowly begins to fade. Right company, in any form, helps to inspire people toward maintaining their spiritual discipline and developing right understanding. Right fellowship is a form of God's Grace. This is important because, although our inner teacher is always working, we do not always want to follow it. The inner teacher of another, at just the right time, may give the right positive reinforcement for our own inner spiritual direction. Right fellowship supports, reinforces, and stimulates the inner teacher. It helps to create a situation in which there can be an exchange of teachings and presence among equals. Surrounding ourselves with good company is an extremely critical part of building a spiritual sanctuary. In this age of increasing mass Enlightenment, it becomes an even more important principle.

The attuned awareness of the inner teacher, plus right fellowship, can be said to equal what is known as the Guru's Grace in the Eastern spiritual disciples. People often go to a guru to be awakened, but with the heightening awareness and energy of spiritual seekers in general, the awakening of the Kundalini may occur as a result of the increased energy that happens in a group meditation or even a spiritual group gathering such as a worldwide meditation for peace. We may awaken each other by simply transferring this energy to each other. This energy comes from God's Grace of right fellowship. Muktananda once made this point in a humorous way by telling us how his dog, who had accumulated energy from being around him, gave Shaktipat to the veterinarian. People often attribute this increased energy and Grace exclusively to the teacher, guide, or guru who is focusing the group rather than to the result of the total group spiritual energy. God's Grace comes in many forms and ways. It can come through the increased cosmic energy of the outer teacher, through the prana of an individual person, through such practices as meditation and fasting, or through reaching a critical point intense enough to awaken the Kundalini spontaneously. It can come from the heightened prana of a whole group, or from a combination of the pranic energies of the inner teacher, outer teacher, and of a meditation group.

World peace is a function of our inner peace. By our state of meditation we create peace by Being peace. For the whole world to be elevated to a state of transcendent awareness, it requires all of us to participate in creating peace on Earth. The author believes this mission of world peace is becoming a planetary expression of God's Will. By building a spiritual sanctuary out of the world, everyone's spiritual evolution will be quickened. We will be brought closer to the quantum leap in consciousness that we, as all of God's children, will someday make. By serving world peace, we are serving the development of inner peace for everyone. By giving our Love to the world, we become that Love. As Love we become the spiritual sanctuary that we seek. To foster this state of world peace, the author founded the Peace Everyday Initiative – creating peace by Being peace. The practice is for people worldwide to meditate for forty minutes per day at sunrise or sunset, linking together in the thought form of peace and visualizing the planet surrounded in Light. (More information is available at www.peaceeveryday.com.)

Right Livelihood

Right livelihood is our alignment with God's Will. We are already perfect. What we really seek is to become the Divine expression of our inner perfection in the world. This is the essence of right livelihood. The more the cosmic energy flows through us, the more we attune to God's Will and are able to be involved in the right work for who we are. We become the creative expression of the Divine Will. In this process, the second chakra awakens and our mind merges in the evolutionary creative energy that was always ours.

Right livelihood is the subject for a book in itself, but there are a few guidelines in creating the spiritual sanctuary that are important to consider. The first is the reminder that although right livelihood is extremely important, our highest function is to rest totally in the awareness of our Transcendent Reality as our primary awareness. Eventually we reach the stage in which it makes little difference to our spiritual state how much time and energy we put into our worldly work. However, for all but those in the most advanced stages of spiritual evolution, too much time and energy spent in work may dull our growing experiences of the Truth. We may find ourselves becoming self-willed doers rather than Being in the state of Grace. As doers, we become attached to the rewards of our work, and in that attachment, the ecstatic experience of our transcendent Beingness is lost. By working too many hours we can become depleted of mental and physical energy. In this depleted state it is harder to remain awake. The famous nineteenth-century saint Ramakrishna advised people to keep one hand on God's foot and the other hand in the world. Shivapuri Baba advised us to do our minimum duties correctly and keep our minds on God. Traditionally, service to others helps to balance our creative work. For some it becomes the most creative and evolutionary expression. Mother Theresa was an inspiring example of this.

Right Relationship

As Love, and only as Love, can we live in right relationship with our mate, children, and all others around us. Unconditional and unrelenting Love is the sole building block of the spiritual sanctuary. In building right relationships it is also necessary to organize our time, space, and energy intelligently so there is enough for individual, couple, family, and societal expressions of this Love. People often think about communication problems when we think of right relationship, yet in one of the author's roles as a family therapist he rarely sees a communication problem. People communicate their fear of intimacy and of Love quite well – through contractions of the heart, avoidance, and acts of retribution. It is very difficult to keep the heart open in the face of rejection and hurt that another projects to maintain a safe intimacy distance. This is the crux of the third chakra issue: How do we rise above the emotional hurt, imbalance, and power struggles to the state of balanced and compassionate emotional sensitivity that reflects the higher awareness of the third chakra? We do this by keeping the heart open no matter what pain we may feel. It is this wound of the heart that leads us into the awakening of the fourth, or heart, chakra and to the awakening of the other spiritually oriented chakras. As we do this, it becomes easier to be in the awareness of the Truth of who we are and to see this play of Truth in all our everyday interactions, turning them into valuable lessons as gifts of God.

If we allow our heart to contract, our subtle bodies then also contract and become misaligned. This contraction then decreases the pranic life force available to us. The chemistry of stress sets in and the aging process starts again. But most important of all, we shut ourselves off from the cosmic energy that is the Love energy of God. It is the source of our spiritual life. It is the source of spiritual awareness. This is the price we pay for the ingrained habit of contracting our heart. As Love, we become the spiritual sanctuary. Without it, the sanctuary survives as a frail shell of intellectual awareness.

Attunement to Mother Nature's Natural Laws

Part of our spiritual sanctuary is already present, waiting for us to notice. It is in the natural laws of the universe, but we are rarely in tune with them as a support for our sanctuary. The Essene communities knew the value of harmony with the natural laws and spent much time studying, Being in Communion, and ultimately living in harmony with them. As a result, not only was their spiritual life enhanced, but they attained very high levels of health. It is reported that it was quite normal for them to attain ages of greater than 120 years.[14] If we are not attuned to these natural laws, our individual thoughts and actions will not be in balance. This harmony is necessary for full health and spiritual life.

This is particularly important because modern society is significantly out of tune with these natural laws on almost every level. We are so out of tune that we may just destroy the whole planet under the delusion of protecting ourselves. The problem is that these societal thought forms are so strong that it is very easy to be swept along by this unconscious wave of disharmony. We have become so disconnected from natural synchrony with universal laws that we need to go to the very source of these laws to begin to regain our attunement. The source is the pure, undifferentiated awareness, which is the Source of All. By merging our awareness in pure consciousness with meditation, we can avoid a distortion in the manifestation of pure awareness into thought and action. The practice of meditation is the main tool for this harmonizing of our awareness. As this practice deepens, the awareness maintains itself in our awake life without formal meditation. At this point we tend to act spontaneously in communion with these laws. We become as the law rather than under the law.

For most people this state of Communion is an idealistic form of sanctuary that is rather difficult to attain or sustain. Nevertheless, by meditating regularly at least two times a day, we will build a spiritual sanctuary in which our lives will become more and more harmonious with these universal laws. The whole process is helped by living in some connection with Nature. It is more strongly reinforced if we are able to live outside of an urban setting, but even attuning to a simple indoor garden in the middle of the city can be helpful.

Once we begin to understand these laws, it is very helpful to do as the Talmud suggests, "to build a fence around the Torah."[15] This means that we create certain self-warning signals or listen to feedback from the right company gathered around us that tells us if we begin to act disharmoniously. One of the dangers in experiencing higher states of awareness is that we begin to feel we are above any concepts or laws by virtue of our direct contact with the Source. The issue is that we are also in direct contact with the tremendously disharmonious societal forces that are always pulling us into disharmony. Swami Prakashanada Saraswati, a spiritual uncle to this one, would emphasize that we are not totally free from the urges of the body and mind until we leave the body. A great many of the gurus who have come to the West, as well as the various leaders from all religions, have fallen into disgrace because they have assumed they were above needing a fence to warn them when they were being drawn away from unity with the universal laws. They just assumed that whatever they did was in harmony. That fence in Eastern spiritual traditions is called dharma, or righteous life. In the West it is called the Ten Speakings (Commandments). The Ten Speakings have several levels of interpretation. When one says "Thou shalt have no other gods before me" (Exodus 20:3), it can mean that we should always be immersed in universal God Consciousness rather than the diverse consciousness of money, power, sex, and other forces of the temporal world. "Honor thy father and thy mother, that thy days may be long upon the land" (Exodus 20:12) can be interpreted to mean to honor the natural laws and the cosmic laws so our life will be long and spiritually fulfilling. These are concrete statements of universal laws that act as guidelines for those who are not fully in touch with the direct Source. It is optimal to live our life as the Love-inspired, spontaneous manifestation of these universal laws; this is the firm and joyous foundation of the sanctuary.

The important thing is not to create a fearful, contractive tyranny out of a self-righteous, blind application of our own projection of what we consider the "literal" meaning of these laws. How we live by these laws is a function of our own spiritual evolvement at any point in time. There is no right way forever. It is not that simple. Life is not static. It is more important to be harmonious with the spirit of the law. This requires some intelligence, discrimination, and right understanding. It was on this basis that Jesus acted to break with the strict interpretation of the written law and heal on the Sabbath. But to maintain the sanctuary, we need to create a feedback system in order to wake us up if we begin to wander. Ultimately, the feedback system is to *know the Way by Being the Way.*

Alchemy of Bodily Health

The physical body is the final aspect of creating a spiritual sanctuary for the alchemical chemistry necessary for human transformation. We have considered our sanctuary from the spiritual, mental, and emotional aspects and now need to include the body as part of what this one calls Whole Person Enlightenment. The purpose of the understanding shared in this book is to create a synthesis of the relationship between the physical body, the emotional-mental body, and the spirit in spiritual life. It is to give an outline for how to increase awareness in our life so that we may extend beyond the inner spiritual experiences of perfection to become the manifestation of that perfection in our ordinary daily life.

By maintaining the practices of right diet and fasting, we help to turn the body into a better superconductor of the cosmic energy. This cosmic energy or prana comes from God and is the immediate experiential "Face of God" that we can know in every moment of our life. The experience of this cosmic Love force uniting us with the resonant experience of the macrocosm is bliss. As we clear the toxins and blocks from our system with diet, fasting, and other sources of natural and vibrational healing such as homeopathic remedies, herbs, flower essences, and gem elixirs, our body becomes more highly organized. As this occurs, we can more easily feel and be attuned with the direct force of God coursing through us. We do not need our Kundalini to be awakened to have an experience of this attunement. We may experience it as one of those sacred moments of Divine inspiration, ecstasy, and Love that so many of us have had at some time in our lives. It may be a moment of a quiet and subtle sense of attunement during which our body, mind, and spirit feel totally harmonious with all of God's creation such as what may occur while watching a beautiful sunset. It may be a continued experience of joyous well-being. It may be the experience of the awakening or energizing of the power of the Kundalini. Although these experiences occur more frequently with proper diet and fasting, this does not mean that by diet and fasting alone we become Enlightened. It is through the integration of the threefold balancing of body, mind, and spirit that we become aligned, merged, and stabilized in the higher evolutionary spiritual awareness.

Seven Alchemical Healers

There are some basic forces, part of the laws of Nature, that help to transform and maintain the body in the most optimal state. H. E. Kirschner, M.D., calls them "Nature's seven doctors."[16] They are right diet, fresh air, pure water, sunshine, exercise, rest, and of course mental, emotional, and spiritual peace. We have touched on some of these throughout the book, but here are a few more touches to deepen our understanding of the simplicity of the natural laws.

Fresh air, as we discussed earlier, is a direct source of nutrition. In addition to breathing exercises, it is good to take an air bath every day. Air is absorbed through our pores and acts as a detoxifier. Kirshner reports that Dr. Kellogg estimated that each person needs about 3,000 cubic feet of fresh pure air per hour to help us detoxify the toxins excreted from our lungs and skin.[17] How much fresh air are we getting in our sealed-off, high-rise office buildings where millions of us work every day? This is a very simple reason many people are out of harmony with the natural law. It is so easy to do. We are surrounded by all sorts of "normal" lifestyle activities that are disharmonious.

Pure water is another of the seven healers. Because of our national and international persistence in creating chemical and radioactive toxic wastes that seep into our waters, it is almost impossible to find pure water. To get anything near the quality of the fresh spring water that once existed, we have to process the water by distillation or reverse osmosis. In processing, the water becomes unstructured and needs stirring to reoxygenate, and it needs mineral salts, and moon- and starlight to become structured and energized (see Chapter 29 for a complete discussion of living water).

Adequate *sunlight* of 30 to 60 minutes per day on the total body gives it a chance to become directly re-energized. Like plants, we soak up and transmute this nutrient into our energy system. Until we become used to the sun, late afternoon and early morning sun are the easiest to begin with. Although a little sunlight is good, hours of sunlight can be too much for the system and lead to imbalances.

Exercise is another of the seven alchemical healers. There is a simple rule: Use it or lose it. Dr. Kirschner teaches that activity is life and stagnation is death.[18] Exercise stimulates all the internal organs and muscle systems, tones the nervous and digestive system, improves circulation, and stimulates the skin system to release toxins. No equipment is needed. In fact, working out in a smelly, poorly ventilated, and synthetically lit gym deprives us of the benefits of sunlight and fresh air we get during outdoor exercise. Outdoor walking is the best exercise, according to many natural healers. The British educator, George Trevelyan, claims to have just two doctors, his right and left legs.[19] For those who feel more vigorous exercise is necessary, it is interesting to point out that the Ayurvedic system of healing recommends exercising to only 50 percent of capacity. The point is that if we turn exercise into a stress for the body we may get aerobic benefit, but too much physical stress may break down body function. Between 50 and 80 percent of our exercise capacity needs to be reached. The author's own personal practice is to take a fast walk several times per week, use the rebounder daily, and do Yoga asanas daily. In this simple way, many of the natural laws are efficiently acknowledged. The general idea of all these laws is to give the body just the right amount of attention to function optimally for spiritual focus in life. This requires some self-observation along with trial and error, until we find the right balance. Then we can settle into a routine of orderly caretaking and not be concerned about it. Everyone must scientifically find his or her own routine.

Rest is another important alchemical healer. It is so important that God even gave us a Sabbath so we could not misinterpret the message. In everyday work life, it is important to acknowledge this time for regeneration. In the process of kaya kalpa, the idea of complete rest is an integral part of the rejuvenation program. It works. Rest implies a break from all daily routines, responsibilities, irritating noises, and so on. A quiet spot in Nature is good, especially for city people who are cut off from Nature's regenerating forces on a daily basis. Rest can take the form of sleep. There is no magic number for hours of sleep; depending on our constitution, we may need from five to eight hours, or even more, per night. The main idea is the regularity of a good night of sleep. For some, a short nap in the day is helpful; for kapha types (see Chapter 24), it can make them feel worse. For sedentary, intellectually active office workers, physical labor like gardening, hiking, game playing, or periods of silence may be the best rest. For others, just the opposite may be best. This may also be combined with light fasting. Daily meditation before, during, and after work creates a rest that helps wake us up from production mentality and is of benefit to us all.

Although aligning with these basic natural forces seems simple, it often requires some social independence. Children, when they have a recess from school, automatically know what to do: they play. How many teachers do we see outside playing? As a physician, the author attends medical conferences, which are almost always in sealed buildings where participants sit for hours at a time immersed in intellectual activity. At lunchtime, instead of sitting around even longer during a lengthy lunch with everyone else, the author finds some open space where he can exercise, breathe some fresh air, take in some sun, meditate, and eat a light homemade salad. To many, it might seem strange to acknowledge the participation of these natural laws in our life, but they keep us tuned to the life force. After you do this sort of thing for a while, if you do it in a quiet, non-self-righteous way, people become accepting and sometimes even join in the fun. There are many who only need the support of a little good company to let their inner teacher guide them to alignment with the natural laws.

Summation of the Chemistry of Alchemy

The chemistry of alchemy involves the decision to reverse the degenerative life process in the physical, emotional-mental, and spiritual dimensions of our lives. It is a conscious choice to reorganize and re-energize the SOEFs by increasing the amount of cosmic prana coming into our system. To successfully do this, everyday life and the world need to be transformed into a spiritual sanctuary. For this purpose, right diet and fasting, even though they do increase the amount of cosmic energy entering the system, are not sufficient. We need a regular practice of meditation, right company, right understanding, right livelihood, right relationship to significant others and society, and attunement to the heavenly and earthly universal laws. In sum, it can be called right life. It is analogous to Buddha's Eightfold Path, or the meaning of the Sermon on the Mount. In discussing right life and meditation as the path to Enlightenment, Shivapuri Baba, an Enlightened teacher who lived to be 139 years old, taught that three disciplines provide the only cure for the ills of this life.[20] These are the disciplines of the physical, moral, and spiritual laws of the universe. He simply reminded people to be absorbed in God and their duties (the three disciplines) as God. This is what is meant by right life.

It is important to emphasize that there is no automatic list to be followed for right life. It requires a wisdom developed out of personal "trial and error," practice, and meditation. For those who have trouble meditating, doing mantra repetition or quiet contemplation is sufficient. For most of us, some of the most profound understanding of right life grew out of our so-called mistakes. As long as we are willing to witness and learn from our mistakes, right life will develop for us. Shivapuri Baba felt that the biggest obstacles to right life are inertia and procrastination. The normal yet often disharmonious ways of our modern society are so much easier to follow. In this regard, Muktananda used to say that the cemetery was his favorite place because it is a reminder that some day we will leave our physical bodies and lose our opportunity to pursue the spiritual path. Therefore, the time is now. In right life, no part of our existence is negated. It represents the full awakening of the first three chakras. This awakening is the foundation for the stabilized awakening of the awareness of the higher chakras. It represents a major step in the integration of the body, emotional-mental, and spiritual levels of our Being. The combination of right life and meditation is the major process for Whole Person Enlightenment.

Alchemy of Meditation

As prana increases in our total context of right life and meditation, we become superconductors, accumulators, and amplifiers of the cosmic energy. This increase more properly aligns all levels of our Being. Our awareness spontaneously increases because the experience of the prana in itself, as the emanation of God and as the Face of God, naturally increases our awareness of the Divine. This experiential aspect of the Divine reinforces our direct awareness of the non-dualistic Truth of God. At some intangible point in the process, this direct awareness, which we often experience in the practice of meditation, begins to maintain itself more and more predominantly in our waking state. At this point, our mundane daily life is transformed by the awareness we experience in meditation. *Our waking lives are tilled with the awareness of meditation, the direct sublime awareness of God, of Love in every aspect of our life. This is the alchemy of meditation.*

As we increase our meditation practice, there is an increased alignment of the physical and all the subtle bodies with the pure vibration of the cosmic prana. Meditation is the Divine digestive system of the cosmic prana. The clearer a channel we become for the cosmic energy, the more continuous flow of it we have moving through us. This brings us into a continual at-Oneness with the universal life force and therefore Oneness with our own Divinity. The closer we become resonant with that energy, the more we simply become that Divine energy. This increased pure prana aligns the SOEFs so perfectly that we become aligned with the cosmic energy, down to our very RNA-DNA structure. The author feels that the spiral structure of the RNA-DNA double helix reflects the spiral-vortical pattern of the cosmic prana. As Cosmic Consciousness penetrates to our atomic and molecular structure, we cannot help but feel the ecstasy of this unity of the ultimate macrocosm of pure prana with the ultimate microcosm of our molecular structure. One feels totally harmonious on every level of Being. It is a total mind-body-spirit ecstasy vibrating in every atom of our Being with every other atom in the universe. *DNA and RNA are the harp strings; the winds of pure prana blow through, and the sound is pure joy. This is the alchemy of meditation.* The experience of it fills us with Love, harmony, and joy. *Love is the ultimate harmonic of the alchemy of meditation.* The awareness that comes from the continual experience of this total harmonic of Love establishes us in the ultimate holographic, non-dualistic Truth. The alchemy of meditation begins when the ultimate Truth of Oneness becomes our predominant waking state awareness, and we motionlessly dance and silently sing in the sublime joy of Whole Person Enlightenment.

Summary, Chapter 11

1. The chemistry of stress represents an entropy-producing process that dissipates the energy and structure of the SOEFs and consequently leads to an increased rate of aging and increased probability of chronic degenerative disease.
2. The chemistry of stress is the chemistry of biochemical, physiological, emotional, mental, and spiritual degeneration.
3. It arises out of the toxic stress of our personal and world lifestyle. Its common degenerative pathway on the biochemical level is excess free radical production, which results in cell membrane and other biomolecular destruction.
4. On the spiritual level, the chemistry of stress is most related to our first three chakras remaining unawakened and out of balance.
5. The chemistry of alchemy begins with a conscious choice to reorganize and re-energize our disrupted SOEFs by increasing the cosmic energy or prana coming into our system. It requires

aligning ourselves with the natural laws of body, mind, and spirit in order to allow the life force to transmute us.

6. This life force is the God energy, the cosmic pranic energy that is absolutely necessary for us to transcend the chemistry of stress. This energy is the ultimate food.
7. Meditation is the ultimate digestive process of this food. It aligns and expands the subtle bodies so that the cosmic energy can come into our mind-body complex.
8. In order to sustain the alchemy of spiritual transformation, it is helpful to build a personal and world sanctuary of inner and outer peace. Our everyday life needs to be transformed into a spiritual sanctuary.
9. Right life is the foundation of this spiritual sanctuary. It arises from right diet, right fellowship, right understanding, right livelihood, right relationship to self, significant others, and society, and attunement to the heavenly and earthly universal laws. It is the living expression for how we integrate our physical, moral, and spiritual lives.
10. There are no rules for right life. The right life at one point in our evolution is different from the right life at another point. It requires an intuitive and practical wisdom that attunes us to the spirit of the law rather than blindly binding us to the letter of the law. Intelligence, contemplation, and meditation help us to develop our understanding and practice of right life.
11. Right life is knowing the Way by Being the Way.
12. The combination of the practice of meditation and right life is the process of Whole Person Enlightenment. It involves the integration of body, mind, and spirit as a totality in our spiritual life. There is no negation of any part of our Being.
13. The alchemy of meditation begins when the ultimate holographic, non-dualistic Truth becomes our predominant awake state awareness and we motionlessly dance and silently sing in Whole Person Enlightenment.
14. Love is the ultimate harmonic of this awareness.

Chapter 12

Nutrition, Kundalini, and Transcendence

Transcendence

Transcendence is the extension of regeneration. Transcendence is the evolutionary process by which the vortex energy of the Kundalini progressively transmutes us from the gross matter of our bodies to a more refined and highly organized and energized SOEF. It is when the body is liberated from its traditional cellular confinement. It is the physical parallel to the transmutation of our consciousness to the Love of Unity Awareness. Eventually it takes us into complete absorption of our form into the formless ground of Being of God. From the time the Kundalini is awakened, we gradually become more etheric, but even after the total merging of the Kundalini energies, enough of our physical body and chakra system is left so we can function in the world. It is the process of transcendence that explains the physical transcendence of Mirabai, Tukaram, Elijah, Enoch, and Jesus. Our spiritual potentials are awesome.

Transcendence is easier to comprehend in the context of the cosmic cycles of involution and evolution. Earlier we discussed the precipitation of the SOEFs from the faster-than-light virtual energy field into particles moving at the speed of light and finally into our dense human physical form. This is the process of *involution.* The process of *evolution* begins with the awakening of the Shakti Kundalini, which is the residue of the involutionary spiritual Kundalini energy stored below the chakra at the base of the spine. The awakening of Shakti Kundalini starts us on a transcendent evolutionary path, which we call spiritual evolution. A major step in this path is the complete synchronistic merging of the chakras and Kundalini into a single energy. This happens when the level of spiritual awareness and pranic energy in the system reaches a certain intensity. At this point we transcend duality in both our subtle energy system and in our spiritual awareness. The difficulty in discussing this transcendence pattern is that our brains are binary or dualistic, but the states we are discussing are neither the One nor the many. Although the description appears to be linear, it fits neither the linearity of our Western minds nor the circularity of the Eastern mind. The process is spiral and vortical.

Spiritual evolution is happening simultaneously on all levels, yet it culminates in an awakened, aware balance at various stages of integration at different times. There may be no total explanation for this process of involution/evolution, except that it is the play of God. We can partially explain it as the existence of the law of cause and effect on the subtle planes. An analogy is the cosmic vacuum in which energy precipitates spontaneously into matter and then returns to its original state of virtual energy. The process happens in every level of cosmic existence, including our food. In the book *Oahspe,*[1] John Ballou Newbrough used the term "vortexual" for all energy within matter.[2] The energy precipitating from the cosmic prana does so in a spiral whirlpool pattern that resides within matter as the potential subtle energy. For example, at a certain moment during the assimilation process, a dissolution of the material food occurs and "vortexual" energy is liberated. The tendency for the corporal is to disincorporate itself.[3] This is the way transcendence works for all of creation, us included. In the process of transcendence, our physical form slowly transmutes into more subtle physical forms, and finally transmutes into subtle energy forms that are absorbed back into the cosmic energy.

Kundalini Vortex Pattern

The pure prana or spiritual Kundalini is drawn directly into the system through the crown chakra, where there is no subtle anatomy to filter it. It is then drawn into the vortex of the sushumna, which is either a major or minor organizing vortical force in the body depending on whether the Kundalini has been awakened. The cosmic prana spirals down to the heart center, which acts as the center of the sushumna vortex, and then broadens again. The vortex energies of all the chakras are linked to this central Kundalini vortex. The chakras are a less refined energy and draw part of their energy from the Kundalini vortex. Doing so, they deplete the energy of the vortex and hence slow down its spiral energy action. Until the awakening of the Kundalini, the body density regularly pulls energy from the Kundalini vortex downward into the physical structure. Once the Kundalini is awakened, this vortex is increasingly energized by its rising. The crown chakra also becomes more activated and more pure prana comes into the system to further energize this central vortex.

(See the Kundalini Vortex Energy illustration in the color plates.)

When the vortex energy reaches a certain intensity, it begins to draw matter into the etheric, or next level of purified and more tightly organized SOEF energy. It works much like sugar being drawn up into the more tightly organized vortex of stirred water as it is dissolved into this moving vortex. With the awakening of the Kundalini, we begin the first movement toward the transmuting of our physical form back to its Source – the transcendent energy of God. The tendency of the energized vortex field is to transmute everything to a higher level of energy existence. This does not deplete the body energy because it is an open system that draws energy from the physical plane via food. The better superconductor we are for the energy, the more active the Kundalini vortex, and the more the process of transcendence takes place.

Feeding the Kundalini

The food we eat is very important in this process of transcendence. If we eat high-energy, lighter foods such as the biogenic live foods, the Kundalini vortex is more energized and thus more active in transmuting us from matter to energy. The watery fruits and vegetables, because of their higher conductivity and their structured water energy, particularly enhance the activity. The closer we move to pure prana in our food, the easier it is for the pranic energy of the system to be drawn into the upper vortex field. The dense flesh foods and low-energy, *tamasic* foods decrease the energy of the Kundalini vortex. Meat is so much denser than biogenic foods that it does not enter the pranic field as efficiently. It then acts as a sort of metaphoric sludge to slow down the vortex vibration and therefore to slow or reverse the process of transcendence. The sludge effect of meat can be overcome by drawing from the prana accumulated by such things as intense meditation. This is obviously not the most efficient use of our pranic build-up. One of the points of Spiritual Nutrition is that, through eating high-prana foods, eating lightly, and fasting periodically, we become better superconductors and therefore we enhance the efficient use of energy in the system for our transcendence. This approach guides us more clearly to begin thinking about the body as an entity of energy.

Any mental and emotional tension in the system decreases the energy coming into the system by thickening and misaligning the subtle bodies. Because the chakras are not getting the normal energy they need to function from direct external sources, they pull more from the central Kundalini vortex. This too results in a blockage of the transcendence process by depleting the energy of the Kundalini vortex.

Kundalini Merging

In this Kundalini transcendence process, the SOEFs become more and more organized as the energy is drawn up. Our body tends to become more etheric. The increasingly energized Kundalini vortex draws up and transmutes more matter and more energy from the more dense subtle energy systems until the subtle energy of the whole organism is drawn into one energy vortex. This is the point at which the two Kundalini energies – Shakti Kundalini and spiritual Kundalini – merge. We literally become One and experience ourselves as whole and complete. An experiential reminder of this is the almost continual awareness of this one as a single vortical transcendent energy field resonating with and being drawn back up into the cosmic energy vibration. This vortical resonating and merging experience, particularly during periods of silent meditation, seems to penetrate to the very atomic level of one's Being.

At the time of the two Kundalini energies merging, the chakras and the subtle bodies become absorbed into the more purified, powerful energy of the Kundalini vortex. Enough of the chakra energy is left to maintain us on the physical plane, but the chakras lose their predominant role and significance. What is left is the continual experience of the pulsation of the pure prana flowing in the Kundalini vortex. This becomes the central energy source of the physical system. The crown chakra changes at Kundalini awakening from a minor portal of energy entry to that of the most important source of energy in the system. The whole system has reached a higher level of SOEF organization and provides a model that explains the process of resurrection. It may also explain the passage in John 20:17 in which Jesus said to Mary Magdalene, "Stop clinging to me, for I have not yet ascended to the Father," and in John 20:19 and John 20:26 in which Jesus passed through the locked doors of his disciples' dwellings to bless them with peace. What may be happening is that Jesus' SOEF was so highly organized and his physical structure was so nearly transmuted into the etheric level, that he was able to go the next step and make his body totally etheric by the use of his mind. This would allow him to pass through locked doors. By projecting his mind down into the vortex, he could draw up the materials needed into the SOEF to repattern and recreate his own body as needed to serve the Will of God. This is a theoretical extension of our total vortex and SOEF aspects of our new nutritional paradigm.

Transcendence After the Merging of Kundalini into the One

Ever since this one's forty-day fast, there is a feeling that this one is wearing a pulsating skullcap all the time, that the top of his crown chakra has been cut off like the bottom of the skullcap, and the Divine energy is intensely pouring in through it. Muktananda referred to this continual pranic pulsation of the crown chakra when he occasionally mentioned in public lectures that he breathed through the sushumna. Adi Da refers to his transcendent shift to a central vortex energy predominance and the absorption of the basic chakra energy into this central vortex, when he describes an experience in which he felt that the topmost part of his crown chakra was severed and the life current, another name for Kundalini, was no longer bound to the chakras as a necessary structure.[4] This experience of crown chakra severing and subtle cosmic pranic pulsation is a direct inner and outer total transcendent harmonic connection with the pure cosmic vibration. It is but another reminder of our True Formless Reality. It is the ultimate food for transcendence. It is the delicacy of Spiritual Nutrition. It is food from God and the energy of God as God. The unitary Kundalini vortex is so energized by the cosmic prana that we are transformed into shining vortex bodies of Light. It is a basis for understanding the subtle meaning of Exodus 34:28–29: "He was there with the Lord forty days and forty nights; he did neither eat bread, nor drink water.... When Moses came down from Mount Sinai with the two tables of the testimony in Moses' hand, Moses knew not that the skin of his face sent forth beams while He talked with him."

This physical transcendence is not necessarily the goal of spiritual life as much as it represents a total freedom to follow God's Will. In any case, whatever happens, it is enough just to Be.

Summary, Chapter 12

1. Transcendence is the extension of regeneration. It is the evolutionary process by which the SOEF organization of the body reaches a more organized and higher level of energy in which the physical matter of the body is transmuted, or is in the process of being transmuted, to its etheric level. It is the physical parallel to the transmutation of our consciousness.
2. The process of transcendence begins with the awakening of the Kundalini.
3. A central Kundalini vortex of energy is the central mechanism for drawing up energies from more dense states to less dense states. It has enough energy to initiate this function after the awakening of the Kundalini.
4. If we eat high-energy, light, biogenic foods, the Kundalini vortex is more energized and thus more active in transmuting us from matter to energy.
5. The closer we move to pure prana in our foods, the less dense our physical system becomes. This facilitates the process of transcendence.
6. Heavier foods and meats slow the vortex energy and slow the transcendence process.
7. Mental and emotional stress also slows the process.
8. At the time when the two Kundalini energies completely fuse into one central energy, the Kundalini vortex becomes the body's main energy center. It draws energy from the chakras into its higher vortical transcendence.
9. After this time, there is only enough energy and form left in the chakras to maintain the physical body.
10. Once this Kundalini vortex becomes the predominant energy system for the organism, the pure prana entering through the crown chakra becomes a most important source for energizing the system. In some, it may be the only source. These people are dining on the direct nectar of God. This is the ultimate Spiritual Nutrition.

PART II

THE SPIRITUAL NUTRITION PARADIGM

Introduction

The Spiritual Nutrition paradigm fills a gap in the meaning and value of nutrition. It honors and describes the purpose of nutrition, not in terms of health per se, but in terms of how it affects and amplifies the evolutionary unfolding of the spiritual Being. From this perspective, we clearly have an opportunity to think about nutrition in a different way. We begin to understand that what we eat affects the quality of the functioning of our mind, whether our mind is noisy, quiet, at peace, or irritated. Our food choices and the way we lead our lives (including the Six Foundations) are both the cause and effect of our diet and lifestyle. Our food choices reflect our state of harmony with ourselves, the world, all of creation, and the Divine. This view of nutrition is part of a core understanding of what it means to live an integrative, harmonious, and peaceful life on this planet.

In this section, we see how our spirit, our mind, our emotions, our body, and even our genetic expression are affected by the food we eat. Spiritual Nutrition expresses a new paradigm in nutrition and assimilation. This section is an in-depth approach to the psycho-emotional and spiritual aspects of developing an optimal diet for spiritual life. It is a wholeness approach to diet that explores the larger planetary implications of what we eat, including the effects on the ecology, conserving natural resources, world hunger, and world peace, as well as the ethical, moral, and spiritual issues related to diet. The author feels that not only is the vegan, live-food diet the diet of choice for spiritual evolution, but it is the dietary part of the blueprint for enhancing our Communion with the Divine, and for ushering in the age of spiritual Enlightenment. Without the context of the other five Foundations, however, it can result in an imbalanced ego state.

Although one cannot eat one's way to God, the Spiritual Nutrition dietary approach of an individualized, organic, vegan, live-food, high-mineral, low-glycemic, well-hydrated, sattvic (holy), moderate-intake diet prepared with Love is a powerful aid in the process of spiritual evolution.

From the perspective of spiritual life, each of these aspects of diet are examined. Discussion includes the importance of eating live food and how live food is not only the most powerful diet for our spiritual life, but is also vital in communicating with our genes and improving or upgrading the genetic expression to the highest quality of health. We also examine the power of undereating and Spiritual Fasting in the activation of gene expression and turning on anti-aging and longevity genes, as well as enhancing spiritual life. In this section we begin to understand the importance of minerals as frequencies of Light for expanding consciousness. It includes a new understanding of living water in our diet in terms of bringing energy and hydrogen ions into the system. The importance of a low-glycemic diet is discussed. The Rainbow Diet is revisited and we now have, from a phytonutrient approach, an additional way to understand the Rainbow Diet. In addition, for the first time, Ayurvedic principles have been used to develop a whole new level of insight into live foods and more sophisticated ways one can remain balanced and grounded on live foods by using the principles of Ayurveda. The somewhat controversial issue of the importance of B_{12} in a vegan, live-food lifestyle is addressed in a way that makes it very clear that in order to create a healthy, vegan world, we must include, at this point, some natural B_{12} supplementation.

In essence, Part II outlines a conscious approach to an evolutionary diet for enhancing the flow of Kundalini and supporting the process of spiritual Liberation. Not only do we eat to enhance our Communion with the Divine, but we eat as a way of waking up to a new evolutionary state of the Liberated Being.

Chapter 13

The Need for a New Nutritional Paradigm

Through our explorations in Part I, we have begun to see that the modern materialistic-mechanistic view of life falls significantly short of supporting the expanded concept of the human organism as having subtle energetic and spiritual qualities. We have established the human organism as a spiritual superconductor and this illuminates the need for a new paradigm or model that can account for and support this expanded view of the human organism. But, first we need to understand the limitations of the modern materialistic-mechanistic paradigm if we are to be fully able to evolve a new paradigm that reflects the amazing insights that we are gaining about life.

Once we understand the shortcomings of the modern paradigm, then we will be ready to set forth the new paradigm – Spiritual Nutrition – as one that feeds the whole person – body, mind, and spirit. Spiritual Nutrition does not throw away the contemporary paradigm but rather includes it as part of the whole.

Confusion of the Conventional Paradigm

The conventional paradigm of life (and nutrition) has developed from the materialistic-mechanistic view of life, in which living organisms are regarded as physiochemical machines. All the phenomena of life, including nutrition, are thought to be explained solely in terms of physiochemistry. Although the materialistic-mechanistic paradigm has led to a certain amount of success in understanding the molecular structure of our food and bodies, the tremendous diversity of opinions in the nutritional world today suggests that we have not developed a comprehensive understanding of the basics of nutrition. The great twentieth-century mystic, Ramana Maharshi, once said that the most important thing in spiritual life, in addition to meditation, is to eat correctly. This sounds simple, but if we look in our bookstores, there are so many different books on nutrition that the simple act of eating seems quite perplexing. At the Tree of Life Foundation, the author, in his role as teacher and medical practitioner, has observed many people coming with so much confusion about deciding what is right to eat, based on all the different theories, that they have anxiety attacks at mealtime.

There are only three gross substances that we consciously take in to support our life process: food, air, and water. In the past, breathing and drinking water did not take much thought. Before the days of air and water pollution, it was fairly automatic. Food, on the other hand, consumes a lot of our time. We forage in the supermarket or health food store for our food, then we have to gather it, prepare it, bless it, eat it, and digest it. We must also grow it or earn money to buy it. By the time this process is completed, we ought to have a unique understanding of and relationship to our food. Yet in the last 200 years, for most of us, this relationship has remained a mystery. It is especially mysterious when we think about nutrition for the enhancement of our spiritual life. Why is it that we have lost touch? Why is it that we are stumbling around in the forest of nutrition, bumping into the trees representing this new diet or that new supernutrient that will solve all our health problems? Presently, if we are concerned at all, perhaps it ought to be with the loss of our basic instinctual connection with the quality of our food and Mother Earth. With the overload of so many new discoveries in the "science of nutrition," there are so many diverse factual details that we cannot fully keep up with what and how to eat. Our basic conceptual frameworks, our perceptions of the meaning of nutrition, and our own natural instincts have become muddled. We cannot see the forest through the trees.

Basics of the Conventional Materialistic-Mechanistic Paradigm

Where did we start to limit our understanding? A major cause of this confusion about the purpose and function of nutrition is the present exclusive materialistic-mechanistic viewpoint that developed during the late 1780s, when the chemist Lavoisier established the doctrine that life is a chemical function and foods are the combustibles. Food is the vehicle for the intake of calories. The materialistic-mechanistic view, which is still predominant today, was very simple then. The complete process of nutrition was considered a combustion process in which foods were seen as carriers of caloric energy, which, in conjunction with oxygen, is released in the digestive process. One needed simply to count the calories needed and select nutrients with the matching number of calories.

Since the 1780s, we have discovered that nutrition is more complex than simply calories. Food has additional factors – proteins, carbohydrates, fats, vitamins, minerals, micronutrients, enzymes, subtle hormone factors, alkaloids, auxones, pacifarins (natural antibiotic substances), thousands of phytonutrients, and whatever new microfactors have been or will be discovered. These new discoveries have only reinforced our materialistic-mechanistic conceptions of food and the human system. Many people are still holding tightly to the caloric approach of Lavoisier. Calorie counting is still in vogue today.

Lavoisier, who is considered by many to be the progenitor of modern chemistry, also contributed another of the major principles of the presently accepted nutritional paradigm. It is called the Law of Conservation of Matter and Energy. This law states that nothing is lost; nothing is created; everything is transformed. The atom was considered the smallest particle of matter and a constant in Nature. From this law it was assumed that no element could be created and no atom could disappear in Nature. Except for the later observation that this does not hold true for radioactive materials, we are still trying today to comprehend nutrition from the exclusively materialistic-mechanistic point of view. The result of this conceptual approach is an excessive and unbalanced focus on individual nutrients and their interactions. This nutrient-supernutrient focus has served to lock us into materialistic conceptions about food, the human system, and the interrelationship between the two.

The next major step in the development of nutritional materialism took place in 1847, when four great scientists – Helmholz, Dubois-Reymond, Brucke, and Ludwig – met in Berlin to put physiology into a physiochemical foundation. They proposed that the laws of chemistry could completely describe the process of human physiological function. Since this historical turning point, the Law of Conservation of Matter and Energy has been the foundation of physiology, metabolism, and nutrition. It has led to the establishment of quantitative research methods and to the implicit acceptance of the Laws of Thermodynamics as a description of the functioning of the living organism. From this sort of thinking came the popularly accepted statement, made by Ludwig Feuerbach, that "man is what he eats." It is also the basis for the consumerism in nutrition we see today. People tend to consume excessive vitamins, minerals, and amino acids in the hope of making their bodies live longer, perform better, endure more, and be healthier. The implied motto is "more is better." It is the underlying assumption behind calorie counting, nutritional computer printouts, and fad dieting.

The focus on gathering nutritional capital is based on the inaccurate belief that nutrition is additive – that is, to be safe, extras of everything should be taken. This is not to say that, at the beginning of a health program, a person may not need extra nutrients to replenish deficiencies and to rebalance metabolism, but after a few months, as the person's health improves, he or she needs fewer nutrients to sustain good health. According to their particular life stress and biochemical individuality, people differ significantly on how much and what sort of supplementation they need. The author, in the last thirty-five years, has not examined one person who did not need some sort of supplementation.

It is important to note that not everyone has followed this limited materialistic-mechanistic approach. The late Paavo Airola, Ph.D., a significant nutritional mentor of the author's and a man whom many considered a nutritional genius, stressed a personal and historical approach in his consulting rather than a materialistic, computerized focus. Nutritional groups such as the live-food (raw food) movement, sproutarians, and now the holistic health movement, have all, at least indirectly, refuted the narrow materialistic conceptualization of nutrition. In these health movements there is an implicit assumption that we need to look at the subtle energy qualities of food and the human body. This awareness is shared by many healing systems around the world. In the ancient Indian sciences of Yoga and Ayurvedic medicine, for example, subtle body and subtle food energy is termed *prana.* In Chinese medicine it is called *chi.* It is known as *ki* in Japan, *mana* in Hawaii, *tumo* in Tibet, Odic force by Reichenbach, and orgone energy by Reich. The term prana, or Shekhinah energy, is associated with the vital life force in general and will be the main terms we will use.

The new paradigm is what this book is about. It states that food can no longer be seen only as calories, proteins, fat, or carbohydrates, or any material form. *Food is a dynamic force that interacts with humans on the physical body level, the mind-emotional level, and the energetic and spiritual levels. The study of nutrition is the study of the interaction with and assimilation of the dynamic forces of food by the dynamic forces of our total Being.* Before we develop this new paradigm of Spiritual Nutrition, it is important to clearly understand the fundamentals of the old materialistic-mechanistic paradigm.

Shaking the Pillars of the Conventional Paradigm

The materialistic-mechanistic paradigm is based on three principles. The first is Lavoisier's principle that nothing is lost, nothing is gained, and everything is transformed. This, together with the "Law" of Energy Conservation postulated by Mayer and Helmholz, has been refined as the Law of Conservation of Matter and Energy. The second principle is called the Second Law of Thermodynamics. It states that, in the course of Nature, all things break down to their most basic and stable forms, and the total energy in a system moves from more organized to less organized forms or states. This process is called entropy. There is a third implied belief that there is no essential difference between the interactions of substances inside the human body or outside the human body.

In the West, all three of these ideas have been challenged in the last 100 years. One group that attacked this paradigm is the Anthroposophical movement under the leadership of Rudolph Steiner. Steiner was a well-known turn-of-the-century European philosopher, educator, and scientist who stated that the greatest obstruction to understanding the effect of food on the human organism is what people have accepted as the "Law" of Conservation of Matter and Energy. He felt it contradicted the process of human functioning and development. In his lectures in the early 1920s, he insisted that the Second Law of Thermodynamics (the law of entropy) and the Law of the Conservation of Matter and Energy were not valid for what happens inside the human organism. This position is supported by scientists such as the physicist Louis de Broglie, who is considered to be the progenitor of wave mechanics. Louis de Broglie stated that "It is premature to suppose that we can reduce vital processes to the inadequate conceptions of physiochemistry of the nineteenth or even the twentieth century."[1] The deeper Kabbalistic teachings are that both personal and world spiritual evolution work by a process contrary to the Second Law of Thermodynamics.

Biological Transmutation

A significant work recently challenged the concept that the Law of Conservation of Matter and Energy applies within the living system in vivo, or "inside the skin." This work was done by a brilliant Frenchman, Louis Kervan, director of Industrial Hygiene Services, Vocational Diseases, and Industrial Medicine in Paris since 1946. Kervan has been a member of the New York Academy of Science since 1963, and has been on the UNESCO advisory council for scientific research. Since 1935 he has thoroughly documented the phenomenon of biological transmutation. Biological transmutation is the natural "alchemical" process that happens, to a greater or lesser extent, when one element in the body is transmuted into another element. This directly contradicts the Law of Conservation of Mass and Energy.

To better understand this very significant process, and to appreciate its historical and practical perspective, it seems best to look at some of the research that has led up to proof of the existence of biological transmutations. Modern research on the subject dates back to 1799, when the French chemist Vanquelin measured lime in the oats he was feeding hens, and found the hens excreted five times more lime than they took in. Vanquelin could only conclude that the lime had been created, but he could not determine the cause. Interestingly, this was only twenty years after Lavosier's work became public. In 1831, another Frenchman, named Choubard, measured watercress seeds for their minerals and measured them again after they had germinated in an insoluble dish (so that they could not have possibly gotten minerals from any other source). He found that the germinated seeds contained minerals that the seeds did not originally have. In 1875, von Herzeele carried the research with germinated seeds one step further by using a controlled nutrient medium. He concluded that a transmutation of elements had occurred. This work was updated by Baranger, Chief of the Laboratory of Organic Chemistry at the Ecole Poly Technique in Paris, who published results concerning the variations of phosphorous and calcium in germinated seeds. He also concluded that a transmutation of elements had occurred, but was unable to understand how it had happened.

In 1962, Kervan published his book *Biological Transmutations,* in which he describes transmutation as a phenomenon completely different from that of atomic fission or fusion in physics. He considers biological transmutation to be a phenomenon that has not been revealed in the era of modern science, a property that does not take place in the realm of either chemistry or physics. He strongly states that many of the biochemical and physiological processes of life are produced by chemical reactions. However, he refutes the beliefs that chemical reactions are the only processes that take place within the human body and that every observation must be explained in terms of a chemical reaction. Kervan does not reject the laws of chemistry. He does reject the attitude that the laws of chemistry must apply to every domain.[2]

To appreciate fully the meaning of his work and to adjust our minds to these new concepts, the author would like to share some of Kervan's research. Kervan's observations started as a child on his parents' farm in Brittany, France. He noticed that the chickens, which had no limestone in their diets, ate a great deal of mica, a component of silica. When the chickens were killed, one could never find the mica, but inside was lots of sand. Somehow, from all of the mica, they were able to make calcium shells. Later experiments showed that when the mica was taken away, the eggshells became devoid of calcium, and the chickens stopped producing eggs. When the mica was added back into the diet, they began to produce eggs again. The implication is that the mica contains some silicate of potassium, which is converted to calcium by biological transmutation.

In his research in the Sahara Desert, Kervan discovered that the workers ate an excess of salt and excreted far more potassium than they took in. This he observed to be a result of an endothermic reaction (a reaction which uses up heat in the body and therefore is cooling) of sodium plus oxygen becoming potassium ($Na_{23} + O_{16}$:=: K_{39}). (The symbol :=: means "transmutes to.") This then was another example of transmutation – sodium into potassium.

In another observation of biological transmutation, Kervan had noticed a continual production of saltpeter by the limestone walls in his own home. Researching this more closely, he discovered that calcium in the limestone was being converted to potassium (saltpeter) by subtracting a an atom of hydrogen through the enzymatic processes of the bacteria on the walls. In the hens, he had deduced that potassium from the mica was converted to calcium by the addition of a hydrogen $K_{39} + H_1$:=: Ca_{40}. With the limestone (Ca) transmuting to saltpeter (K), he was observing a reverse reaction.

Kervan also researched the black formations on the cave walls and the temples of Banteay Srei in Cambodia. He discovered that the black layer was 5 percent manganese and the temple rocks were 15 percent iron. This laid the foundation for the later proof in a controlled experimental setting that iron minus hydrogen converts to manganese.

Kervan has therefore found several different ways that calcium is created, through transmutation, by the combining of different atoms to make a larger calcium atom. Five chemical reactions to produce calcium proposed by Kervan are offered as evidence that transmutation occurs:

1. potassium and hydrogen-K_{39}+H_1+ specific enzyme :=: calcium Ca_{40}
2. magnesium and oxygen-Mg_{24} + O_{16} + specific enzyme :=: Ca_{40}
3. silicon and carbon-Si_{28} + C_{12} + specific enzyme :=: Ca_{40}
4. sodium and hydrogen-2Na_{11} + 2H_1 + specific enzyme :=: Mg_{24} magnesium and then repeat (2) to get calcium
5. sodium and oxygen-Na_{23} + O_{16} + specific enzyme :=: K_{39} potassium and then repeat (1) to get calcium

This leads to some of the potential clinical applications of his work. Kervan himself has done some research on the use of horsetail grass, which is high in silica (reaction 3), to speed up the calcification of broken bones. His research, using rats and some people, suggests that bone recalcification with silica seems to happen more efficiently than with a direct calcium supplement. In some people, bone decalcification may be caused by a deficiency of the enzyme that transmutes sodium to magnesium (reaction 4). If there is a deficiency in the enzyme that converts magnesium to calcium, then it might be advisable to strengthen the bones with potassium (reaction 1) and organic silica. We may also need to consider that decalcification may occur in some people when salt-free diets (reaction 5) are followed, since the sodium may be needed to transmute into calcium. Another implication of the transmutation work is that pregnant and lactating mothers who do not absorb calcium well might want to try supplementing their diet with horsetail silica, which might be more easily transmuted to calcium. According to Dr. Tru Ott, Angstrom Minerals™ have the highest probability of undergoing biological transmutations.[3]

People who are having trouble raising their blood iron with iron supplements might want to take manganese, as some people in France are doing, which transmutes to iron by a separate metabolic pathway. Kervan may be establishing the existence of a variety of secondary pathways, which the body can utilize via transmutation of elements when it is missing the enzymes or nutrients needed for the main pathways.

Kervan's basic explanation of biological transmutation is that, through the action of enzyme conversion within the living system, particles from one nucleus either combine with those of another nucleus to form a new element, or one nucleus of an element divides into two new elements.[4]

The scientific finding of biological transmutation is completely contrary to the Law of Conservation of Matter and Energy. It involves a process completely different from the process of chemistry, which deals with the displacement of electrons in the shell around the atomic nucleus. It is also different from the process of physics, which deals with fission and fusion and follows the Law of Conservation of Matter and Energy. Biological transmutation is the science that deals with the exchanges that occur between the nuclei of the different atoms in living organisms and results in the creation of new elements.[5] Kervan also points out that through the activity of biological enzyme systems, the process of biological transmutation consumes only one-millionth the energy of the same reactions when duplicated by nuclear physics in vitro (outside a living system).[6]

Nobel Prize laureate Szent-Gyorgyi has commented that biology is the science of the improbable, and physics is the science of probabilities.[7] We are also forced to consider the scientific position of Claude Bernard, who felt that when one is confronted with a fact that is in opposition to a prevalent theory, one must accept this fact and abandon the theory.[8]

The author has raised the issue of transmutation because a comprehensive theory of nutrition and its role in spirituality must include and be able to explain all "aberrant" observations. The current materialistic-mechanistic view cannot account for the observation of biological transmutation. The possible existence of biological transmutation directly challenges the Law of Conservation of Matter and Energy on which the materialistic-mechanistic paradigm is based.

The ramifications of the existence of biological transmutation are very great. Kervan felt that the light of biological transmutation may be a new guide to geologists, biologists, philosophers, and metaphysicians, helping them understand the creation and evolution of our planet.

For our purposes, we do not have to consider the whole evolution of our planet. It is enough to apply these concepts to the development of our new Spiritual Nutritional paradigm. It is significant that the concept of biological transmutation gives an added depth to understanding

Roger Williams's work on nutrition, *Biochemical Individuality.* The point he makes is that everyone has different biochemical needs and, therefore, unique nutritional needs.[9] We can connect biological transmutation with Roger Williams's work by seeing that these nutritional needs are determined by the amount of enzymes available for biological transmutations. Williams's work suggests that the functioning of everyone's cells is a very individualized pattern. It has been this author's consistent experience that the healthier a person becomes, the less supplementation he or she needs. The implication is that the stronger the vital force (health energy), the more energy and ability a person has to transmute. It also suggests that the individualized pattern of transmutation and nutritional needs can change.

If this principle of biochemical individuality is taken to its extreme, it is conceivable that there are some people throughout the world who no longer need to eat food, as is demonstrated in Chapter 8. The observations on biological transmutation provide one explanation for the observed phenomenon of inedia (breatharianism).

Challenging the Role of Entropy in Living Systems

The concept of entropy (reflected in the Second Law of Thermodynamics), as applied to the human system, implies that it is the natural order of things for the body to break down or age. Because of the degenerate lifestyles many people on this planet live, this is indeed the case. However, it is not the natural order of things. What may be more accurate is that what seems natural is unnatural, and what seems miraculous is natural. Kervan conceptualizes the issue of entropy in biological systems as essentially a struggle of the life forces against the degradation of matter.[10] Rudolph Steiner makes the point that one of the main purposes of a nutrient is to activate the dynamic forces in us that directly counter the process of entropy. The implication is that if we maintain our body's life force or body energy at a high level, entropy is indeed overcome, and we do not age. In our world, with all its pollution, we have created a lifestyle that allows us, with few exceptions, to reverse only partially this entropy or aging process. On a more rudimentary level, we can see that individuals who deplete their body energy with degenerate lifestyles tend to age more quickly. The author has noticed with clients at the Tree of Life that those who choose lifestyles and diets that increase their life force often seem to become younger and more vital in their appearance and functioning. Certain practices such as Spiritual Fasting visibly suggest that a youthing process is going on.

Further support for a system's ability to reverse entropy comes from the recent research by Richard Brewer and Erwin Hahn, reported in *Scientific American.*[11] They demonstrate that atomic systems that have decayed or undergone entropy from some ordered states can be induced to recover their initial order. This means a reversal of entropy has occurred. This is accomplished by reversing the motions of some of the particles in the disordered system in such a way that they can remember their original condition or pattern. This is called atomic memory phenomena. Brewer and Hahn support the belief that entropy can be reversed, in certain circumstances, both outside of living systems and within living systems.

The main fallacy, however, in applying the Second Law of Thermodynamics to a living system is that it only holds in a closed system (a system in which energy and matter are neither moving in nor moving out), or in a system formed of elements that are independent of each other. In general, not only can we say that the human system is not a closed system, but through the understanding of modern quantum physics (Bell's theorem) we can say that there is nothing in the universe that does not affect everything else. With this awareness we must conclude that everything is an open system. It can therefore be said that the application of the Second Law of Thermodynamics, or the process of entropy, does not apply with complete accuracy to human systems. Kervan writes that it is not difficult to see that life itself works in complete opposition to the law of entropy.[12] He asks key questions that lead us to developing some elements of our understanding of Spiritual Nutrition. Why is life in complete opposition to the force of entropy? What is the secret? How are human systems able to reverse entropy naturally and therefore not be slaves to the process of entropy?

Summary, Chapter 13

1. The conventional materialistic-mechanistic paradigm of nutrition is focused on the component, additive, and interactive effects of material properties such as calories, vitamins, proteins, and minerals. It is based on three shaky pillars: (1) the applicability of the Law of Conservation of Matter and Energy to living systems; (2) the applicability of the Second Law of Thermodynamics to living

systems; and (3) the belief that there is no essential difference in the interactions of substances inside or outside of the human body.

2. Contemporary scientific findings such as the discovery of biological transmutations, the inability of this conventional paradigm to account for "aberrant" phenomena, and our own intuitive awareness directly challenge this materialistic-mechanistic concept of nutrition as the sole way to understand nutrition.
3. The new nutritional paradigm – Spiritual Nutrition – does not throw away the physiochemical paradigm, but instead interfaces with it at the level of the material body. The materialistic-mechanistic view regains validity as part of an emerging dynamic system.
4. A new paradigm of Spiritual Nutrition is evolving which describes nutrients as a dynamic force that interacts with humans on the physical body level, the mind-emotional level, the energetic level, and the spiritual level.
5. The study of nutrition is the study of the interaction with and the assimilation of the dynamic forces of a nutrient by the dynamic forces of our total Being.
6. The new paradigm is crucial to understanding the relationship between nutrition and spiritual life.

Chapter 14

Perspectives on Diet

The purpose of the remainder of the book is to outline the specific aspects of Spiritual Nutrition that will aid the reader in mapping out an individualized diet that is in harmony with the spiritual and energetic view of the human organism and that enhances the process of spiritual unfolding. This is not a search for the perfect diet, because the only thing that is perfect is beyond the body-mind-I AM complex – the Truth of the Self, the Truth of God in All and as All. We already are this perfection, but we have some blocks that keep us from consistently experiencing this Truth. The perfect diet cannot even make us 100 percent healthy because, although diet affects the mind and the spirit, its primary effect is on the physical body. For diet to be truly effective, it needs to be in the context of a full spiritual life of meditation, good fellowship, right life, Loving our neighbors as our True Selves, and continual Love Communion with God – in other words, the Six Foundations. On one hand, diet is a powerful discipline that can help us balance our bodies, minds, hearts, and lives in general. On the other hand, diet is an expression of our state of Beingness and of our harmony with the universal laws of creation.

The author's intent is to supply enough perspective so that we will be interested in creating an individualized diet that reflects our highest state of awareness and is totally appropriate to our function in the world. This is not so easy because food is the principle interface, on a physical level, between Nature and ourselves. The appropriate eating of food is a means of extracting energy from our environment in a harmonious way, and in today's world, this relationship has broken down, becoming mystified and confused. How else, for example, could we, on a national level, have approved the irradiation of fresh fruits and vegetables as a way of "preserving" them? This represents a complete break with Nature. What seems normal is abnormal and vice versa. It is as if we are banging our head against the wall. When we stop, we discover our headache is gone and it is easier to meditate. Meanwhile, modern technology is studying the physiology of how to live normally while banging our head against the wall. Because most people are normally banging their head against the wall, we are considered abnormal because we choose to stop. We are the funny ones eating "a birdseed-and-grass diet." It is difficult to change our program in the face of this social pressure and our old programmed habits and belief systems. Nevertheless, it is necessary to examine these patterns and be willing to abandon what is no longer appropriate for maintaining our experience of blissful Communion with God, our feeling of well-being, a balanced body energy, and nurturing the spiritualizing force of the Kundalini energy within. Diet itself is not *the* key to spiritual life, but it helps to open the door to Communion with the Divine. To live and eat in a way that enhances this Communion is the guideline.

Diet from the perspective of Spiritual Nutrition is not a religion or an obsessive form of searching for God. It is simply part of a balanced, harmonious life in attunement with the universal laws. The primary goal of Spiritual Nutrition is not a healthy body or longevity; these are by-products. *The primary goal is to eat in a way that helps us more easily nurture, hold, and become better superconductors of cosmic energy, so it is easier to energize the Kundalini spiritualizing force and experience the ecstasy of God within ourselves and in every interaction of our lives.* We develop our practice of Spiritual Nutrition so that when God calls we do not ask for another bowl of ice cream.

Creating our own individualized diet for spiritual life requires some artful intelligence in the application of the new nutritional paradigm and the general principles that are being shared. The process is real and basic, rather than esoteric. It involves some trial and error to see what works for us. *The criterion is simple: Eat what increases your experience of Love and Communion and let go of what diminishes this Communion.* It requires some sensitive attention to our daily life needs and to the general purpose of Spiritual Nutrition: *Instead of living to eat or eating to live, eat to intensify Communion with the Divine.* Let our hunger for the Divine be the overwhelming appetite and guide to our choice of diet. In Spiritual Nutrition, we eat consciously to feed our hungry souls.

Summary, Chapter 14

1. We cannot eat our way to God.
2. The Spiritual Nutrition diet manifests most powerfully in the context of the Six Foundations.
3. The basic guideline is: Eat in a way that increases God Communion and let go of what diminishes that Communion.

Chapter 15

Nutrients: The Many and the One

A New Definition of the Word "Nutrient"

"In the beginning was the word, and the word was with God, and the word was God." (John 1:1) This familiar quotation from the Gospel of John is a key to comprehending Spiritual Nutrition. One of its meanings is that all comes from God and is nourished by the God, or cosmic, force. This is the Ultimate Source of all nutrition. *This cosmic force, or prana, in various levels of density, is the basic nutrient for our bodies, and in this context all levels of energy available to us are considered nutrients.* This includes sunlight and all kingdoms – mineral, vegetable, and animal (not to be eaten, but to be nourished by their Love energy). Once we understand that various densities of prana are the essential nutrients for all life function, we are able to expand our definitions of nutrition and assimilation. It allows us now to appreciate a paradigm of nutrition that sees material food as just one level of energy density in the context of a larger spectrum of nutrients important for aiding our spiritual development (see the figure). It is through this knowledge that we can now understand Sri Nisargadatta's teaching that consciousness is the essence of food that has been digested.

In the Judeo-Christian heritage there are several indications of some who were able to live on the less dense energies. In The Forgotten Books of Eden, Enoch, after returning from his visit to heaven, is quoted as saying, "Hear, child, from the time when the Lord anointed me with the ointment of His glory, there has been no food in me, and my soul remembers not earthly enjoyment, neither do I want anything earthly."[1] In Exodus 35:27, it is said of Moses, "And he was there with the Lord forty days and forty nights; he did neither eat bread, nor drink water." In John

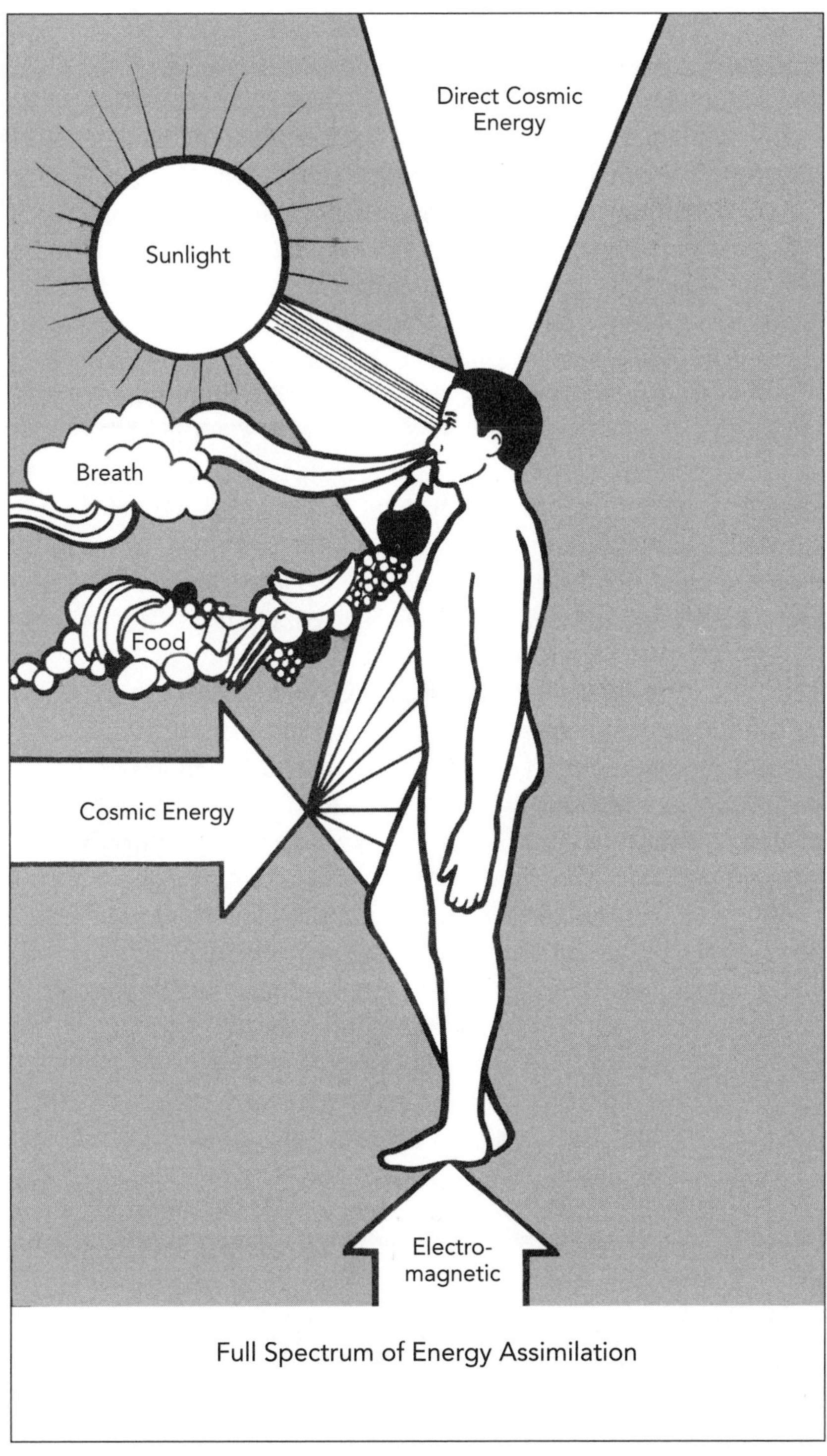

Full Spectrum of Energy Assimilation

4:31, when his disciples said "Rabbi eat," Jesus said to them, "I have food to eat which you do not know.... My food is to do the will of Him who sent me...." Recent documented cases of inedia include several examples of people who, aside from water, were able to maintain their bodies on the less dense, nonmaterial energies alone.

A foundation of the wholistic paradigm is: *Nutrition is what we absorb into our overall body-mind-spirit from the different density levels precipitated from the cosmic force.* It is this principle that allows us to explain how the system is not completely subject to both the Law of Conservation of Matter and Energy and the Second Law of Thermodynamics, or entropy. These two pillars of the old paradigm apply primarily for a system of energy absorption based on the assimilation of solid food as the only source of nutrition. Kervan's work on biological transmutation showed that these laws do not hold (as described in Chapter 14). This does not mean that we should discard the materialistic-mechanistic paradigm because it explains many things strictly on the material level. Rather, it should be included as a limited part of our wholistic paradigm.

The Nutrient of Pure Cosmic Energy

There are many major avenues through which different levels of energy are assimilated into the system. At the top of the head is the crown chakra. It is the only place in the whole system that can directly take in pure, unprecipitated cosmic energy. Initially this point of assimilation plays only a small role in the total energizing of the body, but at more progressed levels of the spiritualizing process it becomes an increasingly important source of energy. After the merging of the Kundalini in the crown chakra, it reaches its maximum importance. Muktananda refers to this as sushumna breathing, saying this is where he did his "real breathing." This pure prana moves down through the crown chakra, initially energizing the brain, the central nervous system, and the pineal and pituitary glands.

It is interesting to note that researchers have found that sunlight penetrates the skulls of chickens and directly stimulates their pineal glands. Dr. Richard Wurtman, in a *Scientific American* article "The Effects of Light on the Human Body," states that light is able to penetrate inside the brain of living sheep.[2] If sunlight can do this, it is feasible that the purer cosmic prana can also penetrate and influence our core brain structures. From there it moves down the spinal cord and sushumna. It has both a direct spiritualizing effect on the body-mind-spirit complex and an energizing effect on the chakras and their associated nerve plexus, endocrine glands, and organs. This downward spiritualizing energy is the spiritual Kundalini. As the system becomes a clear conductor of this energy, it is better able to energize the system and gain the potential to awaken the Shakti Kundalini stored in an inactive state below the base of the spine.

Stepped-Down Cosmic Energy as a Nutrient

The other portals of entry are avenues for stepped-down cosmic energy. This energy is the primary life force energy for activating and regulating the life functions of the body. One important way this life force enters the system is through the chakra systems after it is stepped down through the seven subtle bodies. The more synchronized these subtle bodies are, the more easily the cosmic force can pass through the subtle bodies and energize the system. The larger mind, or total ego, is the sum of the function of the seven subtle bodies. When it becomes harmonious, as during meditation, more cosmic energy is assimilated into the system. In this indirect way, we can say that *meditation is the key digestive process through which the life force is taken into the system.*

Delicious Sunlight

Another important source of the life force is sunlight. Light is the least dense form of prana in our universe. It carries the full spectrum of rainbow stimulation to our system as it filters through the subtle bodies and is taken in by nervous system receptors in the eyes and the skin. The nerve receptors in the eye translate this full-spectrum information into optic nerve impulses that conduct it to the various brain centers: pineal, pituitary, and the rest of the endocrine system. Through these systems it indirectly energizes and activates our whole organism and regulates body cycles and rhythms. It was once generally held that humans are immune from the cyclic hormonal regulating effects of light as seen in lower animals, in which the visible spectrum regulates the reproductive cycle and other daily and seasonal rhythms. Brody cites that research by Dr. Alfred Lewy, a psychiatrist at the National Institute of Mental Health, has disproved this assumption. He has shown that exposure to a bright light can turn off the production of melanin in humans.[3] He and others have done exciting research to show that light therapy is a specific treatment of choice for Seasonal Affect Disorder (SAD).[4] People with SAD become depressed as the days get shorter. They become irritable, sleepy, anxious, socially withdrawn, and disinterested in work and play. Exposing them to ultrabright lights three hours each morning and evening, or five hours in the evening, alleviated their symptoms in two to four days. Preliminary studies have suggested that when workers do not receive enough light or the right kind of light, they develop such problems as increased fatigue, decreased performance, decreased immune defenses, and reduced physical fitness. From the health point of view, Dr. Blackwell at Ohio State University found that worker productivity increased 11.7 percent when employees worked under full-spectrum (similar to sunlight) bright lights.[5] Dr. Hollwich of the University Augklinik in Munster, Germany found that fifty people blinded with cataracts experienced a reduction in amplitude of the adrenal and blood cell rhythms and in the basic regulatory system activity involving the hypothalamus, pituitary, and adrenal cortex.[6] When their cataracts were removed these abnormalities disappeared. Other researchers, such as Dr. Alain Reinberg in Paris, have discovered some strong indications that the menstrual cycle in women is also influenced by light.[7]

Clinicians and researchers such as Dr. John Downing (M.S. in vision psychology, Ph.D. vision science, and Ph.D. in optometry) are also discovering that light is broken down into different bands of the spectrum, each with a different healing effect. Dr. Downing, in a personal communication, has shared that the spectrum follows the basic chakra color spectral breakdown and that each of these colors activates different parts of the body.[8] He finds the most effective clinical application of this is accomplished by beaming one of several specific bands in the red spectrum through the eye to activate and heal different aspects of the sympathetic nervous system. For the parasympathetic nervous system, he has found that different bands in the blue color spectrum are healing. The specific band in either spectrum varies with each individual, because the sunlight-to-eye-to-optic nerve-to-brain-to-endocrine system represents a chain of colored light activation that parallels the specific color association with each chakra and its associated system. Illustrative of this color-to-organ and chakra association is the *Scientific American* article mentioned earlier, by the light research pioneer, Dr. Richard Wurtman.[9] He outlines the specific pathway for light as it affects the ovarian function in rats. Sunlight transmission moves through the optic nerve;

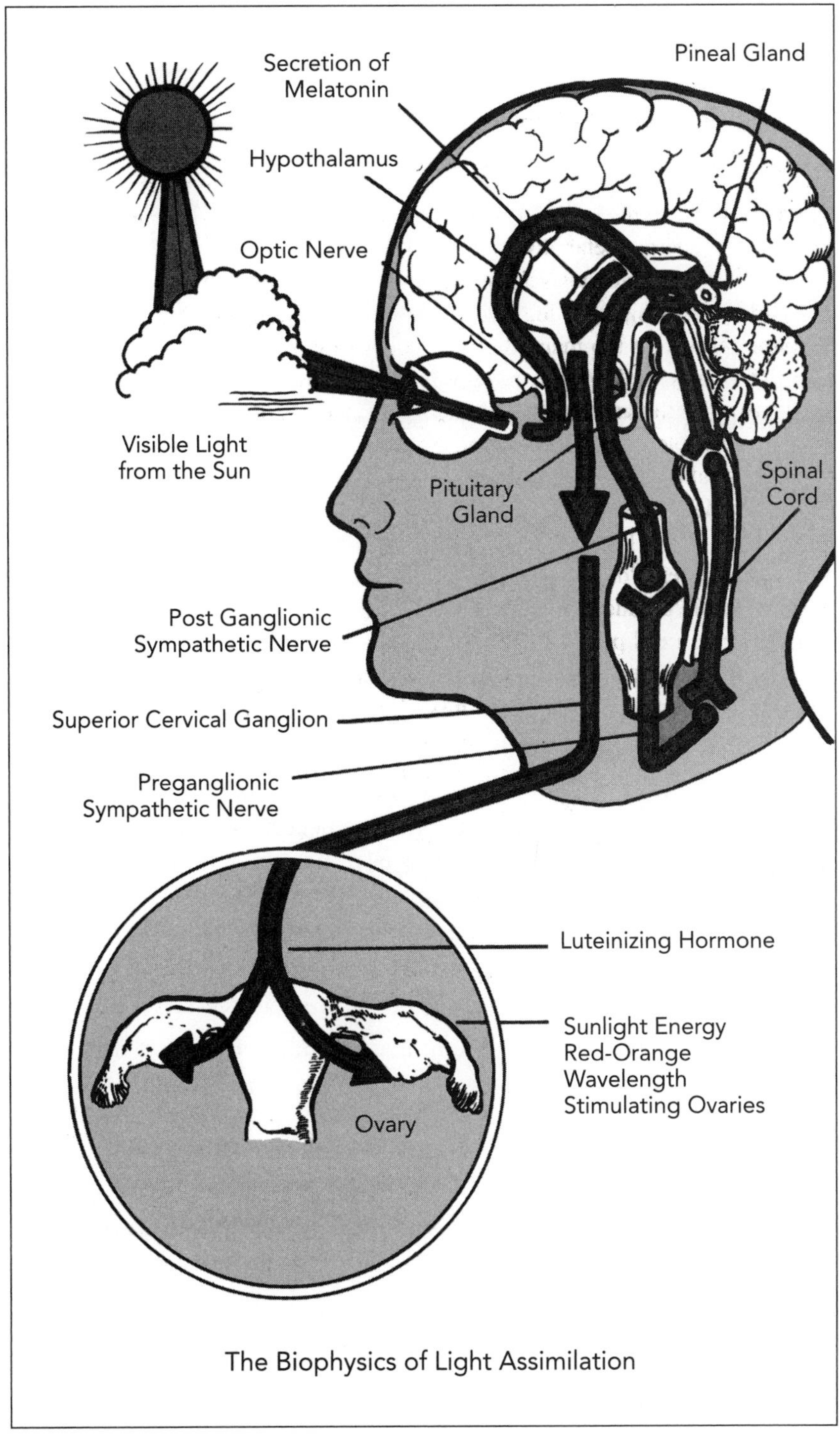

The Biophysics of Light Assimilation

part of it goes to the vision centers in the cortex, and part goes to the hypothalamus and superchiasmic nucleus, which is the body's internal clock. From there it travels to the spinal cord and up the superior cervical ganglion to the pineal, which sends hormonal messages to the hypothalamus, which then releases a hormonal message to the pituitary. Finally, the pituitary gland releases a luteinizing hormone to stimulate the ovaries (see the figure). Researchers have found that light in the orange-red wavelength specifically stimulates this ovarian cycle in rats. It is interesting to note that the sexual function is associated with the second chakra, whose primary color is orange.

Skin receptors take light in directly. Melanin in the skin, like the rods and cones of the eye, is able to absorb the radiant energy of sunlight and convert it to sound or vibrational energy and back again.[10] This energy can be transmitted as resonant energy or transformed into enough heat energy to affect metabolic processes, and, as we well know, sunburn. Sunlight energy is necessary for the production of vitamin D, and it regulates the production of melatonin, a neural hormone produced in the pineal. Research suggests that melatonin induces sleep, inhibits ovulation, and modifies the secretion of other hormones.[11] Frank Barr, M.D., has hypothesized that melanin is centrally involved in the control of almost all physiological and psychological activity.[12] Needless to say, the nutrient of sunlight directly affects us in many important energizing ways. It is possible that as our diet becomes more refined, sunlight subtly becomes an even more important source of direct life force. Currently it is estimated that humans need about thirty minutes of sun per day to maintain good health. During the summer it is best to sunbathe in the morning or late afternoon. During winter, sunbathing is best done at midday. Avoid using sunscreen during this time. Since a major entry point of sun energy into our system is through the eyes, it is best not to wear glasses, contacts, or sunglasses during this time. Although the eyes are the major entry point, the more we get a complete sunbath on our skin the more sun energy is absorbed. It is even possible that the red blood cell hemoglobin in our capillaries at the surface of the skin absorb sunlight directly, just as the chlorophyll in a plant does, and that these energized hemoglobin biomolecular structures could be directly taking this sunlight energy to the rest of our system.

"Vitamin O"

Another major source of nutrient energy is oxygen. In some modern Yoga teachings, it is said that approximately 90 percent of the energy utilized by the body is from oxygen taken in by the lung and skin systems. In the absence of oxygen, our physical bodies can only survive a few minutes. We can live without water for a few weeks and go without food for months. "Vitamin O" is our most important nutrient. This form of energy intake is the most commonly used meaning for the word prana. It is the life force that many experience when they walk into a forest and smile as they inhale the vibrant air. In forests and unpolluted bodies of water, the energetic field of the air has been enhanced. The oxygen molecule has been resonantly excited. When we take it into our lungs, its energy is transferred to our bodies. If the air has been circulated through air conditioning or air ducts, out of contact with the sunlight, polluted, or irradiated, it loses energy and less of this resonant life force is available to us. This oxygen energy comes into the lungs, which surround the heart chakra and act as a balancing point between the upper and lower chakras. Yogis and health practitioners in the West have observed that when the breath is steady, the mind becomes calm. This observation suggests an important link between the breath and the mind. Eighty percent of the oxygen we take in goes to the brain. This high degree of oxygen to the brain adds to the downward flow of the spiritual Kundalini energy and may partially explain how different pranayama exercises are used to excite the Kundalini.

Oxygen is also taken into our systems directly from our food. Steven Levine, Ph.D., has recently developed a hypothesis relating oxygen deficiency in the tissues (anoxia) to chronic disease, and a high rate of oxygen intake, relative to food intake, to good health.[13] In a simple analogy to a battery, he points out that oxygen is the positive terminal and that the foods we eat are a source of vibrant, negatively charged electrons. The electrons move from the negative pole, or food, in a living current of energy to the positive oxygen pole. Trace minerals, iron, manganese, zinc, and other electron carriers are essential for the conduction of this bioelectricity through the cytochrome oxidase system and through our antioxidant system. Vitamins A, C, and E, selenium, and various antioxidant enzymes such as superoxide dismutase and glutathione peroxidase serve to protect this electron energy flow from being disrupted by free radicals, which steal electrons from the system. These free radicals come from external pollution and from internal pollution that results from a poor diet that includes such things as irradiation-caused radiolytic foods. During this process of electron movement and transfer to the oxygen pole, metabolic energy is released, helping to fuel our normal metabolic processes. Optimal quantities of oxygen are required to draw this living current. On the other hand, it is important that we eat fresh, natural foods that are vibrant with high electron energy. These foods are those that still retain the high-energy carbon-hydrogen bonds that have incorporated activated electrons in their bonding as a result of electron activation from photosynthesis. It is this sunlight energy stored as activated electron energy in the carbon-hydrogen bonding that we find in organic, whole, live vegetarian foods. These foods make the most powerful current with the oxygen pole. This last statement implies the superiority of plant food over animal food. It is highly possible that the direct photosynthesis energy of the carbon-hydrogen bond is either altered or lost for humans when it is metabolized first by the animal, and that the animal gets all the benefit of the direct sunlight plant energy. With the current state of our ability to measure heat release from carbon-hydrogen bonds of plant and animal tissues, we may not find any perceptible difference in energy release on a material level. But subjectively, the difference is easier to perceive.

If there is a decrease in oxygen in the system, there is less power to pull electrons to the oxygen pole of our bioelectric current, and the bioelectric current diminishes in power. Therefore, our task is to maintain a high oxygen level in our tissues. In our polluted and stressful environment, this is not easy. We are starving for oxygen in our office buildings as we increase insulation to save fuel energy costs. The rapid planetary deforestation is decreasing the local supply of oxygen, air pollution combines with and ties up oxygen in the air, and the combustion of our automobiles and industries takes it from the local ground level atmosphere. Stress causes oxygen deficiency within the organism. For example, stress from toxic environmental substances in our air, water, and food uses oxygen for detoxification. Chemical pollutants, chlorine in water, and fumes from combustion of petrochemicals from our cars all require that we use our body supply of oxygen to protect us. Emotional stress produces excessive adrenalin and related adrenal hormones, which require oxygen for their metabolism. Physical trauma reduces circulation, and therefore the amount of oxygen to the cells is reduced. Bacterial, fungal, and viral infections require our body immune defense cells, the phagocytes, to produce controlled free-radical forms of oxygen to combat them. This cell-mediated activity is the main defense against many pathogens, including the yeast candida albicans.[14] Our activated immune phagocyte cells increase their oxygen utilization by as much as 50 times when they are destroying foreign invaders to our system.[15] This, of course, draws oxygen away from its main function, which is the oxidizing of our foods to produce metabolic energy.

Poor diet is another form of oxygen stress. Foods that are excessively acidic such as meat, coffee, carbonated drinks, and alcohol create acidity in the system. This acidity is an excess of hydrogen ions (H+) in the system, which deplete oxygen by combining with it to create water. In doing this, they short-circuit the system so that the full energy-producing movement of electrons going to the oxygen pole is reduced. When less oxygen is available for metabolism, there is a build-up of lactic acid, and our cellular environment becomes progressively acidic, resulting in the destruction of cellular function. According to Dr. Levine, hypoxia, or lack of oxygen in the tissues, is a fundamental cause of all chronic degenerative diseases.[16] Low tissue oxygen has been associated with candida albicans infections and the degenerative disease of cancer.[17]

Eating foods high in oxygen content seems to be associated with good health. Water is 85 percent oxygen, so we benefit by drinking water and eating foods with a high water content, such as fruits, which can be up to 90 percent water. The next highest oxygen-content foods are carbohydrates, which are slightly more than 50 percent oxygen by weight. This is computed by using the chemical formula for a carbohydrate, which is CH20. The molecular weight of carbon is 12, hydrogen is 1, and oxygen is 16. These foods are vegetables, grains, seeds, and nuts. Seeds and nuts have fats and proteins that lower the oxygen content, but are still high in complex-carbohydrate content. For example, sesame seeds have three times the carbohydrate content of red cabbage, mung bean sprouts, green snap beans, and many other fruits and vegetables.[18] Proteins contain an average of 25 percent oxygen. Fats have the lowest oxygen content, an average of about 12 percent. Although we need some unsaturated fatty acids for cell membrane formation, they steal oxygen. Another problem with fats, especially animal fats, is that most pesticides, herbicides, and other environmental toxins are fat soluble, so they increase our environmental toxin load and divert body oxygen for detoxification. For these reasons it is better to consume foods that contain essential fatty acids rather than nonessential fats. Avocados and sesame seeds are examples of these beneficial fats. We need 10–15 percent of foods that contain high amounts of unsaturated free fatty acids.

It is important to get the right ratio of oxygen-to-food density. Dense foods are those which have a high molecular weight and therefore are physically heavy for their size. Dense foods in this context also refers to foods, such as fats, which require a lot of oxygen to break them down completely for our oxidative energy metabolism. Fatty foods are the densest by these two criteria. Concentrated proteins such as meats, fish, and fowl are the next densest. They are like putting a big log in the fire; they require much energy to ignite and burn. If we eat too many dense foods, we run out of oxygen to oxidize them efficiently and we get more free radical by-products as part of the metabolism.[19] With an excessive fat-to-oxygen ratio in the system, the oxygen supply is disrupted and diverted and we see the formation of toxic oxygen compounds called "oxitoxins," which include free radicals and lipid peroxides. Lipid peroxides are incipient free radicals. This appears to be the mechanism that explains how a high-fat diet results in cardiovascular disorders. Proteins, in excess, represent "dirty fuel" and require excess oxygen to help us eliminate their nitrogen by-products. Proteins are not really designed for energy production, but we do need proteins for their essential amino acids. Again, we have to find a balance, and 10–15 percent protein in the diet may be quite sufficient for the optimal protein-oxygen mix. Carbohydrates are the best foods to eat for energy production because they burn evenly and require less oxygen to extract the metabolic energy from them; they are the small logs in the fire that burn easily. This awareness has already seeped into athletics and fitness; athletes regularly practice carbohydrate loading to maximize energy for competition.

Research in Japan by Kazuhiko Asai, Ph.D., has shown that an unusual mineral oxide called organic germanium greatly increases the supply of oxygen to the system and catalyzes many of the detoxification functions of oxygen.[20] Asai has found germanium to be of much help in treating cancer, hypertension, endocrine insufficiency, asthma, and Raynaud's disease.[21]

Other ways to increase the oxygen in our systems include placing more green plants in our workplaces and homes and doing moderate aerobic exercise five times per week. This can be anything from fast walking to sacred dance for approximately 20 minutes per session. We can also use antioxidant supplements or eat foods high in both the antioxidant vitamins A, C, and E and key antioxidant enzyme cofactors such as zinc and selenium. Such foods include blue-green algae, wheatgrass, seeds, nuts, and complex carbohydrates.

Breathing Exercises

One of the most important ways to increase oxygen in the system is through breathing exercises. Over thousands of years, Yogis have developed breathing exercises (pranayama) to energize the system, to calm the mind for meditation, and to activate the Kundalini energy directly. This subject is too vast for this book, but there are some simple breathing exercises that will greatly enhance our "Vitamin O" intake. The purpose for these exercises is to help us become aware of how to take a full breath and how to get a full oxygen meal. We breathe all day to stay alive, but most people are using only about 10 percent of their breath capacity. When up to 90 percent of metabolic energy comes from breathing, it merits at least some of the attention we pay to eating our physical food.

Exercise 1: Deep Breathing in All Segments of the Lungs

1. Place your hands at the diaphragm level with little fingers on the lower edges of your rib cage. Inhale into the area that is covered by your hands. This fills the lower lobes of the lungs. Sometimes it is thought that abdominal breathing, in which we move the diaphragm in and out, is filling the lower lungs. This is not the case. The lower lobes extend to the bottom of the rib cage, not into the abdominal cavity. To fill the lower lobes, it is best to focus on the lower rib cage.
2. Breathe in with the sound of an AAH in your mind and exhale with the audible sound of AAH. One benefits maximally if both the inhale and exhale are to the count of seven.
3. Repeat this three times.
4. Place your hands over your breast area and inhale. As you inhale, feel the resonance in your lungs as the middle lobes fill.
5. Inhale to the sound of UUU in your mind and exhale with the audible sound of UUU. Again, inhale and exhale to a count of seven.
6. Repeat three times.
7. Place the thumb part of your hand over your collar bone and inhale into the area under your hands, filling the upper lobes.

8. Inhale to the sound of MMM in your mind and exhale with the audible sound of MMM. Each inhale and exhale is to the count of seven.
9. Repeat this three times. In all three of these inhalations, try to expand your lungs as far as possible.
10. After you have practiced each breath for three rounds each, do three cycles of the breaths in sequence to make a complete AUM (OM) sound with each breath.

As we work with our breath, certain emotions may come up. In some of the Ayurvedic medical teachings anger, hate, and envy are said to be held in the lower lobes. The middle lobes are said to store the emotions of attachment and greed. Fear, sadness, and grief are said to be stored in the upper lobes.

Exercise 2: A Full Breath Rhythmical Cycle

This is the application of the Exercise 1 breath to a breathing cycle. It can be done for six to twenty minutes; a good average is fifteen minutes. It provides a complete oxygen meal. Because many people become energized with it, the best time to do it is in the morning or after returning home from work. If you do it before going to bed, you may become too energized to fall asleep immediately. It is also good for reoxygenating after prolonged time in low-oxygen atmospheres such as air travel.

1. Sit comfortably in an upright position, with your spine straight.
2. Begin the Exercise 1 breath with two counts of time in each lobe position, for a total of six counts on the inhalation. At the end of the inhalation, hold your breath for three counts, and then exhale over six counts. As with the inhalation, there should be two counts for each section of the lung.
3. At the end of the exhalation, hold for three counts and begin again.

The cycle is six counts inhalation, hold for three, and then six counts of exhalation, hold for three counts, and begin the cycle again. Once the timing becomes natural, you do not have to count.

In this exercise, do not force your breath. It is better to inhale and exhale in a relaxed way.

If the air is not too polluted, this exercise is best done outdoors.

With the incoming breath, think about taking in positive energy; with the exhalation, think about discharging negative energy or negative thoughts from your system.

Sexual Energy

One of the most important energies to be considered is sexual. It is both an internal and an external energy. The subject of sexual energy is too vast to ignore or explore in depth in this book. But there are some clarifying points needed for a balanced perspective. As an internal energy, it is stored in its raw physical form in the sperm and egg. The Tao calls this energy form *ching*. Sexual energy is a special form of what the Taoists call chi, or prana. It is powerful enough to recreate a total human organism. It is estimated that in a lifetime of the healthy male enough semen is produced to generate a trillion human lives.[22] When this energy is activated, all the senses are enhanced and men and women feel sexual energy as power or passion. The sperm and egg cells begin to vibrate and create an increased field of sexual magnetic energy. Most of us have experienced this. In the springtime, when Mother Nature is sending off the energy of creation, these sexual cells and sexual energy resonate with her and increase their energy fields.

When we are in good health, sexual energy is always regenerating for us to use. In Taoist teachings, sexual energy and cell production consume 25 to 40 percent of the raw energy taken in through food, sun, Earth, air, and other subtle systems. Every organ and gland contributes nutrients and energy from their SOEFs to produce the sexual seed. In men particularly, excessive loss of semen depletes the total body system of its most precious nutrients. Although men are usually the focus of this concern, the author, in clinical practice, has found a close correlation between the health of the women, their level of sexual energy, and their fertility. A physically depleted female will often complain of low sexual energy and will have difficulty becoming pregnant.

Sexual relations between two people who are in Love, especially if there is not excessive loss of semen, is a powerful way to replenish and balance the sexual energy. There are a variety of books on this subject. *Taoist Secrets of Love* by Mantak Chia is particularly clear on this subject. It is important to increase our ching, or sexual energy, because it can be transformed into creative and spiritual energy. In our Freudian-Reichian culture, the awareness of transformation of sexual energy into creative work and even spiritual energy has also been established. The

Taoists teach that sperm energy is subtly mixed with the prana or chi of the vital organs and refined into spiritual energy. Sexual energy is considered an intermediary link between the raw biological energies and our spiritual energy. This energy is always being transformed automatically and voluntarily into creative and spiritual energy. Yogis also teach that sexual continence aids the evolutionary power of the Kundalini. It has been my experience that there are certain times in the unfolding of Kundalini in which this is more important than others. The process of the Kundalini unfolding usually lets people know automatically when it is the correct time to be celibate. Self-imposed sexual repression as practiced by such diverse groups as Christian and Hindu monks, Yoga renunciants, and striving, excessively disciplined couples on the spiritual path may actually block spiritual unfolding physically, emotionally, psychically, and mentally. In many couples who have imposed this discipline upon themselves as an external practice, it often causes a certain amount of stress and relationship imbalance, which wastes more energy than it might gain. In the monks, priests, and renunciants, the sexual repression often causes personality imbalances and hypocritical sexual activity. Newspaper stories and lawsuits about the Catholic church have emphasized this point.

There is a way to maintain the natural flow of Love energy on the spiritual, mental, emotional, and physical levels without causing the problems of sexual repression and sexual imbalance. The way is to let go of our false concepts of the way things should or should not be, including the issue of celibacy. A survey by Jack Kornfield found that of fifty-four teachers of different traditions, thirty-nine had sexual relationships as part of their lives.[23] The great modern-day saint, Sri Ramana Maharshi, pointed out to his disciples that although celibacy may be an aid, the real issue is where the mind is focused. He taught that the real celibacy is living in God; it is living in the awareness of the bliss of the Self. The main issue is where the mind is focused. He joked that a monk living in the forest thinking about being married is not different from a married person idealizing about being a celibate monk.[24] The question of whether the concept of celibacy is right or wrong is not the issue. Whichever way best helps to keep one's mind on the transcendental Self is the issue. Celibacy for people who are very undisciplined in their sexual lives can be a practice that will help them gain some control in their spiritual and personal life. There may be times in the unfolding of the Kundalini energy that it is best to be celibate temporarily. This then is not so much a conceptual practice, but an attunement to one's own energy flow and needs.

The way for a partnered person is moderation. Overindulgence in sexual life can deplete or imbalance our body energies. The other key word is *balance.* Some people, with their constitutional needs, are thrown out of balance by too limited sexual activity. For some couples, a frequent exchange of sexual energies may prove to be both balancing for each individual and for all the levels of their relationship. The medieval alchemists and Kabbalistic traditions emphasized the importance of marriage, because the sexual union creates a full cosmic cycle that helps maintain the energetic and spiritual balance of the aspirants. The balanced exchange of sexual energy between two equally evolved spiritual partners can be a powerful way to co-commune with God. Both male and female will be energized by such a divine exchange. Certain Taoist or Tantric approaches that allow for the exchange of sexual energy and Love between two people and yet which conserve the semen may be the middle path that is needed for balance. In the Taoist teaching, these practices are best done as an expression of Love between two people in a long-term Love relationship rather than as a sexual technique to increase spiritual energy.

A major difference between sexual energy and raw energy such as food and sunlight is that sexual energy is created and stored within our own bodies. We can draw on it at any time. Sexual energy is a more refined energy because it is made within our system so it is easier to absorb and utilize than our raw energy sources, which first must be assimilated into our energetic systems. In the transmutation and refinement of sexual energy into spiritual energy, the path seems to be from the sperm and egg energy to the meridian energy, which brings it to the chakras. These refine it and transfer it to the Kundalini energy moving in the sushumna.

Energy from the Earth's Geomagnetic Fields

The electromagnetic field energy of the Earth is another source of energy input into our energetic system. It is usually absorbed through the feet. The Taoists describe a point on the sole near the upper center of the foot, called *yung-chuany,* through which it is specifically drawn up. Lying on the ground can also be a way of recharging. In the Essene and Taoist traditions, the earthly forces are thought of as rebalancing forces to the heavenly forces. The yung-chuany represents the roots of the Tree of Life penetrating into the Earth, or yang, forces with its branches extending to the heavenly, or yin, forces.

The Earth connection has an important grounding effect. With people whose Kundalini forces seem too strong, the author will often recommend working in the garden. When meditating, however, it is best to have an insulator such as a wool meditation pad between ourselves and the Earth, or the energy generated in meditation will be drawn off into the Earth. Recently, scientists have observed an Earth electromagnetic pulsation called the Schuman resonance, which pulses at 7.83 hertz per second. NASA discovered that when electromagnetic pulsing devices that recreate this Schuman resonance were installed in spaceships, the astronauts had less illness. Some people feel that one of the causes of jet lag is that we fly too quickly through the Earth 's magnetic field. Research using Schuman resonance pulsing devices to create a constant magnetic pulse in air travel has found that they decrease the incidence of jet lag. The author tries to spend a certain amount of daily time exercising barefoot on the Earth. It is a force of Nature about which we would benefit by having more knowledge. For example, recent Russian work on geomagnetic energies has shown that the growth of children varies with the geomagnetic area in which they live.[25] It is possible that geomagnetic forces have more effect on our energies than we can imagine.

The Densest and Tastiest Nutrient

Although our physical food is the densest nutrient and may only supply 10 percent of our energy needs, it occupies much of our interest. Before reading this book, the reader may have thought it was the only nutrient. We have been playing with our concepts of food for thousands of years. In the Spiritual Nutrition paradigm, it is important to ensure that the food we eat supports our spiritual lives.

Summary, Chapter 15

1. The ultimate nutrient is the God force or cosmic energy.
2. A foundation of the wholistic paradigm is that a nutrient is what we absorb into our overall body-mind-spirit from the different density levels of energy that have precipitated from the pure cosmic energy.

3. The pure cosmic energy is a primary nutrient that we all take into our system through the crown chakra. As our bodies are transformed spiritually, we become open to more of this pure energy.
4. Our system regularly steps down this pure cosmic energy into seven spectrums of energy through the seven subtle bodies. In this way the proper frequency of energy is directed to each of the seven chakras, which are the main intake portals for and are energized by condensed cosmic energy.
5. Sunlight is the least dense form of cosmic energy in our material universe. It is absorbed primarily through the eyes and the skin.
6. "Vitamin O" (oxygen) is necessary for the basic support of our physical bodies.
7. Sexual energy is absorbed in the loving exchange between two people.
8. Geomagnetic forces comprise a poorly understood source of energy, which primarily enters through our feet or any other direct contact with the Earth. They help us keep grounded. The density variations of the Earth's geomagnetic fields also have some unknown effects on us.
9. The tastiest and densest form of energy that we absorb is in our food. This is what we commonly referred to as nutrition before reading this book.

Chapter 16

Food for a Quiet Mind

Our food choices reflect the ongoing harmony with ourselves, the world, all of creation, and the Divine.

GABRIEL COUSENS, M.D., *CONSCIOUS EATING*

When Ramana Maharshi, one of the most famous Self-realized sages of modern India, was asked what the most important aid to meditation was, he replied a pure vegetarian diet. He quoted the ancient Chandogya Upanishad D II 26.2: "When food is pure, the mind is pure, when the mind is pure, concentration is steady, when concentration is achieved one can loosen all the knots of the heart that bind us."[1] Yoga tradition, as emphasized by the Chandogya Upanishad, teaches, "The mind is made of food." It says that the food we take in is divided into three parts: The gross part becomes excrement, the middle portion becomes flesh, and the subtle essence becomes the mind. So we cannot ignore the role of food in our consciousness, even if we are Enlightened like Ramana Maharshi. Ramana Maharshi is quoted in his book, *Be As You Are:* "Of all the restrictive rules, that relating to the taking of sattvic food in moderate quantities is the best; by observing this rule the sattvic quality of the mind will increase, and that will be helpful to self-inquiry."[2] Vegetarianism is one of the main pillars of purifying the mind. It is part of an ancient wisdom, which is also known as Sanatana Dharma, natural way to Enlightenment, or Yoga Dharma. It continues its importance in our modern times.

Yoga and the Kabbalah are spiritual paths that offer models for understanding the optimal nutrition for spiritual life. Traditionally, Yoga is taught as that which "links together" and is most commonly defined as

"Union with the Divine." The goal of prophetic Kabbalah, as with Yoga, is Deveikut, or God-merging. They are complete paths for establishing one's higher awareness. For this exalted purpose, Yoga requires controlling and silencing the mind, not simply developing bodily flexibility or moving and building prana. In Kabbalah, one goes beyond the mind to Chochma (the direct apperception of non-dual, subjective reality of God). The mind is not at all easy to control, as we all know from our ongoing stream of mental activity. The mind can most easily enter into silence only when it is pure, clear, and full of energy. Otherwise, it naturally falls into its normal pattern of disturbance.

We cannot look at the mind in isolation, either. The mind and body are organically interrelated and our bodily condition strongly influences how we think. Therefore, Yoga includes purification of the physical body as an aid to purifying the mind. The tremendous energy required for such inner transformation is provided by prana, through which we can access deeper levels of vitality through various pranayama (breath) techniques. The foundation of Yoga is purification or detoxification of body, mind, and prana. Although Kabbalah is more focused on purification of the mind, the need for a healthy body is recognized. The great Hasidic master, Israel Baal Shem Tov, who lived in the early 1700s, is quoted in *Tzava'at Harivash:* "When the body ails, the soul too is weakened, and one is unable to pray properly, even when clear of sins. Thus, you must guard the health of your body very carefully."[3] The great physician, rabbi, and philosopher of the twelfth century, Moses Maimonides, said "For it is impossible to understand the subject of wisdom and to meditate upon them when he is ill . . . the welfare of the soul can only be achieved after obtaining the welfare of the body."[4] A deep teaching about the importance of the body health on the spiritual path comes from Rabbi Yose, a Mishna sage of ancient times who said, "Let all your deeds be for the sake of Heaven." Pirkei Avos 2:17 (a highly respected Hebrew text) implies that all we eat and how we live is for the sake of Heaven. It affirms this one's principle guideline for diet for spiritual life, which is that *we eat to enhance our Communion with the Divine.* This teaching is current language that aligns with the teachings of the physician-rabbi-Kabbalist Moses Maimonides in his text *Hilchos De'os,* that we "must avoid that which harms the body and accustom [oneself] to that which helps the body become healthier and stronger."[5] In the ancient language, Moses Maimonides points out *we need a healthy body in order to have the energy to emulate the ways of the Divine.* Proverbs 11:17 says, "A person who does Chesed deeds (of Love) does good to himself." This ancient teaching can be interpreted that the good people do for themselves in terms of diet and lifestyle empowers them so they have the health, strength, and resources to give to others. *The basic teaching of Spiritual Nutrition is to eat and live in a way to enhance and sustain our Communion with the Divine for at least as long as it takes to be Liberated.*

Patanjali, in the Yoga Sutras, the classical compilation of the ancient Yoga school, defines Yoga as chitta vritti nirodha. *Chitta* refers to the mind in the broadest sense and includes the subconscious, conscious, and superconscious aspects of the mind. It is closely connected to prana, which is the energetic aspect of chitta. *Vritti* refers to mental activities of all types from physical to spiritual levels, from deep sleep to sensory perception. *Nirodha* means to inhibit, reduce, resolve, control, or eliminate. The practice of Yoga helps us reduce our disturbed thoughts and control our mental activities even at a subconscious level of sleep and dream. To achieve this requires extraordinary concentration, discipline, and work on all three levels of body, prana, and mind that can take years, if not lifetimes, to accomplish. From this perspective, *the optimal diet for spiritual life is that which stills the vrittis (activity of the mind).* This same principle holds true for moving from Binah (I AM consciousness) to Chochma (non-dual awareness of I AM THAT). I AM consciousness is Beingness; a subtle sense of the ego self. I AM THAT is when all sense of individual existence disappears and one is completely identified with the whole.

From this perspective, Yoga has two stages. The first is purification of body, prana, and mind in order to create a clear or sattvic mind. Stage one is the development of sattva. In Kabbalah, it is called kedusha, or holiness. Stage two is the transcendence of sattva to realization of the Self. However, only the pure or sattvic mind is considered capable of realizing the higher Self (Atman or Purusha) or Ein Sof in a lasting manner. In Yogic and Kabbalistic teachings, it is considered rare, if not impossible, to reach the second stage of Yoga or Deveikut without having mastered the first stage. It is easy to conceptually understand the state of Self-realization, the direct apperception of I AM THAT in which we realize that we are not the body-mind-I AM complex and there was never any lack of Union with the Absolute. While it is not rare to get a glimpse of it, to be able to abide in this state is the most difficult thing for all human beings. Lasting Self-realization is achieved by one in many millions of people. Few possess the sattvic or holy consciousness capable of holding any lasting Self-realization, even though it is who we are. Waking up is one thing, staying awake is another.

Enlightenment is the awakening to the Eternal Oneness that Was, Is, and always Will Be. It is the natural, eternal, changeless Truth of the non-dual awareness of the Ein Sof or Paramatman. In other words, *there is not and never was anything to attain.... We have been it all the time.* The purpose of the Spiritual Nutrition lifestyle is to awaken to I AM THAT ... to the cosmic ocean prior to the play of consciousness. It is to help us let go of the delusion that we are Yogis or Kabbalists seeking to attain Union with God. As with the author's teachings about live food ("If it's not broken, don't fix it"), Union was never broken, so it does not need to be fixed – or attained. We no longer need to live as a fish looking for water.

Most are unaware of the disciplined processes necessary for purifying the mind. This can be different from the Grace and subtle effort to transcend the mind, which does not itself require any special practice or complicated techniques. Some of us think that we can just jump into a state of Self-realization and don't need to deal with our prana, a body full of toxins, or a mind weighed down by sensory desires. Those who describe Yoga as a pathless path that requires no rules are correct if one is able to ignore stage one of Yoga, the creation of a stable, sattvic way of Being. In classical India, it was considered that only an extremely rare disciple was able to forego preliminary practices and go directly to Self-realization (anupaya). In the Kabbalistic tradition, it is expected that those who enter the practice are already married and living in an ever increasing state of holiness as preconditions. Shimon Bar Yochai spent eleven years meditating in a cave. Rabbi Yitzchak Luria (the Ari), the sixteenth-century mystic considered the greatest source of modern Kabbalistic understanding, spent six years meditating with his spiritual teacher and seven years meditating and studying in virtual silence, returning home only on the Shabbat, in the process of becoming Deveikut (God-merged). That we Westerners – raised in a culture of sex, materialism and ego, in love with the images and projections of our virtual reality minds – can just easily pop into permanent, non-dual states is a cruel and misleading illusion. It may be convenient to think that we can do away with any physical and mental disciplines and simply be naturally Self-realized in an instant, but it is like believing we are going to win the lottery, giving up our job and waiting for the check in the mail!

The life that produces an inward quiet sattvic/kedusha (holiness) state of mind and body is well defined in Yogic texts as a life based on meditation, chanting, pranayama, service, devotion, austerity, non-violence, asana (Yoga postures), and a sattvic (vegetarian) diet. The same is true in Kabbalah, but with more emphasis on holiness through prayer and mitzvot (practice of good deeds that align us with God and draw the Light). These are regarded as the preliminary way of life for the creation and sustaining ourselves in the sattvic holy state, which is the foundation necessary for Self-realization.

A synergistic view of nutrition is a part of what it means to live in an integrated, harmonious, and peaceful sattvic life on the planet. The body, emotions, mind, and spirit and even our hereditary expressions are significantly affected by what we eat. Sensory inputs from numerous objects, feedback from the motor organs, and other sensors in the body disturb us in many ways, consciously and unconsciously. The Yogic terminology for this disturbed condition of awareness is *vyutthita chitta,* or the disturbed (literally, "provoked") mind. Most of us who come to Yoga from our modern culture of sensation and physical, emotional, and mental stimulation are naturally in a condition of vyutthita chitta. *Samahita chitta* is the concentrated (collected) mind in which body, senses, prana, and mind all function in harmony. A sattvic or holy lifestyle that includes vegan diet, meditation, a balanced, loving, peaceful, non-violent life (ahimsa), right livelihood, and service creates a state of samahita chitta.

The Sattvic Diet

To understand the sattvic diet, it is first helpful to look at the classical descriptions of a sattvic diet. *Hatha Yoga Pradipika* (section 58), the main classical Hatha Yoga textbook, recommends avoiding "alcohol, fish, meat, curds, buttermilk, berries, oil, cakes, asafetida (hing), and garlic." It lists good foods for Yoga: grains, wheat, rice, barley, milk, ghee, butter, honey, dry ginger, cucumber, fine leafy vegetables, green garam (an Indian seasoning), and pure water. Sattvic food, according to the Bhagavad-Gita XSLL.8, is food liked by sattvic people, which promotes longevity, goodness, strength, health, happiness, and pleasure, and is juicy, rich, nourishing, and agreeable. Elsewhere in the Mahabharata, which is where the Gita comes from, the importance of not eating meat is emphasized.

Due to the quality of food production and preparation techniques in modern times, it is important to extend our definition of sattvic food. The equivalent of a traditional sattvic diet today consists of organic, whole, natural fruits, vegetables, nuts, seeds, and grains. A modern sattvic diet emphasizes foods grown in harmony with Nature by organic farmers, on good soils, ripened naturally, and prepared with an attitude of Love. Such foods carry the highest prana and consciousness. A modern sattvic diet does not include junk food, excessively spicy or salty foods, fried food, white flour, white sugar, and other forms of food that unnaturally stimulate your blood sugar or your mind. It avoids meat, fish, eggs, alcohol, highly caffeinated beverages, and often garlic and onion as well. It is careful about, but not necessarily exclusive of, dairy (see "The Place of Dairy Products" in Chapter 17). It does not include genetically engineered foods, irradiated foods, microwaved foods, foods that have been cooked more than twenty-four hours previously, or stale foods. Most restaurant-prepared and fast food would be excluded. The best is natural, organic food home-cooked or home-prepared with Love and consciousness or from organic restaurants based on such ideas.

Diet and the Mind

In Ayurveda it is established that certain foods affect the qualities of the mind in particular ways. These qualities or states of mind are latent in everyone. In Ayurveda they are divided into three categories, called *gunas*. Anyone who is in the physical body is subject to the subtle forces of the three gunas, which are called sattvic, rajasic, and tamasic. A sattvic state of mind is clear, peaceful, and harmonious. It is typified by the pure-living spiritual aspirant. The rajasic state is active, restless, worldly, and aggressive – the mental state of warriors and corporate executives. The tamasic state is lethargic, impulsive, cruel, and morally and physically degenerate. It is typified by our stereotype of the drug addict or thief.

Diet influences the state of mind, and the state of mind influences the diet choice. Members of the traditional warrior class would eat the rajasic diet because it stimulated their minds and bodies into a war-like state. Spiritual aspirants normally choose the sattvic diet and way of life. Consciously or unconsciously, people tend to choose the diet that reinforces and is reflective of their own mental and spiritual state of awareness. The choice of a sattvic diet may either reflect a person's state of harmony or may reflect a person's desire to influence themselves into that state by choosing sattvic foods. The pitfall of pursuing a sattvic diet to create a desired mental state is that it can become a self-righteous religion that traps the aspirants in their own concepts. The object of spiritual life is not to fit a certain conceptual form or way of life. It is simply to Be. In that Beingness, we create a healthy space for evolution into an individualized diet that is spiritually best for that time. In Ayurveda foods are also thought to have three qualities of density: a fine subtle quality that builds the mind, a less fine quality that builds the body, and a coarse quality that is primarily waste matter.

Sattvic Foods

Foods that have high amounts of this most refined subtle quality are called sattvic. These are considered pure foods because they keep the body-mind-spirit complex balanced, clear, harmonious, and strong. A sattvic diet helps one go inward to the Self. They are easy to digest, and their intake does not result in the accumulation of toxins in the system. The intake of these foods helps to keep the mind at peace. These sattvic foods add energy to the SOEFs, rather than draining energy from them for assimilation. Their inherent balanced, harmonious energy is transmitted to us. The experience of a sattvic diet is that of inner strength, harmony, peace, and balance. In the Ayurvedic system, these traditional sattvic foods include all fruits, vegetables, edible greens, grains, grasses, beans, milk, buttermilk, honey, and small quantities of rice or bread preparations. In our present time it is completely vegan.

For our Western bodies, a sattvic diet means at least 80 percent biogenic and bioactive foods (see Chapter 20) and 20 percent cooked or biostatic foods, with a minimum of stimulating condiments. The diet has an abundance of different sprouts of greens, legumes, and grains, immature greens and grasses, fresh fruits and vegetables, raw soaked or unsoaked nuts and seeds, and coconuts. It should be 100 percent organic, grown and prepared with Love.

Rajasic Foods

Rajasic foods are more stimulating to the nervous system. One will often feel some immediate increased energy from eating them. Coffee, tea, tobacco, fresh meats, and large amounts of stimulating spices such as garlic and onions are examples of rajasic foods. These foods will energize us for our worldly activities, but this energization does not always happen in the clearest and most balanced way. A rajasic diet makes the mind go outward. These foods stimulate us to be busy and active, but activity can turn into agitation and restlessness. They tend to push our mind and body beyond its limits. If this is done long enough, we eventually go into imbalance, and disease begins to manifest. An example of this is the coffee addict who needs more and more coffee to keep pumping up to do work. Eventually, the addict becomes more and more physically exhausted until even the coffee will not help. Hypoglycemia, which we will discuss in Chapter 27, is a typical result of rajasic imbalance, especially with the overuse of coffee and sugar. Rajasic foods tend to stimulate the body and mind toward a more competitive, war-like, sensual, and pleasure-seeking way of life. In the traditional caste system, the Brahmins, who were the priests, teachers, and spiritual seekers, were forbidden to have rajasic foods. A rajasic diet was considered the diet for kings and warriors.

Rajasic foods include some biogenic and bioactive foods (see Chapter 20), but they also include flesh foods and many spicy, cooked foods with rich, oily sauces. This diet includes butter, cheese, oils, fried foods, cakes, sugar, and eggs. The taste stimulation of these foods tends to lead us away from our inner cues, moving us easily toward imbalances such as overeating and coffee and sugar addictions. This diet eventually leads to ill health and chronic degenerative imbalances.

Tamasic Foods

Tamasic foods are stale, decayed, decomposed, spoiled, overcooked, recooked leftovers, Genetically Modified Organics (GMOs) (see Chapter 30), irradiated, (see Chapter 30) microwaved, and other forms of processed foods. These processed foods are chemicalized with preservatives, pesticides, fungicides, sweeteners, artificial colors, sulfites, nitrites, and similar chemicals. Tamasic foods create a veil of ignorance and an energy of sloth and decadence. All the fast foods that are so popular today fall into the tamasic category, as does alcohol, which is a fermented, decomposed food, and all other drugs. Any flesh foods that are not freshly killed are considered tamasic; this includes most meat we find in the supermarket. Only freshly killed wild game and fish are considered rajasic. Tamasic foods have no life force left in them. Their SOEFs have been severely disrupted. These foods have only minimal quality left in them, and maximum waste. These foods supply us with toxic chemical breakdown products that affect the functioning of our mind and irritate our nervous system. Because they steal energy from our SOEFs to digest and assimilate, they diminish our life force.

These foods lead more quickly than rajasic foods to chronic, degenerative disease. They tend to bring out the worst psychological characteristics because of the irritable, lethargic, degenerate state they create in us. At some time, most of us have overeaten some tamasic food and have felt raunchy and toxic. This is the tamasic state, a state in which it is extremely difficult to meditate or to be in harmony with Self or environment. A quick assessment of the popular American diet makes it obvious that it is a strong tamasic diet, the results of which are that the U.S. rates twenty-first in life expectancy among the industrialized nations.[6] The tamasic diet may also be contributing to the degenerating moral fiber of our society.

Effects of Specific Food Deficiencies and Excesses on the Mind

The mind and nervous system are specifically affected by certain vitamin deficiencies. For example, thiamine deficiency results in beri-beri, which causes peripheral nerve damage and damage to certain brain centers, causing disorientation, mental confusion, and an off-balance gait. A deficiency of vitamin B_3, or niacin, has been associated with cerebral pellagra, with symptoms resembling schizophrenia. The early work of Drs. Hoffer and Osmond showed that a certain percentage of people diagnosed with schizophrenia overcame the symptoms with high doses of niacin. This indicates the importance of nutrients on the function of the mind.[7] Other researchers have found that high doses of vitamins B_6, B_{12}, E, and C may improve mental functioning in some people. Two new specialties, called orthomolecular medicine and orthomolecular psychiatry, have developed around the world as a result of all these findings.[8] Carl Pfeiffer, Ph.D., M.D., in his book *Mental and Elemental Nutrients,* points to the role of mineral deficiencies such as low zinc, manganese, chromium, and molybdenum, and excesses in copper, iron, cadmium, lead, and mercury, in disrupted mental function.[9] It has been established that body concentrations of toxic metals can cause hyperactivity or mental retardation.[10,11] The point here is that our nutrients, in excess or deficiency, can affect the function of the mind.

Mind function can also be affected by what are now called cerebral allergies. We usually think of allergies as causing only stuffed-up heads, runny noses, and red eyes, but a new medical field called clinical ecology has shown that some people's mental functioning can be disrupted by the foods they eat and the pollutants they breathe. Symptoms include acute and chronic depression, tension-fatigue syndrome, minimal brain dysfunction, restlessness, anxiety, insomnia, hyperactivity, inappropriate behavior outbursts, fear, panic, unreal feelings, personality changes, schizophrenia, psychosis, hallucinations, and inability to concentrate.[12] If we become aware of our inner responses to foods, we are able to avoid the symptoms of food allergies. The book *5-Day Allergy Relief System* includes a good discussion of how to detect and treat these food allergies.[13]

Because of a disharmonious mind and lifestyle, our bodies are shifted into a state of imbalance that may manifest as food allergies or vitamin and mineral deficiencies. For example, by leading a stressful life, we may burn up lots of B vitamins, which need to be replaced in high doses in order to maintain balance. In the long run, the use of high-dose B vitamins to cope with a high-stress lifestyle becomes a rajasic stimulation of our bodies beyond their normal output. It covers up the essential disharmony that is creating the imbalance. For some, the problem may simply be a genetic need for high doses of vitamins according to the principles of biochemical individuality. But for many, this is not the case. This does not mean we should not take high-dose vitamins as an immediate effort to rebalance and remedy the situation. It does mean that we need to look at the causes of the imbalance, make deeper lifestyle adjustments, increase our meditation time, and make health-oriented diet changes if they are merited. In this way we can continue our spiritual unfolding in a solid way.

Hypoglycemia

Because stable blood sugar is important for the normal functioning of the brain and the nervous system, hypoglycemia, said by many to be epidemic in the U.S., is something that needs to be understood.[14] It has been the author's observation in treating many meditators that when their hypoglycemia is cured, their ability to meditate and the steadiness of their meditation improves. When the blood sugar is stable, the mind and emotions are more stable. This alone makes hypoglycemia an important condition of which to be aware (see Chapter 27 for more information).

Diet and Culture

The Greek historian Herodotus, often called the father of history, reported that grain-eating vegetarian cultures surpassed meat-eating cultures in art, science, and spiritual development. He observed that meat-eating nations tended to be war-like and to relate to one another through anger, alienation, and sensual passions. He also commented that meat eaters possessed bravery, courage, and boldness.[15] Rudolf Steiner felt that spiritual progress for humanity depends on a progressive increase in the number of people who follow vegetarian nutrition. He felt that an overemphasis on animal nutrition would eventually pull people away from an interest in spiritual life. There is an implication that one contributing factor to the fall of the Roman empire was the decadent practice of gluttony. Perhaps this was also true in France before the Revolution. An aristocratic dinner served the night before the French Revolution was reported to have nine courses made from one kind of meat that was prepared in twenty-two different ways.[16] When one realizes that an estimated 34 million adult Americans are considered obese, there is some real concern for the spiritual state of our country.[17] There are some hints that in ancient times those involved in the various priesthoods knew about the effects of certain diets on spiritual development and kept these as secrets to maintain their own power over the populations. A remnant of this may be found in India, where the Brahmin priests eat separately from people of other castes. The implication is that the diet of a social group affects the spiritual consciousness of that group.

Food Preparation and the Mind

What we eat is more than nutrients or even the particular energy of the food. We also eat the mental state of those who grew the food, picked the food, prepared the food, and of the one who is eating the food. Food that is grown with Love, picked with Love, prepared with Love, and eaten with Love has a different quality than food that goes through those stages with a different consciousness relating to it. There is a story of a monk who lived a pure life, thought pure thoughts, and ate pure food. A king who had a greedy nature desired that the monk come and stay in his court. The monk agreed to come for a short time. During his stay, however, the monsoon season came and the king insisted that the monk stay until the end of the monsoon. During this whole time, the monk ate the food prepared by the greedy cook of the greedy king. In time, the pure mind of the monk began to be pervaded by greedy thoughts. One day, in an impulsive moment, he stole the queen's pearl necklace. His mind now agitated by this, he insisted that he had to leave. Meanwhile, the whole castle was in an uproar about the stolen necklace, but of course, the monk was not suspected. Once he returned to eating his own food, prepared with pure thoughts and Love, the monk's mind began to clear. After a few weeks, he began to wonder what he was doing with this useless pearl necklace. When it became clear to him what had happened, he decided to return it to the king. The king demanded an explanation. The monk, having returned to his normal fearless state, explained that the food he had been eating in the king's castle, permeated by the king's greedy consciousness and prepared by his greedy cook, had temporarily infected him with greed. Once he returned to his pure food, prepared with Love, his mind became sattvic again and he returned the necklace.

Food prepared with Love and eaten with Love generates even more Love in the person eating the food. If food is prepared with Love as an offering to God and with the consciousness that the person preparing the food, the person eating the food, and the food are one in God, the person eating that food will imbibe that consciousness. In Muktananda's ashrams, food preparers were taught to chant or repeat God's name while preparing the food, so no matter what was prepared, it was always experienced as tasty and filled with Love. This is also true at the Tree of Life Café. The Love programs the water in the live foods with Love that we then imbibe. In cooked food, the water is dehydrated off so it carries less of the Love vibration.

When the author prepares his own food, he goes to the garden to see what is ripe and to what he is drawn. He thanks the individual plant for feeding him and picks it with Love and as an offering to God. Once this harmonious connection is made with Nature, the author is inspired to create whatever meal appears to him based on his inner sensitivity to the food. In this way his relationship with food as an interface with Nature is personal and filled with Love. Food is then not anonymous. In our supermarket and fast-food restaurant world of frozen, irradiated, fried, and multi-processed foods, food loses its roots and the imagery of its source in the Divine Mother. Food lives in a context of Mother Nature's energies of sun, wind, earth, color, and rain. How do we honor our Mother, as the Ten Speakings say, if we eat her offerings without the active awareness that what we are eating comes from her bountiful Earth rather than from a grocery shelf or a fast-food bag? It is powerful to eat everything with the feeling of receiving life. Eating is a way of focusing on all levels of nurturing, which is ultimately Love. Food is a Love note from the Divine.

When food is served anonymously, as in a restaurant, we can connect with Nature and be creating imagery of our own garden. This helps one to connect in a loving way with the Mother's offering. This brings a poetry to the food, which turns it into a conscious experience. The author even did this in his own home, where he ate within 20 yards of the garden from which he just picked the fresh vegetables, and now at the Tree of Life Café, one can still see the garden when eating on the patio. This process is a blessing of the food in a way that honors Mother Nature and our harmonious connection with her. Formally blessing the food with Love and giving thanks to God sets the tone for us to receive the bountiful Grace that is on the table. It helps us be present enough to receive the loving vibrations of each ingredient and the whole. Epicurus became famous as a great eater, but actually he was a great spiritual teacher. One day a wealthy king, having heard of his extraordinary meals, came to visit Epicurus. He was amazed to find him dining on bread and salt. But sitting at his table for the meal he was elevated by the consciousness with which the food was eaten. At the end of the meal, the king so appreciated the meal that he offered Epicurus a gift of anything he wanted. The king received another lesson when Epicurus asked only for a pound of butter. When asked why only that, Epicurus replied, "Just to Be is enough – nothing more is needed." His final lesson to the king was that a good meal depends on the eater and how he celebrates it. After the meal it is also powerful to give a prayer of thanks for being nurtured by the Creator.

From the Essene Gospels comes further lessons in the value of eating to feed the spirit:

> For the power of God's angels enters into you with the living food which the Lord gives you from his royal table. And when you eat, have above you the angel of air, and below you the angel of water. Breathe long and deeply at all your meals, that the angel of air may bless your repasts. And chew well your food with your teeth, that it becomes water, and that the angel of water turn it into blood in your body. And eat slowly, as it were a prayer you make to the Lord. For

> I tell you truly, the power of God enters into you, if you eat in this manner at His table. But Satan turns into a steaming bog the body of him upon whom the angels of the air and water do not descend at his repasts. And the Lord suffers him no longer at His table. For the table of the Lord is an altar, and he who eats at the table of God, is in a temple. For I tell you truly, the body of the Sons of Man is turned into a temple, and their inwards into an altar, if they do the commandments of God. Wherefore, put naught upon the altar of the Lord when your spirit is vexed, neither think upon anyone with anger in the temple of God. And enter only into the Lord's sanctuary when you feel in yourselves the call of His angels, for all that you eat in sorrow, or in anger, or without desire, becomes a poison in your body. For the breath of Satan defiles all these. Place with joy your offerings upon the altar of your body, and let all evil thoughts depart from you when you receive into your body the power of God from His table.
> – Edmond Bordeaux Szekely, *The Essene Gospel of Peace, Book One.* (International Biogenic Society, 1981)

The Spiritual Nutrition Approach

The Spiritual Nutrition approach helps us to develop the highest qualities of peace, Love, compassion, and equanimity. It emphasizes increasing prana and the subtle elements of air and ether that help open the mind and heart and make them more sensitive. The nature of the mind itself is air and ether and therefore the sattvic diet works directly upon it. This way of eating and living also reduces heaviness in body and removes excess weight and toxins that are usually heavy in nature. But following this way also requires that we follow a spiritual lifestyle to be able to sustain it. We must cultivate peace, forgiveness, and compassion, and avoid stress, emotional agitation, and conflict. It is the Way of the Six Foundations.

We see, therefore, that the consciousness of our bodies and minds are both the cause and result of the diet that we eat. Eating, as our most basic and habitual activity, defines not only our physical body but also our emotional state and our human interactions, which usually center around the dinner table. As we progress spiritually, we gain an increased sensitivity not only to the sacred, but also to the food, which is also sacred. We require food that has both high and balanced prana, ojas, tejas (see Chapter 25), and Love as its main ingredients. That is why eating together in a spiritual circumstance is one of the most transformative and spiritual actions that we can do.

In summary, the subtle science of Spiritual Nutrition is the art of selecting food that increases the pranic force for healing and purifying the body and mind, builds tejas, and protects the ojas. It is a diet that calms and creates freedom from the vrittis of the mind. It is a diet that turns us into a superconductor of the Divine. The Spiritual Nutrition diet is the best food discipline to aid our sattvic-kedusha practices of the Six Foundations that help stabilize us in sattva, or holiness. It is a diet that purifies the six koshas and energizes the 72,000 nadis so that the spiritualizing force of the Kundalini/Shekhinah can move more freely through them until we are able to awaken to the realization that we were always the One – we were always free.

We cannot eat our way to the Divine, but we can use our food as part of our foundation for awakening to the awareness of the Absolute. It is less easy to expand consciousness while we eat in an unconscious or harmful way. A sattvic diet helps build the vehicle and develop and expand the mind so that when the Grace of the apperception of Union descends, we are able to integrate it in our consciousness and physical body. It helps us transcend the illusory identity with the body-mind complex and I AM consciousness and merge into I AM THAT awareness. It is the way of eating that allows the Absolute that we are to express itself through the body-mind-I AM complex as the living revelation of the full Light of God.

Summary, Chapter 16

1. Diet affects the spiritual life of whole cultures as well as individuals.
2. In Ayurveda there are three basic classifications of diet: sattvic, rajasic, and tamasic. These different diets affect the mind, body, and spirit in different ways. The spontaneous choice of a particular diet type reflects a person's state of Being.
3. A sattvic diet is the most uplifting, spiritually and physically. It is the diet of choice for most who are on the spiritual path. It takes one inward to the Self.
4. A rajasic diet is one that is stimulating and activating for performing many worldly activities. It is the warrior's or corporate executive's diet.

5. A tamasic diet is a degenerate diet for body, mind, and spirit.
6. An excess or deficiency in vitamins or minerals can affect the functioning of the mind and body.
7. Food allergies can affect our mental and psychological state.
8. A balanced blood sugar aids the ability to meditate.
9. The thoughts of those who gather, prepare, serve, and eat the food affect the subtle quality of the food and the one who eats it.
10. Anonymous food has lost its contact with Nature. By honoring our food as a gift from Mother Nature, we personalize the food in a way that restores our connection with Nature.

Chapter 17

Veganism Is the Key

From a Biblical perspective, veganism (a diet free of flesh, dairy, and eggs) was given as the dietary key to spiritual life right at the beginning of the Torah in Genesis 1:29: "Then God said, 'I give you every seed-bearing plant on the face of the whole Earth and every tree that has fruit with seed in it. They will be yours for food.'" Ten generations later, when Noah was leaving the ark after the great flood and there was no plant food that Noah could find immediately to eat, God said, "Every swarming creature that lives shall be yours to eat; like grass vegetation I have given you all" (Genesis 9:3). This was not a command to eat meat, but a dispensation for the immediate situation. In Leviticus 3:17, the commandment is given that "it is a statute to time indefinite for your generations, in all your dwelling places; you must not eat any fat or any blood at all." This is particularly good advice today, since fat from flesh foods has been implicated in so many degenerative diseases and is a major storage site for pesticides, herbicides, and other environmental toxins that enter the food chain. Before Noah, the first ten patriarchs lived an average of 912 years. In the ten generations between Shem (Noah's son) and Abraham, the average life span dropped to 317 years. Eating flesh cut their life spans by two-thirds.

God's message to Adam was a clear commandment not to kill and eat the animals. At the giving of the Ten Speakings, "Thou shalt not kill" was interpreted by some to mean that one should not kill animals for food. This is certainly what is implied in the teachings of the Essenes and of Jesus, cited in the *Essene Gospel of Peace, Book One*. However, because of the direction given to Noah, we cannot dogmatically claim that the Torah message gives a totally clear moral direction from God about whether or not to be a vegetarian. The original message of the most complete harmony is in Genesis 1:29. It is the guide for understanding the commandment "Thou shalt not kill"; however, this may not be an agreeable interpretation for everyone. In addition, God gave the Hebrews the mysterious raw, high-spiritual-energy food called manna in support of their collective transition to Deveikut.

Although cultural practices have not created the pre-conditions to support the Kabbalistic teaching to be fully vegetarian, Rabbi Kook, a profound Kabbalist and First Chief Rabbi in Israel-Palestine, just before the Israeli nationhood, was a vegetarian and taught its importance. Rabbi Shlomo Goren, the late Ashkenazic Chief Rabbi of Israel, Rabbi Sha'ar Yashuv Cohen Ashkenazic, Chief Rabbi of Haifa, and Rabbi David Rosen, former Chief Rabbi of Ireland, were and are strict vegetarians. The highest percentage of vegetarians outside of India is in Israel. Jesus taught vegetarianism and he and all his disciples, as noted in this author's book *Conscious Eating,* were vegetarian. Other major Jewish advocates of vegetarianism include Rabbi Joseph Albo in the fourteenth century and Rabbis Mar Sutra and Elizer ben Azariah, who both lived around the time of Jesus. The Essenes were a Jewish mystical sect who the evidence suggests may have practiced live-food vegetarianism as early as the sixth century B.C. It was suggested in a biography of Pythagoras, the great Greek spiritual teacher and mathematician, that he studied with the Essenes on Mt. Carmel in the sixth century B.C. and returned Enlightened. After this, although this has not been firmly documented, it was said he taught about live foods, and that he required his students to do a forty-day water fast so their minds would be clear enough to receive his deeper teaching.

Although certain secular Yoga teachers are now saying one does not need to be vegetarian to practice Yoga, the Buddha expressed a clear opinion on this in the Shurangama Sutra: "After my parinirvana (Enlightenment) in the final kalpa (time era), different kinds of ghosts will be encountered everywhere, deceiving people and teaching them that they can eat meat and still attain Enlightenment. . . . How can a bhikshu (seeker) who hopes to become a deliverer of others, himself be living on the flesh of other sentient beings?"[1] Buddhism was originally vegetarian and, according to the Dalai Lama, it should go back to it. It is interesting to note that the Dalai Lama has publicly declared that he is a vegetarian and suggests vegetarianism to his people. This declaration was broadcast on BBC radio as part of the Dalai Lama's efforts to prevent a fast-food chain from opening restaurants in Tibet. The Ahaparinirvana Sutra sums it up: "The eating of meat extinguishes the seed of great compassion."[2]

The science of Ayurveda also teaches that food is the basis of the physical body, which in turn is the support of the mind. Right diet, therefore, is the basis of both physical and mental health and an important foundation for spiritual practice. That is why almost all ashrams, temples, and Yoga centers in India serve only vegetarian food.

The key element to the Spiritual Nutrition approach is veganism. Flesh food (meat, fish, and poultry) increases the animal frequency in the body and it brings into operation more animal-like tendencies such as the vibrations of anger, lust, fear, aggressiveness, and murderous impulses. The energy of a flesh-food diet adds to the impurities of the mind and the nervous system. It communicates the energy of destruction to the cells and brings the energy of death into our auric fields, reducing the flow of higher prana into the body. The lives of the creatures we've eaten weigh down our astral body with their negative feelings of fear and suffering at their time of death.

Some people claim that flesh food is part of their natural diet and so should not interfere with the unfoldment of their higher nature. Sri Yukteswar, the guru of Paramahansa Yogananda, states in his book *Holy Science:* "Can flesh be considered the natural food of man, when both his eyes and his nose are so much against it, unless deceived by flavors of spices, salt, and sugar. On the other hand, how delightful do we find the fragrance of fruits, the very sight of which often makes the mouth water."[3] Flesh food creates a tamasic (dull and heavy) effect on the physical body and mind. It clogs the channels of the subtle body, the 72,000 nadis through which the Kundalini needs to move freely to do its spiritualizing work, and tends to make the mind insensitive. Even Western historians such as Herodotus have suggested that not only violence and crime, but also religious intolerance, are more common among meat-eating groups. Many spiritual teachings support this. The Manusmriti (5.49), an ancient law code of Hindu society, states: "Having well considered the origin of flesh foods, and the cruelty of fettering and slaying of sentient beings, a person should abstain from eating flesh." It also states (6.60): "By not killing any living being one becomes fit for Liberation." The Yajur Veda (12.32) states: "You must not use your God-given body for killing God's creatures whether a human, animal, or whatever."

Vegan Diet and Ahimsa

A key component for creating a sattvic, holy mind is the practice of *ahimsa* – non-violence or non-harmfulness. In the book *Ahimsa,* by Nathaniel Altman, the Buddha is quoted: "Him I call Brahmin who is free from anger, who gladly endures reproach and even stripes and bonds inflicted upon him without cause. Him I call Brahmin who slays no creatures, who does not kill, or cause to be killed, any living thing."[4]

The word ahimsa is often translated as non-violence in the West, but the principle, which literally means "non-harming," has a broader meaning. Ahimsa involves an active stance to reduce the amount of harm going on in the world with a dynamic compassion for all life and, at this point in time, the whole living planet. Ahimsa is acting from an empathetic identification born of a reverence for life that affects every facet of our existence. It involves a personal responsibility to work for the well-being of all sentient creatures. Ahimsa is a practice that strives for less and less disorder and pain in the world, as we do our best to live with increasing harmony, compassion, and Love. In this way we also decrease the vrittis (thought activity) of the mind.

A vegan way of life (no flesh foods, eggs, dairy, leather, or other animal by-products) actively creates six aspects of ahimsa: (1) compassion and non-cruelty toward animals; (2) preserving the Earth and its ecology; (3) feeding the hungry; (4) preserving human life; (5) preservation of personal health; (6) inspiring peace.

Clearly all living involves some harm to other creatures or the environment. Even eating plants may involve ending the life of the plant (which is why some strict votaries of non-violence like the Jains will not eat root vegetables but only fruit, seeds, and grains). But plants are our natural food and are much lower on the food chain than flesh food, so a vegan diet works to reduce the amount of harm in a dramatic way. Veganism causes less overall harm to life because the animals raised for consumption have eaten thousands of plants before they themselves are slaughtered. Just think of all the food that a cow must consume for the steak that one eats.

When we eat, we are biting into the living planet. What we eat is the consciousness of the living Earth. If our eating process is not based on Love and compassion, all of our other actions are bound to suffer. *Anna,* or food, is the first name of God or Brahma in Sanskrit. In the act of eating we are partaking of the entire universe and demonstrating our Oneness with God or Life. Everything in the universe is food, therefore what we eat is God, and therefore feeds our souls. This awareness that food affects our minds is not owned by Yoga alone. The great Greek mathematician and philosopher Pythagoras once said, "As long as men massacre animals they will kill each other. Indeed, he who sows the seeds of murder and pain cannot reap joy and Love."

The eleventh-century Talmudic Rabbi, Moshe Ben Nachman, said about compassion for animals: "For cruelty expands in a man's soul, is well known with respect to cattle slaughters." Isaiah 66:3 states: "He who kills an ox is like he who kills a man." The Quaker leader Thomas Tyron (1634–1703) said: "The violence of killing animals for food stems from the same wrath as the killing of humans."

It is hard to believe that we can end crime, war, or hatred in the world as long as we are killing animals for our food, particularly in the modern era of brutal factory farming. The Mahabharata states: "What we eat in this life, eats us in the life after death." We must not forget the chain of karma:

- Compassion and non-cruelty toward animals are linked morally and spiritually to world peace. Killing an animal for food, even one that we raise ourselves or hunted, is a violent act, which we forget in consuming its flesh.
- Today, cruelty extends beyond the mass killing of animals to the systematic, anti-life, anti-humane treatment of animals, from the time they are born to the time they are "harvested," as if they were a cash crop.
- Animals are deprived of their natural habitat and life cycle for the expediency of the meat industry. Individual killing of animals for food is the first step in the cruelty process.
- The profit-motivated nature of industrializing animals, as if they are inanimate objects and void of any rights, feelings, or soul is the next step in the expansion of cruelty. The way animals, chicken, and fish are treated today is at a level of cruelty that staggers the imagination.
- When eating these animals, we take the vibration of this cruelty and death into our consciousness, often without even thinking of what we are bringing into our own bodies and encouraging in our own environment.

Raising the Sparks of Light

There is an ancient Kabbalistic teaching that says when an animal is slaughtered in accordance with the Divinely mandated laws of *shechitah,* the animal is drawn out of its beastly state into the domain of a life consecrated to the service of the Creator. As the great Kabbalist Rabbi Isaac Luria (the Ari) teaches: "Only a Torah scholar who is God-fearing and eats with proper intent can elevate the sparks of holiness within animals." Rabbi Chaim Kramer, a respected Breslov scholar notes in his commentary to the holy Breslover seminal Chasidic text of Rabbi Nachman's Torah Discourses, Likutei Moharan 37:6 that "when a person eats the meat of an animal which lacks proper ritual slaughter, he also ingests the aspects of animal matter, darkness, foolishness, judgments, forgetfulness, and death."[5] It is also in the Kabbalistic teachings that when a dark, previously human, soul has reincarnated as an animal, there is the additional danger, if one is not holy enough to elevate the dark soul in the meat, that the soul may attach to the meat eater and lower the meat eater's soul into darkness.

From another perspective, Rabbi Yohassen Gershom, a vegetarian Chassidic rabbi from Minnesota, after visiting a modern slaughterhouse, points out that, aside from the cruel way factory animals are raised, no *shochtim,* no matter how sincere, can maintain a spirit of holiness while hundreds of animals are slaughtered under mass production conditions. In previous centuries, an individual prayer was said with holy intention *(kavanah)* on the animals who were raised with Love before slaughtering. With today's cruelty and mass slaughtering, there can be no serious kavanah for the elevation of souls. As Rabbi Gershom asserts, we are now left with the empty shell *(klippah)* of flesh pots without holiness.

Rabbi Yohassen Gershom makes an additional point, according to the Jewish Vegetarians of North America's online newsletter. That point is that the raising of sparks by eating animals is cumulative, not self-perpetuating for all eternity. Each person is born with the service to raise certain sparks and not others. He points out that as we come closer to the time of the Messiah, the process of raising sparks through the consumption of meat is nearing completion. This may be why more people are becoming vegetarian and losing the taste for meat – because there is less need, and there are no longer the proper conditions for raising holy sparks or dark souls by eating meat.

Because of very questionable conditions for proper and holy shechitah, and the holy standards needed to even try to raise sparks by eating meat, there is a high spiritual, as well as health risk, for those who choose to keep eating meat if they are not holy Torah scholars and if ancient shechitah standards are not upheld. As the Torah sages have said, "a boor is forbidden to eat meat" (Talmud, Pesachim 49b). In the Gemora, a part of the Talmud that discusses the *mishna,* or first compilation, of oral Torah, it teaches that a person unlearned in Torah *(am Ha Avetz)* is forbidden to eat meat. The basic message in the Gemora is that the more eating of meat for the sake of physical pleasure does not release incarnated souls within the flesh of the animal. It suggests that one who does not eat meat for spiritual reasons can end up harming souls, and the penalty according to the oral tradition is "measure for measure" (that is, the eater possibly gets incarnated in an animal body in the next cycle).

The principle, according to Kabbalistic tradition, is that human souls can incarnate in any form of matter, including fruits or vegetables, so vegans may perform the mitzvah (good deed) of releasing souls from the vegetables. When one performs a mitzvah using the strength gained from eating the vegetable, the fallen soul trapped in the vegetable ascends with the energy of the mitzvah performed on its behalf.

This again makes the point that only a very, very small percentage of the population, which is the Torah sages, have the responsibility to eat meat, but only if the meat has been properly kosher-prepared. As pointed out earlier, ritually, properly prepared meat in itself is nearly impossible to find today. The spiritually obvious conclusion to this is that only the rare Torah scholar who has access to the rare, properly ritually prepared meat should be eating meat. According to these teachings, when these two factors are added together, only a rarefied, minute number should be eating meat and the rest should be vegetarian.

A student of Rabbi Nachman of Breslov (a great awake Chassidic rabbi who lived 1772–1810) was thinking about becoming a shochet and asked Rabbi Nachman for his opinion. Rabbi Nachman's response is contained in lesson 37 of Likutei Moharan, which explains that the animal's soul is attached to the blood and that the shochet must have true kavanah in using the knife in order to raise the sparks properly. Failure to do so affects not only the animal, but the livelihood of the whole Jewish people. The student decided on a different vocation. Although in previous times meat eating was a stop-gap measure, as Rav Kook points out because people had sunk to such a low spiritual stage, there is no need to continue this heavy level of death vibration. It is now time to move to a vegetarian and vegan diet to uplift the vibration of humanity. A vegetarian diet is associated with the coming of the messianic age.

Vegetarian Rav Abraham Isaac Hacohen Kook, the well-respected Jewish spiritual leader and Torah scholar in the early part of the twentieth century and the first Chief Rabbi of the pre-state of Israel, said that the permission to eat meat was only a temporary concession to the people. He believed it was inconceivable that God would design a perfect plan of harmony for humanity and the Earth and find that it was imperfect a few thousand years later. Rabbi Kook thought that Genesis 9:3 was a temporary concession because people had sunk to such a low level of spiritual awareness that they needed to feel superior to the animals and to concentrate first on improving their relationship with each other. He said that humanity's lust for meat was so strong that if they were denied they might even have reverted to eating human flesh. In this understanding, the permission to slaughter animals was a way to control the blood lust. He interpreted the permission to eat meat as a temporary measure until a more Enlightened era would be achieved and we would all return to vegetarianism.

With the permission to eat meat, animals and people stopped existing in a peaceful harmony. It was a significant shift in the relationship of the human organism to the world ecology.

Based on the following prophesy of Isaiah, it is not unreasonable to assume that in the Messianic Epoch to which he is referring, we all will return to the first dietary law and become vegetarian, which appears to be the original prescription of a diet for spiritual life in the Torah.

> And the wolf shall dwell with the lamb,
> And the leopard shall lie down with the kid;
> And the calf and the young lion and the fatling together;
> And a little child shall lead them. . . .
> Their young ones shall lie down together,
> And the lion shall eat straw like the ox. . . .
> They shall not hurt nor destroy in all My holy mountain.
>
> (Isaiah 11:69)

Vegetarian Diet and Health

Yoga teaches that a vegetarian diet is not only essential for the spiritual life, but is also the basis for good health. Sri Yukteswar notes:

> Various grains, fruits, roots, and for beverages, milk and pure water openly exposed to air and sun are decidedly the best natural food for man. Other foods are unnatural to man. Mixed with the blood, they accumulate in the excretory and other organs not properly adapted to them. When they cannot find their way out, they subside in the tissue crevices by the law of gravitation, and, being fermented, produce diseases, mental and physical, and ultimately lead to premature death."[6]

Animals may be our friends, but they aren't if we eat them. In Genesis 9:3 it says not to eat the fat or the blood of animals. Blood is often filled with adrenaline because of the fear the animal experiences as it and those around it are being slaughtered. When we eat the flesh we take in fear-associated adrenaline. This adrenal-fear energy blocks the awakening of the first chakra into the feeling of trust, and stimulates our system in a way that is adverse to the inner stillness of meditation.

People who eat meat are also at a higher risk of various viral, bacterial, fungal, and parasitical infections. Toxoplasmosis is one of these. There is now the possibility of Mad Cow Disease (which arises through giving vegetarian animals infected meat in their diet!). Twenty-thousand cases of e-coli from meat occur each year (250–500 are fatal). Camphlobacter and salmonella bacteria are on the increase. Salmonella infections can be found in 30–70 percent of chickens. Camphlobacter infection is found in 80 percent of chickens and 90 percent of turkeys; this bacteria causes intestinal infections similar to salmonella. In one study of monkeys fed from leukemic cows, 100 percent of the monkeys developed leukemia after one year. This may explain why in Denmark, where there is a high rate of leukemia in cows, there is also a high rate of leukemia in children.

Flesh food, being at the top of the food chain, has about fifteen times more pesticides and herbicides than vegetable food.[7] Dairy products have about five times more pesticides and herbicides than vegetarian food.[8] Fish contain high amounts of toxic PCBs,[9] a major water contaminant from pesticide runoff. Shellfish accumulate about 70,000 times the concentration of pesticides and herbicides as the water around them.[10] Fish can accumulate more than 3 million times the PCBs present in the water in which they live.[11] PCBs are found in 100 percent of all sperm samples in humans.[12] PCBs are considered one of the main reasons that the average sperm count in the American male is 50–70 percent what it was thirty years ago, and possibly 15–25 percent of male college students are sterile, compared to 0.5 percent thirty-five years ago.[13] We also have the problem of mercury toxicity from ingesting fish.

There are also many problems associated with eating flesh and animal produce such as milk and eggs. For example, Dr. Saenz, a pediatrician, reported in the February 1980 edition of the *Puerto Rico Medical Association Journal* that an epidemic of premature sexual development was connected to the eating of hormone-rich animal products. The segment of the population primarily affected were female children ages one and up. Infants and young children began to develop mature breasts, uteruses, vaginal bleeding and other signs of puberty. This was related to the consumption of whole milk, beef, and chicken because the animals were given estrogen to increase their weight. The doctors found that once these foods were removed from the diet the symptoms disappeared in a short time.[14]

High amounts of concentrated protein foods, and flesh foods in general, do not "burn cleanly," partly because of their nitrogen content. The nitrogen is metabolized into uric acid, which has a toxic effect when an excess is deposited in the tissues. Our bodies are able to excrete only eight grains of uric acid per day, but one pound of meat leaves a residue of eighteen grains of uric acid.[15] Eating flesh foods makes it relatively easy to build up a uric acid excess in the tissues. One reason some people like meat is that it has an initial stimulating effect from the uric acid, perhaps because its structure is similar to that of caffeine. Meat protein is also very low in oxygen. A diet high in meat seems to be related to a disruption of mental function, and in some cases has been found to either exacerbate or cause schizophrenia, according to the research of Dr. Yuri Nikolayev of the Moscow Institute of Psychiatry. The Russian researchers have had some interesting success in stopping the symptoms of schizophrenia with water fasts.[16] When people revert to high meat intake, their schizophrenic symptoms often return.

The main toxic and degenerate effect of a high-protein diet is from eating meat rather than vegetarian protein. Statistics clearly show that vegetarians suffer less from chronic degenerative disease and cancer and have longer life spans than non-vegetarians. For example, in a study of Seventh Day Adventists, who are the largest single group of vegetarians in the United States, the risk rate of colon cancer was 1.0 for strict vegetarians as compared to 2.7 for beef eaters.[17] A study comparing mortality from breast cancer among strict vegetarian Seventh Day Adventist vegetarians and those Seventh Day Adventists eating meat more than three times per week showed that the vegetarians had half the rate of mortality.[18] Seventh Day Adventists had 40 percent less coronary disease, one-quarter the mortality rate from respiratory disease, and a general mortality rate of 50–70 percent less compared to non-vegetarians living in the same American society.[19] The longest-lived people around the world – Hunzkuts, Bulgarians, East Indian Todas, Russian Caucasians, and Yucatan Indians – are either vegetarians or eat very little meat.[20] Only 5 of 154 Bulgarian centenarians eat meat regularly.[21]

Not only do vegetarians live longer and actually have (according to at least ten research reports) more endurance than meat eaters, they are less subject to the health problems that meat eaters experience. According to Herodotus, the great historian, the longest-lived people in history were the Pelegasians, who ate a live-food diet of nuts, seeds, fruits, and vegetables. Their average age was 200 years. This is called ahimsa for our own bodies. The eating of flesh foods significantly increases major chronic diseases like heart disease, hypertension, cancer, kidney disease, and osteoporosis. The risk of colon cancer for meat eaters is four times greater than for vegetarians. According to the 1961 *Journal of the American Medical Association,* heart disease would be reduced by 97 percent if people would switch to vegetarianism. Vegetarian women have one-quarter the rate of breast cancer as meat-eating women. Vegetarian women have one-fifth the rate of osteoporosis as meat-eating women and one-half the rate of osteoporosis as meat-eating men. Twenty-six percent of meat eaters manifest high blood pressure, compared to 2 percent of vegetarians.

The spiritual and health ill-effects of a meat-based diet were dramatically clarified by the Enlightened Being Swami Prakashanada Saraswati in 1986 when he said:

> Every animal that is slaughtered for human consumption brings the pain of death into your body. Think about it. The animal is killed with violence. That violence causes the animal to experience very intense pain as it dies. That pain remains in the meat even after you've

prepared and cooked it. When you eat the meat, then you eat pain. That pain becomes lodged in your body, heart, and mind. That violence and pain which you consume will also eat you. It consumes you so that you must experience the same pain in your life also.[22]

Vegetarian Diet and Blood Types

Some today claim that certain blood types require flesh food because that is part of their ancestral history. While blood type is one factor of many and worth some consideration, it is misleading to base our diet upon it as the main factor. We can find tall and short, fat and thin, slow and fast oxidizers in all blood types. Does this mean that they should all be eating the same food, considering only the blood type? Clearly there are more important factors of structure, weight, and the organic condition of the person than the blood type. Whether one wants to follow a spiritual path and practice Yoga or Kabbalah is yet another consideration. We must also remember that we don't live in the same type of houses nor do the same type of work as our ancestors did, so following their type of diet doesn't make sense either.

Some recent epidemiological research by a medical doctor, published in *The Answer Is in Your Blood Type*, found that type A blood types generally die sixteen to twenty years sooner from cancer and heart disease if they are not vegetarians, compared to those who are.[23] Type ABs follow after that in a shortened life if they are not vegetarian, and type Bs follow after that. Type Os live the longest, whether or not they smoke, drink alcohol, or eat meat. This does not mean they have created a sattvic mind on this meat-based diet. Their average lifespan is 86 years, while the average lifespan of a meat-eating type A is 61, with a high percentage of death from cancer or heart disease. This does not imply that type Os need to eat meat. There is little more than anecdotal evidence to suggest that some type Os need a higher amount of lean protein, which, if they do, can also come from vegan sources. It is interesting to note that several major leaders in the live-food movement are type O, including this one. Whenever the question comes up at a vegan conference of how many participants are type O, the vast majority of these successful vegans are type O. So, it is obvious that many type O people can be successful on a vegan diet. A high percentage of type Os, including this one, do not need to eat a high amount of protein because we are slow oxidizers.

One of the leaders in blood type anthropology is Laura Powers, Ph.D., who is not a vegetarian. She feels that the *Eat Right for Your Type* diet is "pure speculation."[24] Her data, described in *Conscious Eating*, shows the importance of lectins and knowing your blood type. Certain lectin foods, which create a sort of allergic reaction or action like a wrong blood transfusion in one's body, can be detrimental. Avoiding those lectin foods can definitely improve health. The false concept that primitive humans were all type O is further weakened by the work of Dr. Stephen Bailey, a nutritional anthropologist at Tufts University. His research shows that a variety of blood types existed in animals and there is no anthropological evidence that all prehistoric people were only type O.[25] The research by the famous paleontologist, Richard Leakey, suggests that Cro-Magnons who lived 40,000 to 20,000 years ago ate a diet closer to that of the chimpanzee, which was mostly vegetarian.[26] The research by Dr. Steven Bailey and Richard Leaky significantly undermines the wild hypothesis of *Eat Right for Your Type*.

The Place of Dairy Products

Before the industrial revolution, a sattvic diet in India included dairy products. This is also true in the Kabbalistic tradition. Being sattvic, however, depended on good quality milk from cows treated well and raised naturally. Such dairy products are very hard to get in the industrialized world (though some organic farms are making a movement in this direction and should be encouraged in their efforts). A number of Yogis from India have, not surprisingly, found that they cannot drink the milk in the U.S. without getting sick! Ayurveda recognizes that poorly prepared dairy products from badly treated cows increases mucous and toxins in the system and turns milk into a poison, canceling its health benefits. The formula is simple: Good cow's milk is pure *rasa*, or plasma. Bad cow's milk is pure *ama*, or toxins!

In India, the cow is allowed to give milk to its calf first. Only the leftover milk, which is often considerable, is taken for humans. Today, although organic, raw milk is available in several states, it is not even possible to get commercial, free-range, grass-fed, raw, organic cow's milk in the U.S. The dairy industry today removes calves from their mother and slaughters them. The cow knows that her calf is going to be killed and her distress causes toxins to be secreted into her milk. Cows are also mistreated in many ways: confined in pens, milked by machines, produced through artificial insemination, genetically redesigned to produce more milk than is healthy for them, and fed hormones, antibiotics, non-organic grains, fish and sheep parts, and who knows what else. It is really contemptible how we treat this animal, which is like Mother Earth or the Divine Mother in her caring and nourishing qualities!

In addition, we have the possibility of Mad Cow Disease as well as high amounts of pesticides, herbicides, hormones, and antibiotics in the milk. Chemical residues are absorbed into the cow's tissues and even radioactive fallout may be found in the milk. For example, three months after the Chernobyl disaster there was a 900 percent increase in perinatal mortality in the Boston area. This was traced to the fallout of radioactive I_{131} from Chernobyl that the cows (organic cows included) were eating from the grass and concentrating in their milk. Pregnant human mothers were drinking this radioactive milk and it was destroying their babies' thyroid and other metabolic functions. Pesticides and herbicides are found in concentrations 5.5 times greater in milk than in fruits and vegetables. The Mad Cow Disease transmission is not as clear. The spring 2004 edition of *Friends of the Earth* cites several autopsy studies that suggest that 3–13 percent of people diagnosed with Alzheimer's actually have Creutzfeldt-Jacob Disease (CJD) (Mad Cow Disease). Although it is most powerfully transmitted via brain and neuron systems, research in *Friends of the Earth* suggests that CJD can be transmitted by a cow consuming less than one gram of diseased tissue from any part of a cow. Although in 1997 the FDA established some controls, there are significant loopholes such as farmers being allowed to feed cow's blood to cattle, even though research shows the blood can transmit the prions of Mad Cow Disease, and factory farms are still allowed to feed pigs and poultry the remains of slaughtered cattle and the remains of these slaughtered, cattle-fed animals can be fed back to cattle. The Center for Disease Control refuses to make CJD a reportable disease. At least one U.S. company that wants to test all its cows has not been allowed to by the U.S. government, even though more than forty countries have banned the import of U.S. beef and many of them will not lift the ban until all U.S. cattle going to slaughter are tested. In 2003, only 0.001 percent of the cattle slaughtered in the U.S. were tested for Mad Cow Disease. Throughout the U.S. there are also significant reports of "mad" elk, deer, and fish. *Friends of the Earth* suggests there may be at least 120,000 cases of CJD unreported in the U.S.

Cow's milk can serve as a vector for other disease. A study in Denmark found that there was a correlation between an increased incidence of leukemia in cows and of the children who drank their milk. Another study showed that 100 percent of the chimpanzees that drank milk from leukemic cows for one year got leukemia. To this mix we add genetic engineering, which alters the milk in ways we don't yet understand. The milk itself is pasteurized and homogenized, which further weakens its prana. Such milk is a degenerated food filled with fear, the pain of death, and enslavement. There is very little prana in it, very little Love, and little true nourishment. Therefore, there is not much dairy that is a sattvic food. Instead, it is a more tamasic food, which reflects cruelty, pain, and lack of consciousness. This is symbolically reflected in the amount of pus cells per liter of milk. According to Robert Cohen of NotMilk.com, milk in Florida has 633 million pus cells (white blood cells) per liter, which is higher than any other state; the state with the lowest amount of pus cells per liter of milk is Montana with 236 million pus cells per liter. The milk available today, even raw milk from organic cows, is ama (toxic), not rasa (pure). It loses prana, clogs the nadis, and could be high in pesticides, herbicides, antibiotics, hormones, radioactive iodine, and disease vectors including Mad Cow prions. This makes it an unacceptable choice for spiritual or healthful living.

Difference Between Plant and Animal Nutrition

Plant nutrition, when understood as densified sunlight, is distinctly different from animal nutrition. Sunlight, as a cosmic radiation, stimulates the energetic subtle body of the plant and helps to build its structure out of carbon dioxide (CO_2) and water (H_2O) to form activated carbon-hydrogen bonds through the process of photosynthesis, which stores sunlight energy as excited electrons. Taken into our systems, plants stimulate a resonant response from the Inner Light of our higher spiritual subtle bodies, which directly receive the pranic transfer of the stored sunlight. In anthroposophical medicine, this relationship of plant light to the stimulation, formation, and maintenance of the nervous system is important for spiritual development. Rudolf Steiner felt that this outside light was significant because it stimulated the Inner Light as a spiritual process.[27]

When animals eat plants, they benefit directly from this release of light energy into the system. This light builds up the force of their nervous system and its related subtle astral or personality body. When flesh foods are eaten by humans, we not only have to overcome the forces of the animal's biomolecular system, but also of this stronger astral body nervous system. This puts a strain on our own nervous system development and function. This point becomes increasingly important when people have degenerative nervous system diseases. Dr. Swank's diet of low animal fat for the treatment of multiple sclerosis, a degenerative nervous system disease, is an example of the importance of avoiding or minimizing animal food when we are attempting to heal the nervous system.[28] By assimilating the plant energy directly, we stimulate our own Inner Light forces and nervous system. By taking in plant energy indirectly through animal foods, we lose the benefit of this stimulation on our Inner Light and nervous system. As already pointed out, if we do not exercise a biological system, such as our muscles, they weaken. In the same way, eating animal products weakens the nervous system in this indirect way. This is a major difference between plant and animal nutrition. By taking in plant nutrition, we go through the whole stimulation and assimilation process, which eating animal foods does not allow us to do. To digest vegetarian foods requires more inner spiritual Light and digestive power. Over generations of heavy meat eating, some individuals have lost some of this power and may have difficulty assimilating the living plant forces of a vegetarian diet.

Harmony of the Vegetarian Diet

With a vegetarian diet, we avoid the disharmony of killing animals. The vegetables we eat are taken from the ground in their seasonal cycles, in harmony with when they are going to die naturally. Fruits are simply the sunshine gift of the living plant to us. There is a natural harmony between plants and humans. Plants take in carbon dioxide as a product of our respiration and convert it to oxygen and carbohydrates; in this way, we share an important biological life cycle. Each colored plant, as food, is a condensed spectrum band of sunlight color for us to take in for the balancing of our chakras and the physical organ, gland, and nervous systems. When we take in a full spectrum throughout the day, we benefit by having our total chakra system balanced energetically by our plant friends. This is the principle of the Rainbow Diet (see Chapter 26).

Max Bircher-Benner, a world-famous European physician, concluded that the closer food is to the natural sun energy, the higher it is in all levels of nutritional value for the human organism.[29] Plant food is at the top of the nutritional scale and animal food at the bottom.

Steiner clarified another aspect of Spiritual Nutrition in his teaching that plant nutrition connects humanity to initially unrevealed cosmic forces. He felt that nothing clouds the nervous system when nourishment comes from the plant realm, and that it is by the nourishment of plants that humanity can delve into the cosmic interrelationships that take people beyond the constricted limitation of the mundane personality.[30]

Environmental Impact of Meat Eating

In this age of overpopulation, meat eating is an attack on the entire natural world and one of the main causes of environmental depredation and destruction. The land needed to grow grain for livestock takes up 80 percent of the total land used for grain production. Livestock use approximately half of the water used in the United States. Livestock produce twenty times the excrement as the human population, increasing nitrite-nitrate water pollution; the extensive use of livestock is pushing us closer to a clean water shortage. It takes 60–100 times more water to produce one pound of beef than to produce one pound of wheat. In essence, a flesh-centered diet creates need for about 4,500 gallons per day, per meat eater, as compared to 300 gallons per day for a vegan (a diet of no flesh or dairy). In one year's time, a vegan saves approximately 1.5 million gallons as compared to a flesh and dairy eater.

The destruction of the rainforest for grazing land and the resultant greenhouse effect is another example of the deleterious effects of a flesh-centered diet on our ecosystem. An article in the *Vegetarian Times* estimates that current rainforest destruction causes the extinction of approximately 1,000 species per year. For each fast-food quarter-pound hamburger, 55 square feet of the rainforest are destroyed. One hundred species become extinct for 2 billion fast-food burgers sold. The erosion on the land used for livestock in the U.S. accounts for about 85 percent of the 40 million acres of topsoil lost per year. A vegan diet, on the other hand, makes 5 percent of the demand on the soil in the U.S.

The ratio of food productivity per acre from livestock versus vegetarianism shows a tremendous disparity. For example, one acre of land can produce 20,000 pounds of potatoes, but can only support the production of 165 pounds of beef. An acre of grain gives five times more protein than the protein from beef raised on one acre. Legumes give ten times more protein an acre and leafy greens produce twenty-five times more protein than one acre used to raise beef. The grain used to feed 100 cows will feed 2,000 people. Neither our land, water, and atmosphere, nor animal and human populations are safe from the resource-intensive destruction that results from the meat-centered diet. We simply cannot escape the fact that raising animals for meat and dairy has a devastating effect on our entire ecosystem.

Vegetarian Diet and World Malnutrition

The number one health problem in the world today is chronic malnutrition. The United Nations estimates that half of the world's population suffers from malnutrition and 700–900 million people are seriously malnourished. Twenty-five percent of the world's children suffer from the lack of food. Approximately 42,000 children die each day from malnutrition. This comes to 15 million children who die of malnutrition per year, 25 percent of all world deaths. In the last ten years more people have died from malnutrition than from all the wars, revolutions, and murders of the last 150 years.

Approximately 60 million people on the planet starve to death every year. This problem is associated with political and economic factors and natural disasters, but we should remember the impact of a flesh-centered diet on water, land, energy, and other resources. According to nutritionist Dr. Gene Meyer, if meat eaters in the United States simply ate 10 percent less flesh, the resources saved would be enough to feed almost 60 million starving people. Our U.S. livestock regularly eat enough grain and soy to feed the entire U.S. population five times over. More than 80 percent of the grain grown in the United States is to feed livestock. This is 80 percent of the corn and 95 percent of the oats. The total world livestock population regularly eats twice the calories as the human world population. By cycling our proteins through beef, the conversion of beef protein is between one-tenth and one-twentieth that of plant protein. There is a 100 percent loss of complex carbohydrates and 95 percent loss of calories when plant protein is recycled through livestock. In essence, fourteen vegans can live off the land that it takes for one meat eater. A meat diet is clearly out of harmony with the ecological age, and seriously contributes to the environmental problems that can only increase in coming years as the world's population and industrialization increases.

Vegetarian Diet and the Energy Crisis

The vegetarian diet also helps to conserve the world's fuel energy and total raw material resources. For each calorie that we get from beef, seventy-eight calories of fossil fuel are required. Grains and beans require approximately 0.6–3.9 calories of fuel to create a calorie from vegetarian food. In other words, about twenty times more fossil fuel energy is needed to produce one calorie of beef than one calorie of vegetable protein. The raw materials needed to support the livestock industry constitute one-third of the value of all the raw materials consumed in the U.S. The flesh-centered diet is a significant stress on the Earth's ecological balance. The wealthy nations feed more to their livestock than the people of China and India combined consume directly. Two-thirds of agriculture exports go to feed livestock rather than human beings. If every person were a vegetarian it would be possible to give four tons of available grain per year to the world's starving people, and the world population could be fed seven times over. In this context, vegetarianism can be seen as charity because it provides for the poor and the hungry in the way that supports the principles of ahimsa.

Kundalini and Flesh Food

The author's observations in working with Kundalini and diet is that flesh foods act as "intense sludge" to the purifying and spiritualizing flow of Kundalini. Because of this "sludge effect," in rare emergency cases, meat may be successfully used to slow the Kundalini, when people feel the Kundalini energy has become too intense for them. If one wants to slow down and neutralize the spiritualizing process of the Kundalini with diet, a flesh-food diet is the most effective way. However, if one wants to surrender to the process of Kundalini unfolding uninhibited, a vegan diet is most appropriate.

Conclusion

A vegetarian diet is the basic spiritual diet of the Torah. It is the essence of sharing because it allows for more of the Earth's resources to be shared with everyone. It brings peace to the world because it established the habits of peace and the relationship of peace with all of Nature. By living compassionately with all of God's creatures, we develop habits that allow us to show peace and compassion for our fellow humans and the living ecology of the planet. A vegetarian diet is the nutritional blueprint of the Torah. As in the Yoga tradition, because of the contamination and toxicity of dairy, a vegan diet is now the Spiritual Nutrition blueprint of the age of World Peace.

Summary, Chapter 17

1. Because of God's dispensation to Noah to eat animals, we cannot dogmatically say that the Bible commands us to be vegetarian, as it did for Adam. Because of God's message to Noah, the commandment "Thou shall not kill" cannot be said to completely forbid killing animals for food. The choice is ours. The original message of Genesis 1:29 is a vegan diet and waits for us when we are spiritually ready.
2. Statistics show that vegetarians live longer and have lower rates of chronic degenerative diseases such as arthritis, heart disease, and cancer.
3. Plant nutrition, when understood as densified sunlight, is distinctly different from animal nutrition.
4. The light released by the forces of the assimilated plant food stimulates an inner spiritual Light, which enhances our spiritual growth.
5. Although most people can benefit from a complete vegetarian diet, there are some who may no longer genetically have the digestive power to assimilate all their nutrients from a vegetarian diet immediately. The rebuilding transition process may take several years.
6. A vegetarian diet creates more harmony because we do not have to kill blooded life forms.
7. There is a synergistic oxygen-and-carbon-dioxide life cycle connection between plants and animals.
8. Plants contain the full rainbow spectrum of condensed sunlight for balancing our chakras and associated glands, organs, and nerve centers.
9. There is an added danger of eating animal products because of all the hormones, antibiotics, tranquilizers, and other assorted chemicals fed to animals. In addition, animals are at the top of our

toxified food chain, so they concentrate the toxins in their tissues.

10. Animal flesh acts as an intense sludge to the flow of the Kundalini. Because of this, it is an additional treatment for decreasing the energy of the Kundalini.
11. A vegan diet is now the Spiritual Nutrition blueprint of the coming age of World Peace.

Chapter 18

High- Versus Low-Protein Diet

Fact and Fear

The high- versus low-protein controversy is more an issue of fear and confusion than fact. The high-protein approach to nutrition was initially based on nineteenth-century German research that asserted people need a minimum of 120 grams of protein per day. This high-protein thinking lingers today, even though the requirement is now considered by conventional nutritionists to be 60–90 grams of protein each day. But expert research around the world suggests that the real protein requirement is closer to 25–35 grams, and less if the protein we eat comes from live foods. In separate research programs, Ragnar Berg, the well known Swedish nutritionist, and D. V. O. Siven in Finland both concluded that 30 grams of protein is sufficient for good health.[1] Dr. Hegsted from Harvard University and Dr. Kuratsuen from Japan independently found that 25–30 grams is sufficient.[2] Dr. K. Eimer found that when athletes reduced their protein intake from 100 grams of animal protein to 50 grams of vegetable protein, their performance improved.[3] Dr. Chittenden, in extensive studies on soldiers and athletes, found that 30–50 grams per day is sufficient for maximum physical performance.[4]

It is also interesting to note that the average protein concentration in mother's milk is just 1.4 percent, sufficient to supply the human organism with all the essential amino acids and protein needed during the period of most rapid growth and brain development.[5] Apes, considerably stronger than humans, live on a fruitarian diet that averages between 0.2 and 2.2 percent protein, equivalent to the protein concentration in human breast milk. These facts lead one to question: Just how much protein do we really need?

Excess Protein and Degenerative Disease

In terms of metabolic combustion, excess protein in the diet does not "burn cleanly." It has been associated with creating an over-acid system because of the accumulation of toxic protein metabolic wastes such as uric acids and purines in the tissues. Airola points out that overeating protein "contributes to the development of many of our most common and serious diseases, such as arthritis, kidney damage, pyorrhea, schizophrenia, osteoporosis, atherosclerosis, heart disease, and cancer" and that a "high-protein diet causes premature aging and lowers life expectancy."[6] A high-protein diet increases the rate of amyloid deposit in the cells. Amyloid is a by-product of protein metabolism that is deposited in connective tissues and organs. It has definitely been linked with tissue and organ degeneration and premature aging.

The Russians have had some interesting success in treating schizophrenia with fasting and low-protein vegetarian diets. Although they have made a clear connection between a high-animal-protein diet and certain types of schizophrenia, the exact causes are not clear. One part of the brain dysfunction may be related to certain mineral and vitamin deficiencies caused by a high-animal-protein diet. The schizophrenic condition might be related to B_3, B_6, and magnesium deficiencies created by a high-meat-protein diet.[7] A high-animal-protein diet includes twenty times more phosphorous than calcium, which depletes calcium in the system, resulting in osteoporosis and tooth decalcification.[8] The cited data strongly suggest that most people eat too much protein, and that excess protein, especially if it is meat protein, is detrimental to our health.

The Wendt Doctrine

The Wendt doctrine, a result of thirty years of research by Wendt, Wendt, and Wendt, a family of physician researchers, has now received formal recognition by nutritional scientists in Germany. It explains one major factor connecting excess protein consumption to some forms of chronic degenerative disease.[9] The Wendts were able to prove with electron microscope pictures that excess protein clogs the basement membrane, a filtering membrane located between capillaries and cells. It helps regulate the flow of nutrients and waste products between capillaries, cells, and fluid in the tissues they penetrate. The more excess protein there is in the diet, the more protein is lodged in the basement membrane, resulting in a thicker basement membrane with clogged pores. It becomes harder for proteins, other nutrients, and even oxygen to get through into the cells and for waste and breakdown products to get out of the cells. Eventually, the basement membrane becomes so clogged with excess protein that the cells on the inside of the capillary walls begin to store and secrete the excess protein in insoluble forms that accumulate on the inside of the capillaries and arteriole walls, causing atherosclerosis, hypertension, adult-onset diabetes, and what the Wendts term capillarogenic tissue degeneration, the result of clogged basement membranes all over the system. This clogged basement membrane produces cellular malnutrition and results in the anoxia of the tissues. According to Dr. Steven Levine's hypothesis, anoxia is the cause of all degenerative diseases.[10] The key understanding is that excess protein in the diet results in a protein storage disease that slowly chokes off the system. It is much harder to meditate when one is choking on a cellular level and the vitality of the system is slowly dying out.

The Wendts found that this whole process could be reversed by stopping the intake of all animal protein for one to three months, and by eating a low-protein diet. They point out that the basement membrane of a fetus is extremely thin and porous, so nutrients can easily pass in and out. Because there is no protein excess in the fetus, they feel that this membrane lets all nutrients into the cells easily. They hypothesize that if an adult were to eat a low-protein diet, or do extensive fasting, she or he would achieve the same basement membrane porosity, thinness, and permeability as that of a fetus. This would allow excellent assimilation of nutrients into the cells and export of waste products out of the cells. It would ensure the free flow of energy in the system and provide the metabolic energy needed to meditate and stay focused on Communion with the Divine.

Protein Combining Is Unnecessary

One of the most unnecessary vegetarian practices is combining protein at meals. This inaccurate concept is that our system only utilizes protein in its complete state and we must eat all the amino acids at once to supply sufficient protein for our system to use metabolically. This fearful type of thinking comes from the idea that we do not store proteins and amino acids. The Wendt doctrine clearly proves that this is not true.

Research on individuals fasting from all food shows that their serum albumen (a measure of protein in the system) remained constant throughout the fasting period, yet no protein was consumed.[11] This is because of the existence of an amino acid pool that continually sends free amino acids or protein complexes to where they are needed in the system.

In his textbook on physiology, the well-known physiologist Dr. Arthur Guyton describes how this amino acid pool works. He states that under normal circumstances all cells contain more protein than they need. When amino acids are needed somewhere else in the body, the excess protein in the cell is reconverted to the protein building blocks called amino acids. These amino acids diffuse into the bloodstream and either go directly to the cells that need them or to the liver, where they are built into new proteins and sent out into the blood to be carried to the appropriate sites. Food combining to get complete proteins at one meal is completely unnecessary for these three reasons: our amino acid/protein equilibrium system, our cellular protein storage, and the free flow of amino acids in our amino acid pool.

There Is Enough Protein in Vegan Foods

The biggest fear generated by pro-meat eaters and new vegetarians is about not getting enough protein. The real problem is just the opposite: We take in too much protein. According to the Max Planck Institute for Nutritional Research in Germany, considered by Paavo Airola to be the most respected and reliable nutritional research organization in the world, there are many vegetable sources of protein that are superior or equal to animal proteins. The Max Planck Institute found complete vegetarian proteins, those that contain all eight essential amino acids, to be available from almonds, sesame, pumpkin, and sunflower seeds, soybeans, buckwheat, all leafy greens, and most fruits.[12] Fruits supply approximately the same percentage of complete protein as mother's milk.[13] Airola feels "it is virtually impossible not to get enough protein, provided you have enough to eat of natural, unrefined foods."[14]

Twenty-five to thirty grams of protein are more than sufficient for our protein intake. If the protein is taken in its live-food form, even less is needed. In many cases, as our system changes with meditation, fasting, eating lighter, and increasing live-food intake, our basement membranes become clear, more porous, and thinner, so the protein we take in moves into the cells more readily. With reduced blockage, more of the protein we eat pushes itself through the basement membrane into the cells, so our protein needs spontaneously drop. Perhaps over time we might find that the 1.4 percent protein in mother's milk is all we need. The lower limits are not clearly established on the materialistic plane for one who is undergoing a spiritual metamorphosis.

Protein and Spiritual Evolution

What can be said is that excess protein, whether from animal or vegetable sources, slows the flow of the subtle energy in the system and decreases our capacity as superconductors. It acts as a sludge to our body energy in general and specifically to the Kundalini energy. In fact, when the Kundalini energy becomes too intense for some individuals, the author often recommends eating lots of vegetarian protein, even meat on rare occasions, to slow it down. This mild dietary change has worked well for people, and is one way to regulate the flow of the Kundalini energy.

The author first noticed this general sludge effect after he changed his diet to vegetarian in 1972. As the author's basement membranes began to clear, he began to sense when he was eating too many nuts and seeds to compensate for the supposedly low protein of a vegetarian diet. When overcompensating, he would feel toxic, acidic, and sluggish, and it was harder to focus during meditation. Through self-experimentation, the author found the correct amount of protein intake to feel clear and energized. Over the years, as his basement membranes have cleared, he has slowly decreased his protein intake based on this feedback system. The point is that there are no rules. Through self-observation, as our spiritual practices and bodies change, it is possible to determine what our individual protein needs are. A low-protein intake is not the goal or even an idealization. To eat what helps us maximize the flow of energy in the body, the activity of Kundalini, and the experience of our God Communion is the purpose of an appropriate, moderate, low-protein diet.

Protein Requirements Are Individual

The work in *Conscious Eating* makes it clear that some people are genetically fast oxidizers or parasympathetics, which means they need a higher amount of protein and fat ratio to optimize energy production in the mitochondria where the ATP, the biochemical energy molecules, are produced. Other people are genetically slow oxidizers or sympathetic metabolizers, which means they produce the most biochemical energy on a low-protein, high-carbohydrate, moderate-fat diet. There is no one diet for everyone. In *Conscious Eating* there is a self-interview to ascertain this personal dietary information.

Summary, Chapter 18

1. Recent scientific evidence suggests that 25–30 grams of quality protein are sufficient for good health.
2. Excess intake of protein is associated with many degenerative diseases.
3. The Wendt doctrine shows that excess protein clogs the basement membranes of capillaries, not letting oxygen and other nutrients get through to the tissues and cells, resulting in anoxia and cell destruction and death.
4. With meditation, fasting, and a live-food lifestyle, there is a gradual detoxification of the basement membrane, so we assimilate more protein while eating less. Our need for protein gradually decreases.
5. An excess of protein slows the flow of the spiritualizing energy of the Kundalini and of the body energy in general.
6. According to one's individual constitution, one will have more energy on either a lower-or higher-protein diet.

Chapter 19

B_{12}

The work at the Tree of Life and all the author's nutrition books – *Spiritual Nutrition and the Rainbow Diet* (the previous edition of this book), *Conscious Eating,* and *Rainbow Green Live-Food Cuisine* – help provide an optimal situation for everyone to be successful vegans and live-food practitioners. To that end, we address every issue connected with being successful. Breakthrough information has arisen based on new studies and techniques that call for a more accurate assessment of the role of B_{12} in the vegetarian diet. The B_{12} issue is one that is critical to a successful, healthy, vegan, and live-food way of life.

B_{12} acts as a coenzyme whose job is primarily connected to the methylation process needed for the production of phosphatidylcholine, myelin, melatonin, catecholamines, DNA, RNA, cysteine, and normal red blood cells. Several forms of active B_{12} work as coenzymes in the body: adenosylcobalamin, methylcobalamin, cyancobalamin (found in supplements and fortified foods because it is the most stable form of B_{12}), and hydroxocobalamin. There are many natural B_{12} analogues in food, but they do not work as active coenzymes in the body and may actually block the active B_{12} coenzyme function.

Understanding B_{12} Absorption

Understanding B_{12} absorption pathways in humans gives additional weight to the B_{12} issue. The only organisms known to manufacture B_{12} are bacteria, which are found in water, soil, and the digestive tracts of animals and humans (and, consequently, in their tissues or milk). B_{12} is not in honey. In flesh foods the B_{12} is usually attached to a carrier protein for transport or storage. When this protein-bound B_{12} reaches the stomach, the acids and enzymes that are secreted in the stomach free up the B_{12} from the protein it was bound to, and it becomes attached to a specific protein, the R-protein, which transports it through the stomach into the small intestine. Intrinsic factor, a protein complex that transports B_{12}, is also made in the stomach. In the small intestine, the B_{12} is separated from the R-protein via pancreatic enzymes and becomes attached to the intrinsic factor (IF). The IF then takes it to the ileum, the last part of the small intestine, where it is absorbed by special receptor cells designed to receive the IF-cobalamin complex. The IF-cobalamin complex protects the B_{12} against bacteria and digestive enzyme degradation. It makes sure the ileum cells absorb it in priority over the B_{12} analogues. B_{12} absorption may also happen by passive diffusion, which accounts for 1–3 percent of the B_{12} absorbed.

B_{12} from supplements is not bound to protein so it does not need to go through this complicated process. When large amounts of B_{12} are taken in from supplements, it can overcome IF defects, and be absorbed by passive diffusion. It can also be absorbed sublingually (under the tongue) at higher rates than passive diffusion in the ileum.

The average non-vegetarian stores between 2,000 and 3,000 micrograms (abbreviated mcg) of B_{12} and loses about 3 mcg per day. About 60 percent of the total amount of the B_{12} in the body is stored in the liver, and 30 percent is stored in the muscle.[1] The body has a special circulation pattern between the digestive tract and the liver. Through the bile, we secrete 1.4 mcg per day of B_{12} into the small intestine, and healthy people reabsorb about 0.7 mcg. Research suggests that if people have a low B_{12} intake, their absorption rate increases to draw more B_{12} into the system. However, there is still a general potential for slow loss, depending on the variation in this special type of circulation process, known as enterohepatic circulation, before we develop the potential for B_{12} deficiency symptoms.[2] Slight differences in enterohepatic circulation may determine how long one can go before developing a B_{12} deficiency.[3] All this is taking place above the large intestine and has nothing to do with how clean the colon is.

Importance of B_{12}

To understand the significance of this issue, we need to understand a little about the importance of B_{12} in the diet. B_{12} has two main functions.

One is that methylcobalamin is catalyzed by the enzyme methionine synthase to change homocysteine into methionine. When this enzyme is not working or is deficient, the homocysteine in our system increases. Elevated homocysteine also happens with deficiencies in B_6 and folic acid. Recent research has associated elevated homocysteine with the increased potentiality of heart disease, deterioration of the arteries and nerves, increased hearing loss with age, and a 170-percent increase in having two or more pregnancy losses in the first trimester.[4] Other conditions associated with an elevated homocysteine are Alzheimer's disease, neural tube defects, and increased mortality. When the homocysteine is elevated, it appears to be a nerve toxin, as well as a blood vessel toxin. The second major function of B_{12} is as a coenzyme using 5-deoxyadenosylcobalamin in the enzyme methyl malonyl-CoA mutase in the conversion of methyl malonyl-CoA to succinyl-CoA. The succinyl-CoA is part of the energy production at the mitochondrial level in the cells that are the energy factories of the cells and therefore the entire body. This is one of the reasons B_{12} deficiency may lead to low energy.

One of the major symptoms of B_{12} and folic acid deficiency is macrocytic anemia. Folate, also called folic acid, is needed to turn the uracil into thymidine, an essential building block of DNA.[5] This DNA is needed for production of new red blood cells and for red blood cell division. B_{12} is involved in the pathway that creates methylcobalamin. This B_{12} also produces a form of folate needed to make DNA. So, if there is no B_{12}, folate can become depleted and DNA production slows down.

Accurate Measurement of B_{12} Levels

Another little side part of the conversion of methyl malonyl-CoA to succinyl-CoA is that when the B_{12} is not available, the methyl malonyl-CoA level increases and is converted to methyl malonic acid (MMA), which accumulates in the blood and urine. *Since B_{12} is the only coenzyme required in this pathway, MMA level in the urine is considered the new gold standard as an indicator of B_{12} deficiency.* Other causes of high methyl malonic acid are genetic defects, kidney failure, low blood volume, dysbiosis, pregnancy, and hypothyroid condition. The MMA test is important because the progressive medical community no longer considers serum B_{12} levels an accurate measurement of appropriate amounts of B_{12}. In other words, a normal serum B_{12} may not mean that B_{12} levels are healthy. We need a urinary assay of MMA to really determine the answer. This is an important point, because when the author first wrote about B_{12} in *Conscious Eating*, the establishment of the MMA assay as the gold standard had not taken place yet. Some of the author's statements at that time were based on the world research, which was using serum B_{12}. A serum B_{12} of 200 pg/ml (picograms per milliliter) or more was considered adequate. As a result of the new gold standard and what we know about MMA and homocysteine, it is now agreed that the B_{12} serum levels should be around 340–405 pg. In some cases, as much as 450 is needed to maintain a normal homocysteine level. Therefore, to be optimally safe, serum B_{12} levels lower than 450 may be considered as indicating a B_{12} deficiency.

B_{12} Deficiency

A variety of symptoms of B_{12} deficiency are important to vegans and live-foodists. The first is low energy. It could be a reason why some people just don't feel well on these diets, besides not getting the right protein-carbohydrate-fat mix for their constitutional type. There are specific neurological symptoms, often described as "subacute combined degeneration." Some of this damage can be almost irreversible, if it becomes chronic. This nerve system degeneration affects peripheral nerves and the spinal cord. Some of the typical neurological feelings include depression, numbness and tingling in the hands and feet, nervousness, paranoia, hyperactive reflexes, impotence, impaired memory, and behavioral changes. These B_{12} deficiency symptoms are consistent with those suffered by the famous fruitarian Johnny Lovewisdom, who lead a short-lived, vegan community in Ecuador. He suffered from weakness, partial paralysis, and after a few years, was unable to stand or walk. Similar symptoms happened in another short-lived, fruitarian community in Australia. Other B_{12} deficiency symptoms include: diarrhea, fever, frequent upper respiratory infections, infertility, sore tongue, enlargement of the mucous membranes of the mouth, vagina, and stomach, macrocytic anemia, and low white blood cell and platelet count. These symptoms should not be confused with a "healing crisis."

Two of the major possible causes of nerve damage caused by B_{12} deficiency are: (1) a lack of methionine available for conversion into S-adenosylmethionine (SAM) because of lack of sufficient B_{12}, causing a lack of SAM, which is needed for production of the phosphatidyl choline needed to make myelin sheaths (coating for the nerves);[6] (2) the accumulation of propionyl-CoA (a 3-carbon molecule) resulting from the inability to convert methyl malonyl Co-A to succinal Co-A (4-carbon), creating an excess of 15- and 17-carbon chain fatty acids, which are incorporated into nerve structure and alter nerve function.[7] Some of the causes of B_{12} deficiency are low dietary intake of B_{12} and/or poor absorption, which usually comes through loss of intrinsic factor and/or a lack of stomach acid.

Consistent research over the last decade has shown that vegans and live-food practitioners of all ages and sexes have a much higher risk of becoming B_{12} deficient.[8–21] There are more than fifteen studies on vegans and an additional three studies on live-food vegans. The most dramatic was a study done by Dong and Scott on eighty-three subjects at a Natural Hygiene Society conference. Of the non-B_{12}-supplementing, primarily live-food vegans, 92 percent were B_{12} deficient. This likelihood seems to increase with the amount of time as a vegan. There are no studies that show that vegans do not get deficient over time. This does not mean that everyone becomes B_{12} deficient within six years – it may not show up for years. One case study by Bernstein[22] in 2000 describes a man in his eighties who had been vegan for thirty-eight years and reported excellent health. Over a period of a few weeks, however, he began to be emotionally erratic, depressed, confused, and incontinent, and lost motor skills so significantly he could barely stand without help. He was diagnosed as having senile dementia. But, fortunately, his B_{12} was tested and found to be so low it was not detectable. After one B_{12} injection he could sit without help by the next morning. The incontinence stopped within forty-eight hours, and by the end of one week his mental state returned close to normal.

B_{12} deficiency is particularly hazardous for newborn babies, especially babies of vegan live-food nursing mothers who are not using B_{12} supplementation. Since 1980 there have been 130 reports of serious B_{12} deficiency in the infants of vegan mothers whose primary food was breast milk and the mother did not supplement her own or the baby's diet with B_{12}. Lack of B_{12} in the mother's diet has been shown to cause a severe lack of myelin in nerve tissue.[23] B_{12} supplementation in infants has shown a rapid increase in B_{12} values, but the question is whether there are some long-term developmental problems, even if the B_{12} values are returned to normal. Von Schenck, in a review of twenty-seven cases of infant B_{12} deficiency done in 1997, suggested that in many there was permanent damage. Seven were followed for twelve years after diagnosis. Five of these seven had abnormal neurological development twelve years later.[24]

Vegan pregnant mothers need to supplement with B_{12} during pregnancy and the breast-feeding period. Goraya, in 1998 in India, reported that many infants had a B_{12} deficiency among breast-fed infants in low socioeconomic status. Some, but not all, responded to B_{12} therapy.[25] The conclusion is obvious: Prevention is the key concept. In contrast to the average adult storage of 2,000–3,000 mcg of B_{12}, newborns of mothers with normal B_{12} have about 25 mcg. Studies have shown that the milk during the first week of life does contain large amounts of B_{12}.[26] The B_{12} storage in infants at birth is normally adequate to last the first few weeks of life.[27] Afterwards, they must get it from breast milk or other sources. If a vegan or live-food mother is already B_{12} deficient during pregnancy, the baby may be born with seriously low B_{12} levels and develop clinical signs of deficiency as soon as two weeks.[28] The general research suggests that even among non-vegetarians, B_{12} can be insufficient in infants, and that perhaps *all* breast-feeding mothers should consider B_{12} supplements for themselves and their infants during the time of breast-feeding. This lack of B_{12} in the mother's diet during pregnancy has been associated with a lack of myelin production.[29] A B_{12} deficiency in a baby takes somewhere between one to twelve months to develop. It often manifests as failure to thrive and slow developmental progression. The babies are often lethargic, lose their ability to use muscle adequately, have tremors, and even their sensory attunement decreases; they also have irregular macrocytic anemia.[30,31] There is some question, even though the values return to normal, that children with a sustained B_{12} deficiency before starting B_{12} supplementation may have sustained abnormal neurological development.

The good news, as supported by at least one major study in the United Kingdom in 1988 that studied thirty-seven vegan children, is that normal growth and development takes place in children who were breast-fed for six months at a minimum, when there was B_{12} supplementation.[32] Other studies have shown that young and teenage children who were supplemented with B_{12} were found to grow normally.[33,34]

Adults who were vegetarian without B_{12} supplementation for more than than six years usually had lower B_{12} than non-vegetarian adults in the general research. In one study of adults by Crane et al.[35] in 1994, 81 percent of the vegan adults had a B_{12} lower than 200 pg and 19 percent of those 81 percent were less than 100 pg. That corresponds with the percentage of adults found to be low in B_{12} in most vegan and live-food studies. In the author's clinical experience, meat eaters as well as vegans and live-fooders tend to have a fairly high rate of B_{12} deficiency, although meat eaters have less incidence. Among vegetarians and vegans, a high proportion is below 200 pg. In one study, 62 percent were below 200 pg, and 19 percent below 100 pg.[36] The 1982 study, reported by Dong and Scott,[37] of live-food vegans with eighty-three subjects from the Natural Hygiene Society showed that 92 percent of the vegans had a B_{12} lower than 200 pg, and in 53 percent it was lower than 100 pg. The World Health Organization (WHO) considers B_{12} deficiency to be lower than 200 pg, using the old criteria. The rates of B_{12} deficiency tend to increase over time on a natural hygiene diet. Another study in Finland in 1995, reported by Rauma et al.,[38] examined B_{12} status of long-term, 100-percent live-food vegans and found that 66 percent of the subjects had a B_{12} lower than 200 pg. One study done in 2000 by Donaldson[39] at Hallelujah Acres on primarily live-food practitioners, but with some B_{12} supplementation via nutritional yeast, showed only about 15 percent of the people were lower than 200, and none of them less than 160. The supplementation with nutritional yeast was 5 mcg of B_{12} from one tablespoon of Red Star Vegetarian Support. Repeated studies on vegans in a variety of different world regions all showed a significant B_{12} deficiency in vegans who did no B_{12} supplementation, especially if they were vegan for six years or more. Some of these studies included: in Australia with Seventh Day Adventist ministers by Hokin and Butler in 1995,[40] in Thailand in 1988 by Areekul et al.,[41] in 1990 in Israel by Bar-Sella et al.,[42] by Tungtrongchitrat et al. in 1993,[43] Crane et al. in 1994,[44] and in China in 1998 by Woo et al.[45] There seemed to be an increase in B_{12} deficiency over time. When vegans took B_{12} supplements, there was no significant difference between the vegan and non-vegetarian B_{12} levels.[46,47] This is also true with elderly, B_{12}-supplemented lacto-ovo vegetarians versus non-vegetarians.[48,49]

Many non-vegetarians also have a poor B_{12} status because there are many other factors that can cause B_{12} deficiency. They include: malabsorption or inadequate intake of protein, calories, or B_{12}; radiation exposure; drugs and a variety of toxins; paraminosalicylic acid; alcohol; pancreatic tumors; failure of the small intestine to contract and move food, associated with bacterial overgrowth; oral contraceptives; fungal infections; liver and kidney disease; tobacco smoking; B_6 or iron deficiency; and mental stress.

B_{12} in Food

Up until this time, many of us have felt that additional supplementation for live-food practitioners with sea vegetables or probiotic formulas was sufficient protection against B_{12} deficiency. This does not seem to be the case, according to research. Among macrobiotics, who primarily cook their food, we see a very high percentage of children actually having growth retardation due to low B_{12} intake. Many of us have felt that spirulina, aphazonimom-flo-aque (AFA), and all the sea vegetables had enough active B_{12} to avoid a B_{12} deficiency. Although the research is not fully in, we do know that, as pointed out in *Conscious Eating*, these substances do have human active B_{12}. The problem is they also have a significant amount of analogue B_{12} that competes with the human active B_{12}. This analogue amount was not measured in the author's studies that were presented in *Conscious Eating*. Using the MMA excretion approach, which is now the gold standard, research showed that when people used dry-roasted and raw nori from Japan, the dry-roasted nori actually made the MMA status worse, which means it actually reduced the B_{12} level. Therefore, dry-roasted nori could possibly worsen a B_{12} deficiency. Raw nori seemed to keep the MMA at the same level, meaning it did not harm the B_{12} status, but the research showed it did not particularly help it either. No food in Europe or the U.S. that has been tested shows it lowers MMA. Research absolutely has to be done to answer this question fully. The author is hopeful that the gold standard level of research in the future will reveal an authentic, natural, B_{12}, vegan food. Already, Vision Industries, Inc., is interested in doing this level of B_{12} research with AFA.

Many vegan foods have been suggested that may have active B_{12}, but few are proving to actually raise B_{12} levels or prevent its loss.[50,51,52] The research has shown, for example, that tempeh (cultured soy) does not supply human active B_{12}. Research in both the U.S. and the Netherlands has confirmed this.[53] One paper, by Areekul et al. in Thailand in 1990,[54] showed that tempeh from one particular source in Thailand did have some B_{12} analogue, but that fermented soybean did not contain B_{12} and *Klebsiella pneumoniae* was isolated from the commercial tempeh starter. Other foods such as barley, malted syrup, sourdough bread, parsley, shitake mushrooms, tofu, and soybean paste, had some B_{12} in them but did not seem to alter B_{12} status. Amazake rice, barley miso, miso, natto, rice miso, shoyu, tamari, umeboshi, and a variety of nuts, seeds, and grains did not contain any elements or even any detectable B_{12} analogue. The author's study using the earlier gold standard test of using B_{12} active bacteria to determine human active B_{12} did show indeed that arame, dulse, kelp, kombu, and wakame had significant human active B_{12}. But research suggests they have higher analogue concentrations, which may cancel their human B_{12} effect. A study done in 1991 by Miller found that serum B_{12} appeared to be unrelated to consumption of wakame, kombu, and other sea vegetables or tempeh in macrobiotic children. Other researchers feel that it is possible that raw nori, not dry-roasted nori, is a source of active B_{12}. Other studies have shown that dulse did have a certain amount of B_{12} analogue per serving.

Until research is done to see if these actually lower the MMA levels, we can't assume that because a food has human active B_{12} it will help avoid B_{12} deficiency, because the actual non-human active analogues may be blocking the human active B_{12}. The same question arises now with AFA, spirulina, and chlorella. So, until we actually do the urine MMA test of these, to see if it MMA is affected, it is reasonable to eat these foods, but not count that they are actually going to raise your human active B_{12}.

Getting B_{12} in a Less Tasteful Way

There is one exception to this lack of vegetarian B_{12}, which is that we do produce B_{12} from bacteria in our large intestine. But since this B_{12} is produced in the area below where B_{12} is reabsorbed, it is really not available for absorption. Some people have argued that many species of lower mammals do not need B_{12}. This is true because many species that are primarily vegetarian animals eat their feces. Human research also has shown if you eat your feces, you will get enough B_{12}. (The author does not recommend this practice). Dr. Herbert conducted research in England in which vegan volunteers with a documented B_{12} deficiency were fed B_{12} extractions made from their own feces.[55] It cured their B_{12} deficiency. So, there is a natural vegan way to do it. It may not be the most "tasteful way," however. The issue is not whether one has a clean bowel. B_{12}-producing bacteria grow in the bowels, but humans do not normally absorb B_{12} from the large intestine.

Some have theorized that organic foods, in various regions, would improve the B_{12} tests by lowering the MMA levels. Unfortunately, there has been no research to show that washed or unwashed organic food has made a difference in lowering the MMA. One study, by Mozafar[56] in 1994, has shown that when B_{12} analogues are placed in the soil with cow or human manure, the plants do absorb them. Unfortunately, many soils in the U.S. and around the world are deficient in B_{12}. Many animals, aside from eating their own feces, will ingest a variety of eggs, insects, small vertebrates, or soils. For example, gorillas, who are the closest to vegan of all the species, will eat insects and sometimes their feces. So there are ways to do this for vegans, but again, they may not be pleasant to consider. The author would love, at this point, to come up with a "tasteful" alternative.

The Need for More Research

The author's serum B_{12} of 600 pg may have thrown off his conclusions when he wrote his summary in *Conscious Eating* in 1990. The author may have been within that 20 percent of vegans and live-food practitioners who don't seem to be affected within the first six to ten years. But he remains more concerned about the other 80 percent who are B_{12} deficient and the approximately 50 percent whose B_{12} levels have sunk to less than 100 pg over six years.

These overall conclusions are not finalized. Although there is not enough research to prove there is absolutely no vegan food that increases human B_{12} in the system, there is enough to suggest that preventive supplementation be taken to prevent B_{12} deficiencies. It is a possible suggestion that large amounts of dulse, raw nori, and an algae called *cocolithophorid algae,* also known as *pleurochritias cartera,* may provide sufficient human active B_{12}. Unfortunately, these have not been fully tested with the gold standard. It took thirty years to prove that smoking cigarettes causes cancer, but as with smoking, why wait thirty years to find out?

Healthy Levels of B_{12}

The next question is, what is a healthy level of B_{12} in the blood serum? The answer is that a serum level of 340–405 pg keeps the homocysteine level within normal range and 450 pg may give optimal coverage for most everyone. For a general framework, the following healthy levels may be of interest. The normal serum homocysteine level is 2.2–13.2

micromoles/liter. The normal adult urine MMA is 0.58–3.56 micromoles/liter.The normal level of B_{12} for breast milk is 180–300 pg per ml. The normal urine level for children is 820–11,200 micromoles/liter of MMA. The normal serum B_{12} level of children is 160–1,300 pg per ml.

Using the MMA test, elevated MMA was found in subjects with a B_{12} up to 486 pg. This is a really important statement, because up until this time, most of the studies in the world basically say anything above 200 pg is not considered deficient. That was somewhat why *Conscious Eating* suggested that B_{12} in many vegans and raw foodists was low normal, but still within normal. Using the urine MMA test, studies show that without supplementing with B_{12}, vegans have higher homocysteine levels than lacto-ovo vegetarians and non-vegetarians, which means they are deficient in B_{12}. The good news, of course, is that B_{12} supplementation will reduce these high homocysteine levels back to normal range.

Supplementation of B_{12}

The research conclusion is: *It is a reasonably safe bet that about 80 percent of the vegan and live-food population, within six to ten years, runs the risk of a subclinical or clinical B_{12} deficiency and increased homocysteine levels.* Over a thirty- to fifty-year span, that portion could reach 100 percent. An even higher percentage of newborns run this risk. Out of concern for all, particularly for the author's fellow live-food practitioners and vegans, *it is well advised to supplement with an actual B_{12} human active supplement,* especially during pregnancy and while breast-feeding. There are vegan B_{12} supplements, which allow us to be fully successful vegan, live-food practitioners.

The author's general recommendation is that, if you have symptoms of B_{12} deficiency, start with a 1,000-mcg injection once per week for one to two months or an oral administration of 1,000 mcg per day for four to eight weeks. After about two months of the oral, the dose can be cut in half. One month later, one can even cut that in half again. Nutritional Red Star yeast is a B_{12}-fortified food that significantly cuts the B_{12} deficiency rate down to 15 percent in one study, but as a yeast it can activate candida infection. The safest and healthiest approach is to do the supplementation approach with a B_{12} living extract.

The art of supplementation for B_{12} is relatively simple. The minimal need is about 6 micrograms per day. We lose 3 mcg per day. At the Tree of Life we have an activated high-cellular resonance B_{12} supplement that has 6 mcg per one-half teaspoon. The author recommends a minimum of one-half teaspoon two times per day in water. This liquid form is ideal for children. The author feels that a smaller daily intake better mimics how the body assimilates B_{12}. Chewing a B_{12} tablet or letting it dissolve in the mouth is also a simple way. Crane et al. in 1994 suggested a 100–500-mcg tablet at least one time per week if the tablet was chewed. Those who chewed a 100-mcg tablet one time per week for six weeks brought their B_{12} from a below-normal average of 116 up to 291. Those who swallowed it without chewing, raised it from an average of 123 to 139. B_{12} supplements made of cyanocobalamin are damaged by prolonged light exposure.[57] Because of vulnerability of smokers to cyanocobalamin, oral supplementation with methylcobalamin (dibencozide) and adeosyl cobalamin (coenzyme B_{12}) can be used. Hydroxy cobalamin is also a good form of supplement but is primarily in the injectible form. The Tree of Life uses this form for injection. Research shows that it is retained in the body more than cyanocobalamin. Methylcobalamin and adenosylcobalmin require 1,000–2,000 mcg per day for adequate supplementation.

Another question that is relevant to B_{12} supplementation is how much is safe. The Institute of Medicine has not set an upper limit of safety for B_{12} intake. Other researchers suggest that B_{12} intake of 500–1,000 mcg per day is completely safe and that the cobalt and cyanide contribution in 1,000 mcg of cyanocobalamin are toxicologically insignificant.[58] However, people with cyanide metabolism defects, chronic kidney failure, and smokers are safest to use another form than cyanocobalamin. This is because they may have compromised cyanide detoxification ability. There is not, at this time, any significant evidence that cyanocobalamin is harmful to vegan smokers. It is more of a theoretical consideration.

Some people eat according to their philosophy and belief of what they feel is natural. This may cause problems. For example, the black Hebrews, a group of African-Americans who have migrated to Israel, have horrendously high levels of infant B_{12} deficiency, with a certain amount of B_{12}-deficiency-related deaths, as well as adult B_{12} deficiency. They did not believe in taking supplements. Data in a 1982 study by Shinwell and Gorodischer[59] showed that, of the infants who were breastfed for three months and then were given diluted homemade soymilk for three months to one year, a significant percentage had protein deficiency, iron anemia, zinc deficiency, and B_{12} deficiency. Among the twenty-five infants with this condition, three were dead on arrival, and five more died within a few hours of hospital admission, despite treatment. Serum levels were low in nine of fifteen cases, and undetectable in three. This is a not very good example to show the world how we want to treat our children. We can make those choices. There is a theory of what it means to be natural, but there is also a theory of what it means to be healthy.

What is meant by being successful is in being completely healthy, which includes having no B_{12} deficiency and no elevated homocysteine levels. It is the author's medical opinion as a holistic physician, nutritionist, vegan since 1973, live-food vegan since 1983, and as a person committed to supporting all those who choose to become healthy live-food vegans, that it would be wise to incorporate some B_{12} supplementation in your diet. It is more natural to be healthy than it is to be anything less than that. It may be the first time in history since the Garden of Eden that as a culture we have the capacity to healthfully follow the vegan teaching of Genesis 1:29.

Summary, Chapter 19

1. B_{12} is critical for optimum health and well-being.
2. Approximately 80 percent of children and adult vegans and live-food practitioners become B_{12} deficient after six to ten years without B_{12} supplementation.
3. Infants with B_{12}-deficient breast-feeding mothers may become deficient in as short as two weeks and suffer irreparable damage.
4. The author strongly recommends B_{12} supplementation for all vegan and live-food practitioners to maintain optimal health and well-being.

Chapter 20

The Light of Live Foods

Live Foods

The Spiritual Nutrition diet is a special type of spiritual vegan diet aimed at helping us transcend body consciousness, clean the koshas, calm the vrittis of the mind, clear the nadis, and expand the prana. For this reason, Spiritual Nutrition is more disciplined than a regular vegetarian diet, generally lighter, and includes Spiritual Fasting and the taking of primarily live foods (uncooked roots, leafy vegetables, fruits, nuts, and seeds). These are called the food of the *rishis* (sages) or ancient Yogis, as well as the probable diet of the Essenes.

Live foods are raw and uncooked foods, naturally fermented foods such as sauerkraut and miso, and dehydrated foods, in which the food temperature does not exceed 118°F. They are foods that have their natural enzymes intact and have not been processed by irradiation, pesticide use, microwave, artificial additives, GMOs (genetically modified organics), or cooking (heated above 118°F through boiling, baking, frying, broiling, toasting, etc.). Live foods are rich in prana, which brings the prana force not only into the body, but also into the mind, helping to purify the 72,000 nadis and expand consciousness. Live foods are the most powerful foods for enhancing the flow of Kundalini/Shekhinah energy and cleansing the nadis through which the Kundalini/Shekhinah flows on the subtle plane. A kedusha-sattvic diet helps us become superconductors of prana. As the prana in our body increases, these nadis naturally open, allowing us the deeper perception of Truth and reality as Oneness.

Wholeness of Live Foods

The wholeness of live foods is not only health-producing, but non-reproducible by science, which tends to fragment nutrition. Live foods mean wholeness. It is the holographic wholeness of the food, the complete energy pattern of the food, that brings another quality and power to it.

Cooking, and other forms of processing such as microwaving, irradiation, and genetic engineering, destroy the quality and components of the food (and we still don't know the full extent of this destruction). Cooking is not only risky business, but it significantly diminishes the amount of nutrients, vitamins, minerals, proteins, fats, organic acids, and other lesser-known phytonutrients such as bioflavonoids, which are key components for activating positive gene expression. Because the phytonutrients are active in live foods, they play a significant role in gene regulation. A high percentage of phytonutrients are destroyed when foods are cooked. It is interesting to note that phytonutrients form an integral part of the Rainbow Diet (see Chapter 26).

Effects of Cooking Foods

Whether we should cook our foods is a controversial issue. For many, like the author until about 1983, it is not even an issue, because we assume it is natural to cook most foods. Some suggest that everything be cooked, others say fruits or grains should be cooked, and still others say 100 percent raw foods is the way. By applying all levels of the Spiritual Nutrition paradigm, including its material aspect, we can gain some perspective on this subject.

We need to examine the effect of cooking foods on ourselves and on the food. During normal cooking, enzymes are destroyed, the active forms of vitamins and minerals are partially destroyed, pesticides and fungicides break down to form toxic compounds, and there is an increase in free radicals. Cooking foods also coagulates 50 percent of the protein, according to the Max Planck Institute. Also, eating foods that are too hot can actually disrupt the digestive enzymes in the mucosal lining of the stomach. Eating cooked foods also causes an immediate increase in our white blood cell count.

Importance of Biologically Active Enzymes in Our Diets

On the physical level, all our life processes depend on the functioning of enzymes. They are the physical agents of life, important for digestion, for detoxification from internal pollution and external ecological pollution, for repairing DNA, for maintaining our immune systems, and for all our metabolic and regenerative processes. It is estimated that there are 75,000 to 100,000 different enzyme systems in the body.[1] Dr. Ann Wigmore calls enzyme preservation the secret of life.[2] Dr. Howell, the pioneer of food enzyme work in this country, says the quantity of enzymes we have in our systems is the equivalent to what we call life energy or vitality, and thinks of our enzyme level as indicative of our health status.[3] There is some interesting evidence associating enzyme reserve with longevity and vitality. For example, the amylase in human saliva is thirty times more abundant in the average 25-year-old than in the average 81-year-old. The total enzyme level in young beetles is twice that in old beetles. Fruit flies, grasshoppers, and rats all have more enzymes when they are young.[4] After chronic disease in humans, the enzyme content is depleted.[5]

Raw, natural foods come loaded with the active enzymes needed for much of their digestion. They are released the moment we begin to chew and break down cell walls in the food. This is similar to the finding that unprocessed carbohydrates such as grain and raw sugar cane have the right amount of chromium to act as a cofactor in their assimilation. When these are commercially processed into such products as white flour and white sugar, they lose much of their chromium, so in order to assimilate them, we must draw from our own body's chromium stores.[6] Over time, this results in a tissue chromium depletion, just as eating cooked foods results in an enzyme depletion.

Enzymes

Enzymes contain the power of life itself. Eating a live-food diet helps maintain the quality and quantity of our enzyme pool, and thus helps promote longevity. Enzymes are living proteins that direct the life force into our basic biochemical and metabolic processes. Enzymes even help repair our DNA and RNA. Enzymes transform and store energy in the body, they make active hormones, and they participate in their own productive cycle. They dissolve fiber and prevent clotting, they have anti-inflammatory effects and even analgesic effects, and they prevent edema. In *Conscious Eating,* it is explained how enzymes can help build and enhance the immune system, help to heal cancer, multiple sclerosis, and rheumatoid arthritis, and minimize the effect of athletic injuries by decreasing recovery time. Enzymes, of course, are needed for digestion. Live-food enzymes have been proven to have an anti-aging effect, life-extension effect, anti-degenerative disease effect, and a high vitality in the food. Enzymes work with the cellular structure in the cell nucleus in the cell mitochondria, which are the energy factories in the system. Some enzymes move freely in the body as they are needed for digestion, or in the serum of our blood, and are carried to different parts of the body. Many of these mobile enzyme systems, particularly the proteases, are bound to transfer proteins in the serum "alpha-globulins." These alpha-globulins transfer enzymes and other molecules through various parts of the body to regulate all of the body processes.

When we process foods by heating them above 118°F (or boil them for three minutes), there is 100 percent enzyme destruction.[7] The enzymes destroyed by cooking are those that predigest the food in the "food enzyme" or cardiac stomach (the upper part of the stomach) for the first thirty to sixty minutes of the digestive cycle. Eating primarily live foods enhances this predigestion. This means that fewer of our own (endogenous) digestive enzymes from the stomach, pancreas, liver, and small intestine are required to complete the digestive work. There is evidence that the amount of endogenous enzyme secretion will decrease or increase depending on how much is needed.[8] This is important because of what Dr. Howell calls the "Law of Adaptive Secretion of Enzymes,"[9] which means that enzyme energy goes where it is needed in the body. Dr. Howell believes that enzymes represent a certain amount of energy as well as an actual amount of enzyme molecules. If less enzyme energy is needed for digestion, there is more available to enhance other bodily processes. For example, if we are injured or sick, we often experience a drop in appetite because the primary need for the enzyme energy is for fighting the illness and for bodily repair.

An article in the *Journal of Medical Hypothesis* estimates that each cell has 90 million methyl groups at birth.[10] All aging and mental and physical degeneration, including cancer, are marked by a loss of methyl groups. Expression of oncogenes (cancer-causing genes) and anti-cancer genes are associated with the loss of methyl groups at the cell level. The average loss is 1,800 DNA methyl groups per cell per day, limiting lifespan to 65–70 years. If the loss could be cut to 1,200 methyl groups per cell per day, lifespan could increase to 95 years because DNA would function better. When we cook our food we destroy our proteases (proteolytic enzymes) and this creates a need for more hydrochloric acid (HCL) to be used for digestion. The organic betaine hydrochloric acid (trimethylglycine) is a primary donor of methyl groups. Therefore, cooking foods indirectly results in an accelerated loss of methyl groups because less HCL is available to donate methyl groups because it is being used in the digestive process. Therefore the degeneration (aging) process is speeded up. With age, stress, and chronic illness, the store of enzymes in our body decreases. This is because enzymes, so critical for our health, are used up in stress and acute and chronic disease situations. As our enzyme pool diminishes with age, our ability to perform the tasks to keep the body healthy also diminishes. When enzymes decrease in concentrations in the body, the aging process accelerates. Remember, enzymes are protein complexes that are made by our DNA. Therefore, when youthing genes are activated (as we will see in Chapter 21), they also activate enzymes that maintain our health and well-being. One clear way to preserve the body's store of enzymes is to eat live foods, because foods in the natural state are loaded with enzymes, and these enzymes are then taken through the body to build up our enzyme reserves.

By eating foods in which the enzymes have not been destroyed, we maintain a continuous exogenous enzyme input into the system and therefore decrease the endogenous depletion of enzyme energy. There is strong evidence that the excess enzymes released from live foods or even from enzyme supplements, can be absorbed into the system to increase our enzyme content and energy. In this way, a live-food diet can actually add enzyme energy and material to the system. There are three main methods, on the physical plane, for maintaining or increasing enzyme energy in the system: eating a live-food diet, adding enzymes as a supplement, and fasting. The result of conservation and an increase of enzyme energy in the digestive area is that more enzyme energy is available for our vitality, body detoxification, metabolic function, dissolution of scar tissue and crystallized deposits in the tissues, digestion of excess fatty tissue, and regeneration. This increased vitality and health make more energy available to be present in our spiritual lives and more available to be transmuted into spiritual energy. This is one way live foods enhance spiritual life. Although certain illnesses can be turned into an important spiritual growth time, it has been the author's general observation that people with low physical vitality have less energy available for their spiritual focus.

One of the most dramatic illustrations of the importance of live foods for health and vitality is the famous study by Francis Pottenger, M.D.[11] – a ten-year, four-generation study of 900 cats. Half the population was fed a diet of raw meat and milk; the other half was fed cooked meat and pasteurized milk. The cats that received the cooked food developed degenerative diseases similar to those found in our society. With each generation, there was an increase in congenital bone and other abnormalities and a decrease in immune and endocrine function. By the third generation the cats fed only cooked food were sterile and quite congenitally deformed. The conclusion was that some heat-sensitive qualities were missing from the cooked meat or pasteurized milk, and the only factors we know that are completely destroyed by pasteurization are biologically active enzymes. The study suggests that the absence of enzymes in cooked food made the difference.

In terms of the Spiritual Nutrition paradigm, cooking, freezing, and irradiating destroy the physical structures of enzymes and other nutrients and disrupt and disorganize etheric SOEF patterns. To revitalize these nutrients for absorption into the system, their SOEFs must be re-energized and reorganized. To do this, energy must come from our overall SOEF system. Drawing energy from our SOEFs increases the entropy and the aging of our system. Enzymes represent special high-energy vortex focal points for bringing SOEF energy into the physical plane for all general functions as well as for biological transmutation. The more viable enzyme systems we have, the more avenues are open for us to be energized and revitalized in this way. Although it is not the common belief of allopathic doctors in the U.S., the world literature strongly indicates that enzymes in their fully active form can be absorbed across the small intestine, primarily through the Peyer's patches, and go directly into the blood. Studies suggest that 40–70 percent of the proteolytic enzymes can be absorbed this way.

The Energy of Live Foods

A tremendous amount of extra energy is available in live foods. One of the studies that most demonstrates this was done in Russia by Dr. Israel Brekman.[12] The experiment was simple. He fed the same mice cooked food and live food at different times – same food, same mice, with the only difference being that the food was either cooked or uncooked. He measured the amount of energy and endurance the mice had when they were eating only live foods, and when eating the same amounts of food in its cooked state. The mice had three times more energy and endurance on the live food than when they were eating cooked food. If nutrition were a simple matter of calories, there should be no difference in endurance and power between eating the live and the cooked food. However, there clearly was a difference in the effect. This is because foods are not simply calories. This calorie paradigm, developed in 1789, is completely out of date, even though it is still being used by people in the nutritional sciences.

Food has subtle nutrients, general nutrients, electrical energies, phytonutrients, enzymes, vitamins, and minerals. The electrical potential for our tissues and cells is a direct result of the liveliness of our cells. Live foods enhance the electrical potential in our cells, between the cells, at the interface of the cell membranes, and at the interface of the cells with the microcapulary electrical charges. When cells have the proper microelectrical potential, they have the power to rid themselves of toxins and maintain their selective capacity to bring appropriate nutrients, oxygen, and hydrogen into the nucleus of the cell, as well as to feed the mitochondria. This helps maintain, repair, and activate the DNA. Professor Hans Epinger, who was the chief medical director of the first medical clinic at the University of Vienna, found that a live-food diet specifically raised the microelectrical potential throughout the body. He discovered that a live-food diet increases selective capacity of the cells by increasing their electrical potential between the tissue cells and the capillary cells. He saw that live food significantly improves the intra- and extracellular excretion of toxins, as well as absorption of nutrients. He and his coworkers concluded that live foods were the only type of food that could restore microelectrical potential to the tissues. In essence, then, we can say that by restoring electrical potential to cells, live food rejuvenates the life force and health of the organism.

Living Light

From another perspective, Kirlian photography has been a very useful way to validate our understanding of the bioelectrical potential of foods. Different researchers have found that an luminescent field, a natural radiation field surrounding living organisms, takes the form of a coronal discharge we can see with Kirlian photography. The Kirlian photography clearly shows that livefood has a much stronger auric, luminescent field than cooked food. Some research even shows that a person eating junk or cooked food has a much smaller field than when he or she changes the diet to eat whole, natural live food. This leads us to the original point, which is that all living organisms are made of patterns of resonant energy or subtle organizing energy fields. This energy is reflected in the functioning of each cell, and the electrical field of the cells maintains the integrity of the biological system. We can think of the electrical luminescence in the Kirlian photography as a measure of life force in the cell. The stronger the life force of the cell, the stronger the electrical luminescence we see in the Kirlian photograph. In essence, the electrical luminescence represents the pictorial sum of the electrical potential of each cell. The obvious conclusion is that the healthier our electrical potential of each cell in the tissues, the healthier we are.

Dr. Joanna Budwig from Germany, who has degrees in medicine, physics, pharmacology, and biochemistry, is one of the first researchers to combine an in-depth knowledge of the quantum mechanics and physics with an in-depth knowledge of human biochemistry and physiology. From this lofty scientific position, she has concluded that not only do electron-rich foods act as high-power electron donors, but they also act as solar-resonant fields in the body to attract, store, and conduct the sun's energy in our bodies. She theorizes that the photons of the sunlight, which she calls "sun electrons," are attracted by sun-like electrons resonating in our own biological systems, especially in the double-bonded electron cloud found in our lipid systems and in the omega-3 fatty acids such as we get in flax seed. These sunlight electrons, called "pi-electrons," have the ability within our molecular structure to attract and activate the sun photons. Dr. Budwig believes that the energy we absorb from these solar photons acts as an anti-entropy, or anti-aging, factor. As a result of her theory, she believes that live foods, and particularly flax seed, which contains three highly active electron clouds in the double bonds, helps bring a tremendous amount of pi-electrons into the system. On the other end, people who eat refined, cooked, highly processed foods diminish the amount of solar electrons energizing the system and reduce the energy down from the amount necessary to create a high-electron solar resonance field. Dr. Budwig feels that processed foods may even act as insulators to the healthy flow of electricity. In other words, the more we take in solar electrons as a result of our dietary intake of live foods, the better we are able to resonate, attract, and absorb solar electrons in direct resonance from the sun and other solar systems.

Our health and consciousness depends on the ability to attract, store, and conduct electron energy. The greater our store of light energy, the greater the power of our overall electromagnetic field, and consequently the more energy available for healing and maintenance of optimal health. Metaphorically, a strong solar resonance field promotes the evolution of humanity to reach our full potential as human (sun) beings. Light supports evolution; a lack of pi-electrons in the body hinders evolution.

Another very exciting piece of research discussed earlier in this book was reported by German researcher Dr. F.A. Popp in 1984, in a paper entitled "Bio-Photon Emission: New Evidence of Coherence in DNA."[13] He points out the existence of bio-photons, which are energetic phenomena, ultra-weak photon emissions from living systems. Dr. Popp showed that the DNA is an important source of bio-photon emission. Able to measure this emission with a device he called a "bio-photon meter," he found that 97 percent of DNA is associated with bio-photon transmission, and only 3 percent is filled with genetic information. Perhaps this is the function of what many call junk DNA. These ultra-weak photon emissions from living cells and organisms are different from the phenomena of bioluminescence. Dr. Popp found that the healthiest people had the highest amount of bio-photon emission, and that the sickest had the lowest amount. The existence of bio-photon emission is a critical aspect of understanding why it is important to have an abundance of live food in one's diet. Bio-photons are emitted by a variety of forms of macro-molecules including enzymes, chlorophyll, hemoglobin, DNA, and RNA. Dr. Popp found that the foods that generally give off the most amounts of bio-photons are organic, wild-crafted live foods.

The Effect of Cooking on Vitamins and Other Food Components

Research results vary, but most researchers indicate at least a 50-percent loss of vitamin B in cooked foods. Some losses, such as thiamine loss, can be as high as 96 percent if food is boiled for a prolonged time. Biotin losses can be up to 72 percent, folic acid up to 97 percent, inositol up to 95 percent, and vitamin C up to 70–80 percent.[14] Viktoras Kulvinskas estimates that the overall nutrient destruction or loss of bio-availability after cooking is approximately 85 percent.[15] Along with this, the Max Planck Institute for Nutrition Physiology in Germany has found cooked proteins have only 50 percent bio-availability, compared to uncooked proteins.[16] In general, it can be said that cooking foods coagulates the bioactive protein chelated mineral forms (changes their molecular structure so they cannot function properly) disrupts RNA and DNA structure, and produces free radicals in fats and protein.

In *The Essene Gospel of Peace, Book One* by Szekeley, Jesus is quoted as saying, "For I tell you truly, live only by the fire of life, and prepare not your foods with the fire of death, which kills your foods, your bodies, and your souls also."[17]

Cooking also coagulates the bioactive mineral and protein complexes and therefore disrupts mineral absorption. Cooking oils destroy most of the nutritive fats that we need, such as the omega-3 fats; this often creates carcinogenic and mutagenic by-products. Add to this the possible mutagenic effects of food irradiation and genetically engineered foods. There are other, mostly unknown, changes that occur when we cook food. One of them was pointed out by research done at Stockholm University in cooperation with Sweden's Natural Food Association. This showed that the heating of carbohydrate-rich foods (potatoes, rice, cereals) creates a by-product called acrylamide, which is a probable human carcinogen. The research found that a bag of potato chips can contain up to 500 times more acrylamide than is allowed in drinking water by the World Health Organization. French fries sold at McDonald's and Burger King in Sweden showed 100 times the level permitted by the World Health Organization in drinking water. Acrylamide, which has been found to cause benign and malignant stomach tumors, also causes damage to the central and peripheral nervous system. Typical foods that contain high amounts of acrylamide include baked potatoes, French fries, biscuits and bread, and other high-carbohydrate foods.

Cooking food in these modern times has an added danger. Dr. William Newsome of Canada's Department of Health and Welfare Food Research Division, Bureau of Chemical Safety, found that cooked fungicided tomatoes had ten to ninety times more ETU, a mutagen- and cancer-causing compound, than raw tomatoes from the same garden. He found that EBDC fungicides break down under heat to form ETU. He reports that the amount of ETU in chemically treated vegetables is fifty times greater than in the same vegetables served raw.[18] The implications of this, with the enormous amounts of chemically treated foods we cook and consume, are worth considering.

Abnormal White Blood Cell Changes with Cooked Food

In 1930, Paul Kouchakoff, M.D., presented a paper at the First International Congress of Microbiology titled "The Influence of Food Cooking on the Blood Formula of Man." He reported that eating a live-food diet did not produce leukocytosis (an unhealthy increase in the number of white blood cells).[19] Particularly significant about his simple finding was that, since 1846, leukocytosis after eating typical cooked foods was thought to be normal and was classified as such by Wirchow as "digestive leukocytosis" (a beautiful example of scientists studying the normal physiology of head banging). In physiological reality, eating cooked foods creates a pathological response in the body. When foods are cooked, the energy fields are not able to resonate immediately with the body, so the body responds defensively until it can reorganize the SOEFs of the cooked food into patterns it can resonate with and absorb. Kouchakoff also reported that if a food was commercially processed and then cooked, not only did the white blood cell number increase, but there was a change in the ratio of the different white blood cell types to each other.

According to Kouchakoff, the critical temperature for initiating leukocytosis when heating food is approximately 191°F, for thirty minutes. The highest temperature he found before the leukocytosis occurred was with figs at 206°F. Interestingly, the leukocytosis needed as little as 50 milligrams of cooked food to be initiated. An additional finding that should be of interest and relief to some was that if people ate live food with cooked food of the same type, in a 50/50 ratio, the leukocytosis did not happen. He also found that this was true for a mixture of cooked foods and live foods that were not the same, as long as the critical temperature change point of the live food was higher than that of the cooked foods. From the perspective of the Spiritual Nutrition paradigm, these results can be explained by the SOEFs from live foods transferring their energy by resonance to re-energize and organize the disrupted SOEFs of cooked foods.

Food Temperatures and Body Function

If the food we eat is too hot, it can actually disrupt the enzyme systems in our own gastric mucus, as well as injure the gastric mucus directly. A study reported in *Lancet,* the well-known British medical journal, showed that 15 percent of the people tested who drank tea at 122.5°F and 77 percent of those who drank tea at temperatures greater than 137.5°F had gastric enzymatic abnormalities.[20] Dr. McCluskey, in another *Lancet* study report, found that constant irritation of the throat and tongue by hot foods, hot beverages, and alcohol was associated with increased cancer of the throat and tongue.[21] He suggests that we dip our little finger in the hot drink for ten seconds. If it is not scalded, then we can go ahead and drink.

The other extreme is that iced drinks and cold foods can slow down enzyme function and peristaltic action. We have the choice to be harmoniously moderate, eating and drinking foods at room temperature, or at temperatures no hotter than what Jesus calls the "fire of life," which is no hotter than temperatures in Nature. Harmony is accepting and surrendering to Nature's design.

An excerpt from the *Essene Gospel of Peace, Book One:*

> And Jesus continued: "God commanded your forefathers: Thou shalt not kill." I say to you: Kill neither men, nor beasts, nor yet the food which goes into your mouth. For if you eat living food, the same will quicken you, but if you kill your food, the dead food will kill you also. For life only comes from life, and death always comes from death. For everything which kills your foods kills your bodies also. And everything which kills your bodies kills your souls also [the link to Spiritual Nutrition]. Therefore, eat not anything which fire or frost

or water has destroyed. For burned, frozen, and rotted foods will burn, freeze, and rot your body also. Be not like the foolish husbandman who sowed in his ground cooked, and frozen, and rotted seeds. And the autumn came, and his fields bore nothing, And great was his distress.

Youthing on Live Foods

Although in his sixties, the author is still the same optimal weight as in high school forty-plus years ago. The power of a live-food lifestyle including raw, vegan, organic foods, Yoga, and meditation has naturally activated the anti-aging genes. The author has tested this point in doing a variety of strenuous activities, including 600 consecutive push-ups on his sixtieth birthday, and completing the Native American four-year Sundancing cycle, where he was the oldest, or close to it. The author completed three Sundance cycles of four days in the desert without food and water when no one else in the Sundance group of about fifty-two people, including dancers forty years younger, were able to do so. This was strong evidence that this whole live-food lifestyle had created an obviously superior and high-activated youthing gene expression. On the fourth year of the Sundance cycle, for example, the author was the only one to stand from sunrise to sunset for four days and still be attached to the Sundance tree. There is incredible power in the live-food diet and lifestyle. The author's personal experience has been an increase in strength and flexibility as compared to when he was captain of an undefeated football team at Amherst College. At that point, at age 21, the author could do a maximum of seventy push-ups. These are really, of course, just anecdotal points, but they are being shared to make a dramatic point of the regenerative power of an individualized, live-food diet that is vegan, organic, high in minerals, and low in sugar, combined with meditation, Yoga, and periodic Spiritual Fasting. This is the optimal diet for activating the youthing expression of our genes. The author, who has been living this live-food lifestyle for close to twenty-five years, knows of at least forty other individuals who have achieved and sustained high-level energy and wellness on this live-food lifestyle as they age. Although the main point of life is to know *I AM THAT,* a healthy body that can sustain spiritual practices such as the Native American Sundance and hours of meditation certainly helps.

So the question that remains is: Why does the live-food diet give us the best effect in terms of decreasing our caloric intake and maximizing the quality of our food intake? The point from basic nutrient mathematics is that *by eating live foods, we are able to get complete nutrition by eating 50 to 80 percent less food.* What this means is that, when people are eating junk food, they are not getting sufficient nutrition and have to overeat, by as much as twice as much, to get the same amount of nutrition as people eating live foods. Research over the past seventy years, with all forms of mammal and other life forms, shows that the less you eat the longer you live. Recent research by Dr. Stephen Spindler shows that calorie restriction actually turns on the anti-aging genes. This is further discussed in the next chapter. Therefore, this is one reason why a live-food diet is optimal for extending life and preventing chronic degenerative diseases, and for increasing energy, vitality, and youthfulness. It is a natural way to achieve caloric restriction without the experience of restriction.

Application of Essene Food Principles

One of the greatest human experiments on the live-food diet was done by Dr. Edmond Bordeaux Szekely, who over a period of thirty-three years guided more than 123,600 people on such a diet with what he terms amazing results in benefiting the quality of people's health compared to control groups.[22] In commenting on his study, Szekely says that he was on the threshold of great biochemical secrets of life that the Essenes had known thousands of years ago.

From Szekely's book *The Essenes by Josephus and His Contemporaries*, this author was able to extract two basic Essene guidelines about food preparation and eating.[23] These are the keys to these "great Essene secrets." The first is that their diet was raw, living, whole, natural foods. The second was that there was a minimal time lapse between when the food was harvested and when it was eaten. It is called eating in harmony with Nature's laws. The Essenes intensely studied and penetrated the meaning of the laws of Nature, and their eating patterns came as a result of this understanding. There was no storage, processing, freezing, drying, canning, or irradiating. The food was eaten in its full, vital form. They knew that, for a period of time after it was picked, live food contained a vital force from its environmental context of the earthly, solar, and cosmic energy. Over time and through processing, this vital force is dissipated. The SOEFs lose their energy, and their pattern begins to disorganize. Our modem, scientifically accepted instruments cannot detect these subtle energy differences. There are instruments that can measure these subtle energies, but they are not yet accepted by scientists. Because of the limitations in instrumentation, the actual measurable energy released from the carbon hydrogen bonds of live, whole foods and processed denatured foods would probably be the same in terms of actual calories produced. Our bodies get calories, but not vitality, from processed, cooked foods. Raw, live foods build up our SOEF patterns. Cooked, processed foods deplete them. This consideration of SOEFs is a major difference between the materialistic-mechanistic paradigm and the paradigm of Spiritual Nutrition. The only measurement we have is our subjective sensitivity, as when we eat a raw juicy carrot freshly plucked from the garden and compare it to a cooked carrot, or even to the quality of a several-day-old, raw, organic carrot from the health food store.

In the process of developing his health-regenerating diet, Dr. Szekely developed a way of classifying foods that, in terms of the new nutritional paradigm, reflected his understanding of food as having energetic qualities. He saw that using only the materialistic paradigm of food as calories, proteins, fats, and carbohydrates was very limiting. He felt there were four categories of cell-renewing and life-generating foods. The first category he called *biogenic.*[24,25] These are the most life-generating, high-energy foods. They are alkaline producing and energy charged. They are high in enzymes, predigested complete proteins, chelated minerals, nucleic acids, vitamins, RNA, DNA, and B_{12}. These foods, he found, regenerate and revitalize the human organism. In this category, we have all sprouts – soaked and germinated nuts and seeds, sprouted grains, and legumes, as well as the sprouted young wheat grass and other grasses eaten whole or juiced. Sprouting is not a new development. Not only did the Essenes use this technique, but the history of sprouting goes as far back as 3000 B.C. in China with the recorded use of bean sprouts. The process of soaking is used because it activates the proteases, which neutralize the enzyme inhibitors that keep the seeds, legumes, and grains from germinating at the wrong time.[26] Germinating and sprouting increase the enzyme content by six to twenty times.[27] Plant hormones are also activated and phytates are split off, and there is a tremendous increase in metabolic activity. Starches are broken down into simple sugars, proteins are predigested into easily assimilated free amino acids, and fats are broken down into soluble fatty acids. Vitamin and mineral content increases with sprouting; this was one of the original clues of the phenomenon of biological transmutation. Vitamin B_6 is increased by 500 percent, B_5 by 200 percent, B_2 by 1300 percent, biotin by 50 percent, and folic acid by 600 percent.[28] These biogenic foods have the capacity to generate a totally new organism. It is the life force of these foods that is transferred to people and aids their healing and regeneration.

Dr. Szekely's second category of foods is *bioactive* foods.[29] These are foods that are capable of sustaining and slightly enhancing an already healthy life force. Bioactive foods include fresh, unprocessed, raw fruits and vegetables.

The third category is *biostatic* foods.[30] These are foods that are neither life-sustaining nor life-generating; they diminish the quality of body functioning. They are life-slowing foods that slowly increase the process of aging. These are our cooked foods and foods that, although raw, are no longer fresh.

The fourth category he called *bioacidic*,[31] or life-destroying foods. These are foods that have gone through many processes and refinements and are full of additives and preservatives. They rapidly break down life function.

In the Spiritual Nutrition paradigm, biogenic foods increase the total SOEF energy of the system and therefore increase the SOEF organization on every level. This results in a reversal of entropy and the aging process. Bioactive foods bring their own quality SOEF energy to the system; their energy is carried to particular SOEF patterns in our system, to maintain and slowly energize the SOEF pattern of the organism. The biostatic foods require the human organism to give energy to reactivate the SOEFs of the cooked foods so they can be properly assimilated. The result over time is a slow diminution of the total SOEF energy of the organism. This can be offset by other SOEF-energizing activities such as meditating, but is this the best and most efficient way to use our SOEF energy? Bioacidic foods disrupt and de-energize the SOEF patterns, analogous to the Kouchakoff study, in which heavily processed foods not only caused a leukocytosis but changed the white blood cell pattern.

Brekman's research, described earlier, showed that mice that ate live foods had three times more physical endurance.[32] In their whole state, live foods have more enzymes, bioelectrical energy, bioluminescence, bioactive electrons, bio-photons, phytonutrients, higher SOEF energy patterns, and life force energy in general.

When we eat live foods we are consuming the living energy of the planet and fully immersing ourselves in the full energy of food as a Love note from God.

The optimal diet is an individualized, live, organic, locally grown, vegan, highly mineralized, low-glycemic, well-hydrated diet of whole food prepared with Love and eaten with consciousness and gratitude.

The Spiritual Nutrition approach is not a diet; it is actually a way of life in which we live authentically and fully on every level of our Being.

General Recommendations of Raw Versus Cooked

For the treatment of illness, Szekely, along with Paavo Airola, Ann Wigmore, Viktoras Kulvinskas, David Wolfe, and a host of other nutritional experts, recommend a 100-percent live-food diet. When an individual is in generally good health, Szekely, in his study, found that people could maintain themselves well eating 25 percent biogenic, 50 percent bioactive, and 10–25 percent biostatic foods. He allowed this 10–25 percent of biostatic food as a concession, but feels that this should only be lightly cooked tubers and hard vegetables.[33] Paavo Airola has stated that a 100-percent live-food diet would be ideal, but in the recognition that such a diet is difficult for most people to follow, recommends a ratio of 80 percent live to 20 percent cooked as adequate for supporting general health with a little less live foods in a colder climate.[34] Viktoras Kulvinskas feels a 100-percent live-food diet, consisting of 50 percent biogenic and 50 percent bioactive foods, will provide maximum quality health, but concedes for city dwellers and others in transition, that 80–90 percent live food and 10–20 percent cooked root vegetables will provide maintenance health.[35]

The conclusions of the Spiritual Nutrition paradigm, the teachings of the Essenes of eating in harmony with Nature's laws, the message of Jesus in the *Essene Gospel of Peace,* the information about the importance of not destroying enzymes with cooking, the loss of protein bioavailability with cooking, the loss of vitamins and minerals with cooking, the danger of fungicides and pesticides breaking down with heat to form toxic compounds, the increase in free radical production, and the author's observation of the benefit of a primarily live-food diet for spiritual life make it clear that a diet of at least 80 percent live foods with 25–30 percent biogenic foods is adequate for general dietary support of spiritual life.

Conclusion

There is an obvious message here. As we go deeper into the biophysics of live foods, we begin to understand that live food has the highest quality of nutrient concentrates, the highest amount of phytonutrients, vitamins, minerals, bioelectrical energy, biologically active water, pi-electrons, bio-photons, and even the most structured SOEFs. In other words, from the physical to electrical, to subtle organizing energy fields, live foods are superior for our health and well-being than any other type of food preparation. Not only do they allow us to eat less food, but activate our natural inheritance, which is the most optimal activation of youthing gene expression.

When we nourish ourselves with live food, we have the most potent diet for maintaining health and well-being and activating spirit that is available on the planet. Live foods, from this perspective, not only turn us into super energy Beings on the physical level, but superconductors of both electrical energy and cosmic energy, or Kundalini/Shekhinah energy. In this way, they help us enhance our sensitivity to the Divine. The author's clinical experience over the last thirty-five years, with thousands of people in many different groups who have turned toward live food, is that the overall, overwhelming natural response is a shift toward a more spiritual life, whatever one's particular religious tradition may be. Live foods are one of the Six Foundations for Spiritual Life and for Whole Person Enlightenment on every level.

Summary, Chapter 20

1. In cooked foods, 100 percent of the enzymes are destroyed, 70–85 percent of the vitamins are destroyed, pesticides and fungicides break down to form toxic compounds, protein is 50 percent less assimilable because of coagulation, and there is an increase in free radical production.
2. All our life processes depend on enzyme function. When enzymes are depleted, so is our vital force and health.
3. Eating cooked foods causes a pathogenic leukocytosis.
4. If food is too hot, it can disrupt our digestive enzymes.
5. When the physical level of the foods is disrupted through cooking, the energy and organization of the food SOEFs are partially disrupted.

6. The Essene secrets of food preparation and eating are to eat raw, living, whole, fresh, natural foods and to have a minimal time lapse between when the food is harvested and when it is eaten. This is the principle of *authentic* foods (Chapter 30).
7. Foods can be classified into four categories according to their cell renewal and regenerating capabilities: biogenic (raw sprouted nuts, seeds, grasses, and grains), which is cell regenerative; bioactive (raw fruits and vegetables), which maintains cell energy at a high level; biostatic (cooked, but organic), which creates a slow depletion of cell energy; and bioacidic (processed and adulterated), which is cell degenerative.
8. The general recommendation for a maintenance diet for health and spiritual life is 80 percent live and 20 percent cooked foods, with 25–30 percent of the diet biogenic foods.
9. The recommendation for a healing and most spiritualizing diet is a 100-percent live-food approach.
10. A vegan, live-food diet and lifestyle could be the most potent diet and lifestyle for physical, emotional, and spiritual health on the planet.

Chapter 21

Feeding Our Genes: A Key to Understanding Live Foods

The teaching of this chapter is that the foods we eat, or don't eat, communicate with our genes – for better or for worse. Foods do not change the genotype, which is the physical structure of the genes, but the foods we eat do change the way the message in the genes is expressed. In other words, genetic messages can be either turned off or turned on by the nature of our diet. The point is to understand how to turn off messages that result in disease and turn on messages that result in health and well-being.

All of our genetic information is known as the *genotype,* and exists in every cell in our DNA. Gene expression is called *phenotype* – phenotypic expression is the observable, measurable human appearance and behavior determined by genetics. The focus of this chapter is learning how to eat to create the optimal phenotypic expression. The theme is: *Genes do not give rise to disease, but disease rises when lifestyle and diet alter the gene expression in a way that creates disease.*

Gene Transcription and Phenotypic Expression

Although this information may appear relatively new, research in this area has been going on since the early 1980s. According to the book *Inducible Gene Expression,* the concept is that transcriptional regulation is a key strategy to affect the production of new proteins in response to external stimuli. Without getting too deeply into biochemistry and genetics, let's say that gene transcription is associated with how the genes make new enzymes and protein, and initiate RNA and mRNA synthesis. Gene transcription governs the expression of genes – the phenotypic expression. Some of the elements that affect the transcription of genes are called activator proteins, which bind in specific sequences to short DNA sequences connected to the genes. These binding sites are part of larger genetic control units called promoters or enhancers. The activation of these sites, which in turn activate the DNA, ultimately turns on or off the different types of gene expression. These trans-activators are affected by pathways that participate in some sort of signal from outside the cell to the cell protoplasm, and from the cell protoplasm into the cell nucleus.

Research has shown that extracellular stimuli – including changes in temperature, UV light, reactive oxygen species, heavy metals, xenobiotics, and the foods we eat can cause DNA response that will create new proteins, which are the body's efforts to cope with the extracellular stress. The details of exactly how this happens are beyond the scope of this chapter, which is simply to bring the concept to our awareness that *what we eat and how we live affects our gene expression*. However, these details are quite amazing, and the more the author understands about it the more wonderment and amazement he has for the makeup of all life, and in particular the complexity of the human organism. Within the cells, molecular mechanisms for signaling and inducing gene expression act by either repressing expression or activating expression.

Temperature of the body is one interesting area that researchers have studied; a set of genes that are called heat-shock genes are documented.[1,2,3] Studies have shown that the elevation of temperature induces the synthesis of new polypeptides. As temperature rises, the transcription will change to cope. Heat-shock genes increase their transcription rate up to a hundred times within minutes. These heat-shock proteins are referred to as chaperones. Chaperones are a particular class of proteins that reorganize the correct folding of proteins. They also are involved in helping cells "decide" whether to commit suicide. Basically, chaperone proteins are part of the biological mechanism for regulating gene expression. High chaperone levels tend to decrease the amount of toxic-cell and cancer-cell suicides. In other words, low chaperone levels encourage toxic cell and cancer cell suicides. Fasting lowers the chaperone level. This heat-shock protein response can be set off by environmental stresses, physiological stresses, and even non-stressful conditions. The non-stressful conditions include cell cycles and developmental pathways. A cell has the ability to sense the type and severity of a stress and respond appropriately. This ability is reflected in the overlapping pathways when these activations occur in these heat-sensitive genes. Research by Blake *et al.* in 1991 showed that there is even a direct link between the production of adrenocorticotropic hormone (ACTH) in the pituitary and the induction of a set of heat-sensor proteins in the inner cortex of the adrenal glands.

The interwovenness of our bodies' responses and the different organs and endocrine systems that respond is the point here. The environmental cues and responses also include cytokines or growth factors, high concentration of heavy metals, chemical carcinogens, tumor promoters, radiation, and sunlight. The DNA responds by changing what we call the transcription rates of cellular genes, which is mediated by signal transduction pathways to the nucleus, which specifically regulate gene expression by binding to the DNA sequences in what the author would describe as promoter regions. So DNA damage, where there are byproducts of DNA damage, can actually act as a primary signal to the cells to initiate altered gene expression. Some of these responses, even though the extracellular signals are short-term, may actually result in lasting DNA responses. This becomes a potential for the creation of chronic disease. An example of this could be viral gene products from a viral infection, or the activation from steroids and what we now know as retinoic receptors during the process of overcoming inflammation. This gives us a clue to how in some people the normal anti-inflammation program response somehow doesn't get shut off but continues and turns into a chronic disease. One of the most broad-spectrum transcription factors is NF-*KB*. The NF-*KB* factor is a very important regulator of cellular defensive responses to a variety of threatening environmental stimuli including attacks by viruses, bacteria, parasites, physical injury, radiation, oxidative stress, and chemical attacks. These activated transcription NF-*KB* factors express in many genes, not just one, because it is the multiple pathways whose synergistic role is critical in protecting the organism from all sorts of stresses. These proteins that are produced by gene expression have a wide range of activities: antiviral and antibacterial protection, antigen recognition, cellular migration and adhesion, and even red blood cell differentiation and proliferation. It gives us a clue into how even the HIV virus works because these viruses can divert enough of this NF-*KB* for their own purposes and undermine the whole defensive system of the body. NF-*KB* is present in many of the cells of the body, but most important, in the immunological defense systems, particularly in monocytes, macrophages, B cells, and T cells. Ultraviolet light, gamma radiation, x-rays, low oxygen, hydrogen peroxide, and oxidized lipids can cause an activation of the NF-*K*B factor.[4]

Small lipophilic molecules, such as part of the Vitamin A structure and steroids, exert different synergistic effects during the development of organisms, cellular differentiation, and what is known as homeostasis in the adult phase. All these affect, again, the gene expression, or phenotypic expression. One of the key receptors in the DNA is called the peroxisome proliferator activated receptors (PPARs).[5,6] These receptor sites can be activated by a whole variety of compounds, which induce peroxisome proliferation. PPARs are involved in a whole assortment of gene controls that affect lipid metabolism and associated proteins. They are activated by physiological concentration of fatty acids and peroxisome proliferators, including herbicides and plasticizers. In other words, PPARs respond to a variety of signals. These include a variety of drugs, xenobiotics, herbicides, plasticides, solvents and industrial compounds, and long-chain and very-long-chain polyunsaturated and monounsaturated fatty acids. Some of these fatty acids that affect the PPAR activation include: BTA, DHA, eicosapentaenoic (EPA), the decosahexaenoic (DHA), linolenic acid, and arachenoic acids. The monounsaturated fatty acids include oleic acid and erucic acid. Saturated fatty acids include caprylic acid, leic acid, and myristic acid.

The point, again, is that our body is an amazing organism that is actually designed to create a fluid response to a variety of external stimuli and nutrients, with an intricate biology and biochemistry that affects the expression of our DNA. As we put foods into our body, these foods actually stimulate the activation of the PPARs very specifically. The PPARs are a fluid part of our defense system.[7] The function of the PPARs is hypothesized to be very important in the development of early stages of life, especially during the development of lipid metabolism. They are affected by changes in nutrition. Their existence and function implies that nutritional fatty acids act like retinoids, steroids, or thyroid hormones in the control of gene expression. What we eat (and the nature of the fats eaten) does affect our gene expression. The subtlety here again, when we talk about nutrient-gene interaction, is reported in the research described in *Inducible Gene Expression,* which suggests that after glucose gains the phosphorous, a process we call phosphorylation, it becomes glucose-6-phosphate, which can activate the transcription to help glycolic genes at one level and lipogenic genes on the other. This phenomenon seems to be related to insulin as well. The point is that fatty acids, through a well-defined biochemical pathway sequence at the DNA level, participate with different hormones in the regulation of gene expression in direct response to our diet. It is possible that these PPARs are one of the key regulators in the nutrient-gene interaction. Again, without going deeply into biochemistry, the author is simply trying to make the point that what we eat not only affects the genes, but the pathways are well-defined as to how their nutrient-gene expression interactions manifest. This is extraordinarily exciting and reinforces a very simple point: *what we eat feeds our genes.*

Metals and Genetics

One of the most interesting things in our polluted world is the whole issue of heavy metals and heavy metal toxicity. Seventeen of the thirty elements known to be essential to life are metals.[8] These heavy metals are structural and form enzymatic catalytic components; they even act as signal transducers for activation of different DNA expressions.[9] The best example of this is zinc. It is the first trace element to be recognized (in 1869) as a component of an enzyme, carbonic anhydrase. More than 300 enzymes are known to use zinc for proper functioning.[10] Pathological zinc deficiency, as we see as in the autosomal recessive disorder called acrodermatitis enteropathica, can actually lead to death; sufferers must be given high oral zinc doses. Some of these enzymes we refer to are involved in DNA metabolism, as well as RNA polymerases, which, again, activate and help or create new enzymes and proteins from the DNA.[11] Recently it has been discovered that zinc plays an important role as a constituent of proteins that regulate RNA polymerases in multi-celled organisms. Other metals that are absolutely essential to life include cobalt, nickel, copper, and iron.

We have a variety of ways to bring these into our systems, including specific cellular transportation systems and general transportation systems. There is a special gene that helps eliminate the heavy metals called metallothionein (MT), which was discovered in 1957. There are a variety of MT genes: MT1 and MT2 sets. Researchers have defined exactly what chromosome they are on, including chromosome 16.[12] There are also several pseudo-genes. This is an extremely complex set of amino acids; it has sixty-one amino acids, twenty of which are cysteines. These function a lot with heavy metals in general, but more specifically zinc, copper, and cadmium. The important thing here is that organisms that are deficient for these inducible MT genes are much more vulnerable to heavy metal toxicity than their normal counterparts.[13] The heavy metal or MT factors that induce MT synthesis, which is the production of this particular protein from the DNA, are multiple. They include cadmium, zinc, copper, gold, silver, cobalamin, nickel, and bismuth. Hormones that induce MT include the glucocorticoids, progesterone, and estrogen. The catacholamines that induce MT include glucagon, angiotensin, and adenosine. Growth factors that induce MT include insulin and IGF-1. Cytokines and inflammatory agents such as carrageenan, dextran, endotoxins, interleukin-1, interleukin-6, interferon-Y, and tumor necrosis factor all will induce MT production. Vitamins that induce its production include ascorbic acid and retinoate. Antibiotics and cytotoxic agents include hydrocarbons, ethanol, isopropanol, formaldehyde, fatty acids, butyrate, chloroform, carbon tetrachloride, urethan, EDTA, and acetaminophen. Even certain stress conditions, including starvation, inflammation, laparotomy, X-radiation, and ultraviolet radiation, are inducers. All will induce metallothionein synthesis. In other words, this general protein serves to protect our body, not only from heavy metals, but from toxins of all sorts.

These metallothionein (MT) structures are very interesting. For example, MT will bind cadmium much more effectively than it will bind zinc. The various sets of MT are an important part of heavy metal detoxification. There seems to be a definite correlation between the activation of the MT genes and increased ability to deal with the toxicity of heavy metals. It is important to understand that MT, by its ability to bind zinc, may actually moderate the control of certain enzyme systems or RNA polymerases that use zinc. What we see here is that not only do we have a particular system that helps protect us against heavy metals, but also protects the health of our genes. The appropriate supply of minerals plays an important role for gene expression and enzyme function (see Chapter 28). This gene expression of MT is so complicated that it often has more than one function in maintaining the general health of an organism.

Diet and Gene Expression

The type of food we eat has been shown by research to also affect a particular DNA expression. For example, the activation of fat production and of fatty acid synthesis is brought about by switching from a high-fat, low-carbohydrate diet to a low-fat, high-carbohydrate diet.[14] Eating a high-carbohydrate diet is definitely accompanied by an increase in circulating insulin levels. It appears that increased insulin levels increase the transcriptional rate that produces fatty-acid synthase and activates other lipogenic genes.[15,16] Insulin is a powerful effecter on gene expression. Insulin treatment results in a rapid increase of fatty-acid synthase, mRNA, and gene transcription. One study report showed that within six hours of insulin administration, the DNA of animals was induced to create a level of production that was observable in previously fasted mice put on a low-fat, high-carbohydrate diet.[17] In another study, polyunsaturated fats of the n-3 and n-6 families were found to suppress hepatic mRNA levels of several lipogenic genes.[18] These polyunsaturated fatty acids (PUFAs) work on the level of gene production. Researchers have also found that PUFAs exert a negative effect on many genes for the production of fatty acids and could even override the stimulatory effects of insulin, carbohydrates, and thyroid hormones in fat production. PUFAs have been found to suppress hepatic gene expression. Fasting has been found to increase glucagon levels and glucagon seems to act, again, on the gene expression level, to create a downward regulation of fat production. Thyroid hormones also act on the genetic level. Rats that received an administration of thyroid hormone for seven days had their fatty-acid synthase activity doubled,[19] while hypothyroidism reduced hepatic fatty-acid synthase activity.[20]

Another hormone called leptin is a protein that specifically releases fatty tissues that go to the hypothalamus and binds specific receptors that decrease appetite. Researchers found that the administration of leptin to rats consuming a high-carbohydrate, fat-free diet, suppressed the mRNA expression with several lipogenic enzymes. It seemed to be at the same level of suppression of corn oil, which also suppressed lipogenic enzyme expression, while at the same time increasing leptin expression.[21] Research also shows that the growth hormone decreases fatty-acid synthase mRNA by decreasing gene transcription, and mRNA stability.[22,23] Research has also shown that dietary protein and different minerals can affect fatty-acid synthase gene expression as well. Another example of this effect of nutrients on gene expression is evidence that certain fatty acids, such as eicosanoids and vitamins, can actually activate intracellular receptors in ways similar to steroid hormones. Genes, whose expression is activated by insulin, are often negatively affected by contra-regulatory hormones such as corticosteroids. Another example of this principle of the role of diet affecting gene expression is the effect of fasting which is associated with increased circulatory levels of corticosteroids and elevated concentrations of 3-5 cyclic AMP, which creates an effect on the lipogenesis in terms of gene expression. With these examples the author is making a point that dietary factors become important modulators of gene expression.

Alcohol and Gene Expression

Alcohol creates some of the most toxic effects on gene expression. Alcohol apparently seems to affect many of the gene expressions within the central nervous system. Several studies have shown that chronic alcohol exposure alters the expression of both the NR1 and NR2 gene units. These affect the area of the brain called the hippocampus where many changes of the NMDA receptors sub-unit messages of the messenger RNA (mRMA) and protein are observed. The NMDA receptor sites are called glutamate-N-methyl-D-aspartic acid. The overall picture of the research suggests that alcohol affects the regulation of the NMDA receptor sub-unit genes, which may actually contribute to alcohol withdrawal-related central nervous system hyperexcitability. There is also a substantial amount of evidence that acute and chronic alcohol use affects the GABA receptor system.[24] It has been established that the $GABA_A$ receptor sub-unit genes are associated with alcohol. Alcohol affects the $GABA_A$ receptor sub-unit gene expression sites and several brain regions, including the cerebral cortex, the cerebellum, and hippocampus. In other words, research shows that $GABA_A$ receptor sub-unit gene expressions are sensitive to alcohol manipulation. GABA is associated with the valium receptor sites (which are also activated by the commonly used drug valium) in the brain and is a neurotransmitter suppressor unit system in the brain for calming the system. Alcohol also affects glycine, another inhibitory neurotransmitter in the brain, which acts on a strychnine (as in the poison) set of receptors.[25]

Chronic alcohol use has also been shown to alter the expression of the number of dopaminergic receptors.[26] The research seems to suggest that there is a sensitization of the dopaminergic after chronic alcohol intake. Further research shows that alcohol affects the function of the serotonergic system.[27] There are a number of human serotonergic genes affected by the chronic use of alcohol.[28,29] As many as fourteen different serotonergic receptor sites may be affected by the alcohol, with the probable result being a decreased function of the serotonergic nervous system. This includes a decrease in the number of, and density of, post-synaptic 5-hydroxytryptamin receptors in the cortex and hippocampus.[30] Although there are lots of these in the noradrenergic system in relationship to alcohol, there seems to be a strong increase in activity of the brain stem noradrenergic system.[31] Research also shows that ethanol alters the expression of opioid genes.

Alcoholism is associated with low endorphins, and paradoxically leads one to increase the level of social drinking in a futile effort to increase endorphins. Chronic alcohol use also has been shown to create a 30 percent downward regulation and decrease in density of the muscarinergic acetylcholine receptor (mAChR) systems. Chronic alcohol use seems to also cause a decrease in neurotensin receptor density and binding affinity.[32] The point here is that, while we have a decrease in the receptor sites, we're having a decrease in the DNA gene function that produces these receptor sites.

Alcohol and other foods clearly affect the expression of a variety of genes in the central nervous system. Further research, using micro-array chip analysis to examine gene expression in the frontal cerebral cortex of human alcoholics, found selective reprogramming of the myelin-related genes as well as changes in cell cycle genes and several neuronal genes.[33] The use of alcohol is emphasized not only because it is toxic, but because it has been well studied to show how what we eat affects every aspect of our gene expression, including our gene expression in our central nervous system. What we eat affects how we think and how we feel because it affects the genes that regulate how we think and how we feel.

Mitochondrial DNA Expression

Another whole set of gene systems is the DNA in the mitochondria. This is a totally separate set of DNA from the nucleus of the cell. The DNA in mitochondria is determined by the mother only. It is significantly more sensitive to free-radical stress than the DNA in a nuclear system and has far less capacity to repair itself.

Research shows that this DNA is affected by the food we eat. For example, research found that the mitochondrially encoded genes are regulated by retinoic acid, which is a form of vitamin A. These genes include sub-units 5-NADH dehydrogenase.[34] Other nutrients that seem to affect the mitochondrial DNA include thyroid hormone, insulin, vitamin D, and glucocorticoids. There is a definite indication that the fat-soluble vitamins affect mitochondrial DNA gene expression.

Vitamins and Gene Expression

Vitamin D, also known as 1-alpha, 25(oh)2D3, has been found to regulate a significant amount of genes in general, including ATP-synthase, carbonic and hydrase production, genes that regulate carbonic and hydrase production, genes that regulate sodochrome oxidase production, sodochrome B gama interferon, heat-shock protein 70 (discussed earlier), interleukin-6, interleukin-1, interleukin-2 with palothyamine (discussed earlier), prolactin production, parathyroid hormone production, and about thirty other gene functions. It's amazing to view the complexity of the human body, understanding that just vitamin D, and that one form of vitamin D, can have such an effect on so many different genes.

Research on vitamin E is less extensive than on vitamin D, but definitely shows that the tocopherol isomers, such as alpha and delta tocopheranols, have been shown to influence gene expression.[35] The different effects of tocopherol isomers on T-cell production appear to be connected to the regulation of gene expression. Evidence suggests that vitamin E is an important regulator of intracellular signal transduction and therefore an important regulator of expressive gene coating. It appears that most of vitamin E's effect is connected through its control over oxidant-sensitive transcription factors. Vitamin E regulation of genes affects many biological functions, including the vascular, nervous, and immune systems, as well as the diseases that are connected to dysfunction in these systems. The importance of vitamin E in regulating gene expression has implications for the importance of this vitamin in health and disease. Again, what we eat speaks to our genes.

Turning On Our Genes

Now that a scientific foundation is established, we can speak in more general terms about the whole concept of eating and living in a way that activates our healthy genes and turns off our disease-promoting genes. *The principle is that not only what we eat, but how we live and the stresses we create, directly affect gene expression.* The implications of this detailed genetic research are quite exciting. One of the most important elements in this chapter is the broad-stroke statement that we have a potential, under the right conditions, to access all our genetic information at every stage of development, from embryo to adult. The genetic expression of every cell in our body is potentially accessible at any time. The significance of this is that *through proper living, diet, fasting, lifestyle, exercise, and emotional, mental, and spiritual development, we have the opportunity to activate our youthing genes.*

Two pieces of research particularly make this amazing point. Dr. Ian Wilmut, in research completed in 1997, was able to take a mature cell from the udder of an adult female sheep and from this mature cell, he cloned Dolly.[36] His research shows that under the right conditions we can reverse the gene expression of adult cells back to embryonic cell function. The implication is that at any chronological age we have the potential to turn on a younger expression, genetically, of who we are.

Another exciting piece of proof that supports this hypothesis is the treatment of sickle-cell anemia. In 1949, Dr. Linus Pauling, who really is the progenitor of molecular medicine, and his graduate student at CalTech, Harvey Itano, published an extraordinary paper on sickle-cell anemia.[37] They predicted that in the future we'd be able to modify the expression of sickle-cell anemia as a genetic disease.[38] Sickle-cell anemia, which is an inherited condition having to do with one amino-acid change in the hemoglobin structure, causes the hemoglobin to sickle in adults. About 6 percent of children of African descent, according to the author's original research done in Harlem in 1967, have this genetic defect. What happens is the sickle-cell hemoglobin crystallizes in the cell and actually causes the cell to change its shape; a certain amount of sickling of the cells actually cuts into the organs, damages the cells, and damages the organs where these sickle cells clump. It is appropriate to call sickle-cell anemia a molecular disease. In 1994, researchers found that two substances actually do what Dr. Pauling and Dr. Itano predicted. One is hydroxyurea and the other is butyrate. Either one of them awakens the embryonic program of a normal hemoglobin in adults and children with sickle-cell anemia. In utero, fetuses with sickle-cell anemia have normal fetal hemoglobin; it is only after birth that the gene expression for producing the adult hemoglobin emerges with the amino acid defect. When given hydroxyurea or butyrate, the adults with sickle-cell anemia are able to turn on production of a high percentage of fetal hemoglobin – a non-sickling, healthy hemoglobin – in their system. This ameliorates the negative affects of sickle-cell anemia. This is a really exciting message.

What we are saying with these two examples is that by our diet, we are able to turn on the healthiest phenotypic expression of our genetic material.

Lifestyle and emotions can regulate phenotypic expression, upward or downward. From a spiritual point of view, of course, this is important. Taking care of your body, the point of Spiritual Nutrition, is to obtain optimal physical and mental energy to develop your spiritual life. When people don't take care of themselves, they may finally wake up to the importance of spiritual life because their physical body and mental states (as affected by the function of the brain) aren't strong enough to optimize their spiritual pursuits. With this understanding in mind, the importance of eating and living in a way to activate our genes at their healthiest phenotypic potential, gives us the option to maintain our health for an extended period of time to optimize our spiritual life. *Our genes do not themselves give rise to disease as the majority cause. In most cases, disease manifests when people live and eat in a way that turns on the poorest phenotypic expression of who we can be. This is called disease.*

Polymorphic, Pluri-Potential Genes and Individualizing Your Diet

This important concept begins to emerge from the research done in the human genome project, as outlined by Jerry Bishop and Michael Waldholz in their book *Genome*, which describes this breakthrough.[39] The human genome project makes the point that genes are only one part of the story. More important than genetic inheritance is the phenotypic expression. This is the part where we have a choice. As pointed out in the excellent book by Jeffrey Bland, *Genetic Nutritioneering*, scientists have really begun to accumulate an incredible amount of evidence that many diseases previously considered just the luck of a bad draw of genes really are caused from poor diet that creates the poorest phenotypic expression.[40]

Gerontologists are now stating that *75 percent of an individual's health, after the age of 40, is dependent on what the person has done to keep his or her genes healthy and not on the genes themselves.* According to the human genome project there are over a hundred thousand genes and 1.4 million genetic variations. This brings up a whole new principle, that not only are there a lot of genes to affect, but genes are polymorphic, which means there are slight differences in the structure and function of the different genes among people.[41] And as explained earlier, some genes are activated from more than one type of specific protein, so that one message may be translated under one set of conditions differently than under another set of conditions. The principle behind this is that genes are *pluri-potential* – they are affected by a whole variety of different foods and chemical inputs.

This brings us to another point: Even though there are people with slightly different gene patterns, interpreting them is extremely complex, according to current AMA (American Medical Association) research reports. The theory is that even when an individual genome can be displayed on a personal microchip, how that information is interpreted, and the meaning and value of that information, depend on the biological environment in which that human genome is expressed.[42] Knowing that our genes are polymorphic and pluri-potential amplifies the whole concept of a hundred thousand genes in twenty-three sets of chromosomes. These principles are part of the foundation of the author's book *Conscious Eating,* which talks about the importance of individualizing our diet according to our constitution, our lifestyle, and obviously our genetic makeup. One of the leaders in this understanding was the Ph.D. biochemist Roger Williams, who wrote a brilliant book in the 1950s called *Biochemical Individuality.*[43] The teaching in *Conscious Eating,* as in *Spiritual Nutrition,* paraphrases Williams's research conclusions that *nutrition is for real individuals, not a hypothetical "average" person.* So all the RDA (recommended daily allowance) levels, with which the government is trying to minimize our health by assuming there is such a thing as an "average" person, create a great deal of confusion. RDAs don't pay attention to the science that has established the principles of genetic polymorphism and pluri-potential within the human potential.

Williams's concepts in the 1950s were way ahead of the research that proved his point beyond a doubt – that we are not statistical humans. *We are diverse, unique human beings who operate on the principle of biological individuality.* This is the principle that is shared in *Conscious Eating* and *Rainbow Green Live-Food Cuisine,* where it is presented in detail how to eat to enhance your particular biochemical individuality. It is unrealistic for the purpose of this book to cover *all* the details; the author simply wants to give people some idea of the extent of specific support for this concept.

Mind and Emotion Affect Phenotypic Expression

One of the points that take us beyond the point of what you eat or how you exercise is the story of Peter Pan. When J. M. Barrie, the creator of Peter Pan, experienced the traumatic death of his brother, it shut down his phenotypic expression. In his sixties, when he died, he was 4 feet 10 inches and had never gone through physical puberty – in essence, his story was about himself. *The important point is that our mental state and emotional state can significantly alter our phenotypic expression.* J. M. Barrie experienced distress and dwarfism from the emotional trauma of his brother's death. Aside from the extreme response of completely shutting down one's hormonal system and becoming a stress-induced dwarf, other signs of poor phenotypic expression are typically seen by the author in his medical office: low energy, fatigue, unbalanced emotional states, sleep disturbances, chronic pain, inability to lose weight – all signs of a poor phenotypic expression.

One of the points that needs to be continually clarified in this discussion is that the exercise we do, our emotional states, and the food we eat do not actually change the hardcopy of our genes, but, rather, the software expression of our genes. These lifestyle and diet choices modify the expression of the hardcopy of the genes. Although examples have been given of dramatic changes, as with sickle-cell anemia, usually many of these changes take place over time with a consistent, toxic lifestyle. Another point is that what you eat doesn't change things entirely. For example, research shows that only 30–50 percent of people with high blood pressure have the type of blood pressure that is salt-sensitive.[44] Research also suggests that only about 50 percent of the variation of blood cholesterol levels, 36 percent of the variation in blood pressure, and 20 percent of ovarian cancer can be explained by genetics alone; the rest is modified by our gene expression.[45]

How What We Eat Affects Our Gene Expression

The effect of food on our gene expression is very interesting; it can be quite profound. Researchers have found that the amino acids in vegetable protein, although complete, are slightly different than, and offer certain advantages over, animal protein. Vegetable protein has been found to affect many aspects of our metabolism, including the improvement of insulin sensitivity and the reduction of toxic reactions.[46] Simply changing the excess of calories in the diet and improving the ratio of protein to carbohydrates and fat according to your constitution can actually improve the regulation of blood sugar levels.[47] One of the most potent components of food that affects gene expression on the molecular level is phytonutrients. Research on phytonutrients supports the general findings; for example, 82 percent of 156 different published dietary studies found that fruit and vegetable consumption helped protect against cancer.[48] People who eat more fruits and vegetables have about one-half the risk of cancer mortality than those people who are not vegetable eaters.

Diets high in fruits and vegetables are very high in phytonutrients, which include a variety of antioxidants, carotenes, vitamin E, vitamin C, phenolic compounds, and terpenoids that specifically turn on not only anti-cancer genes but anti-aging genes, and anti-inflammation genes. Some of the phytonutrients include: the allyl sulfides in garlic and onions, which are potent stimulators of improved phenotypic expression, antioxidant function, and detoxification; phytates in grains and legumes, which have anti-cancer effects; glucarates in citrus, grains, and tomatoes, which improve the gene expression of detoxification; lignans in flax, which improve the metabolism of estrogen and testosterone; isoflavones in soybeans, which increase activity of estrogen and testosterone; saponins in legumes, which have anti-cancer qualities; indoles, isothiocyanates, and hydroxybutene in cruciferous vegetables, which improve detoxification against carcinogens; ellagic acid in grapes, raspberries, strawberries, and nuts, which improve antioxidant function; and bioflavonoids, carotenoids, and terpenoids, which reduce inflammation and improve immunity. These substances have been shown, according to *Genetic Nutritioneering*, to specifically induce anti-cancer genes, and to turn on and turn off cancer-producing genes. One of the most powerful phytonutrient fruits is oranges, which have more than 170 phytochemicals and 60 bioflavonoids. The combination of these have the effect to obviously modify gene expression in a positive way, as well as create and increase antioxidant expression, anti-inflammatory expression, inhibit blood clots, and activate the expression of increased detoxification systems. There are more than twenty carotenoids in oranges, and these include: lutein and zeaxanthin (very important for vision), crytoxanthin, and beta carotene. These have been associated also with decreasing the incidence of macular degenerative disease. A monoterpine nutrient found in grapefruit is called limonene, which specifically activates the gene expression of a detoxifying enzyme called glutathione S-tranferase. This helps protect against cancer by detoxifying cancer-producing chemicals. Another important one is the glucarate family, found in the whites of the oranges and probably in grapefruit. The glucarates seem to improve our gene expression in terms of protecting against breast cancer. The author recognizes garlic as more of a medicine and not necessarily as a regular food because it has been shown to raise imbalance in EEG studies of the right and left side of the brain. Garlic also has a variety of phytochemicals that moderate gene expression – particularly the sulfur compounds, which help lower blood pressure and cholesterol and boost immunity.[49] Inflammation is definitely affected by our gene expression. The author's favorite anti-inflammatory food is ginger; it has active phytochemicals called gingerols. They have been shown to be quite effective in the treatment of arthritis and other inflammation problems. Used in conjunction with curcumin, these two have been shown to improve gene expression in regard to anti-inflammatory response.[50,51] A very popular flavonoid is called quercetin. Found in apples, onion, and garlic, quercetin helps improve gene expression in relationship to allergy and arthritis.[52] Bioflavonoids, of which quercetin is one, are perhaps some of the most important modifiers of gene expression, in addition to being antioxidants.

This discussion takes us into the whole question of the use of wine and black and Chinese green teas, which are very high in bioflavonoids. The Chinese green teas also contain the class of bioflavonoids called catechins. These catechins are particularly strong antioxidants. Wine has a whole lot of flavonoids. Red wine also has a number of phenolics, the most important being resveratrol and quercetin, which alter gene expression and enhance phenotypic expression to protect against blood clot formation as in heart disease. Resveratrol also has certain anti-aging qualities that are recently being touted to mimic the calorie restriction effect. However, red wine also has the downside of being alcohol. Alcohol does many things to disregulate and undermine healthy gene expression, particularly in the neurotransmitter systems, as well as other systems in the body. Resveratrol, quercetin, and the bioflavonoids can easily be gotten from substances other than red wine. Healthful sources of bioflavonoids include grapes, onion, garlic, and the white inner peel of citrus fruits. The bioflavonoids also promote the activation of the gene expression of phase-two detoxification enzymes in the liver. Bioflavonoids are a class of phytonutrients that contain subclasses, including isoflavones,

flavones, and flavenols. These are very important antioxidants; they affect hormone modulation, anti-inflammatory protection, and gene expression of our detoxification enzymes.

Vitamins and minerals also affect our gene expression. The B vitamins are particularly important in this, especially B_6, B_{12}, and folic acid. These clearly modulate gene activity to protect us against cancer and heart disease, as well as improve brain function. Minerals, of course, play an important role in affecting our phenotypic expression. Zinc is one of the most important of these; it's involved in more than 300 enzymatic reactions. Zinc is important in growth function, immune function, and hormonal development.

Detoxification

Detoxification is one of the most interesting and most important aspects of how to eat in a way that supports gene expression that will protect against the overwhelming amount of toxins in the environment. It is very common for people to come into the author's office and say, "You know, I eat a good diet. Everything is fine. Why am I so toxic?" Well, the author tries to explain to them, research shows that the real toxicity is somewhat related to how effective our detoxification systems are. The research suggests that our detoxification strength in general will vary between three- and five-fold from person to person. One study in Hawaii[53] showed that people with various ethnic backgrounds had a nearly twenty-fold difference in detoxification ability from one individual to another. That is an amazing difference. The data suggests that almost one-third of the variation is associated with diet. The author tries to put people at ease with understanding that if someone is exposed to the same level of toxins as somebody else but has more trouble, what that person must do is work harder to create a better gene expression to amplify the ability to detoxify. The key is that our detoxification enzymes are controlled by our genes.

Some of the nutrients that play a very important role in the detoxification systems include: glycine, B complex vitamins, pantothenic acid (especially because it strengthens the adrenals), chlorine, cysteine, magnesium, selenium, zinc, and glutathione. There are also particular enzymes that are important, one of which is n-acetyl-transferase. One study[54] shows that smokers who have a poor n-acetyl-transferase function have a much higher rate of breast cancer. Lung cancer is much higher in smokers who have a poor level of the detoxification enzyme called glutathione transferase.[55] Once you know that and you want to keep smoking, then you have to make your choices. At least knowing that you have some weaknesses means that you then have the potential to make better choices. The amino acid glycine is kind of a sleeper because most people don't know about its power, but research back in the 1930s found that oral doses of up to 3,000 milligrams of glycine greatly improves the ability of the liver to recover from liver disease and improve its detoxability.[56] One of the most popular phytochemicals today comes from the cruciferous vegetables; this includes the category of substances called glucosinolates – indole-3-carbonal, phenylisothiocyanate, and 3-hydroxybutene. These seem to activate the gene expression for creating detoxification enzymes that eliminate carcinogens from the system. One study, for example, showed that Brussels sprouts increased the particular gene expression for production of glutathione S-transferase.[57] This seems to be connected to a generally low incidence of cancer, especially colon cancer, among people who eat cruciferous vegetables. As we look at the whole issue of detoxification, the bioflavonoids may be at the top of the list as potent phytochemicals for the stimulation of gene expression to create detoxification function. They work at what we call phase-two enzymes in the detoxification system, which has phase-one and phase-two sets. Particularly when concerned with liver detoxification, the bioflavonoids seem to activate the phase-two detoxification.

An interesting concept is the idea of an overload of toxins. If someone says, "I go out and have some food that isn't organic," the author teaches that once in a blue moon it isn't a problem, but to continually eat food that is not organic is to build up "toxic load." The whole issue is how much can we overload our detoxification machinery before it breaks down and loses the ability to detoxify cancer, chemicals, and so forth.

So we have two levels here: We have the ability to build up the machinery by eating certain foods that amplify our detoxification systems and we have the ability of minimizing the toxins coming into our system.

The Anti-Aging Effects of Gene Expression

One of the points we started the chapter with is that we have the potential, through what we eat, how we live, and how we think, to affect the gene expression of our anti-aging genes. An article in *Science* by Dr. Caleb

Finch, a professor at the Andrus Geretonology Center at the University of Southern California, makes this point very clearly. He concludes that heredity plays a minor role in determining long lifespan. The most important role in longevity is connected to lifestyle.[58] One important part of this anti-aging process is a diet high in antioxidants – a diet that's high in carotenoids, flavonoids, zinc, manganese, copper, and vitamins E, C, and A.

The collector's edition of *Life Extension 2004* reports that the phytonutrient resveratrol, which activates sirtuin genes, has been found by researchers at Harvard Medical School and BIOMOL Research Laboratories to activate a "longevity gene" in yeast that lengthens lifespan by 70 percent. It seems to activate one of the same genes as caloric restriction (discussed in Chapter 22). This research has been duplicated in worms and flies. Humans do have their own form of the "sirtuin" genes. It works by increasing the rate of deacetylation. This may also be why resveratrol has such powerful research showing it not only prevents cancer, but may actually be considered as a treatment.[59] Resveratrol stops cancer in a variety of ways, from blocking estrogens and androgens to modulating genes. It has even shown a 30–71 percent ability to block bone metastasis.[60] Resveratrol appears to moderate the body's detrimental inflammatory response to injury of the brain and spinal cord. It has also been shown to protect on many levels, including the antioxidant level, against heart and blood vessel disease.

Resveratrol is classified as a polyphenol. Polyphenols are broken down to subclasses such as flavonoids and proanthocyanidins. Resveratrol is found in organic grapes, pine trees, and other plants such as polygonnum cuspidatum. This expansion of information on resveratrol helps to make the point of the role of phytonutrients in gene control and as antioxidants. When we cook our food, many of the actions of these phytonutrients are compromised or entirely lost. The effects of free radical damage are seen throughout the whole body. It does appear that organs that are very high in oxygen, such as the brain, heart, liver, gastrointestinal tract, kidneys, immune system, endocrine system, lungs, and blood suffer the most from antioxidant stress.

Perhaps the organ, to use the term loosely, that's most affected by antioxidant stress is the mitochondria. The mitochondria require a tremendous amount of oxygen to function appropriately. The rate of aging could almost be measured by the amount of oxygen that the mitochondria are able to receive. Our health protocols at the Tree of Life involve a focus on bringing as much oxygen as possible to the mitochondria. Associated with that oxygen supply and energy production is that mitochondria produce the most free radicals as a result of the energy metabolism. The mitochondria are the source of metabolic energy in the system. Mitochondria have a totally separate set of DNA, which is inherited from the mother only. The mitochondrial DNA does not seem to have the mechanism for repairing itself; therefore, the only way we can protect the mitochondrial DNA, its function, and expression, is to have a body that is very high in antioxidants that are specific for protecting the mitochondria. Those include: glutathione, lipolic acid, coenzyme Q10, superoxide dismutase, and vitamin E. These dietary nutrients help protect the mitochondria from free radical destruction. Understanding that the mitochondria are not only subject to normal oxidation stress and free radical injury by radiation, pollution, and drugs, but diet also has a large effect. When the mitochondria are not functioning well, we see the symptoms of fatigue, low energy, and chronic pain. Dr. Bruce Ames, chairman of the Department of Biochemistry at the University of California, published research that suggests that mitochondrial DNA is about fifteen times more susceptible than nuclear DNA to free radical oxidative injury.[61] The main defense we have for the mitochondria, again, is a high antioxidant input. In an inductive way we can say that the free radical oxidants that are normally produced within the mitochondria as a result of a reduction in antioxidant protection, serve to down-regulate gene expression in the nuclear DNA. If they are not destroyed by antioxidants, they indeed can create an alteration in gene expression from the chromosome messages that result in the nucleus.[62] This is a very important statement of the interaction between the mitochondrial DNA and the nuclear DNA. Substances that alter the gene expression at the mitochondrial level in a negative way include superoxide, singlet oxygen, hydroxyl radicals, and hydrogen peroxide. Luckily, antioxidants play an important role in activating the antioxidant synthase. Antioxidants therefore play an important role in protecting gene expression.[63] The normal reactive oxygen species that are created in the mitochondria have been associated with a variety of chronic diseases, including heart disease, cancer, and Alzheimer's.

Mitochondrial function is not only related to muscle and energy function, but very much related to proper brain functioning as well. Evidence indicates that inflammation in the brain and toxins tend to create a breaking down of the mitochondrial energy production in the brain cells, which causes the cells to die. The term for this cell death is apoptosis. One major pathway of death is when the cells are not able to maintain their function; they shrink, become dehydrated, lose their proper energy production in the mitochondria, and are unable to eliminate the excess oxidants in mitochondria, all of which results in cell death.[64] One of the best antioxidants for the brain is vitamin E, a complex of alpha-beta-theta-delta-epsilon tocotrienols and tocopherols. The tocotrienols and the tocopherols could be the most potent inhibitor of mitochondrial oxidative stress in the brain.[65] Other key antioxidants to protect the brain include vitamin C, the bioflavonoids, coenzyme Q10, and alpha lipoic acid.

Nutritional Practices for Youthing

Now that we have firmly established that what we eat and what we don't eat affects our gene expression, and therefore youthing, we are ready to explore the optimal nutritional practices that will indeed turn on youthing gene expressions. In the author's experience there are four main dietary practices that greatly increase the youthing process – undereating (calorie restriction), veganism and live-food nutrition, and Spiritual Fasting. In the following chapters we will explore these practices, in relationship to gene expression and beyond.

Summary, Chapter 21

1. The human genome research shows us more than 1.4 million genetic variations in the human genome, with more than 100,000 genes.
2. At every stage of development – from embryo to the most elderly – all genetic information is encoded in the gene type and is accessible to any cell at any stage as a potential phenotypic expression. Therefore, we have the potential to activate the highest phenotypic expression at any age.
3. Our genes do not necessarily give rise to disease. Disease arises when lifestyle, diet, and mental stress activate aging gene expression.
4. Genes are both polymorphic in the human population and pluripotential. Therefore, they can act in a variety of ways according to different internal and external environmental pressures.

5. Gene expression is affected by diet, lifestyle, and environmental stresses. Effecters include movement, food, breath, stress, and emotional and spiritual life.
6. Early symptoms of altered, dysfunctional gene expression include sleep disturbances, imbalanced emotions, low energy, and fatigue. These are markers of dysfunctional gene expression.
7. What we eat speaks to our genes, either turning on the youthing genes or turning on aging genes.
8. Food does not change our physical genes or the messages that are embedded in the genes; what food does is change the way the message is expressed.

Chapter 22

Undereat!

There is never enough food to feed the hungry soul.

GABRIEL

The Importance of Undereating

The most important single rule in Spiritual Nutrition is undereat!!! Moses Maimonides (1135–1204 A.D.), Rabbi, physician, and the most celebrated of all Jewish healers, taught, "Overeating is like a deadly poison to any constitution and is the principle cause of all disease."[1] Sai Baba of Shirdi, a great Hindu-Moslem saint of the early 1900s, always gave the advice, "Eat simple and little." Paavo Airola taught that "systematic undereating is the NUMBER ONE health and longevity secret. Overeating, on the other hand, of even health foods, is one of the main causes of disease and premature aging."[2] Jesus, in the *Essene Gospel of Peace, Book One* said:

> And when you eat, never eat unto fullness. Flee the temptations of Satan, and listen to the voices of God's angels. For Satan and his power tempt you always to eat more and more. But live by the spirit and resist the desires of the body. And your fasting is always pleasing in the eyes of the angels of God. So give heed to how much you have eaten when you are sated, and eat always less by a third.[3]

The author's own awareness of undereating was heightened while serving as a physician in India. On Sundays there would usually be a feast, and just as regularly on Monday, Tuesday, and Wednesday people would come in with diarrhea and dysentery. They would be weak and uncomfortable, their lives were disrupted, and they had trouble meditating as a result of their illness. An old Arabic proverb says, "By eating we become sick and by digesting we become healthy." If we are too weak to assimilate the forces and organisms in our food, they overcome us. Those who tended to eat very little at these feasts usually did not get sick because there was less food and fewer bacterial and parasitic forces to overcome. This is one of the secrets of not getting sick while traveling.

One of the most practical reasons for undereating is that it is hard to meditate if our energy is still involved with digesting food. This is especially true if we want to get up early in the morning to meditate and we have eaten too much the night before. What the author discovered was that even while he was in a cycle of meditating six hours per day, as long as he underate the food available (cooked vegetables and chapatis, a flat bread), in no way was his energy for meditation depleted. This rule takes precedence over all other dietary advice. This does not mean that we can make a diet out of undereating junk foods and not deplete our energy. If raw, whole, organic foods are available, they are still the choice for optimizing our diet for spiritual life.

Famous Undereaters

Dr. Pelletier, in his research on longevity, found that cultures in which people led the longest, healthiest lives – the natives of the Vilcabambam region of Ecuador, the Hunza of West Pakistan, the Tarahumara Indians of northern Mexico, and the Russian people of the Abkhasian region – ate low-protein, high-natural-carbohydrate diets that contained approximately one-half the amount of protein Americans eat and only 50–60 percent of the total calories.[4] Airola makes the point in *How to Get Well* that one never sees an obese centenarian.

There are many historical cases of the health and longevity benefits of undereating. St. Paul the anchorite lived to be 113 years, eating only dates and drinking only water. Thomas Carn, born in London in 1588, lived to be 207, and a Mr. Jenkins, born in Yorkshire, England, lived from 1500 to 1670; both ate no breakfast, had either raw milk or butter with honey and fruit for lunch (Carn may have had bread also), and had either raw milk or fruit for supper. The French Countess Desmond Catherine, who lived to the age of 145, ate only fruit.

One of the most famous undereaters is Luigi Cornaro, a Venetian nobleman in the ministry of the Pope, who lived from 1464 to 1566. By his forties, he had nearly eaten himself to death. He was attended by Doctor Father Benedict, who advised him in the arts of natural living and undereating. From that point on, he simplified his diet to 12 ounces of food and 14 ounces of liquid per day, never deviating from this undereating. He was quoted to have said "A word to the wise is sufficient." The one exception to his diet program was at the age of 78 when his family insisted he increase his intake. He increased food intake by 2 ounces and immediately got sick. After this he dropped down to 8 ounces of food and 11 ounces of liquid per day until he died at the age of 102. His writings on undereating can be summed up in two statements: *"The less I ate, the better I felt"* and *"Not to satiate oneself with food is the science of health."*[5] Szekely points out that Luigi Cornaro is a link in the transmission of the Essene teachings.[6] This transmission came through St. Jerome's translation of the *Essene Gospel of Peace,* from Constantine the African, who studied these texts in the monastery at Monte Cassino and who taught the Essene natural ways at the Salerno School of Medicine where Doctor Father Benedict was trained. Part of the transmission of the Essene teachings was Cornaro's emphasis on the practice of sobriety, which he shared with everyone, including the Pope, who became his student. Sobriety, the art of eating in moderation, can be reduced to two simple guidelines: first, to avoid eating more than our system can easily digest and assimilate; and second, to avoid food and drink that disagree with the stomach. Sobriety means to pay intelligent attention to the quantity and quality of foods we eat. In practice, it means leaving the table while still wanting to eat and drink more. An old proverb says, "What we leave after taking a hearty meal does us more good than what we have eaten."

Scientific Evidence for Calorie Restriction and Youthing

Maximum lifespan, which is different from average lifespan, is a measure of who lives longest in any species. Maximum lifespan is the outer limit of lifespan potential and leads us to an understanding about how to turn on the youthing genes and actually reverse the aging process; it is not simply achieving a normal healthy lifespan. It is important to note that in all the calorie-restriction research described here, the animals, in general, were more youthful, vigorous, and energetic, when compared to normals, and showed minimal to no chronic degenerative diseases. It is also important to note that this turning on of the youthing genes and life extension seem to be achieved in a variety of mammalian species. Therefore, it is reasonable to hypothesize that this effect happens in human beings. There is not a single instance in the history of medicine that such broad-spectrum effects in a variety of animals could not be shown to be similar in humans. Obviously, doing double-blind research in humans is a little bit difficult and so we have to fall back on some of the historic examples that were talked about previously.

Dr. McKay, of Cornell University, found in the 1930s that the lifespan of rats doubled when their food intake was halved. Not only did these calorie-restricted rats live longer, but they were more healthy and youthful, compared to the control rats. He found that his control rats, given the normal, eat-as-much-as-you-want diet, became weak and feeble while they lived out their normal lifespan, which was approximately thirty-two months (the equivalent of age 95 in human terms). The calorie-restricted rats at thirty-two months were still alive, youthful, and vigorous; one lived 1,456 days (nearly fifty months, corresponding to age 150 in human terms). When this research was repeated in the 1960s with calorie-restricted rats at the Morris H. Ross Institute, they lived up to 1,800 days, or approximately 180 years in human terms.[7]

In the 1970s, breakthrough research was done by Dr. Roy Walford and Dr. Richard Weindruch at the UCLA Medical Center, where they found that even gradual restriction of calorie intake in middle-aged rats extended lifespan as much as 60 percent.

Professor Huxley extended the lifespan of worms to nineteen times their average lifespan by periodically underfeeding them.[8] Research has also shown that undereating increases the lifespan in fruit flies, water fleas, and trout.[9]

One of the more interesting points about this research, particularly that of Walford and Weindruch, is that it shows that middle-aged mice on a calorie-restricted diet can get significant anti-aging results. In other words, *it doesn't matter at what age you start; you can still turn on the youthing gene expression.*

The next significant breakthrough in this anti-aging work began in the 1990s with Dr. Richard Weindruch and Dr. Thomas Prolla, working at the University of Wisconsin. Using the micro-array gene chip technology, a technique that can measure the expression of thousands of genes at one time, they studied the gene expression in mice, rats, monkeys, and humans. Weindruch and Prolla studied the gene profiles in muscles in normal and in calorie-restricted mice and saw major changes in gene expression between the two groups. Their results were published in the esteemed journal *Science*. This is really the first time in history that scientists could study gene expression. They found that the gene expression was significantly altered by caloric restriction in a way that seemed to slow the aging process. Weindruch and Prolla compared normally fed and calorie-restricted five- and thirty-month-old mice.Their experiments with the older mice showed a significant difference in age-related gene expression when they were calorie restricted. They showed that long-term caloric restriction did slow the aging process.[10]

Dr. Stephen R. Spindler, professor of biochemistry at the University of California, Riverside, using gene technology, studied the expression of 11,000 genes in the livers of young, normally fed, and calorie-restricted mice. Spindler found that 60 percent of the age-related changes in gene expression from calorie-restricted mice occurred just a few weeks after they started the calorie-restricted diet. This is a significant finding, because it indicates that even if it takes years for the full effects of calorie restriction to become expressed, the genetic profile for anti-aging develops quickly when you restrict the diet. Spindler found that calorie restriction specifically produced a genetic anti-aging profile and was able to reverse the majority of age-related degenerative changes that show up in gene expression. He found a four-fold increase in the expression of their youthing genes in short-term caloric restriction and a two-point-five-fold increase in the expression of youthing genes in long-term caloric restriction. He was able to reproduce this with 95 percent reproducibility.

Spindler noted that the caloric restriction not only prevented deterioration or genetic change gradually over the lifespan of the animal, but actually reversed most of the aging changes in a short period of time. In fact, his research only lasted a month with the mice. In another set of research, he found the most rapid changeover from a genetic aging profile to anti-aging occurred in older animals as well as young and middle-aged ones. Again, emphasizing the point that Weindruch and Prolla had made earlier, that it doesn't matter what age you begin, caloric restriction does appear to turn on the expression of the youthing genes, and turn off the expression of the aging genes. We have the full memory of all our gene expressions in all our chromosomes; all we have to do is push the right button to get a healthy expression. This finding suggests (although too soon to say "prove") that calorie restriction could potentially reverse aging and improve and extend lifespan in older animals, and therefore, humans as well. *Spindler's research is perhaps the first to show that caloric restriction could actually turn on the youthing genes and literally reverse the aging process.* The earlier research measured the physiological changes of aging that could be slowed by caloric restriction. An important part of Spindler's research is that short-term caloric restriction can turn on the majority of the anti-aging genes. His impression, from a recent interview in *Life Extension Magazine,* is that if people lose ten pounds, regardless of what their weight is before they start the diet, many of their physiological parameters of health will improve. He found what has already been stated: that weight loss improves insulin sensitivity, improves blood glucose, decreases blood insulin levels, decreases heart rate, and improves blood pressure. He also noted the potential anti-cancer effect.

His research indicated that caloric restriction is pro-apoptotic, meaning it promotes self-suicide of damaged or cancer-producing cells. Spindler, as well as others, feels that this pro-apoptotic effect is because calorie restriction lowers the amount of chaperone proteins. Calorie restriction lowers the level of chaperones and therefore creates more cell death, and particularly more cell death for dysfunctional, potentially cancerous, or mutated cells. If one has a high chaperone level, which tends to occur with age, the cells are less apt to commit suicide, even though they tend to remain damaged or mutated and may be secreting harmful substances to the tissues or even becoming cancerous.

Spindler also found, particularly with older animals, an associated increase in gene expression that created an anti-inflammation effect. The effect of inflammatory stress, as well as physiological stress, seems to happen more with age. He found that a significant amount of this inflammatory gene expression and stressed gene expression diminished with calorie restriction.

In summary, Spindler's results, as published in the proceedings of the National Academy of Science, basically showed: *(1) No matter what age you are, you still get an anti-aging effect with calorie restriction. (2) Anti-aging effects can happen quickly on a low-calorie diet. (3) Calorie restriction of only four weeks in mice seemed to partially restore the liver's ability for metabolizing drugs and for detoxification. (4) Calorie restriction seemed to quickly decrease the amount of inflammation and stress, even in older animals.*[11]

Work by Dr. Berger, described in his book *Forever Young,* was another way that this anti-aging, or youthing principle, has been discovered. He found that if people, through calorie restriction, maintained a weight of approximately 20 percent less than the normal insurance scale weights, one could achieve the calorie-restriction effect, and therefore optimal longevity and well-being.[12] This simplified approach gets away from calorie counting and is the approach that the author often recommends to people.

At this point in time, the only specific anti-aging effect that has been demonstrated repeatedly in all sorts of life systems is that calorie restriction consistently slows aging in all varieties of animals, including various mammalian species. Research has shown that not only does it result in longer lifespan, but it also lowers blood pressure, reduces destructive auto-antibodies that attack the brain, reduces loss of central nervous system cells, strengthens the immune system, slows the overall aging process, lowers cholesterol, diminishes the rate of heart disease, reduces muscle oxygen loss, improves muscle function, reduces free radical damage to body tissue, helps stabilize blood sugar in adult-onset diabetes (and in the author's clinical research even reverses Syndrome X), and helps the body run at peak metabolic efficiency.

The Art of Spiritual Nutrition

The art of Spiritual Nutrition is to take just the right amount of food and drink for our individual needs. It means to consume exactly what is necessary to assimilate the energy and biomolecular structures required to maintain our body as a mature human crystal. It is to eat in a way that completely supports our transmutation into a superconductor for the spiritualizing energy of the Kundalini. It is to eat in a way that best allows us to attract, conduct, store, and transmit the cosmic energy entering our system.

In Part II, we are exploring the qualitative guidelines for this. The quantitative amounts are quite individual, determined only through trial and error. We become both researcher and the one being researched, an approach that helps develop an inner sensitivity to our real biomolecular and energetic needs. Through meditation and fasting, our body is continually transmuting. As we purify on the body-mind-spiritual levels, more cosmic energy is able to enter our system, so we require less energy from Nature via our food. Through fasting and lighter diets, our basement membrane becomes clearer and more porous. As this happens, the nutrients we take in get to the cells more easily so we need less food to obtain the same amount of biomolecular nutrition. This is distinctly different from the concept of minimal eating or progressively decreasing food intake as an obsessive mathematical effort to reach a minimum. That is a deprivation-mortification practice that does not necessarily lead to spiritual growth. It does not have the same effect as the highly intuitive approach of eating the most appropriate amount to maximally stimulate spiritual evolution.

Summary, Chapter 22

1. The most important single rule in nutrition is to undereat.
2. Human cultural studies, case histories, and animal studies have shown that undereating prolongs lifespan.
3. Not to satiate ourself with food is the science of health.
4. The art of Spiritual Nutrition is to be sufficiently attuned to our inner needs and outer life in a way that we know just the right amount of food to eat. It requires us to be attuned to the subtle changes occurring over time and to adjust our diet accordingly.

Chapter 23

Spiritual Fasting

Spiritual Fasting – the Elixir of Spiritual Nutrition

Spiritual Fasting is another powerful force in Spiritual Nutrition. Fasting for at least seven days on green juices, as we do in our Spiritual Fasting Retreats at the Tree of Life, is the most powerful dietary way of becoming a superconductor for the Divine. Done in a full-spiritual context, it calms the vrittis of the mind, purifies the koshas, clears the nadis, and sets the pre-conditions for the awakening of Kundalini. In our Spiritual Fasts there is an intense experience of the Six Foundations and all the cleansing of the koshas is accelerated. As a result of this, about 90 percent of the people who immerse themselves in the high-prana elixir of Spiritual Fasting at the Tree of Life experience a Kundalini/Shekhinah awakening. Kundalini/Shekhinah requires a pranic energy high enough for the Grace of Shaktipat/Smicha l'shefa/Haniha to awaken it. These Spiritual Fasts are the quintessence of what Spiritual Nutrition can be. This is why the Tree of Life Rejuvenation Center has become what many people consider the leading Spiritual Fasting center in the world.

Fasting, practiced as an essential discipline for the attainment of true knowledge, has its history in the spiritual practices of almost all religions. Socrates, Plato, and the Stoic and Neoplatonist philosophers such as Epicteus and Plotinus used fasting to purify the spirit in order to better perceive the Truth. Socrates and Plato practiced ten-day fasts.[1] Pythagoras, the great mathematician, practiced forty-day fasts.[2] Fasting is used in religions such as Judaism, Christianity, Hinduism, Islam, and Buddhism for a variety of different purposes – penitence, propitiation, a preparatory rite for initiations and marriage, mourning, to develop magical powers, purification, health, and spiritual development. In Hebrew, the word for fasting is *tsoum*. It means the voluntary abstinence from food with a religious end. This is a good definition of Spiritual Fasting.

The most important fast for the Jews is the abstinence from food and water for the one day prescribed by the Torah for the Day of Atonement (Yom Kippur). Fasting was prescribed for penitence for sins, and there are fasts of devotion prescribed on Monday and Thursday. Fasts were done to appease God, to ward off punishments, and to seek God's favor. The most famous fasts in the Jewish tradition are Moses' and Elijah's forty-day fasts. Daniel, the prophet, fasted in preparation for receiving his revelations. Esther and all the Jewish people in Persia fasted for deliverance from physical destruction. Judith was said to fast all the days of her life (Judith 8:6). With the exception of these famous fasts, most Jewish fasting was prescribed as part of fulfilling the Torah, until the Alexandrian Jews developed the philosophy that bodily desires interfered with spirituality and fasting helped to release mind energies from the material to spiritual level.

The Essenes, who were ascetic, esoteric, scholarly Jewish communities living near Egypt and the Dead Sea, and who authored the Dead Sea Scrolls, used fasting as an important approach for purifying their bodies and enhancing their Communion with God. The prophet Elijah was said to have founded the Essenes at Mt. Carmel. The name Essene means "expectant of the One who is to come." They were well-known as prophets and great healers. Essene also means healer, and their members were often called *therapeutae*. Many of them lived to be more than 120 years old.[3] The inner core group of the Essenes fasted for forty days one time each year.[4] Jesus was reportedly raised in an Essene community in Egypt after escaping from Herod the Great. He carried the teaching of fasting to his disciples through his own practice of the forty-day fast and other references to fasting for purification and healing of body and soul. He taught in the *Essene Gospel of Peace, Book One* that:

> . . . the word and the power of God will not enter into you, because all manner of abominations have their dwelling in your body and your spirit; for the body is the temple of the spirit, and the spirit is the temple of God. Purify therefore, the temple, that the Lord of the temple may dwell therein and occupy a place that is worthy of Him. . . . Renew yourselves and fast. For I tell you truly, that Satan and his

> plagues may only be cast out by fasting and prayer. [Also in Mark 9:29.] Go by yourself and fast alone.... The living God shall see it and great will be your reward. And fast til Beelzebub and all his evil spirits depart from you, and all the angels of our earthly Mother come and serve you [harmony with Nature]. For I tell you truly, except you fast, you shall never be freed from the power of Satan and all the diseases that come from Satan. Fast and pray fervently, seeking the power of the living God for your healing.[5]

In the two centuries after this, the first Christians practiced various forms of voluntary and prescribed fasting without any set form or rules. The main fasts were the Paschal fast and the weekly fasts of Wednesday and Friday. From 200 to 500 A.D., the practice of fasting came under ecclesiastical discipline. In this process of organized fasting, as in Judaism, fasting lost its character as a voluntary practice, although in both religions, the tradition of voluntary fasting has carried into modern times. For long periods of time the Baal Shem Tov, the Hasidic master, was said to fast during the week and eat only on the Sabbath. The Hasidic master, Rabbi Nachman, was reported to fast from Sabbath to Sabbath as often as eighteen times in one year.[6] According to the Vatican Council II, the Church now only asserts ecclesiastical authority over ceremonial fasting. It encourages voluntary fasting as a legitimate spiritual practice but has chosen not to assert authority over the specifics of the individual fasting practices. There are Christian monks who voluntarily fast as a spiritual practice, as in the practice of Matthew the Poor of the Coptic (Egyptian) Orthodox Church, as a well as the monastic orders of Cistercians, Carmelites, and Carthusians.

In Hinduism, fasting is practiced with the idea of Union with God as well as to fulfill religious prescriptions. The Upanishads, part of the Hindu Holy scriptures, refer to fasting as a means of Union with God. In Hinduism, fasting is used for penitence, before a marriage, before religious initiations, to receive a blessing or a boon from God, and on the new and full moons. The use of fasting in the Hindu tradition is similar to the Judeo-Christian in that it is considered penitence, a time of remembrance and honoring important events, and for sacrifice and Union with God.

Fasting to Enhance Spiritual Life

Fasting allows our physical bodies to turn toward the assimilation of pranic energy rather than biochemical energy. By accelerating the purification of the body, it allows the physical body to become a better conductor of the Kundalini energy. This improves the alignment of the chakras and subtle bodies, which makes it easier for the cosmic prana to enter the body and increases the possibility of the awakening of the Shakti Kundalini. By removing toxins from the system, we not only become healthier, but we remove blocks from the body and therefore enhance the movement of all energy in the system, as well as of the spiritualizing force of the Kundalini. Through repeated fasts we also become clearer channels for the assimilation of cosmic energy into our systems. We also increase our sensitivity to the movement of the Kundalini. The more we are in touch with the feeling of this God Force, the easier it is to be motivated to live in a way that will continue to enhance its development.

Although formally defined as complete abstinence from food and water, fasting, in a larger context, means to abstain from that which is toxic to mind, body, and soul. A way to understand this is that fasting is the elimination of physical, emotional, and mental toxins from our organism, rather than simply cutting down on or stopping food intake. Fasting for spiritual purposes usually involves some degree of removal of oneself from worldly responsibilities. It can mean complete silence and social isolation during the fast, which can be a great revival to those of us who have been putting our energy outward. Gandhi used to observe one day of silence per week. Fasting helps to manifest a healthy body, mind, and spiritual balance and therefore to bring forth the knowledge of God within as Love.

After the first few days of a fast, our appetites usually fade and the attachment to food diminishes. This frees the mind to put more energy on the awareness of our Divine Being rather than our appetites. In fasting, the tight connection between instinct and bodily desires is diminished, allowing us to be free from the physical desires of the body. In this state of renunciation, the mind is free to merge into higher states of Communion with God. This is not done to make the body suffer, because in practical reality the body is also becoming healthier with fasting. It is done because, until we achieve a certain level of spiritual Communion, the desires of the body-mind complex are often stronger than the desire of God Communion. The more we can experience ourselves as free of these bodily desires in the practice of fasting, the easier it is to maintain this freedom in a non-fasting state. Jesus alluded to the power of this when he said, "This kind cannot be driven out by anything but prayer and fasting" (Mark 9:29). Matthew the Poor, a modern-day Coptic monk of high spiritual attainment, who serves as the spiritual father in the Monastery of St. Macarius in the desert of Scete, interprets this statement to mean that by prayer and fasting we are able to drive out Satan (toxins, disease, and bodily desires) from the flesh.[7] Fasting becomes a way to renounce the "pull of the flesh" and enter into the full body Enlightenment of the ecstasy of God Communion felt in every scintillating cell. In this way, fasting is an act of Love.

It is significant that the first act of Jesus after his baptism was to begin his forty-day fast in the desert without food or water. The act of baptism grants fullness of the spirit, and spiritual fullness grants, through fasting, victory over bodily desires. This is the direct teaching of Jesus' forty-day fast. Liberation from bodily and worldly desires then makes it possible to merge in the contentment, fullness, and Love of God Communion. This sequence of baptism, fullness of the spirit, fasting, victory over the bodily desires, and Communion with God is the way that Jesus taught by his own life practice.

The act of fasting, especially the forty-day fast, is a mystical sacrifice of the body. Combined with meditation, which on one level is a sacrifice of the mind, fasting becomes a mystical sacrifice of the ego of body and of mind. At the Tree of Life we teach Spiritual Fasting as a process of mystical death and rebirth. This is the secret of Spiritual Fasting. Our programs include non-invasive detoxifying systems that have minimized detoxification and healing crises, Yoga, two meditations per day including daily Shaktipat and Satsang, and a guided Zero Point Process of the mystical death and rebirth.

There is a significant difference between fasting and Spiritual Fasting. Although people lose weight, cleanse, and purify, Spiritual Fasting begins with a spiritual intention and ends with a deeper experience of the Truth of who we are. When the mind becomes quiet, we become present and through this silence, move into the Divine Presence. In this way we begin to access our Light body, through which we access our cosmic body – as the I AM THAT awareness. Jesus said, "Whoever loses his life for my sake will save it" (Luke 9:24). In his own fasting, Jesus sacrificed his body mystically and showed his willingness to make the ultimate sacrifice on the cross. His sacrifice was not involuntary. Its value was that it was a free offering to God, symbolized by offering his body to his disciples with bread and wine as his blood. Through his forty-day fast and the Last Supper, he was voluntarily crucified before the final offering up of his complete ego-will to God.

The offering of the ego in fasting requires us to reach the level Abraham did when he raised his hand to sacrifice his son Isaac at God's command. It was a partial sacrifice with only the lifting of the hand, but it was total in intent. As with Abraham, we cannot offer anything in place of ourselves when we fast. No money, good acts, or words of renunciation will substitute. It requires letting go of our own body-mind-ego complex. Spiritual Fasting in this inner way overcomes ego and transforms us into the Divine. It is the mystical sacrifice of the body as exemplified by Moses, Elijah, and Jesus. To fast with this understanding leads us to accept the death of the physical body and to overcome our fear of death itself. This is the meaning of Spiritual Fasting. It is not for our health, although it greatly improves health. It is to complete the sacrifice of our attachment to the ego. Spiritual Fasting begins with a sense of Communion with God and usually ends with a deeper sense of that Communion.

Fasting – the Ultimate Way to Reactivate the Youthing Gene Expression

Fasting, particularly Spiritual Fasting, which diminishes the physical stresses of excess food, along with emotional stresses, psychological stresses, spiritual stresses, and environmental stresses, is the optimal setting for activating the youthing genes. Fasting is an accelerated form of calorie restriction, and the results we see are in complete alignment with Dr. Spindler's calorie restriction research findings and the findings of other researchers (see Chapter 22).

The author's first insight into activating the youthing gene expression began with his observations in 1988. It was the transformation he saw in people during the first Spiritual Fasting Retreats. Now he sees this all the time during the transformational seven-day Spiritual Fasting Retreats that happen throughout the year at the Tree of Life Rejuvenation Center, as well as in people doing forty-day fasts, and even extended fasts up to eighty-five days. What he observed was that people were experiencing radical youthing. People with serious high blood pressure – in some cases as high as 200 over 110 – would often, within one week (although sometimes it takes two to three weeks), when they are taken off blood pressure medications, return to a normal blood pressure. After the fast people seemed to then have a slight raise in their blood pressure of roughly five points above where it was during fasting and stabilize there. As a scientist, this one's curiosity was piqued, and the result was a variety of theories for why this happened. The author saw that a number of people were able to significantly begin the process of reversing such chronic degenerative diseases as chronic pain, fatigue, depression, anxiety, digestive disorders, and Syndrome X (see Chapter 27). This doesn't happen every time on a seven-day fast, but it seemed to happen in the majority of the cases. There have been dramatic cases, such as the person who had been hospitalized for five years at a well-known mental hospital in Boston, who arrived on "leave" from the hospital eighty pounds overweight, lethargic, and barely able to walk fifty yards. Over a period of three weeks, her depression dramatically improved and she became energetic, youthful, happy, and full of energy. As her symptoms melted away in her seventy-day fast cycle, she became the extraordinarily beautiful, healthy, young lady she always was underneath, and has remained off all psychotropic medications. This and other examples generated some very interesting questions. A way to explain these results came when Dr. Jeffrey Bland personally presented his outstanding book, *Genetic Nutritioneering*, to the author. Within the first minute of looking at the book, it all became obvious to the author what had been happening: *Through the process of fasting, people were turning on their youthing genes and reprogramming to an earlier stage of their gene expression and returning to health.* It becomes clear that *not only what we eat, but what we don't eat, speaks to our genes.* This breakthrough has shifted the way the author has thought about healing and supports this very ancient process that goes back at least 5,000 years.

Physiology of Fasting

On the physical level of fasting are many techniques and approaches. The goal here is to present a general framework for understanding the process of fasting. The definition of fasting varies. It can mean anything from a dry fast, which is abstinence from all food and water, to a fresh juice fast, to a fast on foods that are one level less dense than we were previously eating. For example, a fast of this latter sort, for a meat eater, would be a vegetarian diet. Another way of fasting is to abstain from that which is toxic to body and mind, and thus eliminating toxins from the system. The physiology of fasting favors healthy cells. Another definition of fasting includes any process that initiates autolysis, during which poorly functioning cells are destroyed, first in the process of fasting, and then the cellular components are broken down and remetabolized. This usually begins after three days of juice or water fasting, which is the classic meaning, as compared to something like a "spirulina fast" or other types of food fasts. These are not really fasts. We stop a fast when the elimination of waste products is complete and the autolysis finishes with unhealthy cells and begins destroying healthy cells. This point is usually indicated by a return of appetite and the disappearance of the white coating on the tongue.

Healthy functioning of the body begins to deteriorate when the normal process of cell regeneration and building becomes slower than the breakdown of unhealthy cells in the body. This is usually connected with the accumulation of toxins in the tissues and cells to an extent that it interferes with the proper nutrition and rebuilding of cells. The Wendt Doctrine of excess protein intake, causing a protein storage disease by blocking the basement membrane, is a clear description of how this works. When the basement membrane is clogged, nutrients, including oxygen, cannot get through to the cells, and waste products cannot diffuse out of the cells back into the capillary bloodstream. The result is that the cells begin to malfunction and degenerate. With excess toxicity and insufficient nutrients, the process of new cell growth slows down. When cells are degenerating faster than new cells are regenerating, we experience aging and disease. It is said that in our industrialized nations many more people die of overnutrition than malnutrition. Fasting helps to clear out the basement membrane so that nutrients can begin to get to the cells and new cell growth can be stimulated. The proteins from the broken down cells are remetabolized and used to build new cells during the fast, so that even without the intake of exogenous protein for cell building, cells regenerate.

During a fast, the eliminative systems of the body – the skin, lungs, liver, kidney, and bowels – become more active. Because the body is not spending energy digesting and eliminating fresh toxins in the system, it is able to direct all its energy toward elimination of accumulated toxins and waste products. The increased release is usually evidenced by foul breath, body odor, dark urine, increased mucus secretion, and foul-smelling bowel contents. Because of the extra energy freed by resting the digestive system and because of detoxification and the fresh minerals gained from a juice fast, fasting has a normalizing effect on the biochemical and mineral balance in the tissues and is a tonifier of the nervous system.

Fasting is probably the oldest healing method known. It is particularly good for rebalancing problems caused by excessive eating. In 1986, the U.S. Congressional Joint Nutrition Monitoring Committee reported that 28 percent of Americans (32 million) between 25 and 74 years of age weighed too much, including 11.7 million who were severely overweight. Fasting for this reason alone is important. Fasting has been used throughout history for healing. Such great physicians as Hippocrates, Galen, and Paracelsus prescribed it. In the U.S., because of the influence of the drug therapy approach to healing and because of a basic break in our high-technology society with understanding the simple processes of Nature, the use of fasting has faded. This has been less true in Europe. In Sweden and Germany there are hundreds of fasting clinics. At the Buchinger Sanatorium in Bad Pyrmont, Germany, where the author studied, more than 80,000 fasts have been supervised.[8]

When to and When Not to Fast

Intentional fasting for short periods of time such as seven to ten days is considered completely safe by many fasting experts. In some Swedish hospital experiments with fasting, patients fasted up to fifty-five days without any difficulty.[9] Paavo Airola states that water fasting up to forty days and juice fasting up to 100 days is generally considered safe by fasting medical experts in Europe.[10] Therapeutic fasts from fourteen to twenty-one days are considered common in European fasting clinics.[11]

If one has any sort of serious illness or acute or chronic disease, it is highly recommended to do any fasting in conjunction with a health practitioner who is well versed in the science of fasting. Those who have a strong vata dosha constitution (see Chapter 24), who are very sensitive to life changes, who lose weight easily and cannot regain it easily, with degenerative diseases from which they are suffering malnutrition or extreme emaciation, or those with wasting diseases should probably not fast. If people insist on fasting with these conditions, it should be done under the supervision of an experienced health practitioner. In general, pregnant and lactating women, people who have not reached full physical maturity, and those who are ten pounds or more underweight should not fast. We should also not fast if we are operating heavy machinery, performing dangerous mechanical tasks, or even have to do much driving. During a fast, our minds and bodies usually become more calm and slower than such tasks normally require for safety.

It is best not to stop a fast in the middle of a detoxification crisis, but gently work our way through it by aiding all the eliminative systems with techniques such as enemas, skin brushing, and foot massage to stimulate organs to eliminate. It is important to stop a fast if an extreme nervous or mental condition manifests or a person begins to enter a cycle of high fevers. These are unusual occurrences.

General Fasting Guidelines

One of the most important aspects of fasting is to enhance all the eliminative channels for the toxins leaving the system. The following guidelines are suggested:

- Take an enema at least once per day. Some clinics recommend as many as three separate enemas per day. Colonics during the fast are excellent as well.
- Brush the skin for 3–5 minutes once or twice daily and follow this with a bath and skin scrub to remove the excess dead cells and draw more toxins out of the system.
- Get plenty of sunshine and do deep breathing exercises to help detoxify the skin and lungs.
- Get moderate exercise during the fast to help activate the system to eliminate toxins. This may include a 30–60-minute walk, swimming, and sacred dance, and 16 minutes per day on a rebounder.
- Practice daily Yoga for moving the lymphatics, as well as general exercise.
- Take short saunas to enhance perspiration, which helps the detoxification process.
- Abstain from sexual activity to conserve energies for healing and regenerating.
- Use flower essences and gem elixirs during the fast to help balance and align the subtle bodies and chakras and to awaken the

chakras. These can enhance the harmony of the body-mind-spirit complex during the fast. Self-heal, silver sword, papaya, lotus, star sapphire, and quartz seem to be the best preparations. Self-heal aids in the natural process of the absorption of prana during fasting. Silver sword aligns all subtle bodies and balances the heart chakra. Papaya is excellent for emotional and sexual balance and allows us to enter the spiritual realms more easily. Lotus stimulates the alignment and balance on all levels of our Being, and is outstanding for fasting and meditation. Star sapphire activates all chakras, especially the crown, and specifically stimulates spiritual opening while fasting. Quartz removes negative thoughts and creates emotional calm.[12,13,14] The gem elixirs and flower essences from Pegasus Products are excellent.
- Drink Tachyon elixir each day to support liver and kidney avenues of elimination.
- Scrape the tongue each day to remove toxins on the tongue.

It is very important to break the fast carefully and consciously. During the fast, the digestive system has shut down and must be carefully restarted. At the end of the fast, the body absorbs everything much more easily, so what we put back into our bodies should be what we really want to rebuild our bodies with. The end of a fast is a very good opportunity to reorganize ourselves around a new quality of diet. A ratio of one day of breaking the fast for each three days of fasting is a broad guideline, though everyone's body is different and this needs to be individualized. One should take a minimum of three days to come off a seven- to twenty-one-day fast. The author recommends breaking a fast in the morning with citrus juice to stimulate the flow of gastric juices and using certain herbs such as ginger and anise to speed up the process of eliminating toxic gas from the system and activate the pybric valve at the bottom of the stomach. Acidophilus is useful for replenishing the bowel flora that is depleted secondarily to the enemas. Trifala is useful for restoring bowel peristalsis.

Types of Fasts

Airola's book stresses the importance of vegetable and fruit juices plus a special alkalinizing broth as the best way to fast therapeutically and for rejuvenation. He points out that this is the approach used throughout

Europe in all the fasting clinics. Kulvinskas is focused more on the water fast for purification and transmutation of the body. Both are correct. There are different levels and purposes of fasting. The concept of different levels of fasting is also a recognition that to fast too severely increases the possibility of a more uncomfortable healing crisis from the toxins that are released. One fast does not necessarily completely detoxify and heal the body. Usually it requires a purification process that takes years. Since the goal of spiritual life is not to see how quickly we can detoxify, picking the most heroic fast first is not always best.

At the Tree of Life we use mainly green juices diluted with water. Some with special permission may do water fasts for short times. In preparation for a juice or water fast, one can practice certain levels of detoxification:

Level 1: Those on a meat diet can abstain from meat one week two times per year.

Level 2: Those off blood meats can switch to fasting three days at one time per month, and twice per year for seven days. This fast can be a mixture of fruits, vegetables, and juices.

Level 3: Those on a lactovegetarian diet can follow the same pattern as level 2, but use only fruit and vegetable juice fasts.

Level 4: Those on a vegetarian diet and using fasting as a spiritual practice can follow a pattern of four seven- to ten-day fasts per year. These fasts should primarily be done with green vegetable juices. The Tree of Life no longer uses fruit juices because they are too aggravating to people with hypoglycemia and candida.

At Level 4 we are entering the use of fasting, meditation, and prayer as part of a spiritual path rather than a simple physiological maintenance of the body. It is important to understand the difference. It is also important to become aware of the risk of one's body becoming too pure in our toxic society. The cleaner the basement membrane becomes, the more sensitive we become to our polluted environment because toxins can move right through our systems. A little mucus in the system, for example, can serve to protect us from being so vulnerable to pollution. If we reach a point of purity that we become too vulnerable, we will not be able to function effectively on the physical plane in serving the Will of God on this planet. What becomes important, as this balance is reached, is to establish a diet that maintains a level of physiological integrity and purity so that the practice of fasting, which on the physical level is to compensate for eating too much and for the toxicity of our planet, can be phased out as a tool for detoxification. If we do not overload the system, the body on the right minimal diet can rid itself of almost any toxin and maintain good health. Once this balance has been achieved, Spiritual Fasting, rather than purificatory fasting, becomes the primary fasting practice if we feel drawn to fasting as part of our spiritual life. The author feels that at least two Spiritual Fasts per year of seven days each is an excellent maintenance approach for body, mind, and soul.

The Forty-Day Spiritual Fast

The forty-day Spiritual Fast is designed to enhance spiritual life and transmute the body. Although people do therapeutic fasts this long or even longer, it is in a different context and with a different meaning. Jesus, Elijah, and Moses, who each fasted for a minimum of forty days without food or water, were not doing it for their physical health. One focus predominated: Communion with God. This is the orientation of the forty-day Spiritual Fast. It is on this fast that we directly confront death and the offering up of our body, mind, and ego to God. The other purifying fasts help in the preparation for this fast. Even so, it is best to prepare oneself by eating just fruits and vegetables for at least one week before the fast, and have one colonic. The general format of the fast can be as severe as a dry fast of no food and water, though this is usually too strict for most people on their first forty-day fast. The author recommends beginning the fast with juice and transitioning to water.

In the first twenty days the most detoxification occurs – this is the time to put emphasis on physical detoxification. Moderate and ample exercise is good. In the second twenty days, lighter exercise is recommended. During the second twenty days a great many more emotional toxic states are released, and it is important to be guided by someone who is familiar with this sort of Spiritual Fasting. The last three to five days of the fast are the most critical, in that our state is clearest and the impressions taken in at this time become deeply imprinted into the total body-mind system. It is best to spend this time in total isolation, preferably out in Nature.

With each forty-day fast, the water part of the fast becomes longer and the green juice part becomes shorter. It is said that many of the inner circle of the Essenes did one forty-day fast per year, accompanied by much meditation and an abstention from worldly activities to maximize the focus on God. After five years of forty-day fasts and living on fruits and vegetables with much meditation and other spiritual practices, it is reported that 1 percent of the Essenes were able to fast on prana as did Jesus, Elijah, and Moses.[15] To live on prana is not the goal, but it does make the point that by a gradual process of Spiritual Fasting and meditation, the body becomes transformed into a perfect superconductor of the prana so that no other form of nutrition is needed.

To do a juice and water fast for forty days each year requires very experienced spiritual guidance and much previous experience with fasting. It should be done with careful consideration. For all these fasts, it is safest to have supervision from an experienced holistic health practitioner.

Personal Experience of the Forty-Day Spiritual Fast

The forty-day Spiritual Fast was profound for this one. There was not any specific idea of what was wanted from the fast except to enhance the Divine Love Communion. It was approached with some degree of curiosity and a clear sense of an inner direction to do it. Creating the time and space for it to happen in the middle of a busy health practice and family responsibilities was one of the first tasks of this Spiritual Fast. The entire fasting process, including the time to come off the fast, required slightly more than two months time. The fast ended with three days of distilled water. The reason for only three days of distilled water was that the fast was primarily a time of retreat and meditation, and when the author is on water for more than three days, the energy for meditation tends to drop.

The energy after the first two weeks of detoxification became high and stable. It was easy to extend the sitting meditation time. After the first twenty days, this one's energy began to move more distinctly inward. Over the next two weeks, the hours of meditation gradually increased toward nine hours per day. During this time, the author took long walks to tone the body. The state of Communion with God, Unity awareness, non-duality, harmony, and Love seemed to be approaching a higher and higher proportion of the waking awareness. The body was clearly becoming a better superconductor. This one could feel the energy pulsing through frequently during the day. Around the thirty-fifth day, this one became aware of the flow of what is called the inner nectar (amrita) in Yoga into the psycho-spiritual system. Physiologically speaking, this is probably connected with the release of the endorphins from the increased prana flowing into the system. This nectar seemed to increase the level of bliss even more. It is a form of inner nutrition.

The critical turning point for the fast was in the last three days on distilled water. This time was spent away from home in total silence in an isolated mountain retreat. To this one's surprise, it was relatively easy to meditate the nine hours per day, which is more than the author had meditated before. Sometimes four hours of continual meditation would go by in what seemed to be a few minutes. The mind became so devoid of thoughts that in meditation, it would simply dissolve into the Light of God for hours at a time. There was no body, no desires, no thoughts, no mind. Only God, unbroken Love Communion with God, for hours. It was clear that the Essenes knew what they were doing. In these last three days of meditation, only the vague sense of a formless I AM consciousness remained as the last bit of identity. This one became a Divine lump in this Communion. Whether formally meditating or just Being, Love existed as the only awareness. Just to Be was totally enough. The flowers bloom, Light radiates, and I AM THAT.

During the times between the merging of the mind into the Light in meditation, the cosmic prana seemed to penetrate down to the microcosmic DNA of the cells. It was a total sense of resonant Unity with the cosmos. The crown chakra seemed fully awakened and activated. The flow of energy into it, which had been increasing over the past eighteen months, was coming into the top of this one's head in an incredible pulseless pulse. The complete crown became one whirling vortex of energy connecting this one with the dance of the cosmos. Since that time, it has never diminished. These three days marked the full opening of the crown chakra. During these three days, this one drank very little water, as this prana and the sunlight became the main food. There was no particular concern keeping the fasting protocol, so not having to drink or move the bowels, this one just rested as a Divine, ecstatic lump. It is possible that if this continued for more than three days this one might have permanently left the body. The wondrous Love Communion with God was so strong that death of the body seemed completely secondary. This was a non-confrontation with death. In transcendence, death is a joke. There is no death for the Transcendent Self;

the body may die, but we clearly are not the body or even the mind. To think we are the personality and body is a case of mistaken identity.

Many spiritual insights and understandings crystallized during this time. It was clear that God had given the gift of three days of Transcendence. Three days of complete moksha. It was also clear that to lie around as a Divine, transcendent lump resonating as the cosmos in unbroken Communion with God is not to be this one's immediate role in this play of the world. To be a free person is to be the Will of God, rather than to be in a particular state, even if this state is the direct ecstatic Transcendence of Total Communion. The body-mind complex has been so sufficiently transmuted by this forty-day fast, that after a few days of fasting and retreat, at any time it is now possible to enter into sustained states of the Divine, transcendent lump of moksha. What then exists as worldly duties are performed in the solid, intuitive, living, transcendent awareness of the Unity, harmony, and Oneness of the world as I AM THAT.

Simultaneously with this Oneness awareness, there is a comfortable working acknowledgment of the apparent duality in which we all live. The motivation for this fast revealed itself as an attunement with the Will of God, rather than as an abstract goal. The author cannot responsibly recommend either for or against fasts such as this as a regular yearly spiritual practice. This is because of a lack of experience in repeated forty-day fasts and the lack of anyone else with current information on such fasts. The experience of this fast was probably much related to many previous years of meditation and spiritual discipline. This account does not imply that simply by fasting for forty days all of us will immediately have transcendental experiences or be sustained in moksha.

In 1995 this one received the intuition to do a twenty-one-day water fast. It was another profound experience, culminating on the twenty-first day with a twelve-hour visionary experience of YHWH. After this powerful initiation into the mantra, it became the active, awakened mantra for Shaktipat/S'micha l'shefa. The four basic Modern Essene principles accepted by all the Essene groups in the U.S. were also received by this one.

In order to provide a deeper insight into fasting, the last book in the author's nutritional series will be on Spiritual Fasting.

Summary, Chapter 23

1. Fasting has its history in the spiritual and religious observations of almost all the world religions. It is very much part of Judeo-Christian heritage as exemplified by Moses, Elijah, and Jesus. Fasting and meditation were a major spiritual practice of the mystical Jewish Essene communities in which Jesus reportedly lived.
2. Fasting in its strictest sense is complete abstinence from food and water. In a larger context, it means to abstain from that which is toxic to mind, body, and spirit. Fasting can also mean to abstain from the densest level of our diet, such as fasting from meat for a meat eater or dairy products for a lactovegetarian.
3. Fasting allows our body to turn to the absorption of lesser densities of cosmic energy rather than the dense biomolecular energy of food.
4. By increasing the amount of cosmic prana entering the body, fasting increases the potential of reaching the critical energy necessary for awakening the Kundalini. The increase in cosmic prana also increases the energy of an already awakened Kundalini.
5. By accelerating the purification of the body, fasting allows the spiritualizing force of the Kundalini to operate more fully in transforming the body.
6. Fasting helps us to overcome the pull of the bodily desires on the mind and makes it easier for the mind to merge in higher states of God Communion.
7. The act of fasting, particularly in the forty-day Spiritual Fast with meditation, is a mystical sacrifice of the body and mind to God. It is a mystical death of the ego.
8. The normal physiology of fasting is based on excretion of toxins and autolysis of dead and degenerate cells. Autolysis does not work on healthy cells until all dead and degenerate cells have been destroyed. The normal time to stop fasting is when this first step is completed.
9. During a fast, we must give extra care to supporting the eliminative systems of the body such as the skin, kidneys, liver, bowel, and lungs.
10. Fasting experts feel intentional fasts of seven to ten days are completely safe. Therapeutic fasts in European clinics of fourteen to twenty-one days are the norm.

11. Pregnant and lactating women, people more than ten pounds underweight, those with degenerative diseases from which they are suffering, severe malnutrition, and wasting diseases ordinarily should not fast.
12. General guidelines for spiritual and for cleansing fasts are given, along with recommended schedules.
13. There is a difference between fasting as a general support to spiritual life and fasting as an active spiritual practice.
14. Discussion of the forty-day Spiritual Fast and the author's experience of such a fast are given, as well as those of a twenty-one-day water fast.
15. Fasting, especially Spiritual Fasting, and a live-food diet and lifestyle including Yoga and meditation are the most powerful and natural ways to activate the anti-aging gene.

Chapter 24

The Ayurvedic Tridosha System

The Spiritual Nutrition live-food diet is qualitatively different from the classic Ayurvedic diet, which aims primarily at balancing the *doshas* to prevent or heal disease. Although classical Ayurveda does not usually recommend a 100-percent live-food diet, we can certainly employ its principles to create an optimal, individualized, Spiritual Nutrition diet for ourselves.

Tridosha Defined

There are many perspectives we can use to help guide our choice of diet. The *tridosha* system of the science of Ayurveda is particularly useful in helping us maintain our awareness of nutrition as the interaction between the forces of food and our own dynamic forces. According to Ayurveda, the five basic elements of creation – air, water, fire, earth, and ether – manifest in the human psychosomatic complex as three dosha essences: *vata, kapha,* and *pitta.* We are all born as a constitutional combination of the three. They govern all our biological and psychological aspects. When they are in balance, they maintain the body in a healthy physiological state. If the doshas become unbalanced, the result can range from a feeling of subtle disharmony in the body-mind complex to the development of disease.

When one dosha predominates as a constitutional force or is the most easily imbalanced, a person is said to have a constitution of that dosha. The word dosha means that which is thrown out of balance. When a person is described as being a particular constitutional dosha, it means that is the dosha most easily thrown out of balance for that person. There are seven basic constitutional types: kapha, vata, pitta, vata-pitta, pitta-kapha, kapha-vata, and kapha-pitta-vata. There are subtle variations of the different constitutional types. Having a feeling for our constitutional type helps us make choices about what foods we eat, when we eat, and how to change our diet with the seasons. The purpose of this chapter is to give enough of a sense of the tridosha system that we can begin to identify our particular constitution as a key in organizing our diet.

Vata Dosha

The vata dosha is roughly translated as air or wind, or ether in the Greek system. It is the principle of movement in the body and the energy that governs biological movement in the body. It is formed of two of the five elements: ether and air. Vata regulates breathing, all movements of the muscles and tissues, the heart muscle, and all biological movements intra- and extracellular, including the single movements of the nerve impulses.

People with a vata constitution are generally thin, with flat chests, and have noticeable veins and muscle tendons. They tend to have dry, cracked skin. Vata people are very creative people who have active, alert, and restless minds. They talk and move quickly, but also fatigue easily. They are quick to grasp things mentally. Their will power is weak, and they tend to be easily knocked off center. They are not mentally stable and tend to be nervous, anxious, and fearful. Their animal archetype is the rabbit, dog, rat, goat, camel, or crow.[1]

When there is an imbalance of vata, it is often recognized on the psychological level as nervousness, fear, anxiety, insomnia, pain, tremors, and spasms. A vata imbalance may also manifest as rough skin, arthritis, emaciation, stiffness, constipation, dryness, thirst, insomnia, excessive sensitivity and excitability, and physical pain. There is a tendency to large-intestine disorders such as excess gas, low back pain, sciatica, paralysis, and neuralgia. Vata personalities are adversely affected by cold, windy, stormy, and rainy weather, which can directly imbalance their nervous system. For example, the author once helped a person with a predominant vata dosha stop her insomnia by having her turn off her fan at night. The wind from the fan was causing a vata imbalance. In general, anything that causes excess, such as strenuous exercise or mental labor, extreme diet, grief, anger, suppression of natural urges, severe weather conditions, or any practices taken to the limit will cause an imbalance in vata.

Vata people enjoy sweet, salty, and sour tastes. They are often thrown out of balance by taking bitter, astringent (dry), or pungent foods. Sesame seed oil on the skin, a little oil in their food, and a stable, calm, soothing environment help to bring the vata dosha back into balance.

In Chapter 25, which discusses how to balance excess prana and vata that may arise from eating live foods, the author defers to this chapter for a more in-depth discussion of vata. The key understanding about vata is learning how to balance one's lifestyle. The idea is to calm and soothe the vata and the prana without having to reactively go to tamasic antidotes such as drugs, like alcohol and marijuana, or flesh food. The answer to this starts with the awareness that as we go on live foods, it requires more thoughtfulness because we are definitely increasing the prana and the possibility for a vata imbalance. The more obvious ways to prevent excess prana and vata is to go slowly and respect the changes your body is going through. Many people on the spiritual path, particularly when they first go on live foods, have a tendency to move too fast and try to go 100 percent before their psyche and physiology are ready. The result is a definite increase in energy, but often more energy than people can handle in a balanced way. There is also a potential for a great release of emotional toxins if one moves to a 100-percent live-food diet too quickly. This can make for a bumpy ride. The main prevention of vata imbalance and a prana excess is to go slow and easy, with a certain amount of sweetness in one's movement, in one's diet, and toward oneself. It is about gentleness toward oneself rather than harshness. This includes avoiding the tendency to over-exercise and push oneself beyond limits. Excess pranayama practice can lead to imbalance because pranayama does not have discrimination – it will just increase prana. If your body is already experiencing increased prana secondary to the diet, excess pranayama may increase prana more than the body is ready to handle. The secret is in being peaceful with yourself: avoiding excess exercise, over-effort, over-scheduling, irregular hours, and not getting enough sleep, which should be between seven and eight hours per night. All these simple practices tend to balance the prana and the vata. When the prana is increased, and the Kundalini is awakened, there is a tendency to burn ojas (life force) faster than we are ready or prepared for. One reason the author strongly suggests the Six Foundations is that they build ojas and, with proper eating, also build the adrenals so that one, in general, builds the internal structure of nadis to be ready to handle the increased amount of live food going into the system.

One of the key principles of this is to eat in a way that balances the vata. Vata is balanced by eating food that tends to be sweet. This is not necessarily a high-glycemic sweet. It could be low-glycemic fruit, such as berries and cherries, or blended foods that are oily and creamy and of a slightly sweet taste. Many of these high ojas- and vata-calming foods include: bee pollen; live foods high in oil content such as avocados or soaked nuts and seeds; sprouted or soaked grains; slightly warm blended greens; raw soups; and blended vegetables. All should be at least room temperature. Herbs that add a certain amount of heat to the system are helpful for balancing vata. These herbs include: ginger; sweet spices such as cardamom, fennel, and cinnamon; asafoetida (hing); and cumin. The idea here is that these herbs tend to minimize gas and bloating, are slightly heating, and specifically balancing for vata. A little bit of pungent spices such as cayenne can be okay. Blended foods are very helpful, as well as raw nut butters, tahini, and oils such as sesame and other slightly heating oils. Sweet vegetables such as beet and carrot (not the juice, but the whole vegetables) are good. Sweet and watery vegetables include: asparagus, cucumbers, dulse, ginger, hijiki, kelp, kombu, all the sea vegetables, okra, sweet potatoes, and sprouts (a certain amount really work well for balancing vata). Finally, certain grains, particularly barley and wild rice, can be included. If one is not on a 100-percent live-food diet, wheat is considered a sweet grain, which can also be balancing, but with wheat there are increased risks of allergy and candida. The author suggests that one stay away from beans as they tend to create gas and therefore aggravate vata, but hummus, for example, can be balancing for vata in mild amounts. Soaked seeds and nuts, particularly in the form of seed and nut sauces and seed and nut milks are excellent for balancing vata. The key taste for vata is sweet, because it satisfies and calms the system. The Ayurvedic system has taught that sweetness is the taste that is closest to the gods. Salt taste adds a little heat. Sour-tasting foods add a touch of acidity, which helps to balance issues. So warm, oily, sweet, salty, watery, "creamy," and soupy cuisine is going to help balance, soothe, and calm vata.

Foods that aggravate vata include: cold foods, carbonated drinks, ice water, an excess of dehydrated foods, salads with light salad dressings, but vata may have the full range of vegetables and salad, particularly if they are combined with high-oil-content food such as avocados, soaked nuts and seeds, or seed and nut salad dressings. Vegetables that tend to produce gas, such as the brassica family (cabbage family) and even nightshades, should be taken in moderation and with an experimental attitude to see if one is affected by these foods in a negative way. Excess roughage should be minimized, or blended into raw soups. If one feels the need for the healing power of cabbage, a little bit of fermented cabbage such as sauerkraut or kim chee can be useful. Moderate- and low-glycemic fruits, including berries, avocados, tomatoes, pears, and a little applesauce, are helpful for balancing because they have a certain amount of sweetness. Excess dry fruits tend to be imbalancing because they are too sweet and because their dryness aggravates vata. Astringent foods, such as unripe persimmons, cranberries, and pomegranates, should be taken in moderation. Apples and pears may have a slight drying effect but can be neutral in their effect on vata if they are taken with warming spices such as ginger or cinnamon. Fruits that seem most balancing for vata seem to be apricots, avocados, berries, cherries, coconut, figs, citrus, melons, nectarines, and plums. Classically some high-glycemic fruits such as bananas and melons have been recommended, but, if you understand the Rainbow Green Live-Food Cuisine (see Chapter 27), the author does not recommend them on a regular basis.

Activities that aggravate vata include over-exercise, drug use, forcing Yogic practices or other spiritual practices, excess pranayama, and lack of sleep. Once we understand these principles of how to calm vata – with moderate or comfortable living that is peaceful and modest in terms of stress, combined with sweet, salty, or oily, watery, soupy cuisine, and not moving quicker than the body is comfortable with in the transition to live foods – we have the best prevention. The author feels that the optimum diet is a 100-percent live-food diet, but feels that people on the spiritual path need to be moderate in reaching that as a way of Being and would best be served by stabilizing at 80 percent and working out a certain amount of balance at that for a period of time before proceeding to more intense levels of the diet. With this practice of moderation, we would see far more people becoming successful with live foods. A small percentage of people, because of their psychological addictive tendencies, need to be on a 100-percent live-food diet to be successful, and those people should do that approach as the number one alternative. If you make it to 80 percent, which so many people can do, you can be successful on a live-food diet with increased chances of minimizing the pitfalls of excess prana and vata imbalance. Although classical Ayurvedic teachings from India do not recommend a 100-percent live-food diet for vatas, by applying the Ayurvedic principles for balancing vata and the use of the full, delicious spectrum of a live-food diet, the author has seen hundreds of vatas be successful on 100-percent live food. One key to this is realizing that live foods in India meant primarily leafy greens, fruits, and raw nuts and seeds, and not the incredible array of smoothies, spirulina drinks, seed and nut milks, soaked nuts and seeds, seed sauces as salad dressings, blended foods, sea vegetables, and bee pollen, which create a powerful vata balancing live-food diet.

Pitta Dosha

The pitta dosha is roughly translated as fire and is experienced as bodily heat energy. It is the force that governs metabolism. It affects digestion, assimilation, and body temperature. Pitta is formed from the water and fire elements.

Those who are predominantly pitta are characterized by strong digestion, large appetites for food and drink, high body heat, and intolerance to heat and the sun. They have abundant perspiration, moderate strength and build, strong body odor, and a more coppery skin with lots of freckles, moles, and blackheads. Their skin is oily, and there is a tendency for their hair to gray prematurely. Hands and feet are usually warm. They crave cold drinks, and sweet, astringent, and bitter foods. Psychologically, people with a predominant pitta dosha have good comprehension and intelligence. They do not overstrain themselves at work. They are, however, ambitious. They have a tendency toward vanity, intolerance, pride, aggressiveness, stubbornness, hatefulness, anger, and jealousy. Their character resembles that of the archetypal tiger, cat, monkey, owl, or bear.[2]

Summer or midday heat will cause an aggravation of the pitta dosha. During the hot season in India, these were the people the author observed to have summer colds, heart palpitations, heat prostration, skin disorders such as hives and heat rash, and general misery from the heat. It was often quite dramatic. The author's son, who is a predominant pitta dosha, was completely healthy through all the seasons in India until the hot season. Within the first few days of 100- to 120-degree temperatures, he became sick, exhausted, developed rashes all over his body, and was barely able to attend school. As soon as the cooling monsoon season began, his health returned completely. Other signs of pitta aggravation are acidity, fainting, excessive perspiration, restlessness, increased thirst and desire for cold substances, paleness, and in extreme cases, delirium. Other causes for derangement of pitta are: emotions of anger, grief, or fear; excess physical exertion; improper digestion or acid system; too much pungent, acid, salty, and dry food; too much mustard seed, sesame and linseed oil, fish, mutton, stems of green leafy vegetables, and wine. Sweet, astringent, and bitter tasting foods help to rebalance pitta, as do moonlight and cold baths.

Kapha Dosha

The kapha principle can be translated as biological water. It is considered to be formed from earth and water elements. Kapha governs biological strength, vigor, stability, and natural tissue resistance. It lubricates the joints, moisturizes the skin, gives energy to the heart and lungs, helps heal wounds, and fills the spaces in the body. Kapha activates the anabolic or growth forces in the body – one reason kapha people tend to become overweight. Kapha manifests as mucus in the chest, throat, nose, sinuses, mouth, joints, and cytoplasm.

People with a kapha constitution have well-developed bodies. They have the type of physical constitutions we may stereotype as football linemen. Kapha people have a slow digestion, made even slower by oily or fatty foods. They do well with pungent, bitter, and astringent foods, which often help to bring them into balance. They are especially thrown out of balance by sweet (which they often crave), sour, and salty foods. Excessively sweet fruits may also cause a derangement. The one exception to this is raw honey, which is considered a main dietary antidote to a kapha imbalance. All dairy products, with the exception of some goat milk products, tend to cause derangement in kapha. Goat milk has slightly astringent qualities that help minimize the kapha imbalance. Kapha people generally are not very thirsty and should not drink the eight glasses of liquid per day that are supposed to be so healthy for everyone.

Exercise is very important for kapha people. They do poorly if they do not get sufficient or regular exercise, or if they nap during the day. It was a relief for the author to discover that his predominant kapha physical constitution was the cause for his need for exercise, not feeling good after day naps, and slow digestion, made even slower with oil.

Tolerance, calmness, forgiveness, and Love are predominant kapha characteristics. They are also characterized as righteous, generous, steadfast in friendship, stable of mind, given to measured and deliberate speech, enthusiastic, and understanding. They have tendencies toward greed, attachment, envy, and possessiveness. Intellectually, they may be slow to comprehend, but once they grasp a concept they retain it well. Their symbolic animal archetypes are bull, lion, elephant, horse, or football lineman (in college, the author was a football lineman). Kapha constitutions are thrown into imbalance in cold and damp weather. For example, during the author's first year in India, his nose never dripped, but within one-half hour of stepping out of the plane into the damp, cold London climate, his nose began to run. Kapha people benefit most from the mucusless diet. Exercise, fasting, and heat are also important treatments for people with kapha dosha aggravation or constitution. Symptoms of kapha derangement are heaviness, drowsiness, constipation, itching, skin disease, dullness, laziness, depression, and excess mucus production.

The Doshas and the Cycles

The seasons, the time of day, and one's age are also forces affecting the balance of the doshas. From birth to the teen years, the predominant dosha is kapha. It governs growth. The most obvious manifestation of this is the tendency for frequent colds and runny noses we see in young children. From the teens to the sixties, pitta tends to predominate. Later, there is a tendency toward vata disorders such as arthritis, dryness of skin, tremors, emaciation, and memory loss. As we get older, no matter what our constitution, we need to shift our diet and life style to adjust for the increasing power of the vata dosha on the body-mind complex (see the figure).

In the daily cycle, kapha forces predominate in all of us from sunrise until 10 A.M. Because of this, those with a strong kapha constitution are most easily thrown into imbalance at this time and do well to

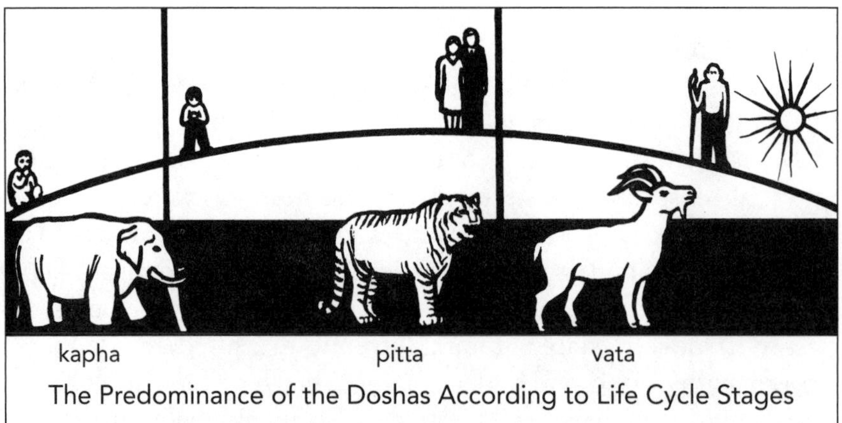

The Predominance of the Doshas According to Life Cycle Stages

avoid dairy products in the morning, eating a light breakfast or none at all. From 10 A.M. to 2 P.M., pitta predominates. This is a very good time to eat, especially for kapha people. However, on a hot day those with a pitta derangement or constitution should eat lightly because pitta is aggravated around noon, when the sun is hottest. From 2 P.M. until sunset, vata predominates. Vata imbalances are often experienced as fatigue and bloating in the late afternoon. Kapha again begins to predominate from sunset to 10 P.M. Because of this, it is better for everyone, and particularly kapha people, to eat about one hour before sunset. If we eat too late, the decreased digestive fire associated with kapha may not be enough to digest food sufficiently. The result is an immediate toxic buildup, which may result in disturbed sleep and difficulty arising early in the morning to meditate. Pitta becomes active between 10 P.M. and 2 A.M., and vata predominates from 2 A.M. until sunrise. Vata creates movement and lightness, and helps to wake people up. This is also a good time to meditate (see the second figure).

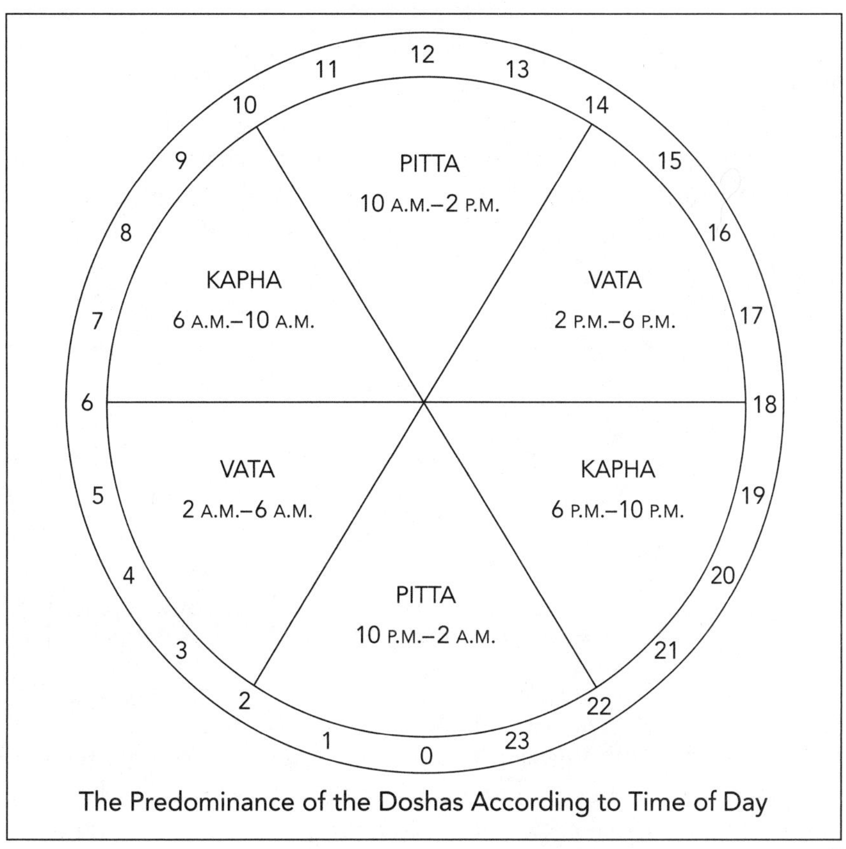

The Predominance of the Doshas According to Time of Day

The cycle of each season has the potential to aggravate a particular dosha. By being conscious of the seasonal shifts of dosha energies, we are able to shift our diets to maintain balanced doshas. This healthy practice of eating with the seasons is not unique to Ayurveda. Elson Haas, M.D., in his book *Staying Healthy with the Seasons,* has described this approach from a Chinese acupuncture point of view.[3] On the equinoxes, September and March 21, and on the solstices, June and December 21, people are vulnerable to health imbalances. During these times, it is harmonious and a good preventive practice to eat lightly and make an extra effort to keep our lifestyles and doshas in balance.

The fall, September through November, is a time of winds. It is a time of decreasing temperature and preparation for winter. During this time vata has a tendency to aggravate. It is important to minimize our exposure to the wind and cold. We can begin to increase intake of foods that have more sweet, sour (acid), and salty tastes, and to increase our intake of rice, wheat, barley, oats, and oily foods.

In the damp cold of winter, kapha is the dosha most likely to aggravate. It is a time when mucus disorders such as colds, congestion, and bronchitis tend to emerge. It is a time to minimize fatty foods, dairy products, and foods with sweet, salty, or sour tastes. The exception to this is a moderate amount of raw honey, which decreases kapha. This is a time to eat more dry, bitter, pungent, hot, and astringent foods, to maintain an exercise program, and not to nap during the day. For example, as a predominant kapha constitution, the author has learned to stay away from cucumbers in the winter, which aggravate kapha, and lean toward vegetables and greens like carrots, dill, radish, cabbage, cauliflower, lettuce, and spinach, which all decrease kapha.

In the early spring, the Ayurvedic teachings describe kapha as becoming liquefied. This is another peak aggravation time for kapha. As a physician, the author has noted a sudden upsurge in kapha disorders such as colds, flus, and bronchitis during this time. This is an excellent time to fast. Fasting, which balances kapha, allows us to clean out the winter kapha build-up, rather than have it clean us out by a kapha aggravation. It is an important time to eat lightly and begin to shift to more fruits, vegetables, and other live foods. The kapha balancing program is still best to follow during this time.

In late spring and summer, as the sun begins to heat and dry the land and our bodies, is the time of pitta aggravation. We see heat rashes, sunburn, burning feet, rashes, heart palpitations, swollen feet, and mental irritability. Sweet, cool liquids, and foods like watermelon are excellent at this time. Foods with sweet, astringent, and bitter tastes help to balance the doshas. Salty, sour, pungent, and hot foods should be minimized. The highest percentage of the diet should be live food, with a particular emphasis on fruits. Cold baths, minimizing direct sunlight from 10 A.M. to 2 P.M., and avoiding excessive physical exertion help to minimize a pitta aggravation (see the third figure).

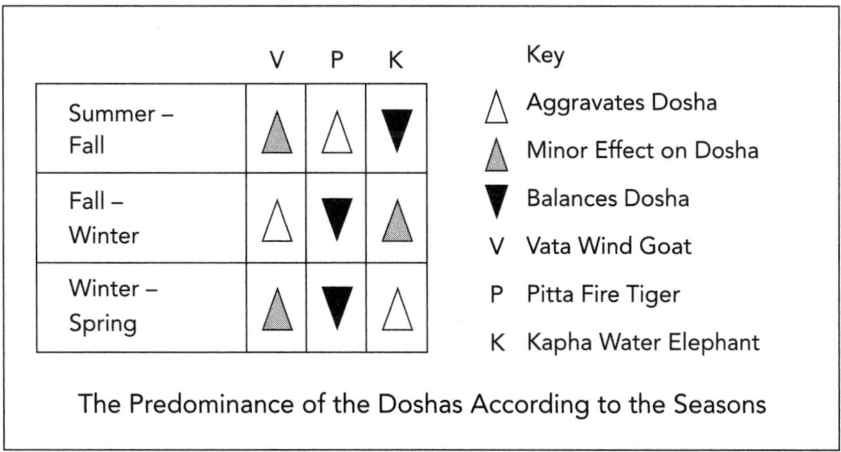

The Predominance of the Doshas According to the Seasons

No Single Diet for Everyone

The descriptive science of the doshas illustrates an essential point about nutrition: *There is no single diet for everyone at anyone time, nor a constant diet throughout the year for a single person.* Kapha constitution people will be aggravated by a diet high in brown rice and salt. Vata people become grounded with brown rice and salty foods. Some vata people can tolerate a little dairy, while a kapha person may become congested from it. There are a few foods that all would do well to avoid. For example, it is best to avoid concentrated processed sweets like white sugar, which are clearly poisonous to the body and mind. Those with a pitta constitution are aggravated by raw honey. However, those with a kapha constitution are balanced by raw honey. For a long period of time, the author avoided all sweets, including honey. In 1984, in the morning, when kapha has a tendency to aggravate, the author occasionally added a half teaspoon of raw honey as an experiment and felt a subtle positive difference. However, because of his teachings of the *Rainbow Green Live-*

Food Cuisine, he does not recommend the regular use of honey to balance kapha, nor does he use honey anymore.

The art of food selection is to become sensitive to the foods that help maintain a dosha balance between our inner constitutional dosha tendencies and the environmental and cyclic effects of Nature on the doshas. What is presented here are single dosha archetypes. In reality, we are a mixture of all three doshas. Sometimes a single dosha predominates, while at other times two doshas are jointly more active, with one slightly stronger than the other. For example, the author is kapha-pitta. Sometimes all three doshas are of equal strength; this is spoken of as being tridosha. In any case, no matter what the combination, we are all affected by cyclic changes and need to pay intelligent attention.

The Six Tastes and Six Food Qualities

Meals prepared Ayurvedically usually contain different percentages of all six tastes because all six together are said to create a harmonious energy and nutrient balance. The six tastes are: sweet (milk, honey, rice, breads, butter); sour (lemon and yogurt); salty (salt) and pungent (spicy foods, ginger, cayenne, and cumin); bitter (spinach and other leafy greens); and astringent (beans and lentils). As we can see in the fourth figure, the energies associated with different tastes aggravate or balance the doshas in particular patterns.

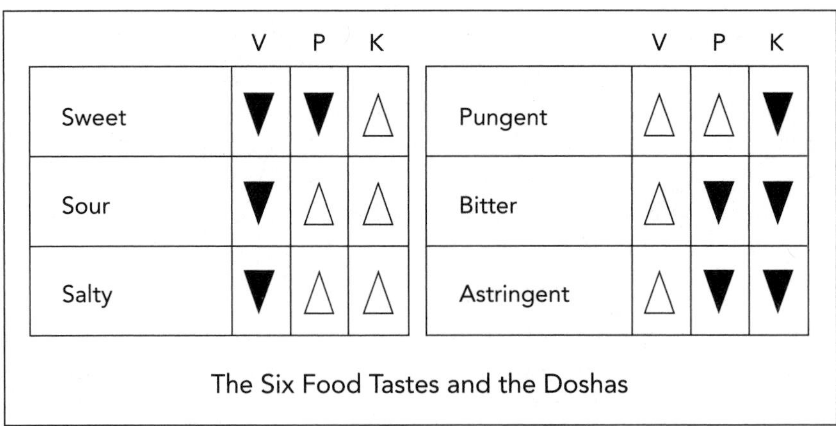

	V	P	K		V	P	K
Sweet	▼	▼	△	Pungent	△	△	▼
Sour	▼	△	△	Bitter	△	▼	▼
Salty	▼	△	△	Astringent	△	▼	▼

The Six Food Tastes and the Doshas

There are also six major food qualities to consider: heavy (cheese, yogurt, and wheat); light (barley, corn, spinach, and apples); oily (dairy products, fatty foods, and oils); dry (barley, corn, potatoes, and beans);

	V	P	K		V	P	K
Heavy	▼	▼	△	Light	△	△	▼
Oily	▼	▼	△	Dry	△	△	▼
Hot	▼	△	▼	Cold	△	▼	

The Six Food Qualities and the Doshas

hot food and drink; and cold food and drink. The fifth figure shows the effect of food qualities on the doshas.

Over the years, Ayurvedic physicians have developed a list of foods and food types according to how they aggravate or balance the doshas. The table on the following pages is a slightly modified list taken from Dr. Vasant Lad's excellent book *Ayurveda: The Science of Self-Healing.*[4]

Perspective on Ayurvedic Tridosha System

To achieve an optimum diet for our spiritual life, we must be attuned to our own constitutional, diurnal, seasonal, and practical work needs. It requires creating a harmony between our inner needs and the external play of Nature. It means not giving up our intuition and power to "this is the answer" diet fads, computer diet programs, any diet system that claims to be the only way to health, or even Ayurvedic lists of the right foods for our doshas. No single system, including Ayurveda, is 100 percent accurate. For example, Rudolph Ballentine, M.D., who uses Ayurveda in his approach, feels that the application of the system is only 80 percent accurate.[5]

Food Guidelines for Basic Constitutional Types

Note: Guidelines provided in this table are general. Specific adjustments for individual requirements may need to be made, e.g. food allergies, strength of digestive fire, season of the year, and degree of dosha predominance or aggravation. (+ means aggravates dosha, – means balances dosha)

Vata		Pitta		Kapha	
+	–	+	–	+	–
FRUITS					
Dried Fruits	Sweet Fruits	Sour Fruits	Sweet Fruits	Sweet and Sour Fruits	Apricots
Apples	Apricots	Apricots	Apples	Apples	Berries
Cranberries	Avocado	Berries	Avocado	Avocado	Cherries
Pears	Bananas	Bananas	Coconut	Bananas	Cranberries
Persimmon	Berries	Cherries	Figs	Coconut	Figs (dry)
Pomegranate	Cherries	Cranberries	Grapes (dark)	Figs (fresh)	Mango
Watermelon	Coconut	Grapefruit	Mango	Grapefruit	Peaches
	Figs (fresh)	Grapes (green)	Melons	Grapes	Pears
	Grapefruit	Lemons	Oranges (sweet)	Lemons	Persimmon
	Grapes	Oranges (sour)	Pears	Melons	Pomegranate
	Lemons	Papaya	Pineapple (sweet)	Oranges	Prunes
	Mango	Peaches	Plums (sweet)	Papaya	Raisins
	Melons (sweet)	Pineapple (sour)	Pomegranate	Pineapple	
	Oranges	Persimmon	Prunes	Plums	
	Papaya	Plums (sour)	Raisins		
	Peaches				
	Pineapple				
	Plums				
VEGETABLES					
Broccoli	Asparagus	Pungent Vegetables	Sweet/Bitter Vegetables	Sweet/Juicy Vegetables	Pungent/Bitter Vegetables
Brussels Sprouts	Beets	Beets	Asparagus	Cucumber	Asparagus
Cabbage	Carrots	Carrots	Broccoli	Potatoes (sweet)	Beets
Cauliflower	Cucumber	Eggplant	Brussels Sprouts	Tomatoes	Broccoli
Celery	Garlic	Garlic	Cabbage	Zucchini	Brussels Sprouts
Eggplant	Green Beans	Onions	Cauliflower		Cabbage
Leafy Greens*	Okra (cooked)	Peppers (hot)	Celery		Carrots
Lettuce*	Onion (cooked)	Radishes	Green Beans		Cauliflower
Mushrooms	Potatoes (sweet)	Spinach	Leafy Greens		Celery
Onions (raw)	Radishes	Tomatoes	Mushrooms		Eggplants
Parsley*	Zucchini		Okra		Leafy Greens
Peas			Peas		Lettuce
Peppers			Parsley		Mushrooms
Potatoes (white)			Peppers (green)		Okra
Spinach*			Potatoes		Onions
Sprouts*			Sprouts		Parsley
Tomatoes			Zucchini		Peas
					Peppers
					Potatoes (white)
					Radishes
					Spinach
					Sprouts

* These vegetables are all right in moderation with oil dressing.

Food Guidelines for Basic Constitutional Types

	Vata		Pitta		Kapha	
	+	–	+	–	+	–
GRAINS	Barley Buckwheat Corn Millet Oats (dry) Rye	Oats (cooked) Rice Wheat	Buckwheat Corn Millet Oats (dry) Rice (brown) Rye	Barley Oats (cooked) Rice (basmati) Rice (white) Wheat	Oats (cooked) Rice (brown) Rice (white) Wheat	Barley Corn Millet Oats (dry) Rice (basmati, small amount) Rye
ANIMAL FOODS	Lamb Pork Rabbit Venison	Beef Chicken (white) Eggs (fried or scrambled) Seafood Turkey (white)	Beef Eggs (yolk) Lamb Pork Seafood	Chicken (white) Eggs (white) Rabbit Shrimp (small amount) Turkey (white) Venison	Beef Lamb Pork Seafood	Chicken (dark) Eggs (scrambled) Rabbit Shrimp Turkey (dark) Shrimp Venison
LEGUMES	No legumes except mung, tofu, and black and red lentils		All legumes OK except lentils		All legumes are good except kidney beans, soybeans, black lentils, and mung beans	
NUTS	All nuts if moderate Soaked nuts		Minimal nuts except coconut Moderate soaked nuts		Minimal nuts Moderate soaked nuts	
SEEDS	All seeds if moderate Soaked seeds		Minimal seeds except sunflower and pumpkin Moderate sprouted and soaked seeds		Minimal seeds except sunflower and pumpkin Moderate sprouted and soaked seeds	
SWEETENERS	Moderate sweeteners except white sugar		Moderate sweeteners except molasses and honey		Minimal sweeteners except raw honey	
CONDIMENTS	All spices are good		No spices except coriander, cinnamon, cardamom, fennel, turmeric, and a little black pepper		All spices are good except salt	

(continued on page 370)

Food Guidelines for Basic Constitutional Types

Vata +	Vata –	Pitta +	Pitta –	Kapha +	Kapha –
DAIRY					
All dairy products in moderation		Buttermilk Cheese Sour Cream Yogurt	Butter (unsalted) Cottage Cheese Goat milk Ghee Milk	No dairy except ghee and goat milk	
OILS					
All oils are good		Almond Corn Safflower Sesame	Coconut Olive Sunflower Soy	No oils except almond, corn, or safflower in small amounts	

Energy Balancing with Herbs

Ayurvedic science has observed that individual foods and herbs have specific energetic qualities that are suggested to us by the nature of their taste. In the author's live-food diet approach, he has added certain herbs to maintain the dosha balance throughout the yearly cycles. For example, as a predominant kapha constitution, he uses ginger, cardamom, cayenne, and cumin as kapha dosha balancers, particularly in the winter when heat is needed. Vata people may want to include the energy of cinnamon, cardamom, cumin, ginger, sea salt, cloves, mustard, and licorice in their diets at the appropriate times. Pitta people would do better to avoid spices except for cinnamon, coriander, and dill.

The use of herbs in this way reaffirms the principle that each food has its own energy essence. Western nutrition's singular focus on classifying foods as simply carbohydrate, protein, and fat increases our sense of separation from food and our disharmony with Nature.

Summary, Chapter 24

1. The tridosha system offers a harmonious diet for spiritual life by helping us identify our constitutional dosha mixture of kapha, pitta, and vata.

2. Nutrition is concerned with the dynamic interaction of the forces of the foods with the dynamic forces of our own bodies.
3. To balance the high vata and prana forces of a live-food diet, it is best to follow vata pacifying practices of slow, moderate, sweet, salty, and sour, rather than transition to a 100-percent live-food diet immediately.
4. We can organize and change our diets according to the dosha energy shifts of the cycles of the seasons, days, and our own lives.
5. By using the energies of different herbs to balance our doshas, we add a useful dimension to the live-food diet.
6. Herbs reaffirm the principle that each food has its own energy essence.
7. On a properly designed live-food diet, it is relatively easy to be successful even as a person with an unbalanced vata dosha.

Chapter 25

Ayurvedic Insights into Live Foods

To clearly appreciate the insight that the Ayurvedic approach to live foods offers, we need to develop an understanding of the subtle levels of the three doshas: kapha, pitta, and vata. These subtle levels are called the three vital essences. For vata, the vital essence is called prana; for pitta, it is called tejas; and for kapha, it is called ojas. The doshas need to be balanced in order to ameliorate or prevent disease. These subtle energy levels – prana, tejas, and ojas – have to do with how to maximize health and spiritual potential. In that context, they are energies more connected to the subtle and causal bodies.

In essence, proper balance and energizing of these vital essences creates positive life force. Prana, a term that most people are familiar with, can be considered the basic vital life force energy. It is also understood as the subtle energy of air and ether, which is, in a sense, the guiding energy behind the psycho-physiological functions and the coordination of breath, senses, and mind. Prana also is a driving force behind deeper spiritual states of consciousness. Tejas is the inner radiance or inner fire. It is also deeply associated with the fire of Kundalini. According to David Frawley in *Yoga and Ayurveda,* on an inner level it energizes and governs higher perceptual capacities.[1] Ojas is the subtle energy of water and earth. It is the stored-up energetic life force of the body, or primal vigor. It involves the integrity and stored energy of protein, fat, and reproductive fluids, as well as healthy gross tissue mass. The amount of ojas a person has correlates with the amount of physical, sexual, mental, and spiritual endurance that person has.

In essence, as we embark on the path of Spiritual Nutrition, the prana, tejas, and ojas need to be balanced. Our physical and subtle physical foundations and balance depends on the strength of ojas. Tejas is the heat and light energy of ojas. Prana is the energy that radiates from ojas after it has been set on fire by tejas. Tejas also can be understood as the fire of the Divine or Kundalini. The term Shekhinah energy can also be used, but for one-system clarity, we will use the term Kundalini in this chapter.

The nadi system, which is the subtle nervous system, interpenetrates all layers of the koshas and takes the spiritual energy into the koshas. The nadis have the ojas as their lining and are the conduit for the tejas and prana. The nadis also intersect to create the chakras. The nadis, in a sense, are metaphorically lined with ojas. The ojas, when it is sufficient, is set on subtle fire by the energy of the tejas or the Kundalini. As the tejas moves through the nadis, it creates a spiritual heat, which people often feel when the Kundalini is awakened. The burning of the ojas by tejas activates and amplifies the energy of the prana. If we do not have enough ojas, the fire of Kundalini, metaphorically and actually, can burn up the nadis. The prana, much like the wind blowing on a fire, also increases the flame of the tejas burning the ojas. This becomes significant when we talk about Spiritual Nutrition because if we do not have enough ojas, which is similar metaphorically to logs on a fire, and we just increase the prana with purifying live foods, asanas, and pranayama, we create a fire that is so strong it rapidly burns up all the logs of the ojas. The result is potential harm to the subtle nervous system, or nadis, which had previously been protected by a lubricant lining of ojas. Once the ojas is burnt up, the fire may burn up the nadis next. Therefore, in Spiritual Nutrition, we emphasize *live foods that sustain and build the ojas.*

The task, therefore, for spiritual aspirants, is to increase all three forces – prana, tejas, and ojas – in a balanced way, so we can have maximal spiritual energy that helps us go to our highest spiritual potential and not deplete the ojas.

The Six Foundations for Spiritual Life, properly applied, protect the ojas, and build the prana and tejas. As explained, the tejas is the inner fire, which really is the Kundalini energy in its activated or non-activated form. The Kundalini is an inner fire, a form of lightning or electrical energy at the subtle levels. The prana, the wind that blows the fire, comes primarily from pranayama, eating live foods, asanas, and other sorts of high-energy practices. The key thing that isn't as obvious is to protect and build the ojas, so as prana and tejas increase, we do not burn up the ojas.

The ojas is sustained and increased by eating a pure diet and by what is called dharmic living. Dharmic living, outlined in the great scriptures, is Foundation Four of the Six Foundations. In this Foundation, we have the yamas and niyamas of Yoga, the Ten Speakings of the Torah, the concept of living in a holy way from the Kabbalistic scriptures, the Eight-Fold Path of Buddhism, and the White Buffalo Medicine way of the Native American path. The holiness also has to do with a balanced mind, balanced emotions, and senses that are all turned toward one thing – God, and experiencing the delight of God in all things.

Building ojas with a diet of live foods requires a greater emphasis on: nut milks and seed milks; nuts and seeds; juicy and oily vegetables, such as avocado; low-glycemic fruits, especially berries, such as goji berries; and other foods with a slight sweetness in taste, like apples, carrots, coconut, and sprouted grains. Goji berries and bee pollen are not only high in antioxidants, but are tremendously rejuvenative. More oily, creamy, soupy types of food, such as smoothies, are all good for building ojas.

To build ojas, it is important to increase the intake of Omega-3 fatty acids. Many people on a low-fat, cleansing, live-food diet become depleted in Omega-3 fatty acids. Lack of short-, medium-, and long-chain fatty acids weakens the physical nervous system and depletes ojas. Purslane, a common herb that grows almost everywhere, is high in the long-chain Omega-3 fatty acids, particularly EPA. Recent research by Dr. Timohir Lelas of Zagreb, through the process of tribomechanical analysis verified the existence of EPA (eicosapentaenoic acid) and DHA (docosahexaenoic acid) in aphanizomenon flos-aquae (AFA) (also known as Klamath Lake algae). Research cited in *Primordial Food* suggests that not only does AFA have EPA and DHA, but that the AFA, probably because of its high levels of alpha-linolenic acid, increases the DHA and EPA in the blood in rats to higher levels than expected by the DHA and EPA in the AFA alone. In other words, AFA amplifies the EPA and DHA levels in the blood. Momoatomic rhodium and iridium have also been found in AFA.[2] These are the only vegan sources we have of EPA. AFA grows almost everywhere. DHA, another important long-chain Omega-3 fatty acid, especially for brain function, is available from a golden algae as well as AFA. An extract of the DHA from golden algae is available at the Tree of Life. Flax seed and hemp seed will provide most of the short-chain Omega-3 fatty acids. Coconut oil is a great oil for building ojas, as are hemp seed and macadamia nuts. Coconut oil increases the conversion of short-chain to long-chain Omega-3 fatty acids by 3–6 percent.

Certain tonic herbs in general, and particularly ashwagandha, shatavari, ginseng, and licorice are good for ojas. These are what Ayurveda calls soma-producing herbs.

Spirulina and chlorella – high in protein, fatty acids like GLA (gamma-linolenic acid, which is highest in mother's milk, second highest in spirulina, and third highest in hemp seeds), sulfanolipids, minerals, and vitamins – are both tridoshic (balance all the doshas) and excellent as ojas builders.

Bee pollen, as the semen of the plant world, is an incredible food for building ojas. It is 20 percent protein (gram for gram, it has five to seven times more protein than meat, eggs, or cheese), is 15 percent brain-building oils and lecithin, has sixty-three minerals and most of the B vitamins, and has vitamins C and E, nucleic acids, 5,000 enzymes and coenzymes, and essential fatty acids. According to the research by Dr. Eric Erickson from the University of Wisconsin, bee pollen causes a positive electric charge. When bees leave the hive, they have a slightly negative or neutral charge; on returning with the pollen, they have a charge as high as 1.5 volts and their bee pollen is charged. Dr. Nicolai Tsitsin, a Russian botanist found that of those in Russia living past 125 years, many were bee keepers whose main food was bee pollen.[3] Much Russian research has shown that bee pollen has powerful anti-aging and regenerative powers. Bee pollen is the ultimate biogenic food and the procreative force of the plant world.

Drinking plenty of structured water with non-heated full mineral salts in ionic form helps to build ojas and prevent dehydration. Crystal energy helps to structure the water (see Chapter 29 on living, structured water).

There are also some physical practices that help to build ojas. These include oleation (rubbing oil on the whole body). Oleation followed by a five- to ten-minute hot shower, and then by repeat oleation is another technique. Basti (oil enemas with or without herbs) is an excellent way to build ojas and decrease excess vata. Herbs that reduce excess vata help protect the ojas. These main herbs can be taken as a basti: jatamansi, brahmi, rose petal, and chamomile. Ashwagandha, licorice, and shatavari can also be used in the basti. The author has been very successful with the use of basti with clients on both short and long fasts for calming the vata aggravations that may occur. One of the most powerful ways to balance vata and build ojas is the ancient Ayurvedic seven-day detox and rejuvenative treatment called *Pancha Karma*. To the best of our knowledge, the Tree of Life offers the only live-food Pancha Karma program in the world, which we have been doing since 1996.

Protecting the ojas by controlling sexual energy may be very important. This does not necessarily mean celibacy; it means appropriate use of sexual energy. People may protect ojas by using certain Taoist techniques, such as retention of semen. It is very clear that excessive loss of semen, or even excessive sexuality, even if you are maintaining your semen, can deplete ojas. A classical sign of low ojas is weakness and fatigue immediately and/or for several days after ejaculation. In such cases, it is advisable to refrain from sexual activity until ojas is restored. Deep yang and yin kidney-building herbs have been very helpful for this. Some teach that this depletion may also occur in women. In thirty-five years of clinical experience, the author has had no woman cite this as a health problem. Perhaps the female depletion happens on a more subtle level. The world literature does suggest that sexual activity can prolong life, so there is no need to be celibate from a health and longevity standpoint. In *The Lancet,* a major study was reported to show men ages 45 to 59 who had sex two to three times per week had 50 percent lower mortality. Similar findings were made in a study in Virginia. The studies on longevity for women were less dramatic, but suggested some longevity benefit, as well as amelioration of menopause symptoms.

Interestingly enough, the Bhakti Yoga of chanting (the Yoga of Divine Love), which is also in essence the Tantric way and in the Kabbalah is experiencing the Light or holiness of the Divine in all things *(azamara),* plays a role for maintaining and building ojas. Proper sleep also protects ojas. It is unfortunate in the live-food movement that the emphasis is often on glorifying how little sleep one can live on. It may be true that live-fooders often need less sleep, but that doesn't mean that less sleep protects the ojas. Many people suffer from depleted ojas by simply overworking and not getting enough sleep. Getting enough sleep is very important for building the ojas. Recent research shows that without sufficient sleep, people have significantly less serotonin in their nervous system, which can be considered the ojas part of the neurotransmitter system. Serotonin creates a neuroendocrine safety net against stress and against heat, similar on a gross level to the role of ojas. Sleep is essential for the spiritual path, particularly going to bed early and getting up early. We need between seven and eight hours of sleep on a consistent basis. More than 100 million people in the United States suffer from sleep deprivation.[4]

Another aspect of living in a holy way that builds ojas is what the Yogis would call control of the senses (pratyahara); this means avoiding most forms of mass media, particularly television, but also excess computer use. A fast from TV involves the not-so-subtle technique of unplugging the television. It is one of the best things we can do to build ojas. TV is filled with outward-moving activities, and it is a prime builder of fear and anxiety. Because of this, TV, like adrenaline-provoking drugs, burns ojas. The overuse of what we call the motor organs, particularly excess talking, also depletes the ojas.

Overworking, over-restraint, overplaying, and excess stress deplete ojas. Building and maintaining ojas means leading a life of moderation. This is hard for younger people to understand, because they have a lot of ojas to burn. For many people, the spiritual path is a long one, and you want your ojas to last and to be regenerative.

Drug Use

The use of drugs depletes ojas and deranges the prana and the tejas. A typical ojas-depleting drug is marijuana; others include peyote, psychedelic mushrooms, LSD, ecstasy, cocaine, heroin, amphetamines, and ketamine. One of the most serious problems associated with these herbal and pharmaceutical drugs is their effect of hyperstimulating the serotonin concentrations through a variety of mechanisms to create neuronal destruction from an excess of serotonin, which then becomes oxidized. In this oxidized form, the serotonin is neurotoxic. A healthy serotonergic system acts like a neurochemical anti-stress system, maintaining balance, resilience, inner strength, and a sense of well-being. For this reason, the author considers the serotonin system a functional part of our ojas and general emotional well-being. When it is depleted, so is the ojas.

Evidence of neurotoxicity has accumulated for cocaine, amphetamines, ecstasy (MDMA), and Redux (a Prozac-like drug).[5] Drugs like ecstasy and LSD can boost not only serotonin, but also adrenaline and dopamine.[6] Clinically, the author can physiologically detect the damage for several weeks after someone has taken ecstasy. Lab studies with animals on neuron affects of Redux show that it destroys the branches of the serotonin neurons called axons.[7] In some cases these animal studies showed neurotoxicity when the drugs were administered just for days at dose levels that humans take for up to one year.[8] If the damage was not too severe, the neurons would sprout new branches.[9] The animals could still function with the destruction. The brain has tremendous capacity and reserve, but neuroscientists suggest that the effects of significant damage may not appear until a later age when the brain's neuronal reserve becomes depleted.[10] Research on Redux by Dr. Vina McCann at the National Institute of Mental Health, published in the *Journal of the American Medical Association,* suggests that neurotoxicity is dependent both on dose level and duration. Redux is often compared to ecstasy as well as Prozac, which both significantly raise serotonin. Studies of ecstasy have shown that when the damaged serotonin neurons sprout new branches, there is a "highly abnormal" brain rewiring that does not follow the original brain pattern.[11] Some of the ecstasy studies, however, have been considered invalid because the researchers used amphetamines instead of ecstasy. The clinical reports of medical symptoms of ecstasy users, however, substantiate the author's concern and warning about the use of ecstasy, so he feels a warning now about its potential danger is as valid as warning about the dangers of cigarette smoking before thirty years of research conclusively proved the toxicity of cigarettes. High amounts of serotonin in the synapses of the neurons can be easily oxidized to form serotonergic neurotoxins.[12] Unfortunately, there is not enough long-term research on any of these drugs individually to make any definitive statements, but it is reasonable to assume that chronic usage or high amounts in one dose have the potential to cause brain damage, at least to the serotonergic neurons, with a concomitant decrease in normal serotonin production and disruption of neuron axons.

Clinical symptoms have been seen in chronic usage of LSD, ecstasy, ketamine, a variety of psychedelic mushrooms, and marijuana. The author has seen many people over the years who have "blown-out" their ojas and other brain functions with these drugs. Symptoms include emotional confusion, memory loss, loss of vital force, adrenal and liver depletion, post-drug depression, psychosis, and a disruption and disorganization of the flow of Kundalini. Kundalini can be disrupted with ayahuasca as well. Some people appear to be untouched by the use of these drugs in the short term, but there remains an unnecessary high risk for too many vulnerable drug users. The most vulnerable are people who have vata constitutions, are vata imbalanced, have been previously diagnosed with mental conditions, have a sensitive nadi system, or are dehydrated. One of the author's sub-specialties is repairing this type of damage as a way to support people's spiritual life, joy, and happiness.

The spiritual life provided by a high-prana diet and lifestyle takes one into the sattvic guna of increased clarity, brightness, and Light of the Divine. To some people, this intensity on spiritual, psychological, and emotional levels may be too intense. Marijuana, peyote, and other drugs that create a more tamasic or numbing state dampen the sattvic effect of a live-food diet. In Yoga, *tamas* is characterized by a veil of ignorance, sloth, lack of discipline, and lack of will power. Marijuana use, seen in this context, may be used as a way to dampen the prana. There are much safer and better ways to decrease vata, prana, and sattva. This does not mean that one may not get some visions or insights from these drugs, but psychedelic drug use is what is referred to in Ayurveda as sattva in tamas, and long-term use of psychedelics has the potential to keep one in the phenomenology of the astral planes and may retard spiritual development on the highest planes of Kundalini, Self-realization and merging with God. The author does not deny that psychedelic drug use has not been a powerful spiritual catalyst and door opener for many on the planet for their first spiritual experiences beyond the three-dimensional plane of so-called "normal life." The question is, does the seeker choose to stay standing in the doorway or to walk through? Proper usage of these drugs in ceremony is common in talk, but rare in practice. The use of herbal or synthetic "consciousness drugs" is not the "medicine" way of the Essene and Kabbalistic paths. Their use is highly likely to be harmful in chronic or long-term use.

At this stage of limited research, ayahuasca does not seem to consistently have any problems with short-term or long-term chronic usage.[13] It is important to keep in mind the case study #1 in Chapter 4 – the subject who took ayahuasca after his Kundalini was awakened and suffered severe imbalances. People have felt they have benefited from one-time or occasional ceremonial use, often at the beginning stages of the spiritual path. Many who have been introduced to spiritual life through drug usage may become caught in the illusion of moving deeper on the path through repeated use. This one knows no Realized Being who supports the use of drugs *for realization,* neither historically nor in the present. That does not mean that ayahuasca taken in its natural setting in the Amazon under traditional shamanic guidance has not been effective in helping people clear up emotional and mental imbalances or helping people connect to the energy of Mother Gaia. Ayahuasca is primarily used by shamans as part of a spiritual healing ceremony. The more important point, however, is that you do not need any dependence on drugs to create these effects or healing. There are many meditators, including this one, who have had such experiences and teachings on a daily basis after the Kundalini awakens. Thinking you need drugs to have this experience creates the illusion of dependency and limits one's freedom to move in any direction in the sacred walk between B'lee mah and Mah in ordinary life. It requires no psychedelics to experience the silent wonderment of "awakened normality" that may be experienced as a result of living the Six Foundations. Once the Kundalini is awakened, the non-causal ecstasy, non-causal peace, and non-causal contentment of life that is our heritage is available regularly. The effect does not "wear off," there is no "trip" to come down from, and there are no side effects. Awakened normality is our natural state. It does not depend on anything outside of us or anything we need to ingest. Freedom is independent of any external conditions. All we need is to be in the silence that allows us to transcend the limitations of the mind and brain. Drugs confine us to the chemistry of the brain and emotions and therefore limit us in this ultimate sense. The awakened life is about being exquisitely present in this world. This is the true miracle. It is not the limited phenomenological world of drugs; it is the real wow of life, as one dances in the Divine Presence and the whole world becomes alive and shares its sacred walk with you. Sai Baba of Shirdi, a great *avadhuta* and God-conscious Being, was so omnipresent that it took an average of one hour to walk fifty yards. Do we really need to travel to Brazil to take some drugs to feel alive? Does this really have anything to do with Liberation? The point the author is raising is not whether drugs, synthetic or organic, are dangerous, or have a high risk-to-benefit ratio, or not whether they are a valid path – but rather, where the path leads? For those who indeed have benefited from them as a door opener, are they a path that leads to full Liberation or perhaps only to the doorway? *Drugs, like the ego of the mind-body complex they stimulate, must be let go if we are to go all the way to the Nothing. Those who dance in the I AM THAT require no props.*

When introduced to other ways of building spiritual awareness, such as meditation and Yoga, often the drug usage significantly diminishes because the seeker has found more sustaining and less potentially toxic ways. As people mature spiritually and have an increasing experience of the non-causal contentment, peace, and joy of sattvic life, drugs gradually stop being considered as a means to evolve spiritually. Once one has the Kundalini awakened, tastes the nectar of sattvic life, and has established a spiritual foundation, drug use simply looks pale. *The vast majority of Eastern and Western recognized Self-realized Beings do not recommend drugs as part of a deep spiritual path to Liberation.* Mostly these drugs stimulate the phenomenology of astral plane experiences and insights, which is not the goal of Liberation.

Once the Kundalini is awakened, the author strongly recommends one does not do any drugs or harsh Yoga practices that force the Kundalini and interfere with the delicate process that has been activated. Simply supporting the Kundalini unfolding with the Six Foundations is enough. The Sacred Feminine has a Divine unfolding pattern all its own that is best respected and surrendered to. It is a feminine pattern of surrender rather than a masculine path of fitting into a pre-set form or forcing with techniques or drugs. The way of Kundalini is gentle and peaceful, and it knows how to help one through blocks in its own unique unfoldment. People who have had difficulty with Kundalini have typically been those who have tried to force the unfolding with drugs, excessive pranayama, or other extreme practices, or who have pre-existing mental disturbances. Aside from this, the author has seen hardly anyone have difficulty if they maintain their foundations of spiritual practice. The issue of drugs and Self-realization is a topic that serious seekers of spiritual Liberation need to honestly address.

Another tamasic and rajasic (activating) substance, and a food that can be used unconsciously or consciously to dampen prana and tejas, and the activity of Kundalini in general, is meat. Dairy today, because of its toxicity, also fits into this category, although historically it was considered a sattvic food. Spiritual Nutrition is about deeper levels of peace. One approach is to make the transition to a high-live-food diet and sattvic lifestyle in a slow and gentle way that allows the psycho-spiritual system to feel balanced and comfortable, so one will not need to counter increased sattva and prana or balance vata excess.

Ojas, Tejas, and Prana in Live Foods

As we begin to understand the subtle levels of kapha, pitta, and vata, manifesting as ojas, tejas, and prana, we have the insight to understand why live food has the highest amount of ojas, tejas, and prana. Vata and prana have to do with the essence of life force, as well as oxygen. As pointed out by David Frawley, a Vedic and Ayurvedic scholar considered an authentic teacher of the Vedas, the traditional Yogic texts emphasize a live-food diet.[14] It is the diet of the ancient Rishis who understood that live foods have the highest prana and that prana helps to expand consciousness.[15] As shown in *Conscious Eating*, live food has more life force energy, or prana. This pranic field is associated with the bioluminescence shown in the Kirlian photography studies.[16]

The principle of tejas is the essence of fire or subtle fire, what one would call electricity, that is in the food, as well as the amount of enzymes. Cooked food has significantly diminished tejas, because the metabolic power of the food, associated with the tejas, is in the enzymes. These are completely destroyed when we cook food for more than three minutes. As pointed out clearly in *Conscious Eating*, live food has considerably higher electrical energy and enzymes, which is the tejas. Live food is also highest in bio-photon energies.[17] These are the subtle radiations of the live food. The electrical potentials are clearly higher in live food,[18] and live food is a powerful source of electrons. All this is disrupted and minimized when the food is cooked. Thus, it is clear that live food has more tejas.

Ojas relates to the water and earth element, or what we might metaphorically call the lubricating nectar of the water and earth. In a sense, the ojas maintains the integrity of the subtle nadis as energy channels for the tejas and prana. The process of cooking destroys the structural quality of the water and disrupts the internal structure of the water in the food. The more structured the water, the greater is its ability to hold the energy in the body. Structured water is important for maintaining the subtle structure of the DNA. Cooking also alters the fat and protein structure that is also part of the ojas. The Max Planck Institute in Germany found that 50 percent of protein is coagulated when cooked.[19] Therefore, when we cook food, we diminish its ojas.

All the types of live food have generally more prana, tejas, and ojas, and therefore are most effective in supporting spiritual life. The typical live-food diet primarily builds the prana, and secondly the tejas and ojas. The Kundalini is the primary builder and activator of the tejas. Green foods such as wheatgrass and sprouts are extraordinary prana builders. Certain live foods, however, like bee pollen, spirulina, and coconut, are exceptional for building ojas. The idea for optimal energetic balance is to add the high-ojas superfoods to your typical live-food diet, so the live-food diet strongly builds the ojas and prana. This unique perspective gives us an insight from Ayurveda into why the ancient great spiritual masters known as the Rishis, as well as Taoist masters, tended to eat not only vegan, but live food, with an emphasis on wildcrafted foods and high-soma herbs and foods.

Solving the Possible Difficulties of a Vegan, Live-Food Diet

Such a diet, using mainly live foods, if not done thoughtfully, as previously explained, can imbalance the vata, the biological air-ether humor. A vata imbalance includes the tendency to get too airy or move too much out of the body. Anxiety, depression, and other forms of emotional imbalance are also symptoms of a vata derangement, along with dry skin, exhaustion, and gas. So we must be careful to keep vata in balance while pursuing such a way of eating. Vata imbalances may increase digestive disturbances and decrease digestive fire. By eating a high-ojas diet and increasing digestive fire with herbs such as ginger, cayenne, cinnamon, basil, and Ayurvedic formulas, such as triketu and agnitundi, such digestive disturbance is minimized.

The bigger mistake with live foods is overeating. Cooking food destroys half the protein, 70–80 percent of the nutrients, and close to 100 percent of many of the phytonutrients. Because of this, we only need to eat one-half as much live food to get the same amount of nutrition. Eating one-half as much food creates significantly less digestive stress. Over time, the fire of the system builds to meet the digestive power needed for live foods. Another factor is that live foods greatly enhance the physical and emotional detoxification process, so when people move to a diet too high in live foods too quickly, they may have a healing crisis caused by the detoxification. For this reason, it is better to move more slowly onto a live-food diet at a rate that your body can handle comfortably. Often people use dead foods to suppress the emotions into dead spaces in the body. Live food adds life to these spaces and brings up the emotions. Moving too quickly onto live foods may bring up too many emotions to handle all at once. Because of this, it is often better to transition slowly.

Not surprisingly, some people, particularly thin or hypersensitive vata types, can have a difficult time with veganism, which makes them feel ungrounded or lacking in energy. They may have tried to be a vegan unsuccessfully and returned to eating meat, which they find makes them feel better and gives them more strength in the short run. Much of this is because people don't know how to be conscious vegans, which requires knowledge of food combining and live-food preparation. While one can be an unconscious meat eater, veganism requires a lot of consciousness to be successful. Most people who fail at veganism do so because they lack the proper nutritional understanding, not because their bodies are not designed for it. They fail to take the vegan food necessary for their body type or the season.

This issue can be resolved in a way that leaves no physiological excuse for not incorporating this way of eating into one's spiritual life. The books *Conscious Eating* and *Rainbow Green Live-Food Cuisine* establish in detail the scientific and Ayurvedic principles for consciously and successfully creating a vegan, live-food, organic, high-prana, and well-hydrated diet. Each one of us is a biochemically individual person and must select a diet that fits our particular body and mind. This includes a diet that balances the doshas (kapha, pitta, and vata) and improves our digestive strength, or *agni,* as described in Ayurveda. But it must be a diet that is also adjusted to whether we are a fast or slow oxidizer, parasympathetic or sympathetic, as well as to climate, life work, worldly responsibilities, and the level of detoxification that we need to be going through at a particular time. It is possible for anyone, whatever constitution and condition, to be successful not only as a vegan but also practicing a predominantly live-food, vegan, organic way of life. It requires the right information on how to do so, as well as making eating a spiritual practice – not just a quick trip to the refrigerator or the restaurant! In general, people with a vata constitution need to eat warm (not cooked), blended, soupy, slightly sweet, salty (full mineralized ionic salt), and sour-tasting foods, and eat according to their constitutional need for a high- or low-protein diet.

In the past, meat eating was often required because of environmental restraints and lack of available vegan food, such as for people who lived in cold climates or high altitudes where vegan food was not regularly available. The technology for successfully creating a sattvic, primarily live-food diet was not accessible, so some people suffered just in trying to become vegans. Balancing the vata and getting the appropriate protein, whether high or low, is easy to do on a live-food, vegan diet. Now we can learn how to balance all of these components, no matter what our psycho-physiological constitution. One cause of difficulty with veganism is a B_{12} deficiency, which up to 80 percent of vegans and live-food vegans may develop immediately or over time. This is addressed in Chapter 19. A B_{12} deficiency often drives people to eat meat. The solution is easy: Simply take a vegan B_{12} supplement. This is much more functional than taking the energy of flesh foods or death into our nadis, chakras, and koshas. For some, low zinc may cause a problem. This is ameliorated by adding more pumpkin seeds to the diet. Adding 1–3 tablespoons of freshly ground flax seeds helps build the Omega-3s. The same is true for hemp seeds, purslane, and Klamath Lake algae. The conversion to the long-chain Omega-3 fatty acids from flax or hemp seeds is amplified by 1 tablespoon of coconut oil per day, from a conversion rate of 1–3 percent up to 6 percent. Golden algae concentrates give high amounts of DHA and purslane supplies the EPA long-chain Omega-3s. Klamath Lake algae supplies both EPA and DHA. For further support on individualizing your diet so that you can partake of optimal Spiritual Nutrition for your own biochemistry, please see *Conscious Eating* and *Rainbow Green Live-Food Cuisine*.

Importance of a Spiritual Foundation on a Live-Food Diet

Once we understand the basic Ayurvedic principles, it gives us a tremendous insight into how to be successful on a live-food, Spiritual Nutrition diet, just as the ancient Rishis were. The Rishis lived their lives in a context that protected the ojas and calmed the vrittis of the mind. The latent vrittis of the mind can potentially be activated by the increased prana of a live-food diet. This is why it is easier to move slowly and steadily onto a live-food diet at a rate that allows you to clear the emotions that may come up. Many men and women in the live-food movement have built up tremendous prana, but because they are not protected by the balance of the Six Foundations, they tend to be spacey, to get off on tangents, and to be imbalanced in their physical, emotional, psychosexual, and spiritual lives. They may have a deep meditation here and there, do physical activities, have sex with a variety of other individuals, emphasize minimizing their sleep, or be workaholic. They don't seem to know what to do with their energy, except to use it up as quickly as possible. This approach often ends up depleting ojas.

Simply increasing prana is not really the full perspective in understanding Spiritual Nutrition. One needs to balance the prana in terms of where it is being directed. In essence, a 100-percent live-food diet without the Six Foundations is like a teenager getting a very fancy racing car, but not knowing how to drive. This is a particularly important teaching for people who are taking this path to reap the benefits of its power, its effectiveness, and for increasing spiritual life. Increased prana, without a larger spiritual context, does not necessarily lead to spirituality. For example, because you are flexible in hatha Yoga or eat 100-percent live food does not mean that you are spiritual. What often happens to people in a hatha Yoga practice, whose focus is primarily physical, is that they increase their potential for becoming ego-inflated because they become ego-identified with the power, looks, and flexibility of their body. It is only in the total context of the full ancient practice Ashtanga Yoga, the eight-limb Yoga (not to be confused with the hatha Yoga practice called Ashtanga Yoga) that it manifests in terms of spiritual life. The eight limbs are the yamas (Do's) and niyamas (Don'ts), asana (Yoga positions), pranayama (breath), pratyahara (sense withdrawal), dharana (concentration), dhyana (meditation), and samadhi (going to the silence beyond the mind). The point is very clear. We need a context of spiritual practices to focus the energy of the increased prana. Although we cannot eat our way to God, in this full context, a live-food diet is the most powerful diet for spiritual life. It is interesting to note that Shrii Shrii Ananda Murti, one of the few realized Beings in modern times who was at the level of moksha, recommended a live-food diet as part of his teachings of the nine secrets of longevity.[20]

It is common knowledge in the general Indian Yoga tradition that asana begins to open up the nadis. As previously pointed out, the nadis not only interconnect the koshas, but also are the channels through which the Kundalini flows, and intersect to form the chakras. One of the reasons we do asana is to open the nadis, as well as build prana. Therefore, whatever we eat will go more readily into the nadis and flow into the chakras and the koshas. The death energy associated with meat enters into the nadis and is even transported deeper into the chakras and koshas. Because of this association between asanas and the opening of the nadis, it is reasonable to assume that if you are not at least a vegetarian and you begin to do asanas and the nadis begin to open, the death energy and subtle toxins of meat, fish, and chicken move more readily into the nadis, the chakras, and the koshas, causing disruption, blockages, and permeating into even our deeper subtle levels with the pain and misery of death.[21] As we understand the subtleties of the spiritual meaning of Yoga asana, we begin to understand that *the deeper purpose of Yoga asana is not only to develop strength, flexibility, relaxation, rhythmical breathing, and ability to sit for meditation, but to open the nadis, rebalance the chakras, calm the vrittis of the mind associated with the chakras, balance the endocrine glands and nervous system plexes associated with the chakras, energize and move the prana or activated Kundalini through the system, increase the flow of prana through the nadis into the koshas for their purification and energization, and expand consciousness.* This is one of the reasons that this author strongly recommends that anyone who is seriously interested in Yoga as a spiritual practice thoughtfully consider following the sattvic diet. This is a diet that is at least 80-percent live food, organic, low-sugar, high-water (remember, water is connected to building ojas), and high-mineralized, prepared with Love.

Summary, Chapter 25

1. The subtle Ayurvedic principles give us useful insights into optimizing the effect of a live-food diet.
2. The key is that live foods not only build prana and tejas, but must also be used to build and sustain ojas.
3. Part of sustaining ojas is to avoid depleting the ojas with drugs or excessive practices or activity.
4. Live foods are highest in prana, tejas, and ojas.
5. When one does Yoga asana, what we eat flows more readily into the nadis and deeper into the koshas. The eating of meat when doing asana brings the energy of death into the nadis and koshas.
6. A live-food diet is more successful when Ayurvedic principles are followed.

Chapter 26

The Rainbow Diet

The Concept of the Rainbow Diet

The vibrations of food are first absorbed visually. The color and arrangement of food create a certain mental and physiological readiness. For example, depending on what foods are displayed, the content and concentration of our saliva changes. This is further augmented by our conscious responses to the aroma and taste of the food. Depending on what qualities of food we need, we become consciously and unconsciously drawn to the tastes, smells, and colors of the different foods. It is to the meaning of the colors of these foods that the Rainbow Diet awareness primarily addresses itself.

The awareness of the Rainbow Diet starts with acceptance that all comes from God and is nourished by the God Force. This force has been described as OM, universal prana, universal consciousness, cosmic force, and virtual energy state. It is the primordial vibration from which all has been created. Everything, including our food, has a natural system of harmonics in relationship to this primordial vibration. In the Rainbow Diet system of harmonics, all foods have a vibrational alignment to the seven main chakras and their colors, and these colors reflect the spectrum of the rainbow.

Four Main Principles of the Rainbow Diet

Here are the four main principles of the Rainbow Diet:

- Each food, according to its outer color, which is its reflecting surface, can be related to the specific color and energy of a particular chakra.

- Different-color foods are specific for energizing, balancing, and healing their corresponding color-related chakras
- Each color food energizes, cleanses, builds, heals, and rebalances the glands, organs, and nerve centers associated with its color-related chakra.
- The purpose of the Rainbow Diet is to help balance, on a regular daily cycle, each individual chakra, its associated organs, glands, and nerve plexus, and the chakra system as a whole.

If we think of plant food as condensed, colored sunlight, we can begin to get a better feeling for the concept of the Rainbow Diet. It does not apply to flesh foods, which primarily stimulate the first chakra. It also does not apply to the colors of junk, fast, frozen, microwaved, and irradiated foods. Red candy is not the same as a red apple. Food is the principal interface between us and Nature on the physical plane, and the colors of our foods are Nature's message or clues about the energy and biomolecular content of the specific color foods she gives us. Through the new paradigm of Spiritual Nutrition, we have arrived at the concept that food is energy as well as material form. The color of food is key to the energy pattern of food and how its biomolecular nutrients will be bonded to specific cells and tissues in our bodies. The color of a food is its signature. As we become sensitive to Nature's efforts to communicate to us through her beautiful colors, we begin to develop a sensitivity to the particular food colors we are drawn to on a specific day as a key to what food energies and nutrients we need to balance our body. The Rainbow Diet is an acknowledgment of Nature's effort to communicate with us. It is also a way to use the meaning of this information in an organized fashion to benefit us regularly through our daily intake of food.

By using the vascular autonomic signal (VAS), a technique for measuring the effect of subtle energy fields on the biological and etheric system of the body, the author was able to support his intuitive idea that the rainbow colors of Nature's foods relate to the harmonics of the rainbow colors of our chakras. The VAS, a pulse developed by the progenitor of auricular acupuncture, Paul Nogier, M.D., is a smooth muscle response of our blood vessels, mediated by the hypothalamic region of the brain. Its function is relatively independent from the voluntary control brain centers and therefore is less affected by subjectivity than are the popular body-testing systems such as kinesiology muscle testing. When an energy field from a substance is good for the body, the VAS is positive, and the tonus of the arterial wall is increased. This increase was labeled by Dr. Nogier as the vascular autonomic signal. Basically, it means there is a change in the VAS arterial pulse when a positive energy field enters the body energy field.

Each food has a specific energy frequency and resonance field, which we have described as the vortex manifestation of its SOEF. The body's energy field and the particular vortex resonance energy fields of each chakra are sensitive to the fields of the living substances put in their proximity. Their responses can be measured instantly by the VAS. Lawrence Bagley, M.D., feels it is a simple technique to place a substance such as an herb, food, drug, or cell salt into the body field and observe the VAS response.

By putting foods of various colors over each chakra, the author was able to determine which colors were most enhancing for each chakra. A direct correspondence was found between the colors of foods and chakras – red foods for the red or base chakra, orange foods for the sexual or orange-colored chakra, and so on. Each food peaked in the intensity of the VAS response at its specific color-resonant chakra. The food also showed a positive VAS, although less marked, at the chakra above and below its specific resonant-colored chakra. This interesting finding supports earlier statements that the chakras are linked as a total system. It also suggests that foods of different shades will affect the system slightly differently. Additionally, the spectrum phenomenon is more general rather than limited to the exact frequency of the basic color for each chakra. Because the author was already testing with the concepts of the Rainbow Diet in his mind and enough research has been done to suggest that even in double-blind studies the minds of the subject and the experimenter can affect the outcome, one cannot say that the VAS approach proves the Rainbow Diet concept, but it does give us some support for the intuitive "rightness" of the approach. It also supplies the reader with another major tool for understanding the relationship between our food and our bodies so that we can develop our own individualized diet.

Different color foods act specifically to energize and balance their particular color-coded chakras. By eating the Rainbow Diet in a patterned way, as described in the next section, we see a regular harmonic balancing of all the chakras as one system. Color healing of chakras and their related systems is not a new approach. It was used in the Golden Age of Greece, in the healing temples of Light and Color at Heliopolis, as well as in ancient Egypt, China, and India.[1] In the United States, Dr. Edwin Babbitt's book, *The Principles of Light and Color*,[2] and the more recent classic work by Dr. John Ott, *Health and Light*,[3] have laid a general foundation for the principles of color therapy in this country. Dr. Wurtman's research in beaming orange into a rabbit's eyes showed stimulation of the rabbit's ovarian function, which is connected to the orange second chakra. For centuries, color treatment has been done through different vehicles of light transport, including water charged with sunlight through a colored filter, direct sunlight or other light source treatment through a colored filter on the body or into the eyes, use of colored metals or gems, and of course, colored foods. Color foods have been used for healing persons of different maladies. For example, red food is used for people with low vitality, which fits with low energy in the first chakra. Red foods are also used to treat people with anemia or a deficiency in the blood vitality. This too is associated with the first chakra. In the Rainbow Diet, however, the focus is not on color therapy as a treatment for disease, but as a natural way through our daily diets to balance and tonify the body, the individual chakras, and the chakra system as a unit. It is for maintenance of health on all levels.

That each food relates to a specific chakra in terms of energizing, healing, cleansing, building, and rebalancing the glands, organs, and nerve centers associated with that chakra is different from chakra healing with colored lights, which is primarily an energizing and balancing effect. For example, rose hips, which are red and therefore particularly important to the first chakra, are high in vitamin C. Vitamin C is important for building and maintaining the connective tissue we need for locomotion, heart muscle tone, ligament function, blood vessel integrity, and adrenal function. The adrenals, which energize our fight or flight response, have the highest amount of vitamin C in the body. Our muscle system supplies the locomotion for survival. The first chakra, red in color, is linked to these survival organ and gland systems. Another example is leafy greens, which are coded for the heart chakra. They are high in calcium, magnesium, and potassium, which are very important for heart function.

Application of the Rainbow Diet

Balance is the key to the Rainbow Diet. The application of the diet is based on the idea that all chakras, even though they have different vibratory rates and different types of awareness, are created equal. All of them must be nourished. The Rainbow Diet calls for the full spectrum of foods for the full spectrum of the chakras throughout the spectrum of the day.

The morning starts with the first three chakras: red, orange, and yellow-gold. Midday is the third through the fifth chakras: yellow-gold, green, and blue in color. Evening is the fifth through the seventh chakras: blue, indigo, violet-purple, and white or gold in color. This sequence aligns with the general pattern for the awakening of the chakras. The daily stimulation and balancing of the chakras by the use of the appropriately colored foods maintains a balance that is important in spiritual life. If we only try to stimulate and charge the "higher" chakras, over a long period of time it is possible to become subtly uncentered or ungrounded.

There are exceptions to this spectral pattern. One is the use of a single color food for limited periods of time to energize a specifically weakened chakra and its associated organs, glands, and nerve centers. There are also times when one wants to activate a specific chakra gently for a short period of time by eating those foods that will stimulate that chakra.

The Rainbow Diet is not a technique for Enlightenment. It is simply a support system to aid in a harmonious and centered spiritual unfolding. It is a whole-person, full-chakra approach to nutrition. It is an organizing principle and a level of food awareness for helping us develop our own individualized diets for spiritual life. The principles of the Rainbow Diet are appropriate for any level of intake of vegetables, fruits, nuts, seeds, and grains. In this diet, white foods, which represent the full rainbow spectrum, can be used with any meal. White foods include vegetables like cauliflower and daikon radish. Although color coding does not apply for flesh foods, one can be a transitional vegetarian, lacto-ovo-vegetarian (the eggshell color is the code), lacto-vegetarian, vegan, or fruitarian, and the Rainbow Diet principles still are very functional.

Let's look at the basics of the Rainbow Diet and the timing of meals.

Morning

Red, orange, and yellow-golden foods are eaten for supporting the first, second, and third chakras. This includes fruits such as apples, oranges, and bananas. Fruits are good cleansers and aid in any unfinished digestion from the night before. The golden colors also include the golden and brown grains such as wheat, rice, corn, buckwheat, oats, and rye.

The yellow-gold color also includes most nuts and seeds such as sesame, sunflower, pumpkin, and almonds. Once nuts and seeds begin to germinate by soaking and sprouting, they become alkaline in their effect in the body and combine well with fruits. These soaked nuts and seeds in the morning are particularly good for people with blood sugar imbalances.

Midday

Yellow-golden, green, and blue foods are eaten for enhancing the third, fourth, and fifth chakras. The predominant color for the midday meal is green. This is the time for eating salads and other vegetable dishes – sprouts, avocados, lettuce, and dark greens. We could also eat fruit meals of green apples, watermelon, or fruits of other colors of the third through the fifth chakras. Although the main color focus is green, it does not mean that minor amounts of other color foods such as tomatoes cannot be included. Carrots, which are in the orange-gold spectrum, also fit in quite well.

Evening

Blue, indigo, purple, gold, and white foods enhance the fifth, sixth, and seventh chakras. Gold is included in the evening because purple and gold are complements, and the crown chakra is associated with golden, as well as purple, Light. The main evening meal's colors are purple, white, and gold. In the context of arising early to meditate, light dinners eaten before sunset are the most appropriate. Common purple foods in the vegetable kingdom include eggplant, purple cabbage, dulse, and beets. Rudolf Steiner said beets stimulate mind-brain function and act as excellent blood purifiers. We can also include some greens and sprouts. The golden foods include the golden grains such as wheat, rice, millet, and oats. Golden nuts and seeds such as sunflower, pumpkin, cashews, sesame, and almonds also fit in.

Extensive food lists for morning and midday colors have not been given because these colors are easy to find. It is also important not to be confined and make an obsessive religion out of it, so the lists have been minimized. The blue-indigo-purple spectrum does not so readily come to mind, so a list of some of the foods has been included.

Gold-White Foods

Grains: different wheat varieties, rye, oats, barley, corn, rice, sorghum, triticale, millet, and quinoa.

Fruits: dates, golden apples, apricots, golden grapefruit, golden pears, kumquat, loquat, oil palm, lady finger banana, breadfruit, cantaloupe, mango, papaya, and pineapple.

Nuts and seeds: sunflower, sesame, soy, wild hazelnuts, filberts, almonds, European walnuts, black walnuts, pistachio, brazil nut, Queensland nut, bambarra nut, and pumpkin seeds.

Legumes: lentils, cowpea, and chickpea.

Vegetables: gold pumpkin, cauliflower, jicama, white asparagus, white radish, and daikon radish, butternut squash.

Herbs: cinnamon, horseradish, caraway, coriander, dill, Spanish onion, yellow or white onions, chives, leeks, scallions, shallots, garlic, and ginger.

Purple Foods

Grains: purple corn and amaranth.

Fruits: bilberry-whortberry, blackthorn berry, black cherry, black figs, spartan apple, durondean pear, all varieties of purple prunes and plums, blackberry, dewberry, raisins, all varieties of purple grapes, mulberry, passionfruit, huckleberry, elderberry and cacao.

Legumes: Canadian wonder bean, black gram seeds, purple kidney bean, climbing purple padded kidney bean, vanilla bean, adulation bean, and purple beans ("green" beans which are purple in color).

Vegetables: eggplant, purple cabbage, beet, purple broccoli, kohlrabi, turnips, purple asparagus, dulse, nori, arame, hijiki, and many purple sea vegetables, sea kale, light purple bamboo shoots, artichoke petals, winter radish, purple potato, olives, water chestnut, Jerusalem artichoke, and purple sweet potatoes.

Herbs: mallow flowers, basil, heather, rosemary, sage, betony, thyme, wild passion flower, marjoram, black pepper, milkthistle flowers, and purple onion,

Blue Foods

Grains: blue corn.

Fruits: blue plum, blueberry, saskatoon berries, bilberry, and cabernet grape.

Herbs: chicory flowers, borage, hyssop, black thorn, brookline flowers, and pansy.

Phytonutrients and the Rainbow Diet		
Colors	Phytonutrients	Foods
Reds	resveratrol, ellagic acid, lycopene, quercetin	tomatoes, red bell peppers, pink grapefruit, cherries, raspberries, red grapes, strawberries, red apples, watermelon
Oranges	carotenoids	carrots, peppers, squash, yams, sweet potatoes, pumpkin, apricots, cantaloupe, mango, oranges
Yellows	flavonoids, limonene	citrus fruits, lemons, grapefruit, oranges, yellow peppers, peaches, nectarines, pears, pineapple
Greens	indole-3-carbinol, thiocyanates, zeaxanthins, sulforaphane, isothiocyanates, lutein	all greens, arugula, kale, lettuce, parsley, watercress, swiss chard, collard greens, mustard greens, beet greens, broccoli, cabbage, brussel sprouts, bok choy
Blues/Indigo	bilberry, anthocyanins	blueberries, saskatoons, grapes, plums, bilberries
Purples	lycopene, terpenes, anthocyanins	raspberries, grapes, strawberries, blackberries, plums, eggplant
Whites	allyl sulfides, quercetin, isothiocyanates	cauliflower, cabbage, radishes, chives, leeks, scallions, garlic, shallots, onions

Phytonutients

The phytonutrient foods all can be taken in a Rainbow spectrum. Included here is a chart to emphasize the Rainbow quality of the phytonutrients.

This is not an all-inclusive list, but certainly gives the imagination a beginning. It is important to note that some plants change color as they mature. Pineapple is an example; in its earlier stages, the VAS test is most active for the green vibration of the heart chakra. As it turns more golden, it tests more positively for the gold vibration of the crown chakra. The outer color at the time the plant is eaten is the main key to use. Some colors do not exactly match the primary color for a particular chakra, but are a combination of colors or fall mid-spectrum between two chakra colors. For example, sesame and sunflower seeds have the strongest VAS response between the second and third chakras and at the crown chakra. These findings indicate a gradual color spectrum transition between chakras. Using this VAS system, it might be possible to select nutrients based on the locations of the thirty-two vertebrae of the spine and their associated organs, glands, and chakras. Such a system, however, does not have the simple clarity that the Rainbow Diet offers.

The Rainbow Diet is a natural and simple approach to nutrition that focuses on a twenty-four-hour cycle. It is easy to eat low- and moderate-glycemic fruits and some soaked and ground seeds and nuts in the morning, a green salad at lunch, and a beet and dulse focused salad or soup for dinner. For people who eat only one or two meals per day, it would be good to create the rainbow cycle with the colors of snacks. With a one-meal-per-day cycle and no snacks to put the other colors into the diet, it is useful to trust your intuition of which of the chakra groups need the most balancing. On some days certain colors will appeal, and on others we may want nothing to do with the those colors.

For the two-meal-a-day person, the same idea holds. If not snacking to get the color spectrum in, then one can develop a cyclic spectrum over a two-day cycle. Eating foods by their colors is like eating a particular color from the sun. It brings us closer to the forces of Nature.

Summary, Chapter 26

1. Everything has a natural system of harmonics in relationship to the primordial vibration of the cosmic energy. This includes our foods.
2. All foods have a vibrational harmonic to the seven main chakras, and the glands, organs, and nerve centers associated with their color-related chakras.
3. Each food, according to its outer color, can be related to the specific color and energy of the same-color chakra.
4. Each food relates to a specific chakra in terms of energizing, healing, cleansing, building, and rebalancing the glands, organs, and nerve centers associated with that particular chakra.

5. The Rainbow Diet uses the full color spectrum of foods and phytonutrients for the full spectrum of the chakras throughout the spectrum of the day.
6. The Rainbow Diet is an organizing principle in helping us develop our own individualized diet for spiritual life. It can be usefully applied to any level of intake of fruits, vegetables, nuts, seeds, grains, and dairy products.

Chapter 27

Low-Glycemic Eating

The author's extensive research over some thirty-five years has confirmed that a low-glycemic diet is one of the key components for good health, optimal gene expression, a healthy living colloid field, stable blood-sugar levels, and a quiet mind. These all support spiritual awakening. The prime purpose of the low-glycemic diet is to prevent the "self-composting button" from being pushed. As briefly discussed in Chapter 6, on the subtle organizing energy fields, negative environmental stresses, acidity, and a high-glycemic diet create a morbid pleomorphic change from healthy cells and protids to viruses, bacteria, yeast, mold, and fungus, which give off microtoxins that begin to break down our living tissue. This self-composting process leads to chronic degenerative disease.

To identify a food as high- or low-glycemic is a statement about how fast that food raises the blood sugar. A low-glycemic food is one that slowly raises the blood sugar and has an overall minimal affect on the blood sugar levels. A high-glycemic food more rapidly converts to sugar and creates a significant elevation in the blood sugar. Typical high-glycemic foods include white bread, white potatoes, and white sugar. Examples of low-glycemic foods include most leafy green vegetables. The determination of the glycemic index of a food requires a sophisticated series of blood measurements of glucose over time after the particular food has been eaten. The average effect of a food on the test subjects is quantified, and the food is then rated on the glycemic index. The glycemic index indicates the glycemic effect of a food on most people.

There are many potential ill effects from a high-glycemic diet besides activating the "self-composting" process that leads to chronic degenerative disease. One of the most serious chronic diseases is diabetes, which has now reached epidemic proportions in all ages of our population. According to the Center for Disease Control and Prevention, there was a 33 percent jump in diabetes in the past decade. There are 17 million diabetes cases in the U.S. 5–10 percent of these are Type I.

Type I diabetes is usually characterized by an early age of onset that includes the destruction of the beta cells of the pancreas, which make insulin. This may have a genetic basis. Some theories suggest that it may be related to an allergy to dairy products that create anti-bodies to the beta cells. It may even be caused by aflatoxin, a mycotoxin given off by candida and other fungal infections. Perhaps there may be multiple causes. Type II diabetes is primarily caused by a chronic excess of white sugar intake. This excess both exhausts the insulin production of the system and also creates insulin resistance. Type II diabetes is relatively easily healed by Phase 1 of the Rainbow Green Live-Food Cuisine and some specific herbs. For Native Americans this healing process has also been supported by the use of indigenous high-insulin foods.

A leading cause of heart and kidney diseases, blindness, and limb amputations, diabetes is the sixth leading cause of death in the U.S., responsible for 210,000 deaths per year. An estimated 16 million people have pre-diabetes.

The following list shows the potential problems that can arise from a high-glycemic diet. The items marked with an asterisk (*) were compiled and listed by Nancy Appleton, Ph.D., author of *Lick the Sugar Habit*, and published in *Health Freedom News*, June 1994.

Hypoglycemia
*Asthma
Depletion and imbalancing of neurotransmitters
*Migraine headaches
Anxiety
*Atherosclerosis
Depression
*Gastric or duodenal ulcers
275 percent increase in PMS
*Periodontal disease
Increase in triglycerides
*Alcoholism
Syndrome X

*Interference with the absorption of protein
Obesity
*Acidic stomach
Diabetes
*Increased cholesterol
*Elevation of low-density lipoproteins (LDL, the "bad" cholesterol)
*Reduction of high-density lipoproteins (HDL, the "good" cholesterol)
Insulin resistance
*Arthritis
Hypertension
Increased inflammatory prostaglandins
*Cataracts
Candida and other fungal infections
*Lowered enzymes' ability to function
Loss of teeth calcium as a result of calcium being pulled from normal blood and bone by sugar combining with it
*Cancer of the breast, ovaries, intestines, prostate, and rectum
Increase in AGES, or glycosylated protein complexes, which accelerate aging
*Increased risk of Chrohn's disease and ulcerative colitis
Hyperactivity, anxiety, difficulty concentrating, and crankiness in children
*Elevated glucose and insulin responses in oral contraceptive users
*Malabsorption in those with functional bowel disease
*Skin aging, due to changes in the structure of collagen
Chromium deficiency
*Impaired structure of DNA
Decreased growth hormone secretion
*Eczema in children
Heart disease
*Increased free radicals in the bloodstream
Weakened immune system
*Emphysema
*Appendicitis
*Hemorrhoids
*Kidney damage
*Disorganizing of the minerals in the body
*Increased fasting levels of glucose and insulin
*Interference with absorption of calcium and magnesium

*Raised adrenaline levels in children
*Varicose veins
*Gallstones
*Tooth decay
*Multiple sclerosis
*Copper deficiency
*Weakened eyesight
*Osteoporosis
*Saliva acidity
*Drowsiness and decreased activity in children
*Changed structure of protein
*Food allergies

A low-glycemic diet helps to create a healthy biological terrain, preventing or reversing self-composting and candida. In the context of Spiritual Nutrition, it is important to give a brief overview of the relevance of the low-glycemic diet, which minimizes high-glycemic fruits, refined carbohydrates, and cooked starchy vegetables. Phase 1 of the Rainbow Green Live-Food Cuisine contains the highest amount of low-glycemic foods, and therefore accelerates the shutting off of the "self-composting button." It consists primarily of raw nuts, seeds, vegetables, oils, and algae. Because of the stresses in our modern environment and our poor nutritional choices in the past, Phase 1 is appropriate for most everyone for the first three months. Some people who are experiencing only mild self-composting can start with Phase 1.5, which includes a minimum of low-glycemic fruits, low-glycemic condiments, and fermented foods. Once the "self-composting button" has been shut off, one can move to Phase 2, which is a maintenance diet. It includes moderate-glycemic fruits, and raw high-glycemic vegetables. It is also important to note that low-glycemic foods tend to be higher in minerals. The table below delineates the foods appropriate for each phase of the Rainbow Green Live-Food Cuisine. In addition, in order to keep your biological terrain, SOEFs, and living colloid field in an optimum energetic state, there are many foods that should be avoided in general; those are listed in the last column of the table.

Rainbow Green Cuisine Food Chart				
Phase 1	Phase 1.5	Phase 2	Phase 2 Minimal Use	Foods to Avoid
Most vegetables (except those listed elsewhere) **All sea vegetables** **Non-sweet fruits** Tomatoes Avocados Cucumber Red bell pepper Lemons Limes **Fats and oils** Flax seed oil Hemp oil Olive oil Sesame oil Almond oil Sunflower oil Coconut oil (butter) Avocado Nuts and seeds Coconut meat/pulp **Super Foods** Klamath Lake algae Super green powders Blue manna Blue-green algae Spirulina **Sweetener** Stevia Yacon root syrup **Salt** Himalayan Celtic	**Vegetables** Carrots (raw, whole) Beets (raw, whole) Hard squash (raw) **Fruits** Grapefruit Raspberries Blueberries Strawberries Cherries Cranberries (fresh, unsweetened) Pomegranates Goji berries **Condiments and sweeteners** Low-glycemic Tree of Life mesquite meal Raw carob **Super Foods** Bee pollen (from New Zealand) **Grains** Quinoa Buckwheat Millet Amaranth Spelt **Fermented foods** Apple cider vinegar Miso Sauerkraut Probiotic drink	**Coconut water** (diluted with other ingredients) **Vegetables** Yams (raw) Sweet potatoes (raw) Pumpkin (raw) Parsnips (raw) Rutabaga (raw) **Fruits** Oranges Apples Pears Peaches Plums Blackberries **Juice** Grapefruit juice (diluted 50% with water) **Condiments and sweeteners** Raw cacao Dark agave nectar	**Cooked moderate-glycemic veggies** Yams (cooked) Sweet potatoes (cooked) Pumpkin (cooked) Parsnips (cooked) Beets (cooked) Rutabaga (cooked) Hard squash (cooked) Summer squash (cooked) **High-glycemic fruits** Apricots Figs Grapes Raisins Melons Mangos Bananas Papaya Pineapple Kiwi Sapote Cherimoya Rambutian Durian Dates **Dried fruits** **Fresh, raw, fruit juices** (diluted 50%) Carrot juice (diluted 50%) Orange juice (diluted 50%) **Seed cheese** **Cooked, organic, whole foods** **Sweeteners** Light agave nectar	**All processed foods** **All animal products** Flesh Dairy Eggs Honey All grains (except those listed) Corn White potatoes Sugar Alcohol Coffee Caffeine Tobacco Heated oil (except coconut oil) Soy sauce nama shoyu braggs Yeast Brewer's yeast Nutritional yeast Mushrooms Peanuts Cashews Cottonseed Bottled juices

Here are some "magic" phase notes that are helpful tips for remembering what to and what not to eat on each phase of Rainbow Green Live-Food Cuisine:

- Phase 1 = Simple – no grains, nothing sweet or fermented
- Phase 1.5 = Includes fermented foods, grain, and low-sweet fruits
- Phase 2 = Higher-glycemic fruits, veggies, and coconut water
- Phase 1 = Okay to eat a small amount of Phase 1.5 fruits or veggies in a large salad
- Phase 1.5 = Okay to eat a small amount of Phase 2 fruits or veggies in a large salad
- Phase 2 = MINIMAL USE of high-glycemic fruit, dried fruits, fruit juice, and carrot juice

Hypoglycemia

Hypoglycemia is an imbalance in the endocrine system that results in significant fluctuations in the blood sugar. According to Paavo Airola, a drop in the blood sugar of twenty points in thirty minutes can be considered hypoglycemia.[1] The rate of the fall of blood sugar is more important than the actual blood sugar level. Stable blood sugar is important for the normal functioning of the brain and nervous system. Hypoglycemia, is considered by many to be epidemic in the U.S.[2] It has been the author's observation in treating many meditators that when their hypoglycemia is cured, their ability to meditate and the steadiness of their meditation improves. This alone makes hypoglycemia an important condition of which to be aware (see Chapter 16 for more information).

Hypoglycemia is usually caused by a disharmony of the endocrine system, especially the adrenals, pancreas, liver, and thyroid. The result of hypoglycemia is an imbalance in the blood sugar with significant drops in the blood sugar in its function as the main fuel for the brain and the rest of the central nervous system. Fluctuations in blood sugar levels disrupt mental function. When the blood sugar drops suddenly, or is too low or irregular, it disorganizes brain function, causing impaired meditation, mood, and spiritual life in general. Hypoglycemia can manifest in a variety of symptoms such as chronic fatigue, exhaustion, weakness, depression, headaches, unexplained mood changes, anxiety attacks, concentration difficulties, transitory mental confusion, and even allergies. Candida, which is stimulated by a high-glycemic diet, also has many of these mental symptoms. A problem surrounding hypoglycemia is that only part of the medical establishment acknowledges that it exists. It was originally described in 1924 by Seale Harris, M.D., for which he was given a gold medal award by the AMA in 1949. Then the AMA officially decided in 1973 that hypoglycemia was a non-disease. An interesting story illustrating this confusion is that of Steven Gyland, M.D. He developed the symptoms of hypoglycemia to such an extent that he had to stop his medical practice. In an effort to diagnose the problem, he was examined by fourteen specialists and three major medical clinics, including the Mayo Clinic. No one diagnosed hypoglycemia. After three years of suffering, inability to work, and seeing a psychiatrist, he discovered the original hypoglycemia paper of Seale Harris. He went on a hypoglycemia diet, and his symptoms disappeared. Interestingly, the medical expert who examined him at the Mayo Clinic publicly claimed not to have seen a case of hypoglycemia in twenty-five years. This claim was made a few years after he had attempted to diagnose Dr. Gyland's problem. If someone does not acknowledge the existence of hypoglycemia, how can he or she diagnose it? Like Dr. Gyland, many clients come to the author, complaining, "I've been to several physicians. All my lab tests are normal. They say I am fine, but I feel miserable." It is difficult to be interested in spiritual life when one is feeling miserable. Often these people have some form of hypoglycemia as part of their imbalance.

Classically, the five-hour glucose tolerance test is considered the procedure for diagnosing hypoglycemia, but some orthomolecular physicians have found that it may give some false normal results. Some people may develop hypoglycemia symptoms during the test but have a normal glucose tolerance curve. It seems that some people are very sensitive to changes in blood sugar, while others may have dramatic shifts in blood sugar and experience no symptoms. The clue to this may be found in Dr. Roger Williams's book *Biochemical Individuality,* which stresses that we have different biological sensitivities.[3] The diagnosis of hypoglycemia requires clinical judgment. In the author's work, a five-hour glucose tolerance test, along with more subtle testing systems such as acupuncture pulse diagnosis, electrodiagnostic testing, and various forms of muscle testing to help confirm the diagnosis, are shown to give reliable results.

Causes of Reactive Hypoglycemia

To understand hypoglycemia, it helps to understand that it is not a disease. It is a symptom of a physiological imbalance in the system which manifests as low or erratic blood sugar. It may be caused by an allergic reaction (to any substance, most often to white sugar), some form of endocrine gland disorder, or even some nutritional deficiency of chromium, zinc, pantothenic acid, magnesium, potassium, or vitamin B_6. Some severe conditions, such as pancreatic tumors, Addison's disease, and pituitary or other brain tumors, are causes, but these are not causes of *reactive* hypoglycemia, which is our focus.

The most frequent form of reactive hypoglycemia the author sees is a subtle or gross endocrine imbalance. It is an imbalance of the glucose metabolism as regulated by the pituitary, thyroid, pancreas, adrenal, liver, and other endocrine glands. A simplified version of the dynamics of the endocrine balance and hypoglycemia will give a feeling for the meaning of hypoglycemia. When we eat white sugar or other sweets, the blood sugar rapidly rises. If the endocrine system is toned, it can compensate for this by smoothly lowering the blood sugar with the carefully timed secretion of insulin to modulate the glucose level. If it secretes too much insulin, our healthy adrenals and liver release more glucose to compensate for the excessive drop in glucose. If the endocrine system is not in balance, it is unable to compensate for the excess stress the sugar has created, and our blood sugar drops too low and we see symptoms. This does not just mean a pancreas disorder of excess insulin secretion. Hypoglycemia is not simply the opposite of diabetes. Quite often, the pancreas is normal, and some other part of the endocrine system is out of balance. It is important to understand that, like our chakras, our glands function as a total system. It may be the adrenals, thyroid, pituitary, ovary, liver, pancreas, or a combination. This is important because the endocrine glands are reflective of the chakra system balance. In some cases of hypoglycemia, the subtle bodies are disordered in a way that the person is suffering from unusual, often frightening, psychic phenomena. Upon treatment of the hypoglycemia, the chakras rebalance and psychic vulnerability and discomfort go away.

In a study by the author on 100 people in 1975–76, reported in *Hypoglycemia: A Better Approach* by Dr. Paavo Airola, only 20 percent had exclusively a pancreas imbalance. An additional 36 percent of those with hypoglycemic symptoms had pancreas imbalances associated with other endocrine imbalances. Exclusive adrenal imbalances caused 25 percent of the hypoglycemia, and an additional 36 percent had adrenal imbalances associated with other endocrine imbalances. In 6 percent, the thyroid alone was out of balance, and 21 percent of the time this occurred in combination with other organs. The pituitary, ovary, and liver were only out of order in combination with other endocrine organs. A liver dysfunction is often the main cause of hypoglycemia in alcoholics or people with hepatitis, but there were no alcoholics in this study.

A useful way to understand the epidemic level of hypoglycemia in the U.S. is to think of it as the endocrine system and the chakra system being out of tune. The high incidence of hypoglycemia is another indication of how important it is for the total chakra system to be energetically balanced. Chronic life stress, which tends to imbalance the chakra system and limit the amount of cosmic energy recharging the chakras, can bring about hypoglycemia. The author has seen fifteen to twenty cases of sudden stress, such as a car accident or even childbirth, precipitate hypoglycemia in people who were already on the edge of chakra and endocrine imbalance. In people who are leading harmonious, sattvic lives and eating a healthy, sattvic diet, there is more resiliency to sudden stresses or even some prolonged stresses, but people living on the edge of their resources are more vulnerable to having their chakras and endocrine system become imbalanced by sudden stress.

Another piece to the hypoglycemia puzzle is the concept of variable sensitivity to the changes in blood sugar. Dr. Buckley, a psychiatrist and clinical researcher, has found that there are glucose-sensitive receptors in the hypothalamic brain center; these act as a feedback system for a specific anxiety center in the brain called the locus coeruleus.[4] When blood sugar drops below a certain point, the glucose receptor center cannot properly control the anxiety center in the locus coeruleus. This results in anxiety symptoms typified by mental and physical agitation, fear, increased heart rate, and irritability. The degree of biological sensitivity of this glucose receptor is a key to how sensitive each individual may be to drops in blood glucose. The determining factor of this individualized sensitivity seems to be a genetic predisposition. Hypersensitivity to alterations in blood glucose, with associated erratic behavior, may be linked with the increasing number of people suffering from unexplained anxiety and panic attacks.

Cause of Epidemic Hypoglycemia

The remaining question is, what causes hypoglycemia, which various reports estimate to be an epidemic of at least 10 percent of the people in the United States?[5] And the evidence for the epidemic of hypoglycemia is mounting. For example, Michael Lesser, M.D., reported that 67 percent of his psychiatric patients suffer from hypoglycemia.[6] In a study of a different population, 25 percent of 5,000 so-called healthy military inductees were found to have blood sugars consistent with the diagnosis of hypoglycemia.[7] The cause for a phenomenon with the magnitude of 24 million people is not likely to be simply vitamin deficiencies or food allergies; it is most likely a stressful, overextended lifestyle and a tamasic diet high in white sugar and other imbalancing stimulants.

Hypoglycemia is the result of living the all-American dream of moving faster, of wanting bigger and better things, and of a highly competitive and aggressive lifestyle that is out of harmony with our Inner Self and Mother Nature. To fuel this lifestyle, we eat processed foods and plenty of instant-energy white-sugar foods. To both relieve the pain of this lifestyle and temporarily energize, we use alcohol, coffee, cigarettes, sweets, and stimulant drugs. Americans consume 125 pounds of white sugar per year per person; this sugar is either hidden in foods or eaten directly, as in our coffee.[8] Paavo Airola once described this as "completely incredible nutritional folly; nothing less than an act of unintentional national suicide."[9] Our bodies were not designed to continually metabolize this high input of refined sugars. The strain of this repeated high sugar intake, like the "normality" of banging our heads against the wall, eventually leads to the headache of a metabolic disorder we know as hypoglycemia. Other major dietary substances that have been linked to creating hypoglycemic imbalances are coffee, alcohol, and cigarettes. Coffee and other caffeine-containing substances like black tea, cola drinks, aspirin compounds, and caffeine-like compounds in chocolate cause an overstimulation of the adrenal glands, which then release adrenaline substances that stimulate the liver to release excess glucose into the blood. This creates a rapid rise in blood sugar in a pattern similar to when white sugar is eaten. Alcohol, particularly in sweet liqueurs and wine, contributes to hypoglycemia. An estimated 70 percent of alcoholics are hypoglycemic. Most do not realize it, but studies have found that blood glucose also increases after smoking a cigarette. All of these toxins act directly to unbalance the endocrine system.

Although hypoglycemia results from multiple causes, the primary epidemic cause is a disharmonious, stressful lifestyle and a tamasic diet high in refined carbohydrates, sugar, coffee, alcohol, and cigarettes. This is why researchers have found that so many juvenile offenders improve their behavior when put on a corrective diet for hypoglycemia. For example, one study found that 82 percent of 106 juveniles on probation had hypoglycemia. On a corrective diet, almost all of them significantly improved in their social function.[10] Numerous studies show that hypoglycemia alters our mental and social behavior toward the tamasic, emotional, mental, and moral tendencies of erratic, violent, and antisocial behavior.[11,12] The lifestyle and diet that create hypoglycemia are some of the first things people who are interested in Spiritual Nutrition would do well to consider changing.

The Treatment of Hypoglycemia

With the appropriate homeopathic and dietary treatment of approximately six small meals per day of a low-protein or high-protein diet (depending on one's constitution) with no sweets or sweet fruit, people heal very quickly. People who are fast oxidizers or parasympathetic (see *Conscious Eating*) need a higher percentage of protein. The optimal diet for hypoglycemia is the Phase 1 Rainbow Green Live-Food Cuisine for three to six months; it is designed to support one's individual constitution. For people who have trouble with a high natural carbohydrate diet, the author recommends that they increase germinated nuts and seeds, which act as pre-digested proteins and help balance the blood sugar. This can be in the form of seed sauces or simply soaked nuts or seeds. The more live foods the diet contains, the quicker the healing. In the author's 1975–76 study of 100 cases, 53 percent of the people had complete symptom relief in three weeks, and 74 percent had absence of all symptoms after one month with the use of herbs, homeopathics, and supplements. The other 26 percent took one to four months to achieve complete healing. All of these cases remained symptom-free on a regular, but healthy, diet at the two- and four-month follow-up. On the diet alone, the healing took an average of six months to a year.

Healing hypoglycemia means not only to have a complete absence of symptoms, but the ability to resume eating only two to three times per day and have sweet fruits, dried fruits, and even some honey in the diet on occasion without having any return of hypoglycemic symptoms. For healing to be sustained, some basic shift in lifestyle toward more harmony with ourselves and Nature is necessary. We need to shift toward a more sattvic diet and lifestyle to sustain real healing and increase our spiritual development.

Hypoglycemia, Meditation, and Kundalini

The author has observed that meditation requires extra blood glucose fuel. Many people seem to increase their desire for sweets after beginning to meditate. Glucose is one of the more efficient nutrients for carrying and transferring prana in the system. The mistake meditators often make is to seek more glucose for the system by eating refined, processed foods laden with white sugar, which is a tamasic food that unbalances the body toward hypoglycemia and a wide variety of other diseases. The Phase 1, 1.5, or 2 of the Rainbow Green Live-Food Cuisine, as previously described, with soaked nuts and seeds, vegetables, and low- to medium-glycemic fruits, will supply a gradual release of glucose into the bloodstream without the ups and downs caused by white sugar. These phases of diet preserve our health much better than eating white sugar. The author has had the opportunity to treat a number of monks and other spiritual aspirants involved in intense spiritual practices who developed hypoglycemia because they did not understand this simple point. In almost all of those who followed the treatment program for hypoglycemia, there was an increase in the ability to concentrate and an improved steadiness of the meditation experience was reported. A steadier emotional, awake, and aware state was also experienced. Once healed, these people were able to stop snacking between meals and return to a normal but more sattvic diet. They were able to incorporate an occasional use of sweet fruits in their diet with no return of hypoglycemia.

When the Kundalini is awakened, there is occasionally a little more pranic energy released than might feel comfortable for a person. One of the main immediate treatments to calm the Kundalini energy is to eat some honey. The author's theory for this is that the ability of the glucose to absorb and transmit prana enables glucose to act as a "pranic energy shock absorber" throughout the system. The Kundalini, when initially awakened, seems to require much from the glucose reserve as it activates and spiritually energizes a person. If an individual does not have enough reserve complex carbohydrate, honey provides extra glucose to keep the nervous system in balance on a temporary basis.

Diabetes and Gene Expression

Because of our horrendous diet of excessive sugar and refined carbohydrates, we are experiencing an epidemic of diabetes in the United States. Research has shown that whenever white sugar has been introduced into a culture, within twenty years there is an outbreak of diabetes. In the United States, this diet is amplified to a major extent. The key to understanding this process is the hormone influence of insulin, which has a tremendous effect on gene expression. It doesn't just control the amount of blood sugar that goes into the muscles; it is also a very loud communicator to the genes. It affects a wide variety of hormones in metabolic functions, including even estrogen in women, the way the body uses calories, and the way the body deposits glucose in the system in fat production.[13] Clearly it's been accepted that poor insulin control influences the gene expression in a way that turns the metabolism into fat storage for calories rather than effective utilization to store energy. This manifests most clearly in what the author considers a classical manifestation of how to eat in a way to give you the lowest phenotypic expression of your genes, which is Syndrome X. Many doctors have thought that the way to deal with diabetes is just to give insulin, but now we have begun to understand that Type II diabetes doesn't have as much to do with insulin as with insulin insensitivity. This is known as insulin resistance.

Syndrome X was first identified by Dr. George Reaven, Professor Emeritus at the Department of Medicine at Stanford University. One of its prime symptoms is insulin resistance. Characteristics of Syndrome X include insulin resistance, elevated insulin levels in the blood, and a switching of metabolism toward fat storage, which results in weight gain and increase of body fat, no matter what the person eats. As body fat increases, paradoxically, insulin resistance also increases. What affects insulin are many other hormones that are at play at the gene level; these include insulin growth factor (IGF-1), human growth hormone, cortisol, somatostatin, serotonin, noradrenalin, and leptin.

What are the keys that regulate these hormones? Minimal stress, excellent diet, exercise, low sugar, and a healthy environment.[14] At the Tree of Life, we have already had several cases of Syndrome X be cured through fasting. A low-glycemic diet with exercise is probably the most important approach to resetting and activating a proper insulin sensitivity at the gene level. This is the Phase 1 diet outlined in *Rainbow Green Live-Food Cuisine*. The research shows that full, unrefined, carbohydrate-rich foods that are very low in sugar, meaning they have a low-glycemic index, seem to be the best for restoring blood sugar and insulin, versus those that are high in sugar and fat.[15] Vegetables that have what is called resistant starch seem to have even a better effect in the control of diabetes and insulin resistance. Interestingly enough, the carbohydrates that we do eat – if they are low-glycemic (mainly vegetables) – seem to have the most positive expression, energy, and function. These low-glycemic carbohydrates influence the regulation of gene expression because they affect the secretion of insulin, glucagon, and other cell-signaling hormones.[16] Another aspect of the diet that seems to be important in improving insulin sensitivity is that it is high-fiber. Again, this high-fiber diet is high in vegetables with a certain amount of fruit; it includes the cruciferous vegetables, carrots, apples, almonds, and foods that are high in dietary fiber. Green juice fasts are excellent for reversing Syndrome X, but not fruit juice fasts. The downside of juicing fruits is that you lose the fiber and concentrate the fruit sugar, which results in an increased level of blood sugar.

Contrary to popular literature, recent research suggests that it isn't simply an excess of carbohydrates that can increase insulin. A high protein intake may also increase insulin resistance. Research by Gene Stiller, Ph.D., found that a protein-enhanced diet may actually increase insulin resistance rather than decrease it.[17] Stiller's research team found that when people consumed a protein-rich diet, their insulin output actually was greater than when they consumed an equal amount of carbohydrate-rich foods. Interesting, of course, is the point that has been made in *Conscious Eating* and *Rainbow Green Live-Food Cuisine* that everyone has to have an individualized diet that will be optimal for them. As pointed out earlier, vegetable proteins and unrefined carbohydrate-rich foods that are low-glycemic seem to be more effective than a diet that is refined, high-glycemic, and high in fat. The unrefined vegetables and grains have a certain amount of soluble and insoluble fiber, which also reduces insulin response. Foods that are high in chromium, vanadium, and magnesium, such as the root vegetables and whole grains, decrease insulin sensitivity.

Another aspect of insulin and blood sugar control is the issue of oxidative stress. The combination of high blood sugar and imbalanced insulin results in the formation of a glucose-protein combination called glycosylated proteins. These proteins create a cross linkage and damage in the tissues that degrades many tissue functions. They have been called advanced glycosylation end products (AGEs). The research shows that the more AGEs that accumulate in our body, the more we are at risk for increased rate of aging.[18] These AGEs also poison the mitochondrial function and cause oxidative stress.[19]

There is a variation of how well we respond to insulin and blood sugar and how we can mediate it. The best defense, of course, is to modify and protect ourselves by eating a low-glycemic diet, getting plenty of exercise, and minimizing the amount of stress and toxins we take into our system, including alcohol and other psychoactive drugs. There is definitely an increase of insulin resistance related to increased genetic susceptibility, poor diet, excess stress, lack of exercise, and exposure to a variety of toxins and drugs of all sorts. The more oxidative stress we create in the mitochondria, the more we damage our organs and the less we are able to handle the organ stress, particularly in the kidneys, heart, brain, eyes, and joints. It's worthwhile to check for insulin resistance. It is inductibly diagnosed at the Tree of Life Health Practice through a five-hour glucose tolerance test which shows the insulin response.

The key point again is that a low-glycemic diet is the most important prevention and treatment for hypoglycemia and diabetes. Other important preventive and healing factors include a moderate fat intake and moderate exercise. Minerals and vitamins that are particularly important for healing insulin resistance include selenium, copper, zinc, chromium, magnesium, and vanadium. Proper amounts of B_{12} are also important for protecting the nervous system against symptoms that occur with insulin resistance. L-arginine (an amino acid) seems to be important for people who have AGEs and free radical aging in general. One research study, at the University of Vienna Department of Medicine, shows that one gram of L-arginine given twice a day to people with oxidative stress as a result of poor blood sugar control produced a significant reduction in oxidative stress. The L-arginine seemed to reduce the amount of damage to the DNA. If someone tends to have obesity, allergies, arthritic troubles, degenerative eyesight, deteriorating mental function, and an increased rate of heart and kidney disease, one needs to pay attention. We need to communicate positively to our genes by controlling blood sugar and insulin through a low-glycemic diet, exercise, and supportive lifestyle and environment.

Summary, Chapter 27

1. The cause for epidemic hypoglycemia is our cultural living of a disharmonious, stressful lifestyle, and eating a tamasic diet excessively filled with white sugar.
2. A low-glycemic diet is the key to prevention and treatment of diabetes, hypoglycemia, the "self-composting" process, and a variety of chronic diseases.
3. Hypoglycemia can adversely affect the flow of Kundalini and the maintenance of a steady meditation state.
4. The Rainbow Green Live-Food Cuisine Phase 1 is the best for treatment, and Phases 1.5 and 2 are the best for maintenance.

Chapter 28

Minerals – Frequencies of Light

Minerals are one of the deep secrets of Spiritual Nutrition. Minerals are frequencies of Light, frequencies of information, and frequencies of creation for the material world in the universe in which we live. The Earth is made of minerals. Our body is made of minerals. Minerals activate all the catalysts for enzymatic reactions in the body. They activate the vitamins. They activate all the organ structures, and in fact, are the basis of all the organ and cellular structures of the body. Minerals are the builders of the system. They are the frequency rates in the system. They are not necessarily the energy makers, however. The human body is composed entirely of minerals and water. The water molecule is the one that acts as a powerful solvent within the human system, bringing in nutrients and washing out waste particles. Without the essential minerals and trace minerals, we could not survive.

Of a total of 90 minerals, there are approximately 23 key minerals, including 16 major minerals and 7 minor trace minerals. These are needed for the body to function at the highest level. The essential trace minerals, as well as major minerals, need to be replaced in the system through water-soluble ionic forms. As early as 1936, the U.S. Senate declared, "99 percent of the American people are deficient in minerals, and a marked deficiency in any one of the more important minerals actually results in disease."[1] This is one of the most intelligent things that has ever come out of the U.S. Senate, and something that was beyond even the scope of medical school. Now, many years later, we are subjected to junk foods, foods that have been pesticided and herbicided, microwaved foods, and increasingly mineral-deficient soils. The situation has only gotten worse. This is why most everyone needs mineral supplementation, whether they are vegan or meat eater. Dr. Linus Pauling, winner of two Nobel prizes, said, "You can trace every sickness, every disease, and every ailment, ultimately, to a mineral deficiency."[2]

For a mineral to be utilized at the intracellular level, it must be in an angstrom-size (that is, so infinitesimal it is measured in units of angstroms), and these particles must be completely water-soluble. It is only the ionic form, or angstrom-size level, of minerals that can enter the cells and activate the proper DNA structures to actuate the guiding frequencies for the function of the body. An angstrom (named after Johan Angstrom) is one-thousandth of a micron, and one-millionth of a meter. The significance of this information is that almost all the mineral supplements on the market are larger than micron sizes. Now, it can get a little confusing, but think about it this way: Particles that are micron in size and larger will be absorbed by the blood, but they are too large to be absorbed intracellularly and inside the nucleus. These larger forms stay in the bloodstream, and eventually become deposited in various tissue locations. Angstrom-size particles travel through the cells, and if the body doesn't need them, it will simply discharge them with no build-up of the minerals to create potential toxicity in the tissues.

We observe that the roots of the plants are designed to break down the soil and utilize and absorb mineral particles, at angstrom-size – that's what they do. With the help of fulvic acid in the humus material, plants are able to take these minerals in, and break them down into angstrom-size, which they use. Once we understand that, we understand that the vegetables we eat transfer angstrom-size minerals from the soil to us via the plants. They do not absorb larger-size particles, because they cannot assimilate them. Angstrom-size minerals are key to optimal mineral absorption. It takes about twelve years for farmland to become deficient of angstrom-size trace minerals. For this reason, farmers would often move every twelve years. These excess minerals of micron-size or larger can cause a variety of problems. The paradox, which is hard to understand, is that while the tissues are full of minerals in a sense, the cell is lacking in the angstrom-size minerals. This is one reason why we can use salt (Himalayan or Celtic sea salt) products for our bodies with amazing results, because they are in ionic angstrom-sizes. If salt isn't in the ionic form, we simply aren't able to absorb minerals into our bodies. Table salt (straight sodium chloride) as well as any heated salt is covalently bonded. It is not available for use in the body and can cause a toxic build-up. This may also potentially apply to salts that are sun dried. The process of sun drying, like many other forms of heating, causes electrons not to be available and the ions to form more tight bonds that make them inaccessible for assimilation. If salt creates a savory and watery feeling in the mouth, then it is still ionic. If it dries the mouth, this suggests that it has converted to the less assimilable covalent form. Although larger mineral forms or covalently bonded salt may help us initially on one level, eventually they have the potential of building up to toxic overload. Paradoxically, one of the most effective ways to pull out these accumulated minerals is to provide the same mineral in an angstrom-size. Angstrom-size minerals act as building blocks for the more than six thousand different enzymes needed for optimal function in our bodies. If we don't have the proper minerals for those enzymes to work in the particular organs that are needed, we do not, in a sense, have the cellular building materials for repair and regeneration of our tissues. For example, in diabetes, because of all the refined foods that are eaten, we have created a deficiency of chromium because chromium seems to be lost from eating refined foods. When we are taking in lots of carbohydrates and need chromium to help metabolize the sugar and to make the insulin work correctly, we are forced to use up our chromium stores and consequently become chromium deficient. When we eat junk foods, or food that is from depleted soils and synthetic fertilizers, we really aren't able to metabolize the sugars and carbohydrates properly. This adds to a diabetic condition. It is no accident that there has been a 33 percent increase in diabetes in the last ten years and a prediction of 29 million to have it by the year 2050. An estimated 16 million people now have pre-diabetes.[3]

In essence, minerals take us to the very formation of life. All qualities of positive or negative health can be traced back to a lack of minerals. In order for us to get adequate mineralization, the minerals need to be in angstrom-size form, which is 0.001 micron. They need to be attached to covalent hydrogen in the water, which will pull them inside the cell. It is at the intracellular level where the action happens. When the minerals reach the nucleus and mitochondria of the cell, there's a transmutation on the cellular level that activates the DNA. The nucleus and the mitochondria are both the energy centers and the creative centers of the cell. Mitochondria also have a particular form of DNA, which is different than nuclear DNA. The minerals activate the primordial DNA. These minerals activate electromagnetic communications both intracellularly and extracellularly that organize the system and communicate about what activities must be done. Some of the DNA frequencies are received in the cell wall. The minerals, and in particular a mineral complex developed by Dr. Tru Ott called Ultimatium™, which is a combination of the platinum group metals, activate small strands of DNA attached to the larger chromosome complexes. These small strands of DNA are like antennae of the DNA. These also need the iridium molecule, which is the key element in Ultimatium™, to send out the proper electromagnetic communication, and to reorganize and heal the DNA structures and the frequencies. Minerals are therefore needed for all levels of intra- and extracellular communication that emanates from the DNA and for the repair of the DNA.

Mineral Depletion in Plant Food

There are specific mineral requirements for cell nutrition. The number one mineral is oxygen. It is the connection of the symbiosis between the plant and animal worlds. It is obvious that calcium is needed for bone production and function of the parathyroid glands. Iodine is needed for the thyroid to function. Iron is needed for hemoglobin production. And so on. The overall generalization is that all disease stems from the weakening of the organism and subsequent parasitic (virus, bacteria, fungus, bowel parasites) infections. Adequate mineralization protects us against this disease process by strengthening the biological terrain. One of the problems we began to face early in the 1920s is plant disease arising from soil depletion. For example, a gray speck on oats indicating deficient manganese, or rosette disease in fruit trees due to zinc deficiency. The point is that plants need proper nutrition, and when they don't get it, they are prone to disease – just like humans. For healthy plant life, corn requires about forty-eight minerals, and wheat and oats utilize about thirty-six minerals. Soybeans, apples, pears, and peaches take more than thirty elements from the soil. Most vegetables, including peas, potatoes, tomatoes, carrots, and lettuce, require more than twenty-five elements from the soil. Repeatedly used ground that is not regenerated gets depleted. The foods that grow in it get depleted as a result, and therefore the humans and animals that are eating those foods also get depleted.

In essence, we can say that the soil in the United States, and in probably most of the world, is overworked and underfed. The result is diseased plants and sick animals. This is the result of the failure to replace the elements taken out during the growing cycles. This can be called the law of soil exhaustion. This imbalance is amplified by creating a glut of food with our high technology, pulling more energy and minerals from the soil than it can offer. The cycle gets worse with the soil becoming further depleted of trace elements and the animals lacking vital essentials for their health. Rain, which was once our friend, and in many ways still is, becomes a problem because the rain further carries the elements from the soil to the sea. The increased soil exhaustion creates exhausted and diseased plants, exhausted and diseased animals, and exhausted and diseased human beings. Roughly it's been estimated, according to *Sea Energy Agriculture,* that Australia loses about six tons of topsoil per square mile, Europe loses 120 tons per square mile, and on a worldwide basis, we lose 4 billion tons of dissolved material that is carried off to the sea from the rivers each year. The soluble elements are washed off first by the rainwater. This is why sodium chloride is so scarce on the land and abundant in the sea.

The Seawater Solution

What is the solution for growing healthy plants again, and therefore well-nourished human beings? Seawater is the most ancient water solution on Earth, and perhaps the most ideal physiologically to remineralize the soils.

One of the most exciting research studies that has been done on minerals was done by Dr. Maynard Murray and described in his book *Sea Energy Agriculture.* Dr. Murray was a medical doctor who truly wanted to get to the essence of what health was about. Murray's thesis, which he stated in 1976 was, "Life is electrical.... There can be no life without a transfer of electrical energy." According to Dr. Murray, the center of life's gravity is the oceans, a repository of minerals from the land, dissolved and carried to Nature's settling basin via streams, both above and below ground. His research showed that we need the right key to unlock the nutrient-rich accumulations of trace minerals. Each cell is a little battery that puts out a current. Without this electrical current, the cells cannot really work and eventually will die. Murray pointed out that life started in the sea. Human blood is about 25 percent seawater, and practically 85 percent of the life on Earth comes from and lives in the sea. Murray's work was to use the minerals in the sea, which added up to ninety trace elements. He used a diluted saltwater mixture in orchards, pastures, and gardens. In his book, he pointed out, "It is possible to build up the immunity to staph, viral, and fungal infections in plants. When we grow corn, wheat, oats, etc. with the sea solids, and feed them to animals, we see changes." Using animal research with species bred to get cancer, and fed food grown with sea solids, he reported that the first generation cut debilitation from 97 percent to 55 percent, a significant drop. "Through each generation sea solids food instill resistance to cancer." Murray's sea solid plants significantly decreased one kind of cancer in mice. Sea solid plants fed to chickens genetically programmed to get leucosis and rats bred to get arthritis manifested significantly fewer of these problems when the foods they ate were produced with sea solids. This foreshadowed the principle of communicating with one's genes, discussed in Chapter 21. Dr. Murray made the startling conclusion that farming has to be the beginning of preventive medicine. We use this saltwater agriculture at the Tree of Life to grow our own "authentic food." We have included the refined procedures of Dr. Murray through the help of his successor Don Jansen.

Dr. Murray began his research in 1936 when he attempted to determine which elements in the sea were the secret to helping plant life. He started with hydroponics. He covered all the plants in a liquid solution, which gave him the opportunity to control which elements would be present in the nutrient development of plants in his experiments. His experiments produced very exciting results. It has now been conclusively proven, on the basis of his work, that the proportion of trace minerals and elements present in seawater was optimal for the health and growth of both land and sea plants. In 1954 he did a controlled crop experiment with corn, oats, and soybeans, growing ten acres each of sea-solid grown and controlled food crop. The food grown with high-sea-solid solutions was also fed to animals in four parts corn, two parts oats, and one part soybeans. Some interesting observations were made. Not only were the sea-solid crops healthier than the control crops, but the effects on the physiology and pathology of the animals fed on the sea-solid foods were amazing. Chickens, pigs, and cattle fed the sea-salt grains matured sooner than control animals, and all resisted diseases better than the controlled. All these animals were able to resist the disease common to their species, much better than the control animals. The experiment showed that pigs fed sea-solid foods carried the health benefits into the second generation.

Experiments by Dr. Murray and based on his work show that once seawater is dried by evaporation, it leaves sea solids that can be brought in as fertilizer to the land. He used 500 to 3,000 pounds per acre. Dr. Murray found that unless a serious rain runoff occurred, a single application of that much would last four or five years, and the plants grew very well. Other research shows that one can dilute the sea solids in freshwater to create dilute solutions containing 1,000–8,000 parts per million of sea solids, for successful results. We know that sodium chloride in straight concentrate seawater will indeed kill plant life on land; however, this does not happen with dilution.

One interesting experiment done in 1940 by Dr. Murray was with peach trees. Every other peach tree was designated for experimental tests, which used 600 cc of seawater per square foot, applied from the base of the trees out to the edge of the foliage to cover the main areas of nutrition. The second and fourth trees were designated the control group and received no application. All the trees were sprayed with curly leaf virus. The seawatered trees remained free of the virus and delivered normal fruit yields. The control trees not only contracted curly leaf virus, but the peach yield was sharply reduced from the norm. The observation period for the test lasted three years, although the spraying with the virus took place only in the first year. The control trees contracted curly leaf virus each year, and finally died, while the seawatered trees retained resistance throughout the three-year test period.

A similar experiment was done with turnips. Half were control, the other half nourished with seawater. The seawatered section of the plot was fertilized with 600 cc of seawater per square foot of the soil. Staphylococcus bacteria, associated with central rot in turnips, were mixed into the soil of the entire plot. After the turnips had sprouted and leaves appeared above the soil, the leaves of both the control and experimental groups were sprayed with the same bacteria. All seawatered turnips grew to normal, healthy turnips, without evidence of center rot. The control turnips contracted the staphylococcus-caused center rot, and died.

Dr. Murray conducted similar experiment with tomatoes, grown hydroponically. He used a sea salt bed where the experimental hydroponics bed received 112 pounds of sea salt to 5,000 gallons of water solution mixture, while the control bed used the traditional hydroponics solution. Both beds were flooded three times daily. Tobacco mosaic virus, lethal to tomato plants, was sprayed on all the plants. The experimental plants did not contract the disease, but all the control plants died of the tobacco mosaic virus.

Resistance to disease in sea-solid-fed plants is paralleled in animal studies. Animals fed sea-solid vegetables were far more resistant to disease. For example, in one experiment C3H mice, a strain of mice bred so that all females develop breast cancer and die from it, were used. The mice were two months of age when the experiment began. The life expectancy of this strain of females was nine months. Each group had 200 C3H mice. Those receiving control food lived a normal lifespan averaging eight months and seven days. The experimental mice, fed food grown on sea-solids-fertilized soil, lived until they were sacrificed at sixteen months. The sea-solid-vegetable-fed mice produced ten litters compared to the expected two or three litters for the control mice. None of the experimental group of C3H mice developed breast cancer. This is a pretty strong statement.

Another experiment was done with Spraque Dally rats. They were divided into twenty-five control and twenty-five experimental rats. The control rats were given normal food. The experimental rats received the sea-solid-fertilized food. They were both injected with cancer (Jensen Carcino-Sarcoma), which is known to be 100 percent lethal. All the rats on the control diet died within twenty-one days of cancer. None of the rats fed food grown on sea solids died of cancer within forty days. Sixteen lived five months until they were sacrificed and found to have no cancer. So this experiment showed resistance against cancer in a high percentage of sea-solid-fed rats.

In another experiment, Jensen Carcino-Sarcoma was injected into fifty-six control rats and fifty-six experimental rats. All fifty-six control rats were dead within twenty-three days; of the experimental rats, two had a cancer take, but it was absorbed and disappeared. Four of the fifty-six experimental rats died of cancer and the remaining fifty-two were sacrificed ninety days afterward, with no evidence of cancer tissue. This is highly significant. All these studies suggest that disease resistance increases when food that is grown in sea-solid-fertilized soil is consumed.

There was an experiment with twenty-four rabbits. Twelve were fed on food grown with sea solids. The remaining twelve acted as control and fed normal food; they were given a high-cholesterol diet for six months. The control group developed hardening of the arteries and all died within ten months. The experimental group did not develop hardening of the arteries.

Another experiment was done with a breed of rats that developed diseases of the eye. The ten eating sea-solid-grown food showed no deterioration of the eyes and bred five litters. Those in the control group all died of secondary eye disease. What we're seeing in these results is that animals grown on highly mineralized food basically took in the appropriate mineralization that created an optimal expression that protected them from disease.

Although this useful research was based on animal studies, the reporting of this research, which was done more than fifty years ago, does not mean the author supports the use of animal experimentation.

It is interesting to note that all land animals develop arteriosclerosis, yet sea animals have never been diagnosed as arteriosclerotic. Freshwater trout develop terminal cancer of the liver at the age of 5 years, yet cancer is never found in sea trout. It does appear that sea creatures have less disease. The whale may be the healthiest creature on the planet; it doesn't even seem to show affects of aging. It is interesting to note that some sea creatures never stop growing. There does not seem to be chronic disease among fish, or it is minimal, compared to what we see on land. The difference between sea and land life seems to be connected to the superior food chain in the sea and the degree of mineralization of the food chain in the sea. In summary, a key to health is proper mineralization on the intracellular level. Our present diets do not have enough nutrients in the proper form to create a complete intracellular mineralization. The result is that the life force of our cells becomes weakened. The cells then are subject to foreign invasion by bacteria, viruses, fungus, and other parasitic forces.

As with animals, so with plants. Field tests have been done in South Dakota, Wisconsin, Illinois, Ohio, Pennsylvania, Massachusetts, and Florida. All the field results were essentially the same. No matter what type of soil was used, production was the same or greater on the soil fertilized with seawater or complete sea solids. Animals fed on the sea-solid-fertilized food crops were consistently more disease resistant than the control group. The sea-solid-nourished garden fruits and vegetables were superior in taste. In general, the produce grown on sea solids seemed to be bigger and tastier than that grown on typical soil.

The message is clear: *A highly mineralized body is a more disease-resistant and anti-aging body.* Plants grown to maturity that do not have the proper minerals have a propensity to compensate. When we take in less than healthy plants, we do not get the proper nutrition. This takes us back to the concept of our inner biological terrain. A weakness of the biological terrain allows the parasitic life of viruses, bacteria, and fungus to take advantage and invade our system. What we are looking at today is that most crops require between thirty-five and forty elements. Fertilizers usually add no more than twelve minerals. In most commercial fertilizers, a maximum of six minerals is provided. Eating food from mineral-depleted soil weakens our terrain and therefore undermines our health.

At the Tree of Life our solution to optimal agriculture is our innovative vegan farming program, which now includes elements of Dr. Murray and Don Jansen's work of high soil mineralization. No animal products are used at any level of our agricultural methods. There has been enough interest in our approach that we now have both an apprenticeship and workshops in vegan farming.

High-Mineral Food Creates Healthy Humans

While sea solids work directly for the plants, they work for humans in a different way. For humans, the elements need to be linked with some kind of carbon in green plants and converted to angstrom-size minerals. As we look at how Nature works, we understand that the role of plants is to convert inorganic elements to organic compounds and create angstrom-size minerals, which can then be absorbed intracellularly in humans. The implication of these seawater studies is that if we are able to restore the mineral content to our food, we have the potential to significantly decrease the incidence of illness, particularly chronic illness. Although disease is more complicated than that, the potential is there to have consistently healthy lives on a foundation of consistently healthy food that is highly mineralized.

When we go the route of studying Nature, we understand what Dr. William Albrecht, one of the nation's leading soil scientists, says: "It shall come to the idea that agriculture can be made an industrial procedure, but the truth is, it is a biological procedure."[4] We need to mimic Nature in our work, not think that we're smarter than Nature. Continued force-feeding of a few chemicals in high-concentration fertilizers upsets the balance of subtle nutrition. This is why the whole pesticide and herbicide approach doesn't work; it does not coincide with Nature. The natural law is: *The more mineralized the soil, the healthier the plants are, and the more disease-resistant they are. The healthier individuals are those who eat the highly mineralized plants.*

Minerals and the Biochemistry of Humanity

Now that we have some appreciation for the importance of mineralization at the ninety-mineral level, which is the maximum amount of minerals available to us from Nature, it is useful to think about minerals as the key to understanding the biochemistry of humanity. This process partly has to do with energy. Minerals carry the vibrations of all life. They are the holistic vibrations of creation. Just as gems are made of minerals, so are humans. It's just that we are a little bit more complex. Bones and teeth are made of calcium and phosphorous; skin and hair are made of silicon. Iron is an important element in the blood. When we lack certain of these minerals, the corresponding body organs and tissues that they energetically support become damaged, impaired, and vulnerable to the disease process. We need our partners, the plants, to process the minerals to angstrom-size so we can absorb the minerals intracellularly. Our primary way of taking in minerals is from highly mineralized plants. Plants, with the help of sunlight, take basic minerals from the earth, air, and water and make them assimilable, in angstrom levels. From a mineral point of view, all disease conditions begin with a mineral deficiency or a toxic substance taken into our bodies. This does not negate the holistic point of view that spiritual and emotional aspects play a role. It's very clear that mineral deficiencies can also be created by an excess of stress and spiritual imbalance. Each mineral has a vibratory rate that supports different aspects of consciousness and spiritual awareness, as well as chakra and organ systems. We are living alchemical Beings who transform the color (as explained in the Rainbow Green Live-Food Cuisine) as well as the vibration for the air, earth, water, and sun, into prana. That energy or alchemy is what allows the vibration of minerals to become the building blocks for our vibratory and physical manifestation. Each mineral has a particular chemical personality and function that, through its vibration, activates the life function of tissues, cells, and organs in a particular way.

It's hard to say which minerals are most important, but calcium, iodine, sodium, silicon, oxygen, phosphorous, and magnesium seem to be the seven most important minerals. In truth, they all seem important. Like all the members of a team, you need every mineral present for the whole system to work. Research reported by Dr. Bernard Jensen and done by the German chemist Koenig[5] tells us the actual weight of each mineral in a 150-pound human body. The important thing to understand is that according to our genetic makeup, some people have a little more of a particular element than others, and that is what makes different constitutions.

The minerals in muscle include potassium, magnesium, chlorine, manganese, calcium, phosphorous, and selenium. Hair and nail minerals include silicon, iron, sulfur, zinc, and chlorine. In skin the highest minerals are silicon, sulfur, sodium, manganese, and copper. In the brain and nervous system the highest minerals are phosphorous, magnesium, potassium, sodium, iodine, sulfur, silicon, calcium, and manganese. In the heart we have magnesium, iron, potassium, calcium, and phosphorous. In the blood the key minerals are iron, copper, zinc, sodium, potassium, and calcium. In blood vessels, magnesium, silicon, and sulfur. The spleen is high in iron, copper, chlorine, sodium, potassium, and magnesium. The highest minerals in the liver are zinc, selenium, sulfur, iron, potassium, and magnesium. The highest minerals in the kidneys are potassium, chlorine, fluorine, manganese, magnesium, calcium, iron, and silicon. In lungs the highest minerals are phosphorous, manganese, and silicon. In the gastrointestinal tract are sodium, potassium, chlorine, fluorine, iodine, calcium, and iron. The key minerals in the bladder are silicon and fluorine. The inner ear requires magnesium, fluorine, iron, and chlorine. The key eye minerals are sulfur and chlorine. The pituitary is very high in iodine, phosphorous, sulfur, and manganese. The pineal is high in phosphorous, sulfur, and manganese. The adrenal medulla is very high in phosphorous, sulfur, manganese, and iodine. The adrenal cortex is high in calcium, fluorine, iron, and silicon. The thyroid and hypothalamus are high in sodium, potassium, chlorine, magnesium, and iodine. The beta cells of the pancreas are high in zinc, manganese, potassium, and chromium. The prostate is high in zinc, silicon, and magnesium. Testes are high in silicon, manganese, magnesium, phosphorous, and zinc.

The major minerals (which are found in higher concentrations in the human tissues) and the trace minerals (which are found in trace concentrations) have their own story and energy to share with us. Much of this interesting information came out of Dr. Don Jansen's classic book, *The Chemistry of Man.*

The following chart shows the minerals found in the organs of the human body. Following the chart are individual discussions of many of these minerals which have the most important impact on human functioning.

Minerals in the Organs																
	Calcium	Chlorine	Chromium	Copper	Fluorine	Iodine	Iron	Magnesium	Manganese	Phosphorous	Potassium	Selenium	Silicon	Sodium	Sulfur	Zinc
Adrenal cortex	x				x		x	x					x			x
Adrenal medulla	x					x			x	x					x	
Bladder					x								x			
Blood	x			x			x				x			x		x
Blood vessels								x					x		x	
Brain and nervous system	x					x		x	x	x	x		x	x	x	
Eyes		x													x	
GI tract	x	x			x	x	x				x			x		
Hair & nails		x					x						x		x	x
Heart	x						x	x		x	x					
Inner ear		x			x		x	x								
Hypothalamus		x				x		x			x			x		
Kidneys	x	x			x		x	x	x		x		x			
Liver							x	x			x	x			x	x
Lungs									x	x			x			
Muscles	x	x						x	x	x	x	x				
Pancreas			x						x		x					x
Pineal									x	x					x	
Pituitary						x			x	x					x	
Prostate								x					x			x
Skin				x					x				x	x	x	
Spleen		x		x			x	x			x			x		
Testes								x	x	x			x			x
Thyroid		x				x		x			x			x		

Calcium

Calcium is one of the key minerals for health. It is the alkalizing mineral of structure and solidity. Calcium has a powerful attraction for oxygen, as well as sulfur, silicon, and carbon. In a 150-pound man, calcium accounts for about 3 pounds, 12 ounces in the body. Calcium is responsible for solidity, as well as movement. It's essential for walking, as well as doing physical and mental activities. Without sufficient calcium in the body, we end up with defective teeth and poor bone metabolism. Its role in the body is similar to its role in soil: It is important for digestion, is a great alkalinizer, and promotes growth and vitality. It also helps with the clotting mechanism to prevent hemorrhaging. Calcium acts to calm the nerves, neutralize stomach acidity, and protect against nervous exhaustion. It helps to strengthen the walls of the arteries and veins. The muscles require appropriate calcium to work correctly. Calcium gives solidity to the body, which is essential during pregnancy for the growth of the foetus, helps heal wounds and scars, prevents scurvy (working with vitamin C), repairs cartilage, soothes the nerves, and protects against tuberculosis, rickets, asthma, and hay fever. It builds and maintains bone structure and teeth. Calcium gives vitality and endurance. A certain amount of calcium is needed to act as a buffer in the system to create alkalinity. It also appears that calcium and glucose attract each other. The more sugar we consume, the more calcium links with glucose and is precipitated out of the solution in our extracellular fluids and blood. In this way, excess sugar corrodes teeth, contributes to stomach acidity, and robs the body of its essential calcium. On the mental level, calcium has a very positive effect upon brain function. It stimulates qualities of love and compassion, expansiveness of intellect, and powers of concentration.

For calcium to be properly utilized, we also need foods that are high in sodium and chlorine. When there is an imbalance of calcium in relationship to sodium, there is a tendency for a general hardening of the body, which is known as calcification. So an excess of calcium, or a deficiency of sodium, can create a precipitation of calcium in the tissues.

Calcium not only builds our physical bone structure and cartilage, but is also useful for relaxing muscles and preventing muscle spasm. Calcium is important for the flow of electrical energy in the system, and it combines with phosphate intracellularly and extracellularly to form an alkaline compound, calcium phosphate. Ionic calcium is an extremely important transport mineral for bringing other nutrients into the cell. Dairy products and table salt can lead to calcium losses in the body, and a variety of research clearly shows that high intake of the wrong calcium such as milk is connected to high rates of osteoporosis. The United States has the highest average calcium intake per person, and the highest rate of osteoporosis in the world. This is because we are getting calcium from the wrong sources and eating and living in a way that undermines calcium metabolism.

A deficiency of calcium undermines the power of memory, and tends to create qualities of selfishness, lack of want for people, and subtle antisocial qualities in the personality. Calcium deficiency may also cause depression, melancholy, mental confusion, and dull feeling in the head, as well as softening of bones, weak teeth, and tooth decay. Calcium deficiencies show up with symptoms of weakness, fear, indecision, lack of will power, tendency to hemorrhage, cramps in the calves, vein fatigue, digestive problems, soft bones, rickets, scurvy, and tuberculosis. Up to 32 percent of the calcium is destroyed in food that is heated above 150°F. High-calcium foods are sesame seeds, dulse, Irish moss, kelp, and leafy greens, as well as most seeds, nuts, and grains.

Carbon

The element carbon is known as the body builder. It brings creativity. It is found in all carbohydrates. It supports all our vital energy systems. Carbon is essential to muscle function and all its metabolism. It is basic to cell birth and death, and key to all protoplasmic functions. An excess of carbon, which in essence, is an excess of carbohydrates, shows up as obesity and laziness, low sex drive, excess acid, high blood pressure, cysts, boils, diabetes, and liver system imbalances. Carbohydrate deficiency in the body creates a sense of emaciation, melancholy, and negativity.

Carbon, in essence, is the principle element of growth. Combined with oxygen, it creates heat, growth, and generation of carbonic acid. Carbon is the basic element of the cell wall structure, and all metabolic energy production. Carbon is present mostly in starches, sugars, and fats.

Chlorine

Chlorine, in its healthy food form, rather than its commercial table salt form, is present in digestive processes and glandular secretions. One of its main functions is as a cleanser in the body. A deficiency of chlorine will contribute to a sluggish liver and glandular and lymphatic swelling. The human body contains about three-fourths ounce of chlorine. Chlorine unites with potassium to work within the muscle system and gives tone to the motor centers. It also can help excite the sexual system. Chlorine helps support the blood cell function, and is obviously important in the formation of hydrochloric acid. It's a cleanser of the lymph, and it enhances peristalsis and circulation. Chlorine helps to heal blood diseases, nervous disorders, poor muscle function, skin inflammation, lymphatic congestion, and congested livers.

An excess of chlorine in the system can create loss of nitrogen, hydrogen, oxygen, carbon, sulfur, phosphorous, fats, and sugars. The result is a tendency toward emaciation. Excess of chlorine also slows brain activity, depresses the reflexes, lowers the blood pressure, causes difficulty breathing, and depresses skin function. On the mental level, a symptom of chlorine deficiency is gloom, low self-esteem, and low self-confidence. Chlorine deficiency can also create a lack of will of the spirit. On the physical level, we see a sluggish liver and lymphatic swelling. In a deficiency of hydrochloric acid, we have gas from fermented foods.

Chlorine is most concentrated in the blood, the lymph, and the pancreas (pancreatic fluid). It helps fight viruses and bacteria. Foods that are high in chlorine include asparagus, avocados, beans, blackberries, brazil nuts, Brussels sprouts, cabbage, carrots, cauliflower, celery, coconut, cucumbers, dandelion greens, dates, eggplant, horseradish, kale, kelp, kohlrabi, lettuce, mangoes, oats, peas, pineapples, raisins, sauerkraut, spinach, strawberries, sunflower seeds, sweet potatoes, tomatoes, turnips, watercress, and watermelon. The vegan diet tends to wash chlorine out of the system; therefore, it is important to bring a lot of chlorine and sodium salts into the system through these foods and natural salt such as Celtic sea salt, Himalayan salt, Krystal™ salt, or Real Salt™.

Natural chlorine in our plant foods is not the same as chlorine added to our water. Chlorine in World War I was known as mustard gas. It is an obvious poison. It has been linked to chronic digestive disorders, acne, psoriasis, seborrhea, and eczema. Chlorine also combines with organic substances in water to form trihalomethanes, which are carcinogens. A study in Canada in 1995 showed that long-term exposure to chlorinated water caused a 34 percent increase in bladder and colon cancer. Research by the National Institute of Health Sciences and Shizuoka Prefectural University found that natural organic substances such as soy, fruits, and green or black tea reacted with tap water to form cancer-causing compounds. Dr. Riddle at Kemysts Laboratory reports that chlorine and chlorination by-products are linked to cancer of the bladder, liver, rectum, and colon, as well as heart disease, anemia, high blood pressure, and allergies.[6]

It is interesting that the increase in arteriosclerosis and heart attack is associated with the practice of chlorinating the water. According to data compiled by Dr. Tru Ott, this heart disease increase has appeared only in countries that chlorinate water, not in countries that did not adopt this practice. A strong association between heart disease and chlorinated water was made by Dr. Price in the U.S. He put fifty chickens on chlorinated water and fifty chickens on non-chlorinated water. Seven months later, 95 percent of the chickens that drank the chlorinated water had arteriosclerosis, while none of the control chickens had any arteriosclerosis. Chlorinated water has also been linked to increased rate of miscarriage and hypothyroid disease, as well as with allergies, asthma, respiratory problems, and destruction of protein. By-products of chlorination include chloroform, which causes excessive free-radical formation, oxidation of cholesterol, and acts as a carcinogen. Dichloroacedic acid (DCA) is another chlorination by-product that has been associated with altering cholesterol metabolism and liver cancer. MX (another chlorinated acid) causes genetic mutations that can lead to cancer. Not only is chlorinated drinking water a problem, but we absorb 6–100 times more chlorine in a shower than by drinking the same water. A basic way to deal with this is to use low-cost chlorine shower filters if your water is chlorinated and filter your drinking water.

The principles of Spiritual Nutrition are to avoid eating or drinking anything that is toxic to our body and mind. This includes chlorinated water.

Fluorine

Fluorine is known as the structure, beauty, and youth element. It is found in the structural system of the body and tooth enamel. It is good for preserving bones. It helps to resist the forces of disease, beautify the body, strengthen the tendons, and knit bones. It works very well in combination with adequate calcium. Fluorine is stored in the spleen, eye structures, and elastic tissues. It influences the deepest internal tissues. One of the most important organs it affects is the spleen, which needs fluorine in order to function. Calcium will combine with fluorine to make calcium fluoride, a longevity compound. People have a lot of natural fluorine in their system to support hard bones and strong teeth. Natural fluorine in the system also helps protect us against virus and bacteria. One reason live-food practitioners have a little bit stronger immune system is that they don't destroy the fluorine in their food by cooking. Fluorine has a cementing quality in bones, hair construction, tooth formation, and integrity of the meninges, nails, bone lining, and sinus wall linings. It is also a purifier. It disinfects and creates resistance to disease throughout the body. It also is an element that helps create beauty and youth. In a sense, fluorine helps us preserve our bodies against aging.

An excess of fluorine in the system can create fear, inflames and enlarges the splenic artery, and may create gas and heart palpitations. A deficiency of fluorine can cause worry, indifference, stress, difficulty getting up in the morning, slow mental functioning, and weakness in the corneal structure, nails, beard, and glossy surface of all the structures. A fluorine deficiency may also be associated with decayed teeth and bones and sclerosis in the brain. It is also associated with the weakening of eyesight, and with difficulty thinking, slow-healing fractures, swollen glandular eyelids, and craving for fatty foods.

Fluorine is an element found in raw fruits and vegetables. When it is exposed to heat, the fluorine tends to be destroyed. Fluorine is an unstable element. When we cook it, heat it, or steam it, fluorine tends to evaporate. The highest fluorine food sources are live green quince, sea vegetables, avocados, black-eyed peas, Brussels sprouts, cabbage, caraway seeds, cauliflower, dates, garlic, greens in general, juniper berries, lemongrass, licorice, New Zealand spinach, parsley, sea cabbage, sea lettuce, spinach, and tomatoes.

Sodium fluoride, used to fluoridate water, is not the same as natural fluoride. Natural fluoride is found in Nature as a calcium-fluora-phosphate. Natural fluoride does help build healthy bones and teeth. It is an organic edible salt. Sodium fluoride is an extreme poison. Dean Burk, Chief Chemist Emeritus of the U.S. National Cancer Institute, is quoted: "In point of fact, fluoride causes more human cancer death, and causes it faster, than any other chemical."[7] As little as one-tenth of an ounce of sodium fluoride can cause death. Sodium fluoride that is put into our water supplies not only does not protect teeth, but is a poisonous industrial waste product from aluminum production. The symptoms of sodium fluoride poisoning as listed in the 1983 *U.S. Pharmacopedia* include tar-like stool, bloody vomiting, diarrhea, faintness, nausea, stomach pain and cramps, excess salivation, skin rash, stiffness, weight loss, mottling of teeth, increased hip fractures, and death. In Kizilcaoren, Turkey, where their village water was 5.4 ppm (parts per million) of sodium fluoride, which is very high, all the inhabitants suffered premature aging. All people older than age 7 had teeth discoloration and the adults had few teeth left. Every single member of the village had some form of bone disease. According to *How to Fight Cancer & Win*, scientists at the Seibersdorf Research Center in Austria have shown that even 1 ppm of sodium fluoride impairs the DNA repair system of the immune system. Other studies have shown that 1 ppm can cause significant chromosomal damage in plants, animals, and humans, and increases proportionately as the sodium fluoride amount increases. At the Nippon Dental College of Japan, researchers found that the fluoride level in U.S. water, which is 1 ppm, can transform normal cells into cancer cells. The American Cancer Institute in 1963 showed that even low levels of sodium fluoride increased the incidence of melanotic tumors by 12 percent to 100 percent. Polish scientists showed that as little as 0.6 ppm of sodium fluoride can create chromosomal damage.

According to the Merck Index, sodium fluoride is a rat and cockroach poison. Sodium fluoride is one of the basic ingredients in Prozac and sarin nerve gas. Neither sodium fluoride nor stannous fluoride, which is in most toothpastes, is safe. A significant amount of research over the past fifty years shows that sodium fluoride shortens lifespan, increases the incidence of cancer, creates mental disturbances, and literally makes humans stupid, docile, and subservient. Humorously, there is no objective, double-blind study that even links sodium fluoride to healthy teeth. It is interesting to note who thought of putting sodium fluoride in the water. It was the Nazis who consciously used it in their concentration camps and for general population control. It was not to help people's teeth. It was to sterilize the prisoners, destroy their mental capacities, and wipe out their will to resist. According to Charles Perkins, a research chemist who spent twenty years researching fluorine: "Any person who drinks artificially fluoridated water for a period of more than one year or more, will never again be the same person mentally or physically."[8] According to Dr. Tru Ott, sodium fluoride inhibits more than 100 important enzyme functions in the body and is associated with approximately 50,000 cancer deaths per year. The number of deaths in fluoridated water areas, according to the CDC (Center for Disease Control), is 5 percent higher than in non-fluoridated areas. It is so deadly that in 1979 a dentist was sued for the death of a three-year-old child who swallowed a fluoride rinse. Sodium fluoride is not only in water, but in Diet Coke at 2.96 ppm and in 42 percent of ready-to-drink fruit juices.[9] This is probably because they are using fluoridated water where their factories are located.

An important part of Spiritual Nutrition is not to drink or eat anything that will impair your physical or mental health, or impair your spiritual will power. This is why the author is making such a point about avoiding all sodium fluoride.

Hydrogen

Hydrogen is considered the hydrating element. Hydrogen is found in secretions, soft tissues, blood serum, lymph, brain, lungs, all the glandular organs, liver, kidneys, spleen, pancreas, and muscles. It prevents inflammation, promotes the transfer of nutrients across cell membranes, moistens lung surfaces for the transfer of oxygen, and helps regulate bodily temperature. Without hydrogen, the blood cannot flow optimally and toxins cannot be removed from the system. A human weighing 150 pounds has about 15 pounds of hydrogen, the highest concentrations being in the lymphatic glands, the liver, blood, kidneys, spleen, pancreas, bladder, and perspiration. Hydrogen is very important for the process of digestion, assimilation, and elimination. It is vital as a carrier of nutrients across cell membranes. Hydrogen can be thought of as having a soothing effect on the body, mind, and soul. Water is one of the main carriers of hydrogen. A symptom of hydrogen excess is puffiness, swelling, edema, water collection under the skin in between the joints, puffy hands, a general sense of puffiness or doughiness in the system, stiff neck, and numbness. People with excess hydrogen are low in energy. Chlorine-carrying foods help reduce the edema tendency, as well as do alkalinizing foods. Eating high-potassium foods helps to reverse the excess hydration.

Hydrogen deficiency can be thought of as similar to dehydration.

When a person is dehydrated, the brain does not work as well, the system becomes irritated, there's a tendency for inflammation, lymph, and the general metabolism becomes sluggish and begins to shut down. Literally, the brain shrinks and the person ages. There is a tendency of inflammation of joints as well. Symptoms of hydrogen deficiency might be dehydration and emaciation, cramps, desire for salty food, and generally dry, wrinkled skin. Proper hydrogen levels in the body help to balance and calm the nervous system, moisturize the tissues, transport nutrients, help with elimination, decrease inflammation, and regulate temperature.

High-hydrogen foods are moisture-carrying foods, with water having a pH below 7.2: citrus, fruit and vegetable juices, apricots, asparagus, blackberries and juice, blueberries and juice, broccoli, Brussels sprouts, cabbage, carrots, carrot and celery juice, chard, cherries and juice, kohlrabi, leaf lettuce, mangoes, papaya, peaches, pineapples, prunes, pumpkins, sauerkraut, sorrow, spinach, strawberries, Swiss chard, tomatoes and juice, turnips, watercress, and watermelon.

Iodine

Iodine is the metabolic mineral. Iodine is very important for the thyroid and a variety of different glands and brain function. It prevents goiter and helps with cell metabolism. Iodine is very important in the body for the assimilation of the key minerals calcium, silica, chlorine, and fluorine. Iodine is important for brain function and teeth and bone metabolism. It is found also in high concentrations in the spleen, blood, saliva, perspiration, and tears. An excess of iodine will show up with the symptoms of nervousness and anxiousness, bulging eyeballs, and acute sense of touch. Psychological symptoms are fear of the future, oversensitivity, and nervous tremor. Signs of iodine deficiency can also include nervousness, but with increased cholesterol, weight gain, restlessness, slow mind, slow metabolism, fearfulness, goiter, awkwardness, much mucus, and heart and lung difficulties. The foods richest in iodine are dulse and kelp. All sea vegetables basically contain all of the minerals of the sea, bringing us a good source of trace minerals in general.

Iodine seems to work as a monitor, or controller, for calcium metabolism. It's one of the key minerals. Iodine has the highest frequency of all of Nature's essential minerals. It supports enzyme systems that help the functioning of certain thyroid hormones and assists in regulating cellular metabolic rates. It may be helpful in protecting against breast cancer. It is important for normal mental and physical development in children because of the importance of normal thyroid in a child's growth and development. Lack of iodine may also be associated with retarded growth in children, poor bone development, bad teeth, and dull mental functioning. As far back as 1915, as many as 90 percent of the American population were considered deficient in iodine. Iodine appears to be one of the minerals that get burned up by stress, and so whenever there's anxiety, tension, and depression, there may be a need for iodine. Iodine acts in the body as a cleanser. It protects the brain by destroying toxins in the blood before it passes the blood brain barrier and increases the assimilation of salts for normal metabolism. Iodine, because it is water-soluble, works with the lymph, travels to every cell in the body, works as a disinfectant, balances the metabolism, and creates electrical balance in the body.

It is best to think about the minerals in synergistic patterns. Iodine is a very good example of that because these key elements work in patterns to make the organs and tissue work in an optimal way. The pattern is just a little bit different for each person. An example of this is cataracts, which seem to be connected to calcium being pulled out of the pattern because of a lack of iodine. Iodine also works in relationship with phosphorous to activate the brain's clarity. Dulse may be a better choice for supplying iodine than kelp because dulse has a little bit more manganese than kelp, and manganese is an important element for the functioning of iodine in the system. Besides kelp and dulse, the foods that are high in iodine are asparagus, blueberries, Brussels sprouts, cardamom, carrots, chervil, chives, coconuts, cucumbers, eggplant, garlic, green peppers, kale, leaf lettuce, loganberries, mustard greens, okra, oats, onions, potatoes, rutabaga, all the sea vegetables, spinach, squash, strawberries, Swiss chard, tomatoes, and watermelon.

Iron

Iron is a key vitality mineral, along with oxygen. It works in combination with oxygen. Without iron we cannot draw oxygen into the hemoglobin. Together with oxygen, iron in the human body builds vitality, magnetism, and optimism. Iron improves circulation, digestion, elimination, perspiration, and tissue oxidation. It also acts to build the immune system against colds. A significant disease of iron excess is hemochromatosis, which has particular life-threatening symptoms that result as iron builds up in the critical tissues of the heart, brain, and liver. Hemochromatosis can be lethal if it is not diagnosed appropriately. It is the result of a gene defect. Signs of iron deficiency, which occur more in women when menstruating, as well as in seniors, include depression and melancholy, poor oxygenation, low vital force in the nervous system and brain, susceptibility to colds, low blood pressure, anemia, poor mental functioning, poor memory, and poor speech.

Close to 57 percent of meat eaters are deficient in iron.[10] Vitamin C, particularly a complete vitamin C, amplifies the assimilation of iron. Vitamin C in fruits and vegetables naturally amplifies iron absorption. This may explain why vegetarians have less iron deficiency than meat eaters.

The foods richest in iron are dulse, kelp, Irish moss, black cherries, greens, blackberries, raisins, and spinach. Perhaps the most potent iron food, however, is chlorophyll. Researchers have found that when people are anemic, high amounts of chlorophyll treats their anemia. This may be because the structure of the magnesium in chlorophyll is exactly the same as the hemoglobin, only that there is iron instead of magnesium. The author theorizes that there is a biochemical transmutation, via Dr. Kervan's enzymatic transmutation theory, in which manganese is converted to iron. The total amount of iron in the human body is about 3.25 grams. Iron is absorbed in the duodenum, or small intestine, and after that the hydrochloric acid in the stomach combines with iron to form iron chloride. Apparently iron is more readily assimilated from live fruit and vegetable juices than from solid foods. The iron from the juices is held in the duodenum long enough for it to be absorbed, whereas the iron in solid foods sometimes passes through the duodenum before iron can be absorbed out of it. In addition to the hemoglobin, iron is found in gastric juices, lymph, bile, eye pigment, hair, and skin. A diet rich in iron, sulfur, potassium, calcium, and phosphorous supplies the minerals that can activate the biologically altered brain and bring it back to normal. People who are low in iron look pale, dry, and anything but healthy. If there is a sufficient iron in the system, there's a glow, a kind of an iron-rich blood glow to the system. There is also an increase in energy and vitality that is associated with enhanced beauty and magnetism. Iron, of course, is in magnets, so it creates a certain magnetism. David Wolfe, in *Eating for Beauty,* lists it as a beauty mineral.[11]

Iron is a very important cofactor in many types of enzymes and is associated with good mental cognition and functioning. Water-soluble iron, in ionic form, tends to increase vitality and general well-being, enhances resistance to infections, and stimulates energy and stamina.

Magnesium

Magnesium, the relaxer mineral, is one of the most important minerals. Magnesium is important for all muscles, heart function, and the digestive system. Magnesium deficiency is associated with a chronic stress state and decreased adrenaline function. More than 80 percent of the population is deficient in magnesium. Magnesium is very important in the treatment of all people with chronic exhaustion, adrenal exhaustion, and depression. It is very important for the optimization of neurotransmitter function.

Almost all the clients seen at the Tree of Life are deficient in magnesium. This is particularly true with people who are experiencing tension, anxiety, adrenal exhaustion, chronic fatigue, constipation, and muscle spasm. Magnesium is very good for muscle cramps and spasm, particularly when people are fasting. Magnesium activates many enzyme systems and is involved in neurotransmitter production. It helps regulate temperature control in the body. It is needed for synthesis in protein. Magnesium is used by the pituitary gland as part of its regulation of parathyroid, adrenal, and thyroid function. It is a key enzymatic mineral used in almost 100 different enzyme systems in the Krebs cycle of making energy in the mitochondria of our cells. Many people who are depressed have a magnesium deficiency; therefore, it is used quite often in the treatment of depression. We don't need a lot of magnesium to get proper functioning; we have about 2 ounces of organic magnesium in our bodies.

Magnesium is very alkalizing to the body, and works as a natural laxative. At the Tree of Life we use it regularly for these two purposes with clients. It also helps calm nerves and improves flexibility, particularly in the muscles, nerves, ligaments, and joints. It has a positive effect on the mucous membranes, nerves in general, and excretory and secretory nerves. It is good for insomnia, as well as to cool the body. Magnesium neutralizes acids in the system. It helps to alkalize the body (or raise the pH level), and soothes and cools the brain and nervous system in general.

An excess of magnesium often shows up as diarrhea. Magnesium excess is like amplifying the common sedative qualities of magnesium, so we start to see symptoms of poor memory, central nervous system apathy, slow reasoning power, and a dull brain function. With a magnesium deficiency we see a hyperactive nervous system, cramps, muscle spasms, anxiety, apprehension, excessive concern about work, tremors in the head, quivering in the voice, and a sense of doom psychologically, as well as depression. We also see shoulder and neck muscle stiffness in the evening. In time, a chronic magnesium deficiency creates an overactive inflammation of the nerves, disrupts mental functioning, undermines ambition, and causes the personality to become scattered and erratic. Women who are magnesium deficient may have difficulty with their menses. One of the main treatments for menstrual difficulties is magnesium and vitamin B_6. One interesting symptom is that tobacco smoke is extremely irritating and debilitating to a magnesium-deficient person. Hatred, jealousy, resentment, bitterness, hostility, and greed tend to create a magnesium deficiency. These qualities are often ameliorated by giving magnesium to the person. Magnesium is synergistic with calcium. It is the combination of calcium and magnesium that helps maintain healthy bones, teeth, and tissues. It activates cell growth, improves tissue elasticity, and relaxes the nervous system. The magnesium helps us feel younger, lose weight, and is associated with an increase in libido. Magnesium in combination with calcium is anti-aging and even helps protect the skin.

Magnesium is highest in nuts, whole grains, unpolished rice, and wheat germ. Generally high-magnesium foods include apples, apricots, avocados, beet tops, berries, black walnuts, Brazil nuts, cabbage, coconuts, comfrey leaves, figs, dulse, endive, greens, spinach, rye, walnuts, watercress, and yellow corn.

Manganese

An important, but lesser-known, element is manganese. Some research suggests it is the motherly Love element, because animals that are deficient in manganese do not have much empathy or connection with their offspring. Generally speaking, manganese is a brain and gentle nerve food element. Manganese helps develop a strong nervous system and coordinates our thoughts. Manganese is also found in the lining of the heart. Often it is stored in combination with lecithin. In a certain way its function is very similar to that of iron. In fact, Dr. Kervan's work shows that manganese will convert to iron (manganese at one level participates in the regulation of iron metabolism because it converts to iron).

Manganese and iron maximize the creation of iron-rich blood. Manganese on its own helps carry oxygen from the lungs to the cells. It is important for skeletal enzyme systems in the body and protects humans and animals against impotence, skeletal and postural defects, and liver, kidney, and pancreas difficulties. Manganese can also help support people with neuromuscular control in cases of myasthenia gravis, multiple sclerosis, and tardive dyskinesia. Manganese also helps elasticity and strengthening of ligaments and muscles. Manganese also appears to have an effect on the digestive tract; it is actually found in and influences the intestinal lining, the lining of the biliary ducts, and the passages in the ducts of the gall bladder and liver. It has been shown to help with bones, hard tissue, and discs, as well as being particularly good for repairing and strengthening slipped discs. Manganese supports the function of SOD (super-oxide dismutase), a very important antioxidant system in the body, particularly important against radiation. It's not just a trace metal, but it's been shown to catalyze the formation of thyroxin (a thyroid hormone). Manganese is an essential element for bone development, a variety of enzyme reactions, fat metabolism, protein synthesis, and cell production. It can stimulate neurotransmitters and improve glucose tolerance. Manganese is needed for the body to optimally utilize protein and carbohydrate molecules. It works in conjunction with selenium to dissolve and eliminate harmful fatty acids and cholesterol, and to support the synthesis of red blood cells in the liver and kidneys. It is associated with helping to heal arteriosclerosis and heart disorders, lower cholesterol, grow a healthy pancreas, and improve vision.

The author first began using manganese in 1970 for treatment of tardive dyskinesia, a side effect of anti-psychotic medications and SSRIs such as Prozac. It is one of the few minerals that seem to have an effect on tardive dyskinesia – a sometimes irreversible condition that manifests as unusual facial twitchings, pill-rolling movement of the fingers, difficulty sitting still, and a general "restless leg" syndrome that covers the whole body.

It is rare to have manganese excess; manganese deficiency is more common. A manganese deficiency is linked to poor growth and impaired reproduction, as well as calcium deposits in the inner ear, which can lead to Down's Syndrome problems. A deficiency of manganese has been associated with vindictive, mean, and sadistic personality characteristics. One of the interesting psychological aspects of manganese deficiency is aversion to doing physical or, especially, mental work. In manganese deficiency the will power is not strong, the mind is just not present, and the ability to make decisions is quite limited. The manganese-deficient person can be easily upset, and is impatient, angry, and quarrelsome. Some paranoia also tends to develop. Doubt, confusion, indecision, ambivalence, and a sense of being overwhelmed seems to haunt the manganese-deficient person. Other signs of manganese deficiency are ailments that are worse at night, much burning and perspiration, headache from motion, swollen glands, depression, aversion to being touched, aversion to working, impatience, anxiety, nightmares, and cracking joints. Without manganese, according to Dr. Jensen, the brain actually shrinks, as do the bones, marrow, and linings of many organ systems.[12] Synovial fluid in the joints dries up and therefore we get bones and joints that crack and creak.

The treatment of manganese deficiency isn't just giving manganese, but includes increasing silicon, chlorine, sodium, potassium, iron, and magnesium.

In summary, manganese helps neurological systems as its main effect. Its helps coordinate thoughts and actions, creates an ability for decisive and clear thinking, and has a general recuperative ability. It improves the memory, enhances intellectual power, and opens the heart.

Manganese is in short supply in our everyday devitalized diet. Manganese is abundant in nuts, seeds, grains, and leafy greens, as well as in natural salts. The foods richest in manganese include almonds, black mission walnuts, blueberries, cardamom, celery, English walnuts, and pignolia nuts.

Nitrogen

Nitrogen is an interesting element as it exists in balance with oxygen. Oxygen has a radical, explosive quality while nitrogen is more restrained. If nitrogen replaced oxygen, we would die of suffocation. If nitrogen were removed from the air, we would burn up from the oxygen. So it's part of a life-giving balance. There are about 3.8 pounds of organic nitrogen in the body. Nitrogen is the critical element in protein. When we talk about nitrogen, we are, in a sense, talking more about protein. What contains nitrogen in our body are albumins, protein compounds, alkaloid agents, and ammonia and its breakdown products. Nitrogen, in combination with hydrogen, oxygen, and carbon, is needed for power and strength and vitality for all organs. In the muscle system, myosin, which is the principle protein in muscle, is made of 17 percent nitrogen.

People with excess nitrogen have a tendency for low heat generation, tender tissues, swarthy complexion, and often faulty oxidation. There is a tendency toward nervous system difficulties. They also manifest lethargy, deep sleep, glandular swelling, loose teeth, and have slow wound, fracture, and bone healing. In these nitrogen-excess people, the liver, kidney, and intestines are overworked, and bones and joints are susceptible to injury. Mental states they tend to have are ones of being unconscious, melancholic, and filled with fears and anxieties. They also suffer from significant absentmindedness, sleepiness, colds, and flus. In general, their immunity is deficient and their body is quite acid. Mentally, high-nitrogen-excess people tend to go into shock from fear, sorrow, failures, operations, and accidents because their nerves are so out of balance and high-strung. In general, nitrogen-excess people tend to eat an excess of flesh foods, as a result of autotoxemia, which in turn weakens their emotional, physical, and immune systems.

Nitrogen-deficient people tend to be the opposite of conservative; they tend to have rash and compulsive behavior and are impatient and quick to judge and act. Their depressions are intense and their tact is minimal. These people tend to have low vitality and an erratic emotional state, as well as mental state. The treatment of low-nitrogen people is not simply increasing protein; they need a certain amount of free nitrogen, which is available in a very nitrogen-rich atmosphere, as exists in a warm humid climate, such as in California, Hawaii, or Florida. Any locations with a low altitude and much vegetation empathetically encourages improved nitrogen metabolism and low nitrogen retention in the body. Signs of nitrogen deficiency are feebleness, numbness, muscular weakness, fatigue, absentmindedness, no sexual energy, hypochondria, lack of desire to work, cracking the tendons, and brain weakness.

Foods high in nitrogen include all protein foods, spices, nuts, almonds, walnuts, beans, lentils, pignolia nuts, dried peas, spirulina, chlorella, and algae in general.

Oxygen

Oxygen is the life of the party. Without oxygen there would be no party. Oxygen strengthens all of our systems – metabolism, mental functioning, cell regeneration, vitality, and anti-aging. Oxygen is the element of enthusiasm and youthfulness. If there's an excess of oxygen, we tend to get excesses of those characteristics such as being too optimistic and expansive. These people tend to be completely led by feelings and instincts because the brain is overstimulated. In oxygen deficiency, on the other hand, we have people who are nervous, stubborn, hypersensitive, and have an increased amount of bacterial and fungal infections, as well as cancer. Cancer is more activated when there is low oxygen in the atmosphere, close to 12 percent, because cancer cells are anaerobic. Low oxygen creates decreased brain function, congestion, bleeding, and a decrease in sexuality. Often people on the airplane fall asleep; one of the reasons is that the oxygen in the cabin is equivalent to about 8,000 feet altitude. Fortunately, the oxygen in the pilot's section is a higher concentration. Oxygen is the main element outside of glucose for effective energetic functioning of the brain. Low oxygen diminishes the senses of sight, touch, and hearing; low oxygen clearly accelerates the process of senility and decreased intellect, and generally slows mental functioning. Oxygen is needed for the mitochondria to produce energy. The person with low oxygen usually has low energy and an increased rate of aging. These people tend to become more stubborn and hypersensitive with poorly functioning mitochondria in the brain and body cells; memory decreases and emotions are imbalanced. This can result in depression, with intense desire to be in the mountains, hills, and the oceans. It can also result in a need for seclusion.

The bottom line is that it is very important to breathe and do pranayama practices (breathing exercises). It is very important when you realize, according to some studies, that by the time you're seventy you can lose up to 50 percent of your lung capacity. This does not apply to people who are doing regular breathing exercises. At the Tree of Life we put a strong emphasis on increasing oxygenation at the mitochondrial level with several non-invasive oxygenation technologies. Oxygenation and maintaining iron levels can significantly slow the aging and senility process.

We have oxygen in all our foods, but generally oxygen is very attracted to the blood through iron; therefore, foods that are high in iron are particularly important for bringing oxygen into the system. Other minerals that activate the oxygen are calcium, potassium, and iodine.

High-oxygen foods would include iron tonics, nuts and seeds, and liquid chlorophyll. Fruits and vegetables in general are also good, especially in a juice form. High-oxygen foods include beets, blueberries, carrots, figs, grapes, green pepper, horseradish, leeks, mustard greens, nuts, seeds, ripe olives, onions, parsnip, raisins, sea vegetables, spinach, and tomatoes and juice. All the greens are high in oxygen, and particularly the watery fruits and vegetables.

Phosphorous

From a spiritual point of view, phosphorous is among the author's top seven important minerals. It is the illumination mineral. Phosphorous, the Greek word, means "Light bearer." Phosphorous has to do with psychic perceptions, idealistic tendencies, humanitarianism, and philanthropy. It has to do with the subjective functions of the brain and the physical brain sensory system – taste, touch, smell. Phosphorous also has much to do with intelligence. Throughout history, phosphorous has been synonymous with intelligence and has been seen as the mineral that helps link the soul with matter. Phosphorous is absolutely essential for spiritual life. The phosphorous for the brain needs to be absorbed from the environment in the form of lecithin; this is different than the phosphorous needed for bone building. High-phosphorous, high-lecithin, vegetarian foods include soybeans and bee pollen, which has 15–20 percent lecithin. According to the scientific literature, the actual process of thinking burns up phosphorous, so those who are doing a lot of thinking or meditating need a much higher phosphorous input. Phosphorous seems to be used in study, memorizing, reading, intellectual functioning, visualizing, and comprehension. With each thought we think, we use up phosphorous. So those who are intellectual need to eat a lot of phosphorous in the form of lecithin, because the activity of all the neurons requires phosphorous. That means people who do a lot of mental work, office work, students, scientists, meditators, and also pregnant mothers require a higher level of phosphorous in their diet.

One of the nutritional principles that people don't really grasp is that minerals, just like vitamins, are literally used up. For example, people under a lot of stress will go through huge amounts of B_{12}, compared to other times in their life when they need much less B_{12} because they're in a stress-free environment. The same thing goes for minerals like phosphorous and magnesium. Intense mental activities of any sort require a tremendous amount of phosphorous. Phosphorous is also used up in telepathy, ESP, and dream work, as well as in mental imbalances such as obsessions, delusions, and hallucinations.

Phosphorous is needed for bone development and semen formation.

In the form of calcium phosphate, phosphorous helps build and repair bone. Phosphorous is needed in DNA and RNA production, and for making ATP (adenosine triphosphate), which is a major way energy is stored at the biomolecular level in the body. Phosphorous is needed for white blood cell production and for metabolic regulation. Some feel that phosphorous, as a Light-bearer, is associated with how strong the aura is around people. Phosphorous is activated by calcium and silicon. About 2 pounds of phosphorous is needed in the body to be most effective.

Phosphorous is found in excess in people who drink a lot of colas and other soft drinks. Excess phosphorous can create an imbalance in people who work from the position of idealism rather than practicality. People who have excess phosphorous spend money excessively, are affected by auto-suggestion, have a mind that is over-working, are excessively excitable, and have a decrease in quality of decision-making, practical judgment, concentration, and will power.

The amount of life stress, plus depleted soils, creates a situation in which minerals are being depleted more from our diets than ever before. With a phosphorous deficiency, weakness is one of the main symptoms. With deficiency there is a sense of being faint, no sexual energy, low appetite with significant hunger, and a desire for cold drinks. There is an intensified nerve pain and a general weakness in the liver system and in brain function. Phosphorous-deficient people tend to have increased migraines, light sensitivity, lung hemorrhages, frontal headaches, and pain in the temples. There's emotional liability, paranoia, fear, a sense of weakness and helplessness, and increased trembling. A phosphorous-deficient person tends to lack confidence and then creates Love and sympathy, to compensate. There is an increased general fear and anxiety, and fear of the future.

High-phosphorous foods include almonds, lentils, carrots, cashews, corn, dulse, kelp, oats, olives, pumpkin and squash seeds, rice bran, sesame seeds, soybeans, sunflower seeds, walnuts, wheat bran, and wheat germ. Bee pollen, which is 15–20 percent lecithin, may be the most potent vegetarian source for lecithin; it is sufficient to supply all the body's lecithin needs. Bee pollen, the semen of the plant kingdom, fills you with the life force energy of Nature. This is important because vegetable phosphorous tends to be primarily for the bones and vegetarian lecithin phosphorous is specific for brain function. It improves physical and mental health. It improves elimination, respiration, circulation, the ability to recover, sexual function, muscle efficiency, heart function, oxygen in the blood, and rate of internal oxidation. In general, bee pollen is healing, expanding to the nervous system, and has been associated as the food of longevity and "food of the gods" for thousands of years.

Potassium

Potassium is the "well-being" mineral. It is involved in secretions, brain performance, cell function, alkalinizing the blood, cell membrane conduction, hair growth, skin activity, fibrin blood-clotting function, muscle coordination, heat resistance, memorization, and the electricity in the body. Potassium is important for normal heart functions, particularly the nerve activity or the rhythm of the heart. Potassium helps with pituitary function and helps in the treatment of some depressions. The most important minerals protecting heart function and against heart attacks are magnesium, potassium, and zinc. Potassium also helps as an analgesic, and is important for brain function.

The human body typically has 3–4 ounces of potassium; muscular people have a higher amount of potassium in the body. Potassium is often good in athletes, or people engaged in long-term repetitive exercise or physical work. Because potassium has a high affinity for oxygen, it increases the tissue oxygenation. One of the most important things with potassium is that it helps relieve edema by helping move sodium out of the body. Potassium and sodium work in conjunction with each other. When there is an excess of sodium, adding potassium tends to recalibrate the system and move sodium out. In this way potassium acts as a diuretic because the sodium takes water with it. Potassium stimulates the kidneys as well and thus acts as a natural diuretic. Potassium compounds act to stimulate all types of fluid, lymph, and detox channels.

Signs of potassium deficiency on the mental level include fears, especially fear of loneliness and death. Potassium-deficient people often feel anxious. Long-term potassium depletion is also associated with depression, violent crimes, and even suicide. Some peculiar symptoms of potassium deficiency include troubled sleep, vivid dreams, and explosive sounds being imagined in the ears. Potassium-deficient people are hungry, and have a thirst that is unsatisfied by water. They lose their ambition. They are very sensitive to weather change. Low potassium may decrease the total amount of oxygen in the tissues because potassium very actively attracts oxygen. Potassium is very important in the autonomic nervous system, the muscle system including both the voluntary and involuntary muscles, and in sugar metabolism. A potassium deficiency is a significant contributor to heart disease, chronic fatigue, and poor concentration. Deficiencies in potassium can result in decreased adrenal and pituitary function. A potassium deficiency symptom is hypersensitivity to touch.

Excess potassium may cause thought confusion, unclear thinking patterns, slowing of the reflexes, and even depression. An excess of potassium may also neutralize some stomach acids.

Potassium works in a dynamic synergy with sodium. This sodium-potassium synergy is important in all the body cells to maintain and restore normal cell membrane, osmosis, and electrical polarization across the cell membrane. Potassium is important for all energy metabolism, as well as nerve impulses, which have to do with getting the rapid firing of the nerves and polarization and repolarization of electrical potential across membranes. Sodium works with potassium as an osmotic pump to move hydrogen and oxygen molecules in and out of the cell. This process is important for creating energy and helps the chemical cellular reactions. In this process, potassium stays mostly inside the cell in the intracellular fluid; sodium is working on the outside in the extracellular fluid. They maintain a dynamic balance. If either mineral is out of balance, the cell permeability and electricity are compromised, and the ability of the cells to absorb nutrients and excrete waste materials is limited. Potassium alkalizes the intracellular fluid. Common table salt throws off the potassium-sodium balance, especially when we are eating high levels of meat and cheese, and are not getting the raw fruits and vegetables that are the main sources of potassium.

High-potassium foods include sun-dried black olives, dulse, kelp, Irish moss, and all bitter greens. Watercress is one of the foods highest in potassium.

Silicon

Silicon is found in Nature as silica, which is a silicon calcium. Silicon is the beauty element. It gives the sheen, resilience, and smoothness to skin, hair and nails. It is also essential for all neuron transmission in the form of electrical impulses through the neurons. It acts as a link between the blood system and the nervous system. People with adequate silicon not only tend to have beautiful skin, hair, and nails, but also have a certain kind of beauty of movement, a sense of charm, and charismatic personality. Silicon is also a protector of the skin, as well as an insulating agent. Silicon is one of the important minerals for connective tissue, hair, ligaments, lungs, lymph nodes, muscles, nails, skin, teeth, and tendons.

While in agreement with its beauty power, the power in its role as a form of crystal energy in the system gives additional insight. Silicon is connected with consciousness. The more silicon we have, the more we have the energetics and radiant flow of the human crystal that we are. After many years of using the Tachyonized Silica Gel from horsetail grass, the author is impressed with its power to help turn us into a tachyonized crystal, particularly working through the lymph and blood system. Tachyonized Silica Gel is a basic builder. It is useful for anyone who has any degree of silicon deficiency. Silicon is very important for flexibility and elasticity, and therefore is good support for the practices of martial arts, Yoga asanas, and gymnastics. Muscle tissue contains at least 2 percent silicon.[13] Silicon is also useful for creating a strong jaw and teeth, and in for preventing cavities. Silicon is the binding element, as well as helping with the flow of electricity and other forms of energy movement in the body. Silicon is needed for plumpness of skin and functioning and strength of basically all connective tissue. The highest concentration of silicon is in hair and nails.

The ratio of silicon to calcium is important. The higher the ratio, the more youthfulness we have. With age, calcium begins to become higher in relationship to silicon. Silicon also controls, along with iodine and sodium, how calcium is used in the system. A 150-pound human contains about 1.5 ounces of silicon. Silicon makes the body alkaline. In partnership with sulfur, silicon works to create healthy hair and nails. Silicon also enhances a sense of well-being and appetite. Joints are made more elastic, eyesight is improved, varicose veins are reduced, complexion improves, and hair becomes more abundant and shiny when silicon is added to the system, therefore we can think of it as a very good mineral to combat aging. It is also associated with lower cancer rates. Chronic sores tend to be healed when there is sufficient silicon.

An excess of silicon may manifest as an overactive intellect, with a tendency for the mind to dominate the emotions. In excess, silicon tends to create overconfidence in people. A peculiar symptom of silicon excess is the craving for sunshine and longing to be in the mountains and the hills.

A silicon deficiency manifests as being sensitive to emotion, bug bites, noise, and loud conversations. It has an acute sensitivity to the ears. A deficiency also tends to have the symptoms of an excessive concern for ethics and principles. The lack of silicon in the bones and joints results in a swelling of the connective tissues, cracking of the joints, and the tendency to degenerate. With deficiency, ligaments are weak, chiropractic adjustments do not hold, and there is an increase in dental cavities, poor eyesight, and lack of mental functioning. According to Dr. Jensen, vaccinations are often harmful to children who are silicon deficient.[14] Other interesting symptoms of silicon deficiency include bleeding, buzzing in the ears, intellectual gullibility and impressionability, and sleepiness alternating with insomnia. Emotional disorders associated with a lack of silicon include schizophrenia and neurosis. A silicon deficiency is associated with a desire for tobacco and drugs.

Most refined carbohydrates have lost their silicon. The foods highest in silicon include barley, bamboo shoots, kelp, oats, rice polish, rice bran syrup, straw tea, and alfalfa tablets. Silicon-rich foods include burdock root, cucumbers, skin of cucumbers, skin of bell peppers, grasses in general, horsetail grass, hemp leaves, marjoram, nettles, New Zealand spinach, nopal cactus, radish, romaine lettuce, and skin of tomatoes, as well as bamboo sap. Nature's First Law bamboo sap has the highest silicon content of any food on Earth. Nuts, seeds, grains, and cereals are high in silicon. Flax seed, sunflower seed, and sesame seeds are especially good sources. Other generally basic sources include alfalfa, apples, apricots, asparagus, barley, beans, beets and beet greens, cabbage, carrots, cauliflower, celery, cherries, corn, dandelion greens, dates, figs, greens in general, horseradish, kohlrabi, millet, nectarines, onions, parsnips, pomegranates, raisins, pumpkin, brown rice, wild rice, spinach, sprouted seeds, strawberries, tomatoes, turnips, watermelon, wheat bran, wheat germ, and whole wheat.

Sodium

Sodium is a fluidity element. It keeps us pliable, limber, active, and useful. It fixes the whole body in many ways by keeping calcium and magnesium in solution. The ability of sodium to keep calcium in solution in the joints keeps the joints and ligaments supple, and helps prevent arthritis. In the nerves, a sodium-potassium balance is needed for the movement of electrical impulses. One-third of the body's sodium is stored in the bones.[15] The lymph system is very high in sodium and the spleen is really considered the sodium organ. In the blood sodium regulates the fluid balance. In combination with iron and chlorine, it makes the blood salty and helps to generate electromagnetism. By regulating the body's sodium concentrations, the body regulates water and hydration levels in various tissues. Sodium is stored in the stomach wall; it plays an important role in neutralizing excess stomach acid. The neutralizing power of sodium in the walls of the stomach and bowel keep those organs from being destroyed by the hydrochloric acid and enzymes in digestive juices. Sodium also helps dissolve mucus in the stomach and neutralizes bacteria in the stomach and intestinal tract. It basically produces an alkaline medium that inhibits the growth of pathogenic bacteria. Sodium seems to feed and activate the healthy bacteria of the bowel. Sodium generally influences calcium metabolism in the blood and also the medulla oblongata secretions in general, the secretory glands, gastrointestinal tract, the cerebral membranes, the stomach, intestinal walls, the spleen and pancreas, and albumin metabolism. For the spleen, the bowel, the gastric secretions, the blood, and intestinal nervous secretions to work properly, they need sodium. Proper sodium, iron, potassium, silicon, and chlorine in the body enhance the sense of fluidity and beauty in the system. Proper sodium not only creates beauty, smoothness, and grace, but also improves memory, favors longevity, and enhances youth. A normal adult weighing 150 pounds has about 3 ounces of sodium in the body.

Excess sodium can create a variation in moods. An excess of sodium may create some degree of congestion in the body, the function of bile may be decreased, and pancreatic juice secretion lowered. Alkalinity problems could happen with any of the foods that are high in sodium or phosphate, potassium, magnesium, or silicon. But this doesn't happen very often because mostly people are too acidic.

Symptoms of sodium deficiency are often melancholy, depression, argumentativeness, a sense of inflamed and overheated nervous system, and faulty memory, with poor intellectual abilities. Some days the person could be apathetic or dull, having difficulties studying or concentrating, with a kind of erratic judgment. In the evening or nighttime sodium-deficient people tend to be fearful. The dreams of sodium-deficient people often include violence, snakes, storms, floods, death, and destruction; often these people wake between 1:00 and 5:00 in the morning. A sodium-deficient person may also have anxiety, fear, restlessness, and even hysterical outbursts.

Physically, a sodium-deficient person may have a disturbed digestion and tend to become emaciated. We may see this more in people who live in hot, dry climates, where sodium is lost at higher rates. A high-sodium diet, combined with high-sulfur fruits, really helps the intestinal tract and digestion and peristalsis and also improves function of liver, pancreas, skin, sexual organs, the nervous system, and brain. The loss of sodium tends to create a precipitation of calcium, and the bones become hard, the joints get weak and stiff, and the ligaments become dry and contracted. With the same principle, when the eye muscles lose elasticity because of low sodium, eyesight can diminish and the eyelids twitch and sting, and become weakened. Classic symptoms of sodium deficiency include a weakened voice, hoarseness, joint stiffness, tender cervical glands, inadequate mucus secretions, stiff hips and shoulders, and the mental symptoms already mentioned. Sodium-deficient people also lose their muscle strength, efficiency, and coordination.

For many of the functions of the body, our bodies really cannot use inorganic or covalent table salt, but we need sodium from our foods or angstrom-size sources. Sodium chloride, if exposed to heat, as in kiln-dried salt, converts from an ionic bonding to a covalent bonding. In this form, it is somewhat toxic to the system. The best sources for elemental sodium are the underground sources of salt, such as Real Salt™ and Himalayan salt. These salts contain about eighty-two minerals. In this ionic form they taste almost sweet and savory and bring the saliva into your system. If they have turned covalent, they usually have a bitter taste and drying sense. High-sodium foods include apples, apricots, asparagus, beets and all greens, cabbage, carrots, celery (one of the best sources), coconuts, collard greens, dandelion greens, dates, dulse, figs, horseradish, Irish moss, kelp, kale, lentils, mustard greens, okra (very high), black olives, sesame seeds, New Zealand spinach, strawberries, sunflower seeds, turnips, and black mission figs (also very high).

Sulfur

Sulfur is the pitta element of fire. It significantly affects brain function, in conjunction with phosphorous and manganese. The metaphysical teaching about sulfur is that it stimulates the link between the soul and the physical body. It aligns and integrates thoughts and emotions with soul expression. It helps to link the soul of humanity and the individual soul with the physical body and the material world. In contrast to phosphorous, which is needed primarily for thinking and psychic phenomena, sulfur is a communicative magnet for thought and action. Sulfur is perhaps more linked to soul intelligence and sensory connection between the higher mind and the three-dimensional world. Besides affecting the mind and the connection of the higher mind or the super-causal mind to the physical world, sulfur has an important effect on the liver and the promotion of biological secretions. Sulfur seems to be needed for healthy protoplasm. Sulfur is also important for healthy nerve function and temperature control in the body. It brings softness to the tissues and helps with stress and asthma, arthritis, inflammation, and constipation. Some research suggests that a high sulfur content in the tissues can speed athletic recovery by 75 percent, especially with the use of MSM (methylsulfonyl-methane, which also helps with hypoglycemia and diabetes).[16] A deficiency has also been associated with muscle cramps, back pain, inflammation, and muscle difficulties. Sulfur helps with producing mental calmness. It improves the ability to concentrate. Sulfur scavenges free radicals, and in that sense it's good for allergies to food and pollens. Sulfuric amino acids such as methionine, cysteine, cystine, and taurine help to protect us from negative affects of radiation and heavy metals. They are used in a variety of detoxification programs. Sulfur minimizes acidity in the stomach, cures ulcers, helps with hypersensitivity to drugs, and improves the body's ability to produce insulin. Sulfur builds up the immune system.

Sulfur is an important mineral for general health and well-being. A 150-pound human body contains about 4 ounces of sulfur. It brings vitality to the system and elasticity to all the connective tissues by helping to build collagen in the system. It is one of the beauty minerals, along with chlorine, sodium, iron, and silicon. David Wolfe considers sulfur the foundational mineral for all beauty.[17] Sulfur is essential for the formation of hair, nails, and skin. For that reason, we can say that high-sulfur foods are basically beautifying foods. Even the fineness of one's hair depends on the amount of sulfur we have in the system. The more sulfur, the redder or lighter the hair is. It also creates more curly hair. Sulfur is needed for collagen synthesis. It helps the skin, hair, and nails from becoming rigid and brittle. In homeopathy, sulfur is used for skin difficulties, and clearly sulfur has a powerful effect in clearing up skin conditions and for skin repair. One of the best foods for this is MSM, in conjunction with vitamin C. MSM may help to undo cross-linkages associated with aging and scarring. Sulfur is one of the four key elements – along with vitamin C, copper, and zinc – that make cells function well and help the skin look young. Sulfur needs vitamin C to activate it. So sulfur works like all the minerals in the proper synergy and proper balance. Although hot sulfur springs are good for skin beauty, excessive bathing in hot sulfur springs can cause other imbalances. According to Dr. Bernard Jensen, inorganic sulfur excess from sulfur pools may result in anemia and imbalances in the nervous system, and may even cause atrophy of vital organs. There is a difference between sulfur we get from food and sulfur waters or sulfur drugs.

Sulfur excess can cause imbalance in the nervous system, with moodiness and a variety of emotional imbalances. Excess sulfur intensifies emotions, but in the morning, excess sulfur can create depression and slowness. Signs of sulfur excess include irritability of the system, changeability, depression, and slowness in the morning. Excess sulfur, particularly through hydrogen sulfide from eating too many sulfur foods, can result in auto-toxicity.

Deficiency in sulfur may be connected to unstable blood sugar. Sulfur is a part of the insulin molecule. For this reason, at the Tree of Life we often give MSM to help with hypoglycemia and diabetes. Sulfur deficiencies can produce irritability, hysteria, imbalanced emotions in general, and cravings for chocolate, sweets, and beer. There is also craving for salads, greens, high-magnesium vegetables, berries, fruits, sweets, black tea, and starchy, creamy dishes. Sulfur deficiencies also create a peculiar craving for fresh air. Sulfur deficiency emotions include excess pride and sensitivity. Anti-establishment feelings, weakened will power, and a mind that works faster than one can verbalize also typify sulfur deficiency. Emotions cycle from depression in the morning to happiness in the evening and a tendency for rage, followed by remorse. Sulfur deficiency symptoms also include a desire for mysticism and beauty, an experience of great bodily temperature changes, and an aversion to getting up early in the morning.

On the physical level, there may be some lowering of the heart energy, hypersensitive bladder with frequent urination, uterine cramps, anemia, and irregular menses. Sulfur-deficient people often experience increasing burning pains and have a sense of dryness in their body.

The treatment for sulfur depletion includes a high-sulfur food diet as well as foods high in magnesium, nitrogen, iron, sodium, manganese, potassium, silicon, chlorine, iodine, calcium, and high-phosphorus fats. Cold air, lots of good outdoor activity, and particularly living in an altitude between 2,000 and 4,000 feet also help. The highest-sulfur-content foods include arugula, kale, cabbage, cauliflower, horseradish, Brussels sprouts, and watercress. Other good sulfur sources include artichokes, asparagus, avocados, bee pollen, black currants, Brazil nuts, broccoli, carrots, celery, chervil, chicory, chili peppers, corn, cucumber, dill, durian, figs, filberts, garlic, hemp seeds, kohlrabi, lettuce, lima beans, mustard greens, mustard, oats, okra, onion, parsnips, peas, potatoes, pumpkin seeds, radishes, soybeans, spinach, thyme, tomatoes, turnips, and turnip greens. Foods high in sulfanolipids include spirulina, chlorella, and aphanizomenon flos aguae (AFA). Sulfur in food is lost with dehydration and heat. One of the possible ways to bring sulfur into the system besides the angstrom sulfur is DMSO and MSM.

Most people find that eating too much sulfur food can cause gas and bloating and a certain amount of excess fire in the system. For this reason it's good to combine sulfur foods with the sea vegetables or fatty foods, including nuts and seeds, which balance the pungent energy of sulfur. Sea vegetables have a lot of potassium and sodium, which tend to balance sulfur in the system. Eating high-sulfur foods with fatty foods like avocado or nuts and seeds creates an interesting energetic balance, especially with the cruciferous vegetables and pungent onions, garlic, and chili peppers.

Zinc

Zinc is very important in the functioning of the pancreas, as well as the male genital function especially prostrate gland, sperm production, and even genital formation. It is highest in the thyroid and sexual organs. Zinc occurs in the highest percentage in the prostrate gland. It is next highest in the kidney, hair, nails, red blood cells, muscles, thyroid, eyes, liver, muscle, aorta, pancreas, spleen, ovary, testes, lung, brain, and finally adrenals. Zinc is important in the treatment of diabetes, because it's connected with insulin formation. Zinc also helps maintain proper blood sugar levels in conjunction with chromium. Some people find zinc helpful in the management of rheumatoid arthritis.[18] Zinc is also important in the healing of arteriosclerosis, along with copper and germanium. Zinc is important in the healing of artery injuries. It can be used in the treatment of lymphatic congestion. Zinc is important for healing bones and wounds. It also works synergistically with vitamin A and sulfur to create strong hair. It is important for night vision, as well as taste and smell. It is particularly good for supporting brain function and helps improve memory and the mental processes. Zinc is helpful in treating people with alcoholism, as alcohol tends to flush zinc out of the system. Zinc is important for normal cell division, repair, and growth. It is needed for the synthesis of DNA. Several of the zinc-dependent enzymes are involved in nucleic acid metabolism including RNA polymerases.[19] Zinc is an important part of proteins that regulate the activity of certain RNA polymerases. These components are called zinc fingers transcription factors and are part of structural factors that bind to regulatory DNA sequences. Zinc is also needed for nucleic acid synthesis. It particularly has its impact on sex hormones, thymic hormones, insulin, and growth hormone. The overall result is that growth and normal development of the sexual energies and organs as part of the larger reproductive system depend on zinc. Zinc is very high in breast milk for the first two weeks and a newborn baby's liver contains three times more zinc as that of an adult, suggesting its importance for development.

Zinc may be the most important antioxidant known. Zinc affects more than 300 enzymes.[20] Zinc plays a role in the enzyme systems needed for the breaking down of old collagen and the synthesis of new collagen. It helps with creating healthy skin and building new collagen. It is needed to support skin beauty. That is why it is very helpful in the treatment of burns. It can even help in DNA repair. A normal amount of zinc helps protect against wrinkling, stretch marks during pregnancy, and signs of aging. Zinc is part of at least 25 enzyme systems in the digestive and metabolic and respiratory systems. Carbohydrate digestion and phosphorous metabolism are also affected by zinc. In the ileum and duodenum, in the small intestines, zinc is absorbed. Zinc does not kill viruses and bacteria, but it stops them from reproducing, therefore it is useful to support the immune system. Zinc quickly dissolves and moves throughout the body fluids, especially saliva and nasal secretions. Because of this, zinc is a tremendous line of defense against infections. Zinc in your saliva, for example, helps stop bacteria growth in the mouth that produces harmful acids that destroy tooth enamel. Because of this, healthy zinc levels in the body are associated with fewer cavities in the teeth. A good healthy zinc level also stops body odor because it eliminates the bacteria.

The body contains about 1.8 grams of zinc. Zinc is one of seventeen minerals that are essential to life.[21] Others include cobalt, nickel, copper, and iron. Zinc often needs vitamin A as a cofactor.

Calcium and phytic acid compete against zinc. This is the problem we have sometimes with the grains, which are high sources of calcium and phytic acid. Zinc also competes with cadmium. Part of the treatment for cadmium toxicity is increasing the amount of zinc.

Symptoms of zinc deficiency include fatigue, along with increased rate of infections and injuries. Low zinc can cause dwarfism and delayed sexual development. Mothers with a zinc deficiency tend to have smaller babies and babies with smaller-than-normal brains. Zinc deficiency has an association with different types of birth defects such as Down's syndrome, spina bifida, and clubbed feet. Zinc deficiency is also associated with Alzheimer's, paranoia, diabetes, PMS, depression, infertility, herpes, acne, obesity, alcoholism, high blood pressure, thyroid problems, hair loss, prostate cancer, and various eye difficulties, including cataracts. Zinc deficiency can cause slow healing. Zinc deficiency can come from high alcohol consumption. Vegetarians tend to run a little low on zinc but consumption of fruits, vegetables, and seeds in high quantities creates significant protection from zinc deficiency. About 60 percent of adults over age 60 are zinc-deficient.[22]

Good sources of zinc include poppy seeds, pumpkin seeds, pecans, cashews, pine nuts, macadamia nuts, sunflower seeds, sesame seeds, beets, and coconuts.

Cobalt

Cobalt is an element that is part of the B_{12} complex and many of the enzymes of the body are enhanced by cobalt. Cobalt is found in the red blood cells and plasma, as well as kidneys, liver, pancreas, and spleen. An excess of cobalt could possibly affect the thyroid function, causing goiter. Angstrom-size cobalt is a good source.

Copper

Copper seems to be involved in all the body tissues. Many of the enzymes needed for metabolism and anabolism use copper. Tyrosine converts into melanin with copper. Copper also has an effect on protein metabolism and general healing. Copper is important in the formation of RNA, and is involved with iron in the formation in the womb. Copper is important for building connective tissue and cartilage because it is needed to activate the enzyme lysyl-oxidase, which is needed for the building process. Copper helps to protect us against joint problems, ruptured blood vessels, and spider veins. These are all symptoms of poor collagen. The copper also helps keep hair from turning gray.

Copper is one of the most important minerals for protecting us from parasite infections. Copper has been found to kill almost all microscopic parasites. There are thousands of different parasites that significantly impair our health. Doses of copper that are too high or too fast can have die-off type of side-effects, however, because depending on the number and different types of parasites in the body, copper can cause a healing crisis as the parasites use toxins as a defense mechanism before the copper kills them. Parasites, as they die, also give off toxins, particularly ammonia that can cause flu-like symptoms. Angstrom-size copper itself is not toxic and that's the copper that should be used. According to Dr. Tru Ott, the way to start a copper parasite purge is to use half a dropper of copper for a few days, then go to a dropper, then to two droppers a day for a period of one month. You can do this twice a year. Another form of purge is a little more sophisticated: At week one, start with one-half dropper each night, one dropper the second night, one-and-a-half droppers a third night, and so on until you reach three droppers a day. The second and third weeks you want to do one-and-a-half droppers a day, and then a half dropper per day for one week. That's a total of four weeks. You repeat the cycle three times, or until all evidence of the parasite infection is gone.[23] Along with the copper, molybdenum is part of the parasite cleanse, at one-half dropper in 10 ounces of water a day. In addition, two droppers of silver in the morning and in the evening, and two droppers of zinc in the morning support this cleanse. Also, a good bowel cleanse would be appropriate for clearing the bowel of parasite conditions. Copper should be taken by itself, at least thirty minutes away from the others and one hour from zinc and molybdenum.

Copper may have a contrary or destructive effect on vitamin C in the body. Excess copper in the system can cause paranoia, Wilson's disease, and deposits in the liver, brain, kidneys, and the corneas of the eyes.

Best sources of copper are whole-grain cereals, almonds, green leafy vegetables, and legumes (beans).

Germanium

Germanium is a unique oxygen-binding mineral. It brings much more oxygen into the system, as well as helps detoxify pollutants. Some people have even claimed that it's good for treating cancer. Sometimes the need for germanium shows up in the treatment of diabetes, high blood pressure, and cardiac insufficiency, because of its ability to bring oxygen into the system.

Good sources of germanium include garlic, ginseng, aloe vera, comfrey, chlorella, and all the high-chlorophyll foods.

Selenium

Selenium is an extremely important mineral as an antioxidant in the system. It plays an important role in the glutothionine antioxidant system. Selenium is a key part of the enzyme glutathione-peroxidase, a very important antioxidant that protects cell membranes from the free radical oxidation where most free radical damages tend to occur. Selenium is also needed for a variety of functions, including development and protection of the lens of the human eye and protection against cataracts. Glutathione-peroxidase helps protect the lens against free radical damage. Importantly, glutathione-peroxidase helps to detoxify thoughts.

Vitamin E and selenium work synergistically together for supporting normal growth and fertility. They work together to support tissue elasticity by preventing the oxidation of polyunsaturated fatty acids.

Selenium protects against many chronic diseases, including heart disease. It seems that in areas where selenium intake is low, the death rates from high blood pressure and stroke are about 300 percent higher than in high-selenium areas. Some research has shown that high blood pressure in animals can be treated with selenium.

Selenium is one of the most important elements in protecting against cancer. Research has shown, for example, that people who are given adequate levels of selenium are less likely to develop cancer than those who receive a placebo.[24] Some claim that cancer rates in general may be reduced as much as 70 percent by taking 200 mcg of selenium per day. The National Cancer Institute agrees with this projection.[25] Japanese women who consume 250–350 mg of selenium have 20 percent of the breast cancer rate as U.S. women. One Arizona study showed a group who took 200 mg/day for seven years had 42 percent less cancer than the control group.[26] It binds with the unstable molecules in our cells and protects against further damage that can create cancer.

Selenium is also associated with improved immunity. Research in Brussels shows that taking 100 micrograms of selenium a day improves overall immune system by 80 percent.[27]

Muscles do contain some traces of selenium, as do the liver and kidneys. The body only uses about 3 millionths of an ounce. Excess selenium can cause hair loss, dermatitis, and muscle weakness. Deficiency of selenium contributes to aging and higher rates of cancer, high blood pressure, and infertility. A selenium deficiency has been associated with anemia, age spots, liver spots, fatigue, muscle weakness, cystic fibrosis, irregular heartbeat, Parkinson's, high infant mortality, and SIDS (sudden infant death syndrome). The biggest problem we face with getting enough selenium is that there is very little selenium in North American soils; therefore, we need to supplement with angstrom-size selenium. Food sources of selenium include bee pollen, especially from Nebraska and North and South Dakota, Himalayan salt, broccoli, tomatoes, onions, asparagus, nuts, and whole grains grown on high-selenium soils. Angstrom-size selenium may be the most consistent source.

Molybdenum

Molybdenum is a lesser known trace mineral. Foods that have vitamin C must contain molybdenum to activate the vitamin C. Molybdenum can protect against tooth decay. It works as an enzymatic agent and plays an important role in iron and nitrogen metabolism. It promotes healthy cellular function. Some research shows that molybdenum may have similar effects as Viagra without the side effects, but it may take several months to manifest this erectile effect.[28]

A deficiency has been associated with increased incidence of cancer.[29]

Angstrom-size molybdenum may be the best sources since it is not found in many common foods.

Vanadium

Vanadium is another trace mineral. It seems to keep blood sugar from rising too high. It supports the absorption of blood sugar into the muscle system and protects against elevated cholesterol, particularly a build-up of cholesterol in the central nervous system. At the Tree of Life, we use vanadium frequently to help with insulin resistivity and Type II diabetes. Kelp and vegetables are good sources of vanadium.

Boron

Boron is the fifth element in the periodic table. Boron is essential for the assimilation of calcium and magnesium in the body, and is a cofactor in the functioning of vitamin D. Vitamin D, once it is activated by sunlight, needs to go through enzymatic processes that transform it to its most active form. These enzymatic processes require boron. Boron is the key mineral in protecting against osteoporosis, supports the immune system, and has an anti-inflammatory effect.

Boron is a micronutrient that has been basically known to promote bone density, but new research makes this one of the most exciting minerals to think about. It has been shown to shrink prostate tumor size, lower the PSA (prostate specific antigen), and actually help prevent prostate cancer. Other research shows that boron can alleviate joint pain and preserve brain cognitive function. Exciting research by Zhang et al., shows that, in a study on the treatment of prostate cancer, those who took the highest amount of boron were 64 percent less likely to develop prostate cancer, compared to the men who took the least amount.[30] They found that the greater amount of boron-rich foods consumed, the lower the risk of being diagnosed with prostate cancer. In a study published in the proceedings of the American Association of Cancer Research, Gallardo-Williams et al. found that mice with already active tumors that ingested high levels of boron had their tumor sizes decrease by 38 percent.[31] The PSA dropped as much as 88.6 percent.

The traditional effects of boron on bone metabolism have been more clearly understood, in that boron is vitally important in calcium and magnesium function and bone metabolism. The main effect that boron seems to have is its ability to reduce the loss of calcium and magnesium in the urine. The net effect of the boron is to raise the ionized calcium levels. Boron's function is to preserve the calcium-magnesium balance in dietary situations of nutritional stress.[32] In general, about 3 milligrams per day of boron protects against urinary losses of calcium and magnesium. Research has also shown that there are increased levels of plasma, ionized calcium, beta-estradiol, and testosterone.[33] Boron seems to have an integrative effect on bone metabolism and vitamin D.[34] Basically, the effect of boron on raising the plasmic calcium may be because of its ability to enhance the effect of vitamin D.[35]

One of the newer findings is that boron seems to have an effect on the inflammatory aspects of arthritis. Research has shown that boron seems to inhibit cyclooygenase (COX) and lipoxygenase (LOX). The newer research shows that these enzymes have an important effect on activating inflammation. Its ability to inhibit those enzymes gives it anti-inflammatory properties. Boron may also work not only by inhibiting those enzymes, but also inhibiting COX2 and prostaglandin E2 (PGE2) by suppressing the nuclear factor kappa beta (NF kappa B), which is a pro-inflammatory cytokine.[36] There is evidence that where boron levels are low in the soil, people have a higher percentage of suffering from arthritis compared to areas where boron is higher in the soil. In areas of the world where the boron intake in the diet is 1 mg (1,000 mcg) or less per day, the incidence of arthritis is 20–70 percent, while in areas of the world where boron intake is 3–10 mg, the incidence of arthritis drops to 0–10 percent.[37] In a study of boron to treat arthritis, 50 percent of the people who received 6 mg per day noticed a subjective decrease in pain on movement.[38] One of the more exciting effects of boron is on brain function. As researchers are beginning to understand that the inflammation in the brain seems to be associated with the pro-inflammatory cytokines and the COX2 and LOX enzymes, they are finding that boron helps with the brain inflammation; it also increases cognition and perhaps even slows the progress of Alzheimer's.[39] It seems to increase people's ability to perform both cognitive and psychomotor tasks. Those who had a boron-deficient diet had less function, and their EEGs were even different.[40]

Levels of 3–10 mg per day of boron are totally safe. Research done in 1904 suggested that 500 mg per day did create symptoms, which of course is considerably higher than anything humans should be taking. Other research has shown that boric acid can cause loss of vitamin B_2.[41] One should be aware of maintaining a good B vitamin intake if you are taking high doses of boron.

Boron is a trace mineral found in non-citrus fruits, such as avocados, apples, pears, plums, and grapes. It is also found in nuts and legumes. People's need for boron can be as high as 9–12 mg per day, although a reasonable dose is about 3 mg per day.

Chromium

The most well-known purpose of chromium is for balancing the blood sugar. Chromium and vanadium both work on glucose metabolism.

They activate the enzymes that are associated with creating the glucose tolerance factor. Chromium is involved in enzymes that are part of the glucose metabolism, for energy formation, fatty acid production, and cholesterol formation. The function of insulin is enhanced by chromium. Vanadium creates a synergy with chromium to help regulate blood vessel function, to reduce hyper-cholesterol levels, and lower blood sugar. Chromium also affects our protein and RNA synthesis.[42]

At the Tree of Life, chromium is used a lot with people who are hypoglycemic, suffer from chronic fatigue, are pre-diabetic, and those who have Type II diabetes. Good sources of chromium include cloves, whole grains, fruits, and vegetables.

Silver

Silver has been proven to kill more than 600 different viruses and bacteria. In a sense, it's a broad-spectrum antibiotic. Silver has a certain frequency charge that shatters anaerobic parasites, but not the normal healthy bacteria in the body, which are primarily aerobic. Some people have reported that silver in the bloodstream speeds the healing process of fractures by 40 percent. Occasionally people with muscle aches, pains, and backaches are improved with silver, probably because these are associated with viral or bacterial infections in the spinal fluid, which traditional antibiotics or colloidal silver cannot reach.

Zinc and silver make a very powerful synergistic team as a secondary immune system. Silver is also effective in controlling warts. Angstrom-size silver is the best source.

Gold

Gold is associated with improved brain function, has an antidepressant affect, and helps with despair, fear, drug and alcohol addictions, melancholy, Seasonal Affect Disorder, circulatory problems, heat flashes, night sweats, and puncture wounds. Gold is one of the greatest remedies for promoting deep sleep and dreamtime. It improves REM sleep. It is amazing how two droppers of angstrom-size gold at bedtime helps many people, especially elders, sleep through the night.

Gold is a pure amalgam, which means it sticks to all the elements. Angstrom-size gold is used by the body to repair DNA damage and thus slows down the aging process. Gold has also been shown to help with many glandular functions. Some anecdotal research suggests that children given ionic gold supplements have improved IQ function and a better learning curve. The best source is angstrom-size gold.

Lithium

Lithium is a mineral salt that has been associated with the treatment of manic-depression at a minimum of 900 mg per day as lithium carbonate. At this level, however, it has been associated with dulling the mental state, dizziness, drowsiness, diarrhea, nausea, excessive thirst, shakiness, tremors, weight gain, a metallic taste in the mouth, and hypothyroidism. Lithium waters have been known since the second century A.D. to be used for the treatment of mania and for depression. Research suggests that in bipolar disorder there is a loss of brain matter, including the hippocampal area. Recent research suggests that it may actually be helpful at lower doses for brain function. There is limited evidence that it may affect serotonin and norepinephrine production in the brain. Other evidence suggests it may inhibit the enzyme inositol monophosphatrase and other enzymes associated with neuromodulation of neurotransmitters. There is also growing evidence that lithium may provide some protection against neurodegenerative diseases including Alzheimer's.[43]

Why lithium is intriguing is that it may be associated with protecting against the neurotoxicity of beta-amyloid plaques and neurofibrillary tangles[44] that contribute to neuron death. In mice studies, lithium inhibited the action of an enzyme called glycogen synthase kinase 3 alpha, reducing the production of beta-amyloid protein by 40–78 percent.[45] Lithium was also found to decrease neuronal death from glutamate-induced excitotoxicity,[46] which has been associated with neurodegenerative disease including dementia. It did this by stimulating the formation of a protective protein called brain-derived neurotrophic factor (BDNF), which develops and maintains healthy neurons. Lithium seems to be associated with neurogenesis, the growth of new neurons. In one study, researchers found a 25 percent increase in the number of dividing cells in the hippocampus area of the brain; this is a strong indication of neurogenesis. Lithium has also been associated with the production of B-cell lymphoma protein-2 (bcl-2) which is known to promote new brain cell growth. In one human study of people with bipolar disorder, lithium was found to increase gray matter by an average of 3 percent after one month of lithium treatment in 80 percent of patients.[47] Angstrom-size lithium is the best source.

Platinum

Platinum has begun to prove itself as a much more effective treatment for cancer than gold. Platinum is useful to get rid of headaches, PMS, cold feet, and general sensitivity. Platinum is also associated with well-being and longevity. Platinum can help with improving sleep and quality of dreams, and has been associated with increased energy levels.

Platinum and gold, in order not to be toxic, must be taken at the angstrom level. The best source is angstrom-size platinum.

Iridium 77

As stated earlier, minerals are frequencies of Light. Iridium is the frequency that connects us with the living field of the cosmos. Iridium is part of a special class of minerals known as *monatomic* minerals. They take us to a different level of mineral use and understanding. They go back thousands of years to the pre-Egyptian time of Sumeria. These minerals are found in certain soils, particularly where meteorites have fallen and are associated with some of the volcanic soil as far back as 60 million years. Some of these soils have as much as 6 percent content of monatomic minerals.

Foods and herbs rich in monatomic elements include grapes, aloe vera, cacao, carrots, pycnogenol extracted from maritime pine bark from France, Essiac tea (the main ingredients include sheep sorrel and Turkish rhubarb), blood root, blue-green algae, and St. John's wart. Another source rich in the monotamic elements is Ultimatium™ a powder or liquid extract made by Dr. Tru Ott.[48] People have also been able to extract monatomic elements from sea water as far back as the time of the Essenes.

What is a monatomic mineral? Without going into a full lesson in biochemistry, we need a reminder that there are three states of matter: gas, liquid, and solid. Solids that have lattice structures, a micro-cluster of a complex of atoms, are called metals. Another phase of solid has ceramic-type qualities; these are non-metallic superconductors. These are the monatomic minerals. In 1989, a nuclear physicist discovered that atoms of some monatomic minerals exist in micro-clusters. Most of these micro-clusters are found with the transition group of precious metals called the PGM (platinum group metals). They can be changed from a metal state into a monatomic state. If there are more than a specific number of these atoms in a micro-cluster, they form a lattice with metal properties. Micro-clusters with less than the critical number of atoms will just aggregate and become monatomic, with ceramic properties. The monatomic atoms are not held in position by electron sharing as they are in metallic structures. For example, for palladium, the critical number is nine atoms. If the number of atoms is nine or fewer, the palladium will be monatomic; if it is ten or more, the palladium will have a lattice formation and act as a metal. Valence electrons, in the outer shell of the element in the monatomic form, are not available for chemical reactions. Because of this they cannot be identified by the normal biochemical means.

One of the unique qualities of the monatomic elements is they become superconductors at room temperature. One of the Spiritual Nutrition teachings is that we are to transform ourselves into superconductors. The key elements that we are talking about are called transition elements; they include ruthenium 44, rhodium 45, palladium 46, silver 47, osmium 76, iridium 77, platinum 78, and gold 79. (The numbers after each element name is the atomic weight of the element.) These are the elements that are part of the PGM group. These are an entirely new phase of matter and we are just beginning to understand them. Their properties include acting as a superconductor at room temperature and levitation. Because they are superconductors, they tend to balance the magnetic field of the Earth, which gives them the power of levitation. This may be a clue to how in ancient times they had the ability to use these elements to levitate some of the eighty-ton rocks used in building the pyramids and other architectural wonders. Monatomic elements don't have a particular specific gravity, because their weight varies widely with the temperature in the magnetic environment. Monatomic elements tend to transmute. The normal nuclei in lattice are in a spherical shape and have a strong nuclear force keeping it round. The nuclei of the monatomic elements are only partially filled outer-orbitals, and become more oblong shaped, because there is a lack of what we call dipole interaction between the nucleus and the electrons and with the surrounding nuclei. This deformity increases the particle distance, weakens the strong nuclear force, and allows an electromagnetic repulsion between the protons, so the nuclei can become more stable. If the deformity creates a two-to-one ratio, this nuclei becomes super-deformed and creates fission. It's possible that some monatomics do not have this super-deformed nuclei. It is the state of easy transmutation that is one of the powers of the nuclei of the monatomic elements. The fluffy white powder quality of the monatomic atoms is because they are not held in place by the rigid lattice structure seen in the metals. The specific gravity of metallic iridium is about 22; the specific gravity of monatomic iridium is about 3, so it's one-seventh as dense.

Some of the claims, going back to the *Egyptian Book of the Dead* for the monatomic minerals, include restoration of youth and vitality, activation of the third eye, connecting to the gateways of other dimensions, opening up the ability to see into the past and the future, levitation, and the potential of ascension. Sir Lawrence Gardener in his book *The Lost Secrets of the Sacred Ark* talks about their use being recognized at a different stages of history, going back all the way to Lemuria, for levitation, transmutation, and teleportation. Scientists and physicists now talk about monatomic material as "exotic" matter. There have been different names for it throughout history. In Mesopotamia it was called *shem-an-na,* which is not too far from what we know as manna in the Torah. The Egyptian term is *mfkzt.* The Greeks regarded it as a gift from paradise and the medieval alchemists, such as Paracelsus, called it the Philosopher's Stone. The Greeks regarded it as having the power of enhancing Communication with the Divine, the power of levitation, and the power of *electrikus.* In Greek mythology, it was at the heart of the quest for the Golden Fleece. Horus, as the Egyptian God of the Dead for the underworld, is somewhat connected to this, as the white powder is symbolized as the golden tear from the eye of Horus. The Emerald Tablets of Thoth, uncovered beneath a pit in South America, refer to the white powder and prophesies associated with it that it would disappear from the Earth and would be restored at a critical time in history. Iridium means iridescent, or rainbow; it is known as the word iris, meaning rainbow. In the Torah, the rainbow is a symbol of connection between Noah and God after the flood, but perhaps it has other meanings as well. The Egyptians worshiped Isis, the seat of the rainbow, where in the ancient temples they did transform gold into the white powder of iridium. Mfkzt is mentioned in the Egyptian pyramid texts of the sacred writings, which were written during the period of the fifth-dynasty pyramid tomb of King Enasx in Saqqara. The author, his mate Shanti, and the expert intuitive Kevin Ryerson, have taken people on several Essene pilgrimages there. The manna was used in a way that allowed the king to live forever with the gods. It was called the Field of Mfkzt. The alchemist Eirenaeus Philalethes, a well-known British philosopher who produced a work in 1667 called *Secrets Revealed,* in which he discussed the secrets of the Philosopher's Stone, made a point that it is not about transmuting base metal into gold, it's about transmuting gold into the higher gold, to its highest level of purity and power. As we now understand it, it is probably transmuting gold into iridium, which is the highest level of the manna. This is the true Philosopher's Stone. In the fifteenth century, the French alchemist Nicholas Flanel wrote in his last testament in November 22, 1316, that when the metal was perfectly dry, it made a fine powder of gold, which is the Philosopher's Stone. They didn't really have the scientific technology to understand that when they transmuted the gold, alchemically it became iridium. The Kabbalist Jacob Boeheme talked about seventy-seven, which is the atomic number of iridium. Seventy-seven is the total number of Divine names. There are seventy-two names of God, plus the five names that belong to the spirit of God. It is, of course, no coincidence that the high-speed iridium has three electron orbits – five on the nucleus, sixty entering, and twelve in the outer ring, making seventy-two plus five, or seventy-seven. This Light powder is referred to in a variety of sacred texts. In Japan it is mentioned in the Shinto religion and the bloodline of the emperor. The Kahunas from Hawaii tell of the *mannahuna,* keepers of the manna. The different Hawaiian island mountains, such as Mauna Lua, and Mauna Kea, were associated with the sacred shem-an-na, from the mythical continent of Lemuria, or Mu. In Ireland, it is also mentioned, considered, and connected with the myth of the Leprechauns. They talk about it as the rainbow mineral, which indeed is what iridium is. It has all the colors of the rainbow. Alexander the Great may have used it to take a metaphysical journey to a place called the kingdom of Ahura Mazda, the Persian god of Light. He took a vision quest following the ingestion of mysterious white powder formed from the metal. This mysterious powder was called the enchanted paradise stone. The monatomic iridium or manna is found throughout history in many cultures. Moving beyond modern physics and attempts to describe monatomic iridium, history shows us that the ancient royalty of many cultures used this white powder to nourish their Light bodies. This is Spiritual Nutrition at its highest level. It is also very good for the health of the physical body.

In *Modern Science,* in May 1994, Miguel Alcudierre states: "It's now known that it's possible to modify space-time in a way that allows us to travel at an arbitrarily large speed by purely local expansion of the spacetime behind the spaceship and an opposite contraction in front of it – a motion faster than the speed of light, reminiscent of the warp drive of science fiction."[49] It just depends on the use of these monatomic minerals. The physicist Alcudierre called this metal "exotic matter" and said that it comes out of the platinum group. It is further described as matter with a property of having a negative ionic energy density, which is different than physical matter, which has a positive ionic energy density. In the May 1995 issue of *Scientific American,* in an article called "The Electric Gene," it was reported that the platinum group elements (PGM) were examined for their effect on human DNA. They report that when certain PGM elements naturally attach to each end of a short strand of DNA (these short strands are like antennae on the larger DNA), the strands become ten thousand times more conductive. In essence, the PGMs turn the DNA into superconductors. The double helix of the DNA becomes a highly conductive axis and the DNA becomes a highly conductive molecule. The *Platinum Metals Review,* a specialized journal, has consistently published articles concerning use of platinum, iridium, and other PGMs in the treatment of cancers.[50] The significance in this is that when the DNA of the normal cell is altered by the cancer energy, it starts producing abnormal cancer cells. This DNA distortion can be reversed by the use of the PGMs. They resonate with the defective DNA and create a healing resonance that helps the DNA to revert to its proper form. This treatment obviously does not involve any surgery, radiation, or chemotherapy; it simply involves restructuring the DNA back to its normal structure. This is one of the points of Spiritual Nutrition: to reset the DNA back to its highest phenotypic expression. Although this has not been made public, research by Bristol, Myers and Squibb has found that ruthenium atoms interact with DNA, correcting the malformation in cancer cells.[51] So these monatomic platinum metals are able to somehow communicate with the DNA and the cells in a way that restructures the DNA and transforms it back to a normal structure. Researchers found that iridium and rhodium also have anti-aging properties and these platinum compounds also interacted with the DNA to reprogram the DNA back to normal. It is also known that the gold and the platinum metals in the monatomic high-spin states can activate the endocrine gland system in ways that heighten awareness, perception, and openness to new levels of perception.

The monatomic elements particularly affect the pineal gland, increasing melatonin production, as well as the pituitary gland, increasing serotonin production and activating the body's junk DNA, therefore potentially activating unused parts of the brain. Researchers have shown that the PGMs comprise 5 percent of the brain by dry weight and are composed of these superconductor monatomic elements. One might theorize that the PGMs offer us human beings the power to further activate our Light body. The biochemistry laboratory at the U.S. Naval Air Defense facility found that each of the 70 trillion cells in the human body communicates with each other by superconductor transmission. Researchers found that a unique substance appeared to be the basis of the cellular communication, and that this substance is the white powder, the monatomic iridium or manna. It could be that this monatomic iridium is, in a sense, the conductor of a 70-trillion-piece orchestra.

One published study on the medicinal use of the white powder by pharmaceutical companies shows that it has anti-viral, antibacterial, and anti-cancer properties.[52] We can theorize it has these effects because it reactivates the healthiest vibration of the DNA and therefore strengthens the immune system against viruses, bacteria, and cancer. From a cellular point of view, when the DNA is out of balance, it is distorted and cannot replicate itself correctly. The ability of the cell to take in the Light and the healing energies through the DNA is blocked. Specialized genes called protooncogenes, which carry the electromagnetic patterns that specify the composition of the proteins that encourage cellular growth and the healthy replication of proteins for the immune system, are disrupted. The result is that these protooncogenes, under stress, transmute into oncogenes, which are carcinogenic or cancer-activating genes. According to Dr. Tru Ott, more than fifty different independent research results show that the high-spin monatomic platinum group attaches itself to the DNA strands of the individual chromosomes in individual DNA in the cells. These short-chain DNA fragments greatly enhance the flow of the superconductive energy. In essence, the monatomic platinum group, particularly iridium, turns the DNA into a cosmic acceptor of electron energy and therefore corrects the system. The importance of bringing electrons into the system is why sulfur emphasizes the importance of water as an electron donor as well as the minerals in general. The cosmic flow of the electrons into the DNA helps to rapidly restore the oncogenes back to the normal protooncogenes, or a balanced state. This is a whole different approach to cancer and health because we are not destroying any cells; we are restoring them to their correct, healthy form. This is the basis of the healing aspect of Spiritual Nutrition, which is that we eat in order to rebalance our genes. Once the flow of electrons to the cell is restored, other chronic disease states may clear up because the DNA is operating at its highest level. The overall effects of the PGMs, as far as we can tell, include stimulation of the pineal and pituitary glands, which are known to secrete more than thirty different hormonal secretions and affect brainwaves formation. PGMs may possibly repair the damaged DNA for more than 100 different disease states by increasing the flow of electrons to the DNA as well as increasing the intracellular communication.

Dr. Ott himself has found increased balancing of his own aura, which is known as the Meisner field, by his use of the white powder. The author's personal exploration with iridium (manna) has noted increased psychic sensitivity and a sense that an additional light bulb has been turned on in the system. Once, in a ten-and-a-half-hour meditation, the author was literally out of the body for four hours, physically walking out of his body. The author had never before consciously experienced that for such an extended time. Generally, people have described an inherent sense of well-being, clarity of mind, and basically a sixth chakra openness and vision. Iridium is best not thought of as a drug, but as a supplement taken in small amounts over time to slowly open the third eye. With some exceptions, a one-time dose may not have much effect except when taken during an intense ceremony.

Much of the information on this exciting breakthrough work has been shared with the author by Dr. Tru Ott, who had discovered an ore containing high amounts of iridium. By putting it through some alchemical processes, he has been able to make the white powder iridium – the Philosopher's Stone. Presently this is available for sacred ceremony. We have used it in our White Buffalo Spirit Dance and other ceremonies. The author's personal connection is through his blood lineage to the Levite priesthood going back 3,400 years. In the symbolic giving of the bread of Melchizedek, it is possible that the bread that Abraham received was the white powder. This may just be symbolic or it may be much more. Bethlehem means house of bread. The author doesn't believe that the ancient mystics were just thinking about physical bread when they were talking about this. In the Lord's Prayer is a request to give us our daily bread. We need to think of it as more than just physical bread, but the "bread of presence," as suggested in Samuel 21:6. In this context it was known in Exodus 25:30 through 35:13 and 39:36, Numbers 4:7,

Samuel 21:1–7 as "show-bread." Exodus 25:29–31 states that the "show-bread" was made by Bezaleel at Mt. Horeb. Bezaleel was not a baker; he was a mystic goldsmith chosen by Yah to lead the building of the Ark. "Show-bread" was to be taken with frankincense. In the historical use of the manna, it is taught that the frankincense amplified the use of the manna. We need to understand, as pointed out by Dr. Immanuel Velikovsky, a Jewish psychologist and philosopher, in his book *Ages in Chaos* that the "show-bread" is obviously not white flour, but is silver and gold."[53] In Leviticus 24:5–7, Bezaleel is mentioned as wiping the bread with frankincense. In Egyptian times, particularly in Karnak Temple where we have visited on our Essene Odyssey Tours, there are a number of cone-shaped items made of what appears to be gold, but their description is the "white bread." This "bread of presence" is also called "*shefa* food." *Shefa* in Hebrew means spiritual energy descending from the Divine Presence. In Exodus 16:15, when the Hebrews asked what manna was: "And Moses said unto them, this is the bread which the Lord hath given you to eat." The manna is being described as being white, resembling seed, with the sweet taste like honey (Exodus 16:31). In the *Egyptian Book of the Dead,* which is perhaps the oldest book in the world, it describes that this is the "bread of presence." It points out that the pharaoh seeking Enlightenment, on death, ate the manna or mfkzt before going into the afterlife. There are continually descriptions of the pharaohs ingesting the manna from as far back as 2180 B.C. It was also known as the "powder of projection," by which it was possible to transmute the basic human ignorance into an ingot of spiritual gold. In Corinthians 10:3 manna is referred to as spiritual food, and as the true blood of Eucharist in John 16:31–41. Revelations 2:17 says that "him that overcometh I will give to eat a certain manna and will give him a white stone and in the stone a new name written, which no man knoweth saveth that he might receiveth it."

Lawrence Gardener suggests, in his book *The Lost Secrets of the Sacred Ark,* that the Ark of the Covenant was a battery, among other things. It was constructed as a battery, to provide energy for the transformation of gold into manna. He traces how King Solomon used the Ark to make the sacred white powder for transformation and the Ark was not actually lost after his time, but continued for many generations, to the time of King Hezekiah. The idea of batteries as we know them today was actually used in very ancient times. The "Iraq battery," also known as the Baghdad battery, is thousands of years old. It was found in 1938 by a German archeologist, Wilhelm Koenig, in a clay jar that was 2,240 years old in the national museum of Iraq. It was attributed to the Parthiens and it actually was a battery. All it required was a little bit of vinegar to make it active. They constructed one in 1957 and reported in *Science Digest* that the battery worked. So the Ark being a battery is not a new idea, because the battery didn't start with Count Alesandro Volta, but started quite a while ago in the time of the ancient Sumerians. There is also a picture of one of these batteries at the Hathor Temple in Dendera, Egypt. One interpretation of the Ark then, which is about as far as we can go, is that it was a tremendous force of energy that obviously did burn people up, was used in battle, was used to levitate, but also quite possibly was used by Moses for his alchemical work in making gold. Lawrence Gardner makes a strong case for this in his book.

This takes us back to the principles of Spiritual Nutrition. In pre-Egyptian times they knew that one of the aspects of the individual is what we'd call the Light body or what the Egyptians mainly referred to as *ka*. They knew that both the physical body and the Light body needed to be fed, and the optimal food was the shem-an-na. Manna particularly stimulates the pineal gland. We can think of the pineal gland as a physical structure linking us to the Eternal Truth. It is the organ of inner perception that helps us rise above the limitations of our earthly understandings. In Yogic traditions it is connected to the sixth chakra. It is the metaphoric third eye, in which all our seeing becomes One. The pituitary gland, which is also stimulated by the shem-an-na, is a cosmic receiver. It channels the selected frequencies through its hormonal secretions to the pineal gland, which then amplifies and sends them throughout the body.[54] The pineal gland in this context has control over what will and will not transmit to the rest of the body and what affects consciousness. We can almost think about the pineal as having certain granules like a crystal in a receiving set. Perhaps what is being activated by the shem-an-na, or the manna, are these granules. It is interesting, as a physician, noting that the Caduceus of Hermes has two wings representing the left and right side of the brain and it has a central pillar symbolic of the sushumna through which the awakened Kundalini travels. The two serpents represent the ida and pingala, and in the center is a Light ball that represents the pineal gland and the merging of Shakti and Shiva into the One at the top. This balance with the two wings, two serpents, and the central pineal is known in some Yogic circles as the swan or pramahansa. The three columns (two serpents and central pole) also represent the three columns of the Tree of Life. It is the symbol that represents the fully Awakened Being. The swan symbol also refers to the Medieval Knights of the Swan, representing the highest of the Holy Grail consciousness, such as Sir Perceval and Lohengrin. Inside the king's chamber, inside the king's sarcophagus, the author has personally meditated and experienced moving into other dimensions as through a worm hole into space. Reports, according to *The Lost Secrets of the Sacred Ark*, confirm that the king's chamber appears to have been contrived as a superconductor transporting the pharaoh into other dimensions. Other research suggests that the manna, or shem-an-na, was very much a part of the king's chamber. According to the first pyramid explorers in the ninth century who entered the king's chamber, they found that everything had a layer of mysterious white powdery substance. This is no accident. Research suggests that King Solomon had rediscovered how to make the white powder and that the manna was in the temple chambers of the Great Temple. At the temple of Serabit el Khadim, they found 50 pounds of the manna. Historical information suggests the manna was taken from there to the Great Temple of Solomon. The Ark and the manna seemed associated, and both have been "lost" at one level. Historical accounts of its presence in the First Temple existed all the way down from King Hezekiah to his grandson King Josiah. It was then hidden before Nebuchadnezzar came to invade and destroy. What was very interesting to the author is that after that (around the time of King Herod), the Essenes were found to be a source of this manna. It turns out that the Essenes of Qumran knew how to make it. Research seems to suggest that the Dead Sea contained in some of its aqueducts high-quality natural gold, and the Dead Sea precipitates have 7 percent gold in the monatomic state with 30 percent magnesium. So it appears that the Essenes were able to use a method by which they were able to take it from the conventional gold that they could get out of the water and transform it into the monatomic form of iridium – manna. They may have learned this technique from their Essene brothers, called the Egyptian therapeutae, who were particularly connected with the Karnak Temple in Egypt. This is particularly interesting to the author as an Essene elder. Dr. Tru Ott may be an Essene because of his spiritual understanding, his insights on water and minerals, and bringing this information back to us.

From ancient times, the manna has had an interesting history. The production of this gold dates back to the time of Hathor, in the Hathor

Temple in Dendera, a little north of Luxor, Egypt. The Hathor Temple dates back 4,500 years ago. The mfkzt, found on the wall of the Hathor Temple, suggests that they were making it that early. It has come from Sumeria, to Egyptians, to Melchezidek. Abraham received "the flower stone" (always associated with the righteous) from Melchezidek. He then passed it down through Moses to the Levite House, as supervised by the priest of Zadok. It was reactivated by the Essene communities and is now being reactivated by the contemporary Essenes. The author gives great thanks to Dr. Tru Ott for bringing this information and the manna back to us for our sacred ceremony. This "bread of presence" is the covenant food of the "righteous" (spiritually strong, holy, and awake – not the moralistic meaning it has come to have). This is the true meaning of Spiritual Nutrition. Seek the food that turns us into full superconductors of the cosmic force, literally and figuratively. Manna is the bright substance of God. It is the mineral essence of Spiritual Nutrition.

Conclusion

The important thing about all the minerals is that they are frequencies of consciousness, frequencies of Light, and frequencies of information, which are all needed for spiritual life.

Certain minerals play a more explicit role in the physical, emotional, mental, and spiritual aspects of spiritual life. The most important mineral for spiritual life is the manna, or iridium, which is specifically geared to expanding consciousness and opening up the pituitary and pineal consciousness of the sixth chakra. Phosphorous is the most important mineral after iridium for meditation, for vision, and for expansion of consciousness. After phosphorous comes sulfur, which is said to stimulate the link between the soul and the physical body and align us to integrate our thoughts, emotions, and spirit with material expression. Sulfur is more linked than phosphorous to soul intelligence. Sulfur works in conjunction with manganese. Manganese has been associated with Love and compassion. Sulfur not only supports expanded consciousness, but is involved and is known, in a sense, as a beauty and flexibility mineral along with chlorine, iron, and silica. Sodium is also a very important mineral for tissue and joint flexibility and proper functioning, as are silicon and chlorine. Oxygen and iron help build the physical prana. Iodine, which is most important for the fifth chakra (throat chakra), mediates the general metabolism. Sodium, as a fluid element, helps keep us limber and active and supports the calcium and magnesium in the body to stay in solution, minimizing stiffness. Magnesium is the relaxation mineral and helps to protect us against muscle spasm and against tension and anxiety. Calcium also helps with the structure and is in relationship to magnesium in helping to prevent muscle cramping and spasm.

Appropriate levels of all the minerals are important for optimal spiritual life. The minerals from the physical level of Yoga to the mental and spiritual levels that the author believes are most important in spiritual life are iridium, phosphorous, sulfur, manganese, silicon, sodium, iron, oxygen, potassium, chlorine, iodine, magnesium, and calcium. It is optimal to be inspired to mineralize on all levels of life, to open up all frequencies of consciousness, that we may transcend limitations and identifications with the mind.

Summary, Chapter 28

1. Minerals are one of the deep secrets of Spiritual Nutrition.
2. Minerals are frequencies of Light, frequencies of information, frequencies of consciousness, and frequencies of potential.
3. Minerals take us to the very formation of life.
4. All qualities of positive or negative health can be traced back to having sufficient minerals or a lack of minerals.
5. There is no life without the transfer of electrical energy.
6. Research shows that minerals are essential for plant life, and therefore essential for human life. The role of plants is to convert the minerals into ionic or angstrom-size minerals for humans to absorb.
7. Manna is the ultimate alchemical mineral; it is the Philosopher's Stone. It is the most powerful mineral for transforming consciousness.

Chapter 29

Living Water

The Mystery of Water

The basic substance on which all life is based is water. Without water, life doesn't happen. So, what is the mystery of water? What is the mystery of the chemistry of life? Any farmer can tell you that even a rich soil, if there is not adequate moisture, will not grow seed. The seed will never germinate without proper hydration. The function of water is to bring active natural hydrogen into the cell, so the cell becomes hydrated and the DNA of the nucleus becomes hydrated. The meaning of hydration is hydrogen-donating electrons. This is the secret of water. When we understand this principle, choosing what water will best serve us becomes very simple. One other function of water is its role as a universal solvent to eliminate toxins out of the body and out of the cell. Water also acts as a harmonic communicator through its structure, so that the cells can communicate between each other and intracellularly, through patterned frequencies that the water is able to transmit.

Water, H_2O, contains the two critical elements of life: hydrogen and oxygen. The hydrogen molecule comprises 97 percent of the universe. Why is the hydrogen molecule that is charged to donate electrons so important? Because the chemistry of life depends on the flow of our electrons. Nobel Prize laureate Szent-Györgyi said it very simply: "All of life depends on a small trickle of electrons from the sun." These electrons are stored in water, in live foods, and in the almost magical monatomic element called iridium. As previously discussed, monatomic iridium turns us into a cosmic conductor of free electrons. It is the free electrons that establish, maintain, and create life, as well as create all energy happening intracellularly, extracellularly, and at any level in the body. In essence, a key to understanding nutrition is electron flow. Live foods have the most electrons of any food. Water, when it has a pH of 7.2 or less, has biologically active natural hydrogen, and therefore the most electrons.

The secret to the chemistry of life is the flow of hydrogen-donating electrons and how it affects all intracellular processes. DNA needs the electron energy from the hydrated water to repair it. The flow of hydrogen into the cells from the natural water helps bring oxygen into the cell in the form of H_2O. The flow of hydrogen, which is electron-donating, activates the cytochrome oxidative system in the mitochondria of the cell to make ATP. ATP is the source of biological energy. The biological transmutation principles, discoveries of Dr. Louis Kervan, discussed in Chapter 13, are all based on the flow of hydrogen, and therefore electrons. Once we understand this basic principle that water has to do with hydration (hydra), and that the hydrogen it brings into the system subsequently releases electrons into the system for all energy systems to work, we are then ready to understand the principles of water. Water that is high in hydrogen, and therefore electrons, works as a powerful antioxidant. Water in this context is the universal antioxidant.

Natural water is a high-hydrogen-donating water, such as you see in pristine rainwater. When you distill water, you free up the natural hydrogen in the water, so you can hydrate the cells. Total dissolved solids (TDS) tells you the amount of minerals and other frequencies in the water – pesticides, herbicides, and so forth. Eliminating the discussion about the problem of contaminants in the water, and focusing on the minerals in the water, we can understand the research of Dr. Tru Ott, who the author acknowledges for the insights he so generously shared on water. Dr. Ott's research seems to indicate that if the TDS is greater than 50 ppm (parts per million; also commonly notated as mg/l – milligrams per liter), those total dissolved solids interact and trap the electrons so they cannot be used to transfer to our cells. At a TDS of 200 or above, we would have only a minimal availability of free hydrogen and electrons. Water with a TDS of 200 or greater usually tends to be alkaline. With a TDS of 50 or less, hydronium ions gets formed, resulting in H_3O; this is more actively an electron-donating hydrogen input. This piece of information makes it clear that the most natural and healing water is the most hydrogen-donating water – the water that has the highest amount of electrons. "Mature" distilled water is optimal because it is the highest hydrogen-donating water. Mature water is distilled water that has been restructured in a highly energetic way. The water-maturing process is outlined later in this chapter. Distilled water that is not matured is aggressive water. It is the most powerful natural solvent on the planet. It will pull out toxins and heavy metals, but may also leach much-needed minerals from the body. It does not have the potency, life energy, or safety of mature water.

Once we understand this principle, we can then begin to understand why certain beverages are not particularly conducive to our electron input. For example, caffeine drinks bond to hydrogen and therefore prevent hydration, similar to carbon monoxide (CO) binding to hemoglobin and therefore not allowing the oxygen to function. Carbonated beverages create a similar situation, because they create a chemical acidity that is not a natural hydrogen and they bind the hydrogen. They also create a false acidity by creating a carbonic acid. The implication is that you cannot simply add hydrochloric acid or other acids to water and assume the result will be a hydrated water. Chemicals added to water do not necessarily create a natural hydrogen in the water. Herb tea is a nutritional drink, but not necessarily a hydrating drink. This is because herb teas have a high TDS and the hydrogen ions and electrons are bound up. This doesn't mean that herb teas are bad; it simply means that they are not hydrating. They are for nutritional and herbal effects, not for hydrating. This is an important clarifying point. For example, live juices are very good because they have many minerals and they are hydrating. But they are not necessarily as hydrating as mature distilled water.

In contrast to chemical acids, there are natural acids – lemons, limes, apple cider vinegar, and grapefruit – that are very high in natural electron-donating hydrogen. They acidify the cell cytoplasm inside the cell around the nucleus. Outside the cell, in the extracellular fluid, we have alkalinity, while inside the cell, in the cytoplasm, we have acidity. This polarity between the inside and outside of a cell is normal and healthy; it is what drives the osmotic pressure and creates an electrical gradient. Our saliva pH measures the extracellular pH, and it will become alkaline when we take something like apple cider vinegar, because the vinegar makes the extracellular fluids alkaline, because it is donating its hydrogens to go intracellular, so the intracellular protoplasm becomes more acidic.

Hydration, which requires a TDS of 200 or less, is much more effective when the water has a TDS of 50, or even lower. Healthy water increases alkalinity of the extracellular fluid and increases the acidity of the intracellular fluid. The biggest cause of DNA malfunction is dehydration, which is a lack of hydrogen ions. Hydrogen-deficient DNA is more likely to mutate, and therefore cause cancer. It needs the high electron input to replicate accurately. If the cells are dehydrated, they are unable to supply that electron demand of the DNA. DNA strands are nucleic acids, and therefore inextricably tied to hydrogen molecules and acidic (hydrogen-replenishing) water. When we become toxic, we create an O_2 starvation because the toxicity builds up in the cells and the electrical differential across the cells becomes weakened. The result is that the oxygen cannot get in with the activated water, because there is not enough electron-filled hydrogen inside the cell to draw the oxygen.

The acid-alkaline discussion has a variety of paradoxes, but natural acids and alkaline-producing foods create an increase in hydrogen in the intracellular environment, also known as the cytoplasm. It is the cytoplasm that uses the hydrogen ion to hydrate. Alkaline water also has a hydrogen, but it is minus the electron, and therefore forms a hydroxyl ion, a powerful free radical that, in essence, oxidizes the system. Oxidization increases aging and degeneration. In other words, the alkaline water's hydroxyl ions are electron takers, not donors. The alkaline water, however, may give you a feeling of energy because, as cells are destroyed from free-radical oxidation, they give off energy. Unfortunately, this is short-term energy. This is why some of the research in Japan has suggested that there are long-term deleterious effects from drinking alkaline water, particularly water having a pH of 8.5 or higher. The important point here is not getting confused about the word alkaline. Alkaline water isn't our friend. Naturally purified, acid water is our friend, and it creates an alkaline extracellular fluid and an acid intracellular fluid. As the hydrogen moves intracellularly, it brings oxygen with it and therefore increases the respiration inside the cell and also within the mitochondria. The mitochondria definitely need oxygen to function properly.

The difference between intracellular and extracellular acidity is important to understand. Acid-producing foods, such as meat, alkalinize the cytoplasm and actually deprive the DNA of the hydrogen ions that DNA needs for replication. Meat acidifies the extracellular fluid and alkalinizes the intracellular fluid, which is just the opposite of the direction we want to go. When people (often those with cancer) are told that they are very acidic (using the word "acidic" in the more common way), it is referring to the acidity of the extracellular fluid, not the intracellular fluid.

Research done by Phelps and Kokoschinegg[1] suggests that the temperatures at which water is best structured and carries the most amount of information seem to be at certain points, or "windows." The best known window is at 4°C; another window is at 37.5°C, which is basically body temperature.[2] Some people suggest it is best to leave water out overnight, so it will restructure itself in the moonlight and the cool night temperatures. This is what the author does. It is a beautiful and simple alchemical process. Some people, particularly those who have a kapha constitution, have a little bit of a stress when drinking cold water, so the 37.5°C, approximately body temperature, is a comfortable drinking water high in structured energy.

Often people have extracellular fluids that are quite mineral depleted. The least expensive way to ameliorate this is with ionic salts such as Himalayan, Celtic, Krystal, or Real salt. These salts are non-heated salts. They have ionic bonding. All heated salt becomes covalently bonded. Covalently bonded salt is difficult for the body to absorb intracellularly.

Now that we understand the basic principles of water, let's look at it from a broader perspective. Every function of the human body is connected to the osmotic flow of water within and among cells. This concept of osmotic flow, which means that energy moves from higher points of ionic concentration to lower points of ionic concentration across an energized membrane, is one of the main ways things move in a biological system. It is one of the primary methods of mineral and nutrient transportation at the cell level. It is also the way toxins are removed from cells. The benefits of water are best achieved if the body receives pure mature water on a consistent basis. Pure water is natural high-hydrogen-donor water, 7.2 pH or lower. With age, the body dehydrates if pure, mature, electron-rich water is not given on a regular basis. The work by F. Batmanghelidj, M.D., described in *Your Body's Many Cries for Water,* shows that the ratio of water inside the cell to the water outside changes from 1.1 to 0.8 with age.[3] As the water inside the cell decreases, the mineral concentration of the cell decreases as well, which means we begin to demineralize at the same time we begin to cellularly dehydrate. Along with this process is a decrease in our thirst sensation, so our thirst mechanism does not alert us that we are dehydrating. The only way we can usually reverse or prevent this process is to do the obvious: Drink at least two quarts (64 ounces) of pure water each day. The ratio of intracellular to extracellular remains 1.1 if we remain hydrated. That means even if we don't feel thirsty it is important to drink. Drinking can actually make you feel thirstier. Once we understand these water principles, it becomes clear that carbonated water, caffeine, soda pop, coffee, beer, and alcohol actually dehydrate us. They rob the useful hydrogen from our cells, thus dehydrating us intracellularly.

Functions of Water

The human adult body is approximately two-thirds water – 50 percent of our body weight. In utero, the fetus body is 90 percent water. An infant's body is 75–80 percent water. If we don't hydrate appropriately with H_2O, our water content may drop as low as 40–50 percent with age. One of the main common compounds in the body is water. Fat is 20 percent water, blood is 80 percent water, bone 25 percent, kidneys 80 percent, liver 70 percent, muscles 75 percent, skin 70 percent, and brain 85 percent. This is very important when you realize that 85 percent of the brain is water, and when the brain starts to dehydrate, the neurons dehydrate and shrink. This is a significant contributor to senility.

Water has many important functions in the body beyond its role as a solvent and transporter of substances. The flow of electrons extracellularly to inside the cell activate a string of critical biochemical reactions. For example, these biochemical reactions stimulate seeds to sprout,

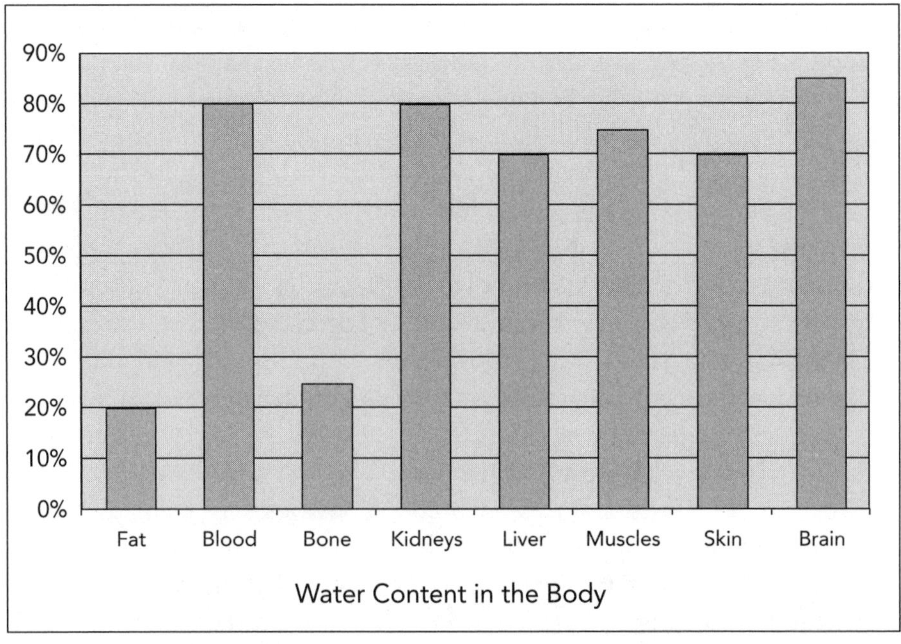

Water Content in the Body

which in turn create an active healing biochemistry in the body, which causes us to feel happy and healthy.

Water acts as a universal solvent, and that is partly how it produces life on the planet. Water's ability to act as a solvent is what makes nutrition work for all living substances. Plants absorb nutrients when they are watered, just like water dissolves nutrients so they can enter our bloodstream. This is basic information, but it becomes clearer, as research has shown, that water acts as a medium that transfers and relays the tiny frequencies of information of DNA from one cell to another. If our water is polluted, meaning what is entering us is polluted with a set of negative frequencies, such as pesticides and herbicides, the water can't really relay accurate intracellular and extracellular information. So, if we are consuming water that is contaminated, it not only brings in poisons but it blocks adequate frequency information extracellularly and intracellularly to and from the DNA.

Water, acting as the solvent, has an electrical and mineral content that helps to regulate all the functions in the body. This is disrupted by dehydration and toxic wastes, which block the information transfer. This disturbance causes a distinct loss of electrical flow and breakdown of the cellular reactions. Dehydration also creates a build-up of extracellular acidity and toxemia, which greatly impairs the electrical energy differentiation between the cells. Because of this, it disorders the intra- and extracellular gradient. Toxemia and extracellular acidity leads to oxygen starvation, damages the DNA, and accelerates aging. It increases free-radical damage and the extracellular acidity blocks the flow of hydrogen into the cells.

Water has many important properties besides its role as a solvent and as a way of bringing nutrients to the cell. As we begin to understand the electrical power of water, we see that the osmotic flow across the cell membrane actually generates hydroelectric energy. This is associated with the flow of electrons coming in with the hydrogen. This electrical energy is stored as ATP and GTP, which are the basic units of biological energy in the body. The hydroelectric energy generated by the hydrated water crossing the cell membrane barrier is also used to produce ATP and GTP. Water has, in a sense, subtle adhesive qualities that help in the bonding and stabilization of the cell membrane structures – it sticks the solid structures of the cell membrane together. Water also has a hydrolytic role and is important in all water-dependent chemical reactions of the body. These are called hydrolytic reactions. It is this hydrolytic role that helps dissolve and free up certain chemicals in the system, and that allows seeds to grow. When the seeds are watered, water activates processes through the hydrolytic role it plays.

A wonderful quality of water is its role as an antioxidant. The beauty of this is that its antioxidant powers reach all water compartments, which is essentially the entire body. The high-electron charge of healthy water brings electrons into the system so they are able to destroy free radical activity. High-electron water neutralizes the negative effect of free radicals, which crave electrons and end up taking them away from cell membranes, causing them to disorganize, thus accelerating the aging process. Water is, in essence, not only the universal solvent, but a universal antioxidant.

Dangers of Dehydration

Water, particularly in the neurons, serves as a way of transporting neurotransmitters to the nerve endings to use for neural transmission. These waterways exist in the neurons and are called microtubules. When the cells of the brain are dehydrated, these microtubules become blocked. Proteins and enzymes work more effectively in water that has a minimal amount of viscosity. This is particularly true for the receptor sites in cell membranes. When these receptor sites, which are three-dimensional molecular formations, become dehydrated, the water develops a higher viscosity, and proteins and enzymes are not able to work at the same level of efficiency both inside and outside the cell. In this way, the solvent power of water regulates all metabolic activities in the body.

When we understand these principles, we begin to better understand what we call the symptoms of dehydration. One is dyspepsia, also known as stomach pain. This results because the cells in the lining of the stomach need to be hydrated and flushed between meals to get rid of acids and to develop a certain level of alkalinity. When we are dehydrated, or we don't drink before meals, we actually cause a thinning of the stomach cell membrane buffer zone and it does not adequately protect our stomachs from the acidity that is naturally secreted. Another symptom of dehydration is rheumatoid pain (or arthritic pain), which has to do with any sort of joint pain because the joints are lubricated by water. The water creates a small film of water that helps lubricate the interface of the joint. During dehydration this lubricating film of water evaporates and the joints rub right on each other. Back pain, particularly lower back pain, and sciatica are often the result of the intervertebral discs becoming dehydrated. These discs normally create a space cushion between the vertebrae by virtue of how much water they can hold. When the discs are dehydrated, 75 percent of the upper body weight that they cushion against begins to bear down on the intervertebrae spaces and put pressure on the intervertebral nerves. This often causes muscle spasms. Usually a few days after we rehydrate, the pressure on the nerves begins to alleviate. The relief of sciatic pain for example, may happen within an hour of rehydrating. Sciatica may be an important sign of dehydration. Heart pain, or angina, is another symptom. When the body is dehydrated the blood flow to the heart is reduced. Headaches and toxic build-up and contracted blood vessels are another symptom, along with dry tongue and constipation. One of the main causes of death in airplanes is dehydration, which causes clots in the legs, which then can migrate to the lungs as pulmonary embolisms.

It is estimated by some scientific sources that 75 percent of Americans are chronically dehydrated. In 37 percent of Americans, the thirst mechanism is so weak from the dehydration that it is mistaken for hunger. In fact, one of the best ways to lose weight is to drink when you are hungry. One glass of water at bedtime can shut down midnight hunger pangs for close to 100 percent of dieters. This both treats the dehydration and gets to the cause of excess appetite, which is mistaking the thirst mechanism for hunger. The disruption of the metabolic system in the body is so significant when we become dehydrated that even with mild dehydration, the metabolism will slow down as much as 3 percent. Dehydration is probably the number one trigger of fatigue in the daytime. A 2 percent drop in body water can so significantly dehydrate the neurons and the passage of neurotransmitters in brain function that we can become fuzzy-headed, develop short-term memory difficulties, have trouble with basic math, and lose focus on the computer screen. This is with only a 2 percent drop. A glass of water can significantly reverse some of the process of dehydration. A study at the University of Washington showed that drinking five glasses of water a day decreases the risk of colon cancer by 35 percent, the risk of breast cancer by 79 percent, and the risk of bladder cancer by 50 percent. This is a significant statement about the importance of water. Dehydration is something that may happen with age, so one of the main anti-aging treatments is drinking adequate water, which is about a half gallon (64 ounces) per day for a 150-pound person.

Best Types of Water for Drinking

When water flows across the cell membrane, it creates hydroelectric energy. As it crosses, it creates a cell membrane electrical differential. The movement of healthy water into the system actually brings energy into the whole system. Energy transmission is not only from the hydrogen ions crossing the cell membrane barrier, but also from the minerals and electrolytes in the water. Although the main idea of drinking water is not for the mineral content, since we can add the minerals in a variety of ways, it is important to remember that all too often high-mineral-content water (high TDS) contains carbonates, nitrates, nitrites, THMs (trihalomethanes), pesticide residue, and other assorted contaminants that are explicitly not good for our system. Electrifying the water may actually activate these deadly pollutants.

Because 20–40 percent of the bottled water in the U.S. is actually tap water (as noted by the Natural Resources Defense Council), this may not be as good a choice as the bottled water label suggests. Carbon-filtered water may vary from marginal to excellent.

Reverse osmosis filtering is good; it doesn't necessarily get all the TDS out or destroy the toxic patterns in the water, as does distilling, but bringing the reverse-osmosis-filtered water TDS level down to 200 makes it second best to mature distilled water. A TDS of 100 is good and 50 is excellent. It will optimize the health quality of the water. Other downsides to reverse osmosis are that the filter membranes really need attention, the process wastes a lot of water, and it is not as good at removing arsenic, nitrites, nitrates, THMs, and fluoride as distilling.

Cosmic Meaning of Water

For someone who has done the Native American Sundance four-year cycle, in which one goes without water or food for four days in the hot desert, water has taken on a new meaning. One develops a very, very strong appreciation for the meaning of water as the source of life. It was during the Sundance that the desire to understand the secret of water was definitely enhanced. In essence, water is like the Divine Presence in living creatures. It vibrates within all life as the blood of Nature that takes on many forms: a glass of water, the vast oceans, turbulent mountain streams, or even the blood in our bodies. Water and life are synonymous. Yet, playing different roles, it remains one essence – moving as the play of consciousness. Symbolically, water may be considered the movement of consciousness on the planet. It is the foundation of life on the Earth and resonates in constant harmony with the universe, holding the solar energy of the sun and stars, the lunar energies, and the energies of the Earth. In that process, water changes its properties. Depending on what energies it absorbs and carries, water can be either a benefit or a harm to people, making them well or ill. It can give off positive or negative energy, healing or disease-producing energy.

Some, such as the great medieval physician Paracelsus, pointed to the incredibly important effects of water for healing. For millennia, water has been seen as a healer. The healing mystery of the *mikvah* (spiritual purification pool) existed for centuries before John the Baptist, the famous Essene teacher who used the River Jordan as a mikvah and who popularized the practice in a way that was incorporated into the Christian tradition as baptism. These uses of water for healing relate to the transformative powers of water to wash away negative vibrations, or karmas, and rebalance our system. The great researchers of water, such as Viktor Schauberger and Johann Grander, have established a three-part understanding of water that clarifies its importance: (1) Water is a carrier of information, both of energy and of specific vibrational information. (2) Water retains that information. Through distilling, we have the ability to erase this information. (3) Water can transfer information. Johann Grander, the inventor of Grander Water, established a very important technique, or system, that not only brings new information in, but prior to that, erases all harmful information that is in the water.

That water is a carrier of information, especially structured water, has been pretty well established, both on a physical level as well as an intuitive level. Water, even if the actual molecules of a substance are not there, as we have learned from homeopathy, can still hold a positive or negative vibration. For example, even if we have filtered out chlorine and fluorine, which are poisons to the system, the water structure still holds their vibration. Until these messages in the water are erased, they may work in a negative way in the system. Such approaches as distilling or the Grander water technology appear to be able to erase all the negative information in the water, which includes the negative information of pesticides, herbicides, chlorine, fluorine, and pathogenic bacteria that have put their vibration into the water. Then, as with the Grander technology, we need to establish a healthy vibration. That healthy vibration is why mature distilled water and the Grander water have been successful in bringing health to people. This healthy vibration information carried in the water is not only for the human body, but actually can help transform the water information in ponds, lakes, and rivers back into a healthy information system that will bring those dead, contaminated waters back to life. This ancient and recent understanding about water has also been made graphic by Masaru Emoto in *The Hidden Messages of Water.* He found that healthy, life-giving, healing water makes beautiful hexagonal crystals, whereas pathogenic water will either not crystallize, such as with chlorinated water, or will make partially deformed crystals.

To deepen our cosmic appreciation of water as it relates to humans, we need to know a little bit more about the chemistry of water. What we need to understand is that water's two hydrogens and one oxygen create what is known as a dipole, the positive pole being the hydrogen atoms, and the negative pole being the oxygen atom. Even though the total molecule is electrically neutral, the water molecule has an inner structure that is in a sense polar. This is why the water molecule is called a dipole. This dipole effect allows water molecules to connect to each other through the hydrogen bonds. Research shows us that usually a water hydration shell, or structured water, has 300–400 water molecules connected together through the hydrogen bonds. This structure is critical for human life because that is how energy is carried. So we really can't say that the formula for water is H_2O. It is really, in a sense, a single, very big molecule, H_2O times 400. The molecular weight of water is not 18, but probably closer to 7,200. Water in its liquid state is a super-molecule. If it were simply the single molecule called H_2O, it would be in a gaseous state. This is the basic physics of water. Because of these hydrogen bonds that link the molecules, water is identified in Nature as a liquid. When we boil water it acts as a foreign body in the system because the body can't recognize it. It is too disorganized. This was the conclusion of the work done by Paul Kouchakoff in 1930.[4] Clean, healthy water as a super-molecule communicates the physical vibrations of the whole cosmos, as well as the spiritual vibrations from the mystical point of view.

The minerals in water become what are known as ions, and the water molecules act, in a sense, as an insulator around them. The more minerals we have, the higher variety of information we have. Information in water is a vibrational frequency. The author had the honor of working with the great crystal researcher, Marcel Vogel, who proved with his scientific instruments that you could send Love into the water and actually create a frequency pattern. You can also send hate into water and create a pattern. This has been validated pictorially in *The Hidden Messages of Water.* Water carries emotions and consciousness. Water also carries the information from pesticides, herbicides, and a variety of toxins that we put into the environment. The more information that is in the water that is dissonant, the more confusing the information becomes. This information is protected by a water molecule coating that some call a "hydration envelope." Chemists term the number of molecules that surround an ion the "hydration number." The higher the TDS, the less clear the information is.

Tests by Engler and Kokoschinegg in 1988 found that not only does water have a structural memory, but it has a structural variability.[5] Because of this structural variability, it can store information over a long period of time. For example, if a drop of water comes through the air as a raindrop and it hits a polluted environment, it will take on the energy of that water pollution, whether it is sulfur dioxide or nitrates. When it hits the rivers, it takes this information into the river and introduces a vibration of pollution. This pattern is one of the ideas of homeopathy: we dynamize it, we dilute it 1:10 or 1:100, and potentize it. We activate the energy by percussing it, which increases the communication of energy. The dilution and activation of river water may mimic this homeopathic procedure and amplify the toxicity of polluted water.

Heating water creates chaos, so the water is less structured. Because of less structure, its ability to transfer information is decreased and the memory is partially erased. The body, in its deepest way of working, does have ability to sort out and protect itself against negative vibrational energies, including negative vibrational water. Samuel Hahnemann, the founder of homeopathy, was very clear about this when he talked about illness as an alteration of information that occurs at a very subtle level.

In summary, water: (1) can carry both positive and negative information; (2) has a memory; (3) has a memory that can be erased; and (4) can transfer that vibrational information. From these insights we understand at another level how to prepare our drinking water, as well as the importance of properly prepared water so that we are not taking in all the negative vibrations of the environment.

Blessing Water

In the Kabbalistic teachings, water is the Light of God made manifest in the physical plane. In this context, water pollution is a worldwide phenomenon and represents both a spiritual and physical crisis. The external water pollution in the oceans, lakes, and rivers mirrors the inner physical and spiritual pollution, as well as our global spiritual crisis.

For thousands of years, Kabbalists have used pure water for physical and spiritual cleansing. This is the mystery of the mikvah water purification ceremony, which usually takes place in a cosmic womb – a sacred pool of running water or a clean stream. Kabbalists have used this ceremony for thousands of years. It connects us to the force of all natural waters and all mikvahs on the planet. In more modern times it was made famous by the Essene John the Baptist, in the River Jordan (we have actually done a mikvah in the River Jordan on our Essene Odyssey Tours). The water's metaphysical and cosmic essence acts as a cosmic solvent to cleanse physical, emotional, mental, and spiritual impurities. Kabbalists teach that water can heal, rejuvenate, and even hold the secret to immortality. Unfortunately, the blood of centuries of war, religious persecution, and environmental pollution from our greed-based economic and corporate systems have disrupted the spiritual powers of water.

One of the ancient and mystical seventy-two names of God, *VAV MEM BET,* has the power to restore water to its original Divine state. The author's choice to release the power of this sacred name, which normally is only released to Essene and Kabbalistic students, is based on the world crises of spiritual and physical pollution. This is a powerful mantra used to rectify the water. The more people who use this prayer, the more opportunity we have to create a morphic field of holiness that will be carried in the power of water throughout Nature and resonate in every living being. Although Kabbalists have a particular prayer over water that energizes it, any loving prayer works. This is also true with our food. As explained in *Conscious Eating,* live food contains structured water, which can best hold the vibration of the prayer, while cooked food is dehydrated and whatever water is left after cooking is disorganized by the heat. So bless the water and food with your Love and appreciation of the Divine. This is the essence of Spiritual Nutrition. This is the essence of food preparation and the essence of water preparation. Our fundamental physical essence is water. So this VAV MEM BET blessing and blessing the water with Love and gratitude literally vibrates on some level in all living beings.

The brilliant work by Masaru Emoto, published in *The Hidden Messages of Water,* supports this approach in a very graphic way.[6] His pictures of water crystallization of healthy water show that water becomes a spiritual message of the cosmos, which is Love and gratitude. This pictorial research shows how water is linked to the fundamental vibration of the human soul. The more we use water in this cosmic way, the more we participate in the collective healing of the planet. In African traditions, if there is too much fire energy (war, hate, greed, violence) in a community, water is used to bring balance. The cosmic healing power of water is known in almost all cultures.

Water is a physical mirror of the soul; it reflects what is in people's souls and the expression of the soul. For example, water exposed to the great classical musical works formed beautiful crystals, but when exposed to hard rock, it became so disorganized it could not even form any crystal shapes. Emoto has concluded from his pictures that when geometric crystals are formed, the water is in alignment with the healing frequencies of Nature and life itself. He found that crystals do not form when the water has been polluted, as in tap water that has been chlorinated. The water in almost all the major cities in the world will not crystallize for this reason. Water exposed to prayer and thought forms of Love and gratitude form beautiful hexagonal crystalline forms. This is also true of unpolluted water found in pristine areas of Nature. When we purify and bless our water, we create water that creates beautiful life force as hexagonal crystals flowing throughout our bodies, blessing every cell and amplifying our healthy soul energies. This blessing is circular because the purer our soul energy, the sweeter the water tastes and the more energetically nourishing it is. Based on the ancient Kabbalistic understanding that we are all One world soul, whenever we bless our water in a conscious heartfelt way, we send out messages of peace, Love, and gratitude, which are linked to the cellular water in all people and in Nature. As we resonate with our mature water we resonate with water everywhere and in that process resonate with all souls and the very soul of the planet. We are actively creating a morphogenic field that unifies the world as One soul knowing its Unity as the Divine Presence.

High-Vibration, Restructured, Mature Water

If we study Nature, we see that rivers, in a sense, self-organize and energetically recharge themselves through spinning motions. In that process, water as the universal solvent, melds with or pulls in nearly every element. Hydrogen, the main ingredient in water, accounts for 97 percent of the molecules found in all the universes. Before our culture lost its ability to sense subtle energetics, water was always seen as central to the shamanic sacred rituals, such as in the mikvah in the Jewish-Kabbalistic-Essene tradition. The idea of drinking sacred waters when visiting an oracle or shrine is part of many cultures, such as the ancient mythology of the Sumerian goddess, Inanna, who had a vase in place of a heart, from which wonderful waters flowed. The idea of going to holy water centers that have been blessed for healing seems to be in many cultures. Dr. Viktor Schauberger (1885–1958), an Austrian who worked in the forest service (and who, one assumes, had much time to be in and think about Nature), is considered the grandfather of understanding water in our modern age. Copying Nature, Dr. Schauberger developed a whole new level of water technology called implosion technology. He understood the ways of Nature and then copied them. Schauberger taught that water is a living, rhythmic substance. He also taught that water needs to be "matured." Water in the high-energetic mature state gives everything needed for life. If the vibrations of water are imbalanced and, in a sense, immature or polluted, water can be diseased and create harm to fish, plants, animals, and humans. Following Schauberger's thinking, we understand that when we still water by damming it, bottling it, or cooking it, the water begins to deteriorate and lose its structure. It becomes gross, degenerate, and therefore potentially harmful to us.

The most structured water is water that is moving, dense, and at 4°C or 37.5°C. Schauberger favored 4°C as the optimum. Wild rivers have this kind of quality. They are cold, they are swirling, and they form there own homeostasis, or equilibrium. When we dam a river, we block the flow of its energy. Because of our lack of culture as human beings, we develop short-sighted engineering projects that cut forests, create dams, and tamper with the circulatory system of our planet. The result, of course, is imbalances that create floods, droughts, and extreme weather problems.

Nature is also mimicked in our own bodies. In May 1998, a short newspaper article in the *Daily Mole* in England reported that medical scientists, in conjunction with aeronautical engineers, at the Imperial College in London,[7] were able to observe that the blood swirls as it rushes through our arteries. In other words, Nature has even designed our internal water systems with vortexes and internal twists in our arteries to mimic and recreate the vortical energies. This system of vortexes gets out of balance and is destroyed when our flow is blocked by a build-up of cholesterol and calcification in the arteries. One of Dr. Schauberger's most interesting observations was that the subtle qualities of water affect humans emotionally, mentally, and even spiritually. Depending on the water, it can either bring an increase in our sense of well-being or a deterioration, not only individually, but to a whole society.

As proven by Dr. Thomas Narvaez, there is a certain energy factor that he called the "vitality factor." It can be increased or decreased in water.[8] This is another way of saying what people have known for thousands of years: Our thoughts not only affect our bodies, but also the physical and emotional bodies around us. Water not only carries information in the sense of frequency information, but, as reported by Dr. William Tiller, Professor Emeritus from Stanford in the Department of Material Sciences, and his co-researcher Walter Dibble, Jr., water is really multidimensional. Dr. Tiller discovered that water can act as a transducer of energy from the subtle frequency domain into the material plane. This means that water is able to transfer prana. High-prana water will transfer energy to those drinking it. The work by Dr. Glen Rein also validates the idea that non-electromagnetic energy – in other words, prana – can be stored in the water, and can later communicate with living cells for healing and building energy. Healing water is high-prana, structured, positive-energy water, as contrasted to diseased water filled with physical pollutants, pesticides, PCBs, and so on, along with negative thoughts, mechanized in a way that minimizes the prana.

We now begin to understand the importance of mature water. It carries emotions and thoughts, as well as prana. When we mature water we are amplifying the positive emotions, the positive thoughts, and the prana. Another way of saying this is that poor water systems, in a sense, compromise the liquid memory as well as water's function as an energy transducer from higher realms down to the three-dimensional realm. A negative example of this is research done by Dr. Schweitzer, who documented the observation that when we buy water in plastic bottles that have been exposed to fluorescent lighting, our lips dry out and become chapped. In other words, the fluorescent lighting on the plastic bottles changes the structure of water such that it actually becomes toxic to us.

Part of understanding this maturing is to understand the process developed by Viktor Schauberger, called implosion technology. To understand implosion, we have to get a little feeling of the opposite – explosion technology. Explosion technology is usually how we access, or convert, the energy stored in our natural resources, to heat our homes, drive our cars, and produce electricity. Explosion technology is how we combust gasoline to drive our cars. We explode atoms to create atomic energy. This is certainly wasteful and dangerous, as well as inefficient, because we lose most of the chemical energy stored in the fuel in this conversion process. Most of this energy is lost through friction resistance, which creates a whole lot of heat. Implosion technology is different because it is based on vortex energy – the same vortex energy described in other parts of this book – and on reversing the flow of the vortex. It, in a sense, is a suctional process in that it causes matter to move inward in a spiral vortex form. It mimics the way Nature works with energy. It also mimics a bathtub, in which the water spirals down the drain. This is vortical energy. Our location in the Earth's rotation will determine the spin direction of these vortexes. This is called the Coriolis Effect. The vortex characteristic is that the outside of the vortex moves slowly, and the center moves faster. The vortex action increases the energy present.

Various experiments (Dr. Franz Popel at Stuttgart Technical University in Germany, in 1952, Alexandersson in 1966, and Coats in 1996) have confirmed this implosion idea.[9] This vortex energy causes a drop in temperature and an increase in density. The vortex motion is the secret for keeping water healthy and disease-free. This is why we observe in Nature that water is spiraling, meandering, crashing, and moving around. Obviously, this suctional force is generated not just in water, but in tornadoes and hurricanes and dust devils, and so forth. It can build very strong energies. Nature doesn't have a lot of straight forms, and these vortexes and spirals help reduce resistance to the flow of things.

The Water Maturing Process

At this point it is helpful to discuss the process of "maturing" water. The first step is to distill the water (even if it has already been reverse-osmosis- or carbon-filtered). The research shows that when you distill water, you destroy its memory. Distilled water is like rainwater in the sense that it has been heated and destructured. Because of the heating of the water, most of the frequencies of possible toxic chemicals are destroyed. Distilled water has the least amount of toxic frequencies of any water. Distilled water is what Viktor Schauberger called "immature" water.

The second step is to restructure (mature) the water to bring it to a state of maximal aliveness and structure it so it will hold new healthy frequencies. Viktor Schauberger suggests that we place the water in an opaque egg-shaped container. The author suggests using clay (glazed or unglazed) or glass (optimally, opaque glass) rather than plastic or metal, which are not as energetically appropriate. The egg shape is effective because it doesn't have corners and crevices where energetic stagnation can occur. (The Tree of Life Foundation's Awakened Living Shoppe can special order beautiful egg-shaped clay vessels for maturing water. However, you can also use a cylinder-shaped glass container that can be purchased locally.)

As the next step, the author suggests adding twelve drops of Active Ionic Minerals™ to 1 gallon of the distilled water. The Active Ionic Minerals™ include fulvic acid, which works in Nature to help plants take in minerals from the soil at the angstrom level, which humans can use. One wants to add enough to create an optimal TDS of 50 – twelve drops per gallon. The mineral component most closely mimics a river-soil-bank energy contribution to water. It also helps to cluster the water and build its electrical charge. As an alternative, one can also use a minimal "smidgen" scoop of ionic, unrefined salt mined from deep salt deposits from ancient ocean beds, such as Himalayan salt (called Krystal Salt™) or Celtic sea salt. This minimum amount of minerals makes the TDS slightly less than 50 and helps to turn the water into an electron-active, hydronium (high-hydrogen), conductive water. The minerals at 50 TDS create, activate, and maximize electron donation to the body. The minerals must be angstrom-size to be absorbed intracellularly. These Himalayan salts are ionic minerals existing at the angstrom or smaller than angstrom-size and are readily assimilable into the system. The twelve drops of Active Ionic Minerals™ (or smidgen of raw salt) brings a certain polarity and electrical energy to the water, while keeping the total TDS less than 50. The 50 TDS is enough to actuate the bioelectrical, antioxidative, and life force energies, without compromising the water's hydrogen molecules' ability to release electron energy. The point to remember here is that the best way to get our minerals is not from water, but from food. The role of water is to bring hydrogen into the system to hydrate the system intracellularly, to eliminate toxins, and to amplify the osmotic process. When the hydrogen moves in, toxins move out.

Next in the restructuring process, add twenty-five drops of Crystal Energy™. Created by Dr. Flanagan, Crystal Energy™ is actually physical micro-crystal clusters that restructure water from its blank state into a highly structured form.

Now, rapidly stir the water with a long wooden spoon until a vortex in the water is created for a few seconds, and then very abruptly stir in the other direction. Then change directions again. This abruptness creates a certain chaos that mimics water in Nature hitting rocks. Creating a vortex in the water energizes the water in a way that brings both electromagnetic and pranic energy into the water we drink. The convection of the spiraling movement keeps the liquid fresh.

Now that the water is restructured, the next step is to bless it and bring in higher etheric energies to the water. This brings new healing memory to the water, filling it with increased prana and energy, helping to erase any possible leftover toxic memory. The blessing of the water can be something simple like placing your hands on the container and saying "I bless this water." The water will then give you whatever you need for your highest physical, emotional, mental, and spiritual needs. As discussed earlier, Kabbalists bless water with VAV MEM BET. Blessing with Love and gratitude in your own way works just fine. These blessings create healing frequencies in the water that are then amplified by the structure, the prana, the electrical energy, and the biomagnetic energy of the water. This is the secret to creating mature, living water.

Next we let the water mature outside for about eight hours overnight, where the evening cools it off to the more concentrated level and it's nurtured by moonlight and Earth energies. Viktor Schauberger recommends keeping it out of the sunlight because he observed that sunlight makes mature water lose its energy. After maturing overnight, storing the water over a Tachyon Silica Disk™ adds more energy and brings the tachyon energy of the cosmos into the water. One can store the water in a refrigerator or in a cool place away from the sun.

This is a little bit of work, but this water ceremony brings you in contact with Nature in a profound and meaningful way. There are mechanical vortex energizers that can create vortexes. Even though it helps the people who don't want to, or can't, do the work, they run about $350 and are not necessary.

The process of culturing immature water into a mature, high-pranic, living, structured water is designed to mimic Nature in its pure state. The distilled water, which is essentially pattern-free, is like the rain falling into the river where the swirling vortexes and curves suck in the pranic energy and the river water is mineralized in its path. The Active Ionic Mineral™ mix, with its fulvic acid, comes from and mimics the soil humus and other humic materials, beneficial bacteria, carbon, and the leaching into the river from the topsoil. Then we bless it like the ancients who purified and healed themselves in the healing waters as our experience of Yah's Grace. We leave it overnight where the rays of the moon, stars, and Earth further energize it with prana and the forces of Nature.

This is the holy secret of cultured, structured, mature water. This is a secret of Nature. This is a secret of how mystical cultures worked in relationship to the wonder of Nature on this planet. As we do this water maturing process, not only are we culturing the water, but we are culturing ourselves to higher ways of Being and living in the world that honor the Divine gift of life and put us in right relationship with it. This process helps us participate in our own healing process and drink our own blessings.

Summary of the Water Maturing Process

1. Distill the water.
2. Place the distilled water in an opaque clay or glass egg- or cylinder-shaped jar.
3. Add 25 drops of Crystal Energy™ and 12 drops of Active Ionic Minerals™.
4. Stir the water in the egg-shaped or cylindrical, opaque container several times in one direction and then the other, with quick reversals.
5. Place hands on the container and bless the water.
6. Let the container filled with water stay outside overnight in view of the moon and stars.
7. Keep the water out of the sun.
8. Store in a cool place over a Tachyon Silica Disk™.
9. For those of you who love esoteric approaches, if there is a favorite place on Earth that you want to connect with, place a pebble from that land inside the egg and it will give off the vibration of that land into the water.

Summary, Chapter 29

1. Water is a carrier of hydrogen ions at a pH of 7.2 or less, in which the hydrogen ions are able to transfer electricity into a living body for its healing effects.
2. Alkaline water carries the hydroxyl ions that are free radicals. These, in the long run, destroy the cells.
3. A total dissolved solids (TDS) measure of 200 is the minimum one needs for healthier water; the optimum is a TDS of 50, where the hydronium ions of water, which are H_3O, are produced. They give us even more electricity.
4. Water carries both the physical, as well as the structural, information of pesticides, herbicides, chlorine, fluorine, and so on. The best way we can release the patterns from the water and access the physical contents in an efficient way is with water distillation, which not only physically removes the contaminants, but destroys the memory of water so that it doesn't act as a negative remedy on us.
5. Water is most structured at 4°C or 37.5°C. In that structured state, which is our biological state as well, in our cells, it holds memory, information, prana, and blessings. Maturing water gives us the ability to erase the negative information and input positive information. This is the secret of many of the "magical waters" that are available today. A simple technique for doing this, for bringing healthy mature water into our system, is water distillation followed by restructuring it with the Active Ionic Minerals™, Crystal Energy™, vortexing it, blessing it, and letting it sit outdoors overnight. Cultured, mature water is filled with Love, gratitude, and healing vibrations.
6. Water is that great communicator of consciousness. What we drink affects our consciousness and our physical, emotional, and mental state. If we want our physical, emotional, and mental state to operate on the purest level, it helps to put in high-vibration water that is as pure as we like our mind to be. By drinking water filled with Love, gratitude, and healing energies, we create a morphic resonance field that creates Love and healing in other people and in all the water bodies of the planet.

7. Healing waters are high-pranic, well-structured, positive-energy waters that are an energetic reflection and transmitter of the cosmic, planetary, and individual soul.
8. Without water there would be no life on this planet. Healthy water brings life and uplifts the spirit. It is the reflection of the wonder of the planetary soul. Polluted water brings disease and misery. It too is a reflection of the planetary soul.

Chapter 30

Go Organic – Authentically

Organic foods are produced without using genetically modified organisms (GMOs) or toxic chemicals. Organic production methods are vastly superior to commercial, chemical-based agriculture in producing foods with optimum nutrition. Foods produced by organic farming practices exhibit improved vitamin and mineral nutrition, as well as superior taste, shelf life, phytochemical and antioxidant content, and stronger and more organized SOEFs.

Investigations are showing that wild-crafted foods (foods harvested from wild plants) have the highest nutritional content, with organic foods next, and conventionally grown foods last. The USDA periodically publishes data on the nutritional content of food. Historically, since the 1940s, each publication of this data shows a decline in the average nutritional content of food. Wheat, for example, used to average a protein content of 19 percent in the 1940s, but today it averages about 12 percent. The same trend exists for fresh fruit and vegetables and other foods. This decline of nutritional content, even of whole, fresh foods, is accompanied by additional losses from cooking and processing. There appears to be a strong correlation between the onset and trend of this decline in nutritional content of foods and the introduction and increasingly heavy reliance on chemical fertilizers, pesticides, deep tillage, gene manipulation, and other practices of conventional agriculture. These practices have been well-documented as leading to a decline in soil quality and loss of topsoil and fertility. Further evidence of this relationship between conventional practices and the decline in nutritional content of foods is the fact that, on a fresh-weight basis – the critical way to look at nutrition for consumers of raw food – organic foods have about twice the vitamin and mineral content as conventional foods. On a dry-weight basis, this difference in nutritional quality is less obvious, so scientists tend to use the dry-weight comparison to support their claim that foods produced by chemical-based farming are not statistically different from organic foods. However, this obscures the fact that food is living nutrients and life-force energy, while food ash is burnt residue and not food. Humans are biologically designed to consume food!

Organic food production plays a very important role in healing our world. Its focus is getting toxic chemicals out of agriculture. Organic farmers are performing an incredibly valuable service to society through their efforts to reform food production methods to better conform to Nature and to protect the environment and human health.

Authentic Food

Going beyond the focus of getting chemicals and GMOs out of our food, *authentic food* production focuses on enhancing the biological quality of food. So we are talking about a new set of concepts that do not dictate what one shouldn't do in order to be considered "organic." Authentic food has to do with what we can do to add energy to food and soil, by Love and devotion in its production. This allows us to absorb the highest energy from our food, which is the main way we derive energy from the planet. Authentic food lifts food to a new level and quality.

The term *authentic* has to do with farmers who are more concerned with quality than with mass production, even if it is organic. It identifies fresh, organic food produced by local growers who want to focus on what they are doing instead of what they are not doing. The concept of authentic goes right down to the fundamentals of how food was offered in the past. These principles are:

- All food is produced by the growers who sell it.
- Fresh fruits and vegetables are produced within a 50- to 150-mile radius of the place of their final sale.
- Seed and storage crops are produced within a 300-mile radius of their final sale.
- The growers' fields and greenhouses are open for inspection at any time, and the customers themselves can be the certifiers of their food.

- All of the agricultural practices used on the farm selling "authentic" are chosen to produce food at the highest nutritional and vibrational qualities.
- Soils are nourished as they are in the natural world, with farm-derived organic matter, minerals, and particles from ground rot.
- Green manures and cover crops are included with the broadly based crop rotations to maintain biodiversity.
- A pest-positive rather than pest-negative philosophy is involved, recognizing that pests appear when there is an imbalance and focusing on how to correct the cause of the problem rather than treating the symptoms. This is a holistic approach to farming. The goal, of course, is vigorous, healthy crops that are endowed with inherent powers to resist pests.
- Any authentic farm or garden land is a zone free of genetically modified organisms.

The definition of authentic farming obviously stresses local, seller-grown, fresh, organic food – concepts that are not so easy for agribusiness to adopt. This supports the health of the ecosystem, our bodies, and the local economy. Because many of us to do not have access to authentic foods in contemporary society, one solution is to grow your own. For most people at this point, it is appropriate to at least shift to buying organic food from your local health food store. Although authentic food is at the cutting edge beyond organic, the organic movement plays an incredibly important role in the healing of the planet. It is of prime importance that everyone go 100 percent organic.

Living Soil

The entire world's food supply depends on the quality of the soil. Topsoil is the foundation for the food chain, especially of the vegan diet. The plants we eat receive their nourishment from the soil. So if the soil has been depleted by overuse or poisoned by chemicals, the nutrient content in the plants we eat will suffer. When plants have depleted nutrients and life force, we will too. On the other hand, living soil, soil rich in microorganisms with strong SOEFs, will yield plants that are full conductors of the cosmic prana. Eating these plants will harmonize with and strengthen our SOEFs and health in general.

Unless we pay attention to our harmony with our topsoil, we humans, who are created out of the dust of the Earth, will return much sooner to personally refertilize it.

Pesticide Pestilence

Presently more than 20 percent of the pesticides currently registered in the U.S. are linked to cancer, birth defects, developmental harm, and central nervous system damage.

Let us understand, pesticides are designed to kill living creatures, and human beings are living creatures. The organic movement is one of the most important things we have to begin to rectify the destruction of our soils, the very high rate of cancer in children and adults, and the literal poisoning of the planet. The only people who benefit from this pollution are the corporations that profit directly from the sale of chemicals and indirectly from the suffering of others.

Some research has shown that when children are put on an organic diet, there is a 50 percent cure rate of hyperactivity, without doing anything else. This is not surprising since most pesticides and herbicides are neurotoxins, and developing nervous systems are more vulnerable to these brain and nervous system poisons. More than 12,000 children in the U.S. are diagnosed with cancer every year. Cancer is now the second leading cause of death, after suicide, for children under age 15. These high cancer rates in children were unheard of before this era of pesticides, herbicides, and genetically engineered food.

One of the most significant effects of an organic vegan diet is the tremendous health benefit of stopping the chronic poisoning from pesticide intake. Unless one eats organic fruits and vegetables, one is continually exposed to pesticides. One of the most important pathological effects of these toxins, besides initiating cancer, is the varying levels of neurotoxicity to the brain and the rest of the nervous system. These have more subtle symptoms such as reduced mental functioning, decreased mental clarity, poor concentration, and, the author believes, hyperactivity and Attention Deficit Disorder (ADD). Some recent research has linked a higher rate of Parkinson's disease, a brain disease, to those people who have a history of higher pesticide exposure. So we do have some very suggestive evidence that the use of pesticides and herbicides really affects our mental function and brain physiology, including increasing the incidence of Parkinson's. This is not exactly a surprise when you realize that pesticides are *designed* as neurotoxins. Does it surprise us to think that we are biologically similar to the pests that we are trying to eliminate? Our nervous systems are more sophisticated, and may take longer to poison, but it still happens.

Scientists can pretend to discern "safe" levels for an individual chemical, but in fact, there are no "safe" levels. Certain categories of dangerous chemicals, such as those that cause cancer and disrupt nervous system and hormone function, need to be immediately discontinued if we are to survive as a species.

The amazing observation is that pesticides do not even achieve their stated purpose, yet we still are willing to risk our lives to use them. Dr. David Pimentel of Cornell University, an entomologist and one of the world's leading agricultural experts, estimates that more than 500 species of insects are now resistant to pesticides. It is no accident that crops destroyed by insects have nearly doubled during the last forty years, in spite of an almost tenfold increase in the amount and toxicity of insecticides.

Even on a cost-benefit versus health approach, the use of pesticides comes out on the negative side of things. According to Dr. Pimentel, pesticides cost the nation $8 billion annually in public health expenditures, not to mention the unmeasured losses from groundwater decontamination, fish kills, bird kills, and domestic animal deaths.

In summary, pesticides can affect every living organism. Humans are no exception. The more detrimental effects of pesticides, herbicides, and fungicides include: cancer, nervous system disorders, birth defects, and alterations of DNA; liver, kidney, lung, and reproductive system problems; and an overall disruption of ecological cycles on the planet. Pesticide usage is a major public health problem worldwide. Pesticide usage not only leads to disease, but directly destroys the life force of the soil. It reflects a consciousness that is completely out of touch with the laws of Nature.

Protecting Against Food Chemicalization

We have the power to refuse to consume what is detrimental to our health and to the planet. Since there is very little real control and monitoring by the U.S. government or by the chemical companies, the responsibility for our health lies with us, as it always has. Let us put our money where our mouths are. Buy organic produce whenever possible.

Buying organic not only helps us avoid pesticide poisoning, but also supports the organic farmers who are rebuilding the soil. The more organic farmers there are, the less the organic produce will cost. According to a study at Tufts University, organic produce has a nutrient content approximately 88 percent higher than commercially grown produce. Other studies suggest organic food has even higher percentages of nutrients than commercially grown food. This means that, by buying organic produce, we actually get more for our money and for our health.

The good news is that many people are listening. The total of organic products sold has grown at a rate of about 20 percent per year in recent years, and many supermarkets now stock organic products. Please support this positive shift in the supermarkets, and buy organic foods.

We have the power to restore the world to one that is aligned with the healing harmony of the universe. Let us do it.

Genetically Engineered Foods – "If It's Not Broken, Don't Fix It"

Genetically engineered (GE) foods provide a more significant threat to our subtle worldwide ecosystems than even pesticides and herbicides. John Hagelin, an award-winning quantum physicist and candidate for president on the Natural Law Party ticket, said, "When genetic engineers disregard the genetic boundaries set in place by Natural law, they run the risk of destroying our genetic encyclopedia, compromising the richness of our biodiversity, creating a genetic soup. What this means for the future of our ecosystem, no one knows." Dr. John Fagan, internationally recognized molecular biologist and former genetic engineer, says, "We are living today in a very delicate time, one that is reminiscent of the birth of the nuclear era, when mankind stood on the threshold of a new technology. No one knew that nuclear power would bring us to the brink of annihilation or fill our planet with highly toxic radioactive waste. We are so excited by the power of a new discovery that we leaped ahead blindly, and without caution. Today the situation with genetic engineering is perhaps even more grave because this technology acts on the very blueprint of life itself." When you do not know what you are doing, and you insist on meddling, you have the potential to create a great deal of damage. There is an old saying, "If it's not broken, don't fix it."

More than two-thirds of food on grocery shelves contains genetically engineered ingredients. In 1996 and 1997, there were nineteen genetically engineered products on the market. Now there are more than thirty. These ingredients clearly have not been adequately tested for their impact on human health. The dangers of GE foods – also known as GMOs, genetically modified organisms – are multiple.

Once a gene is inserted into an organism, it can cause unanticipated side effects. Mutations and side effects can cause GE foods to contain toxins and allergens, and to be reduced in nutritional value.

GE foods have potential to damage the ecosystem, harm wildlife, and change the natural habitat. Our plant and animal species have evolved over millions of years, and introducing genetically engineered species upsets the delicate balance of the ecology.

Gene pollution may never be able to be cleaned up.

The use of GE crops increases pesticide pollution of food and water supplies. Approximately 57 percent of the research done by biotechnology companies is done to support development of plants that can tolerate larger amounts of herbicides.

GE foods may cause unpredictable, permanent changes in the nature of our food. The essential problem is that the genetic structures of our plants and animals have been nourishing the human race for thousands of years. Because genetic engineering is far from an exact science, the new genetic structure of a plant could give rise to unusual proteins that could really cause a problem for humans and our health.

GE foods may be missing important food elements or have changes in the nutrient ratios. Genetic engineering may accidentally or intentionally remove or deactivate substances in food that the engineers may consider undesirable in food. The engineered food, or the missing substances, may have qualities that we do not yet understand.

The use of GE foods results in decreased effectiveness of antibiotics. It is now commonplace in genetic engineering to introduce antibiotics in genes as a marker to indicate that the organism has been successfully engineered. These gene markers have the potential to create bacterial mutations that are resistant to antibiotics and therefore undermine the effectiveness of antibiotics.

Harmful effects may not be discovered for years, in the sense that we do not have an idea of what can potentially happen as we introduce these GE foods into our diet. There are no long-term studies to prove the safety of genetically altered foods.

GMOs can have unanticipated negative ecological impact. For example, some genetically engineered bacteria looked like they were useful in one limited way, but independent researchers have discovered that they are capable of making the land infertile. If it is not obvious, it should be – we cannot predict the effect of a new microorganism on the ecology and the environment. "If it's not broken, don't fix it."

GE foods may create newer and higher levels of toxins in the environment. Many plants produce a variety of compounds that are toxic to humans or alter the food quality. Generally speaking, these toxic elements do not cause problems in the levels normally found in plants, unless we consume those plants in large quantities. The practice of combining plant and animal species in engineered foods has the potential to create new and unpredictable levels of toxins. Even the FDA and the EPA now classify as insecticides certain corn and potato strains that are engineered to produce toxins that will kill insects. These plants are no longer even classified as vegetables!

One of the biggest problems with genetically engineered plants is their presumed ability to tolerate unlimited pesticides. In the '60s, the "green revolution" created higher crop yield at first, but then serious problems surfaced over time. With large-scale use of high-yield seed, higher levels of fertilizers and pesticides had to be used. Both of these inputs are costly, ecologically devastating, and damaging to the health of farm workers. The aggressive use of monoculture production destroyed the diversity of local ecologies, affected traditional crop varieties, and led to permanent loss of crop diversity. Because the need for increased irrigation used groundwater supplies faster than they were replenished, a soil erosion problem developed. Then, after a few years, those "disease-resistant" crops began to become infected. Since the green revolution (over the last forty years), the use of pesticides in some places has undergone a nearly tenfold increase and the crops destroyed by insects have nearly doubled. There are now more than 500 species of insects that are pesticide-resistant.

These crops, because they are commercially grown, are less nutritious. Some studies have found a reduction in IQ of up to ten points in the generation of children brought up on these "green revolution" foods. Genetically engineered crops – because they are so strongly tied to a monoculture approach, chemical fertilizers, herbicides, and pesticides – will probably cause an increase in all of the health and mental health problems associated with the "green revolution," and possibly on a grander and more serious scale, because the gene pool will have been disrupted.

The possibility of the danger of eating GE foods and/or foods that contain genetically modified substances was highlighted by the research of Dr. Arpad Pasztai, a senior scientist at the Rowett Research Institute in Aberdeen, Scotland. He fed genetically engineered potatoes to rats. The rats developed smaller hearts, livers, and brains, and had weaker immune systems. Some rats showed significant brain shrinkage after only ten days of eating genetically modified potatoes. This the most significant piece of data on the health dangers of GMOs – and an ominous warning.

Public relations hacks for GE foods talk about the importance of "feeding the world's hungry." This is a cruel joke. The GE crops are primarily intended as feed for livestock, not to provide nutrition to people. Contrary to corporate public relations spiels about producing more per acre, genetically modified soybeans, for example, actually produce approximately 4 percent less than conventional varieties, according to the research of agronomy professor Ed Oplinger at the University of Wisconsin. His study covered soybean yields in twelve U.S. states. Other studies with Monsanto's transgenic soybeans showed 10 percent less productivity, compared to conventional varieties.

Part of the argument against genetically engineered food and for going organic is the importance of preserving heirloom seeds, which contain the original seed genetics. Heirloom seeds also work on a deeper energetic soul level. They contain the entire history of a people and of a land. These seeds nourish our souls and strengthen our connection to the land. They are bred for nourishing people, not for making money. This shamanistic, Earth-based understanding is in sharp contrast with the intent of the genetic engineering corporations.

So why does the corporate world push a technology that breeds ill health, is a danger to the world ecology, does not feed the world's poor and hungry, and is actually less economically productive per acre? Robert T. Frailey, when he was Co-President of Monsanto's agricultural sector, put it bluntly: "It's really a consolidation of the entire food chain."[1] GE foods are created not because of health or productivity factors, but because they are patentable and give international corporations an opportunity to try to control the food chain and the world population that depends on it for sustenance.

Irradiated Foods – Another Biohazard

Irradiated food is a biohazard. Irradiating food completely disorganizes the energetic field. (This is also true of microwaved food.) Although it is claimed that irradiation kills all the infecting bacteria, even *E. coli,* the bacterium most often cited when arguing for the use of food irradiation, has evolved new forms that are radiation-resistant. In other cases, irradiation does not get rid of the toxins that the bacteria produce. Botulism is one of those cases where the toxin produced is worse than the bacteria itself.

There is no solid evidence to show that eating irradiated food is safe, but there is some evidence to show that it has specific dangers. Food is irradiated with gamma rays. The gamma rays break up the molecular structure of the food and create free radicals. The free radicals react with the food to form new chemical substances called "radiolytic products." Some of these include formaldehyde, benzene, formic acid, and quinones, which are known to be harmful to human health. In one experiment, for example, levels of benzene, a known carcinogen, were seven times higher in irradiated beef than in non-irradiated beef. Some of these radiolytic products are unique to the irradiation process and have not been adequately identified or tested for toxicity.

Irradiating food destroys somewhere between 20 and 80 percent of the vitamins, including A, B_2, B_3, B_6, B_{12}, folic acid, C, E, and K. Amino acids and essential fatty acids are also destroyed. Enzymes, of course, are destroyed, as are the bio-photons.

In addition, food irradiation plants are unsafe. Radioactive accidents have already happened at the few food-irradiation plants that exist in this country and worldwide.

In attempting to determine what to do about food irradiation, the FDA reviewed 441 toxicity studies. The chairperson in charge of new food additives at the FDA, Dr. Marcia van Gemert, testified that all 441 of the studies were flawed. The FDA, however, determined that at least five studies were acceptable under 1980 toxicological standards. The Department of Preventive Medicine and Community Health of the New Jersey Medical School found that two of these studies were methodologically flawed. In one of the five studies, animals eating a diet of irradiated food experienced weight loss and increased miscarriages, possibly due to radiation-induced vitamin E deficiency. The remaining two of the five studies used irradiated food at levels below the FDA-approved 100,000 rads and thus cannot be used to scientifically justify food irradiation at the level the FDA approved. Nevertheless, with none of the five studies supporting the use of food irradiation, the FDA has approved the use of food irradiation in our food supply. This includes vegetables, fruits, spices, and a variety of flesh foods.

This book is not intended to focus on the issue of food irradiation, except to say that it significantly decreases the quality and energy of food. With the Spiritual Nutrition approach, which avoids food irradiation, we can have a healthy diet that will sustain our lives and the quality of our own DNA.

Going Organic

The poisoning of our global environment is a threat that has to be faced directly. If we are to stand up to corporate practices that threaten the health of farmers, rural communities, consumers, and ecosystems, we must vote with our mouths. By refusing to eat irradiated foods, commercially grown pesticided and herbicided foods, and genetically engineered food, we are making a very clear statement to the corporations and the governments that are influenced by corporate donations. We are saying that we, the public, will not buy your story or your food; we will not support the poisoning of the plants and all living creatures on this Earth. For this reason, the author cannot stress strongly enough the importance of going 100 percent (or close to 100 percent) organic in our food choices. At the Tree of Life Café, we guarantee 100 percent organic live food.

There is no shortcut to health and happiness except by following the natural and spiritual laws of life to the best of one's ability and present knowledge. Humanity and all sentient beings are sustained by the same radiating Light of the universe within and without us. If we are to be in harmony with this Light as it comes to us through the natural interplay of earth, water, air, and fire via the vegetable kingdom, then it is essential to choose to eat organic, authentic agricultural products that are grown in the fullness of this Light. We should be very cautious when we attempt to tamper with Nature.

By eating authentic, organic, whole foods the way Nature has given them to us, we have a sound way of eating that begins to bring us back to health, for ourselves and for the planet.

Summary, Chapter 30

1. Eating organic and authentic foods is a powerful way to protect our health, our children's health, and the health of the planet.
2. Genetically engineered foods are a potential danger to our personal health and the ecological balance of the planet.
3. Contrary to fraudulent public relations marketing, genetically engineered crops are less productive per acre than organic crops.

Note: The information presented in this chapter is a condensed version of Chapter 4 in *Rainbow Green Live-Food Cuisine* by Gabriel Cousens, M.D.

Chapter 31

A Conscious Approach to an Evolutionary Diet

Purpose of Diet

To design a diet for ourselves requires a clarity of purpose. Just as an architect does not design a building without the purpose of the building in mind, to transcend the unconscious gobbling of our food we also need a perspective of what we want from our diet. Six purposes of diet have been developed in this book. We practice Spiritual Nutrition to:

- Aid our spiritual unfolding in the context of the Six Foundations.
- Increase our ability to assimilate, store, conduct, and transmit the cosmic, heightened, evolutionary energies now being generated on our planet and the intensified energy released by our own spiritual development, so that these energies either activate and increase our energy potential for the Kundalini awakening or further support the already awakened Kundalini that acts as a spiritualizing force in our body-mind-spirit complex.
- Maintain, purify, and honor the body as the physical aspect of the spirit and as the temple for the spirit in a way that keeps our minds clear and our bodies physically able to cope with the demands of the spiritual process of Whole Person Enlightenment.
- Balance our individual chakras, balance the chakras as a whole system, and directly aid our meditation process.
- Use the process of developing an individualized diet for spiritual life, which we call the art of Spiritual Nutrition, as a spiritual practice in itself.
- Honor and enhance our food as a main interface between

ourselves and Nature, bringing us into harmony with Nature and its universal laws, and with the ecological issues of food and peace on our planet.

Foundations of the Spiritual Nutrition Approach

There are several key nutritional aspects to the Spiritual Nutrition approach that can be of benefit to most everyone. To review, they are:

- Live foods – raw, whole, unprocessed
- Veganism – diet free from flesh, dairy, and eggs
- Undereating – calorie restriction that supports optimal phenotypic gene expression
- Sattvic, holy diet that quiets the mind
- Low-glycemic – minimizing high-sugar foods
- Organic – foods that do not contain chemical pesticides, herbicides, or fertilizers, and are not genetically engineered or irradiated
- High-mineral – taking in the necessary frequencies of Light
- Well hydrated – foods high in the hydrogen offered by structured water
- Individualized to your constitution
- Spiritual Fasting – green juice fasting in the context of meditation and spiritual practice, several times per year

Our Own Individualized Optimal Diet

There are many factors affecting our development of an individualized diet: our dosha constitution, the principle of biochemical individuality expressed as fast- or slow-oxidizer and parasympathetic or sympathetic types, the seasons, the political and social climate, our age, the amount we meditate each day, the level of our Kundalini energy, our degree of physical activity, the level of predictability of our daily needs, our state of digestion and general health, our present stage of detoxification, and our present diet. This is why computer diets have limited value. There is a biological computer system, however, that is effective – one that gives us the answers in terms of our appetite, tastes, food desires and aversions, instincts, impulses, and intuition. It is the computer of our own inner sensitivity. As with any computer, we have to learn how to work with it consciously. In this computer the data of our own direct experience as to what, when, how, and how much we eat is the most important. There is no one diet for everyone. Books such as this one can only be guidelines for where to start in our personal exploration. To do this effectively, we must become our own laboratory with ourselves as the researcher as well as the subject being researched. *Conscious Eating* and *Rainbow Green Live-Food Cuisine* have detailed discussions on how to individualize one's diet.

As in any experiment, we have to limit the variables to obtain clear data. Four basic variables are the time we eat, the environment in which we eat, how much we eat, and what we eat.

Regular timing of meals is important. Regularity helps the body adjust its physiology to those times. Some people recommend no breakfast, a big lunch, and medium dinner. Others, such as certain groups of Buddhists, do not eat after 4 P.M. The author once met a French healer who discovered an ancient system that dictated we could eat a large meal in the morning, and another large meal for lunch, and we would have excellent health as long as we did not eat or drink anything after 2 P.M. He had hundreds of case histories to support his point. Most systems agree that between 12 noon and 2 P.M. is the time to have the main meal, or even the only meal, of the day. It is the time when the pitta, or digestive forces, are the strongest. The author has found if he eats more than a minimal supper or eats too late (later than one hour before sunset), it is harder to get up early in the morning for Yoga, pranayama, and meditation. But three or four hours later, when he is finished meditating, his body is hungry. The key to timing is not to listen to the experts but learn to eat when we are hungry and drink when we are thirsty. The corollary to this is to refrain from eating and drinking when not hungry or thirsty. We have to discover for ourselves when and how much to eat at a particular time of day. The general recommendations for the timing and amounts can serve as a starting place for our experiments in self-observation. A stable mental and emotional environment is also important for obtaining clear information. By not eating when emotionally upset, by daily meditating before meals, and eating in a calm, quiet environment, we help the emotional factors influencing digestion to become consistent.

How much we eat, another important nutritional factor, is part of the art of Spiritual Nutrition that requires particular attention. No matter what we eat, if it is excessive, we will not get clear information about that particular food. It is good to allow time for complete digestion between meals so we can observe the whole digestive process of the food. Unless we have hypoglycemia, it is good to allow at least four to five hours between meals. How good a food is goes beyond the immediate taste. It needs to be good for us in the whole process of digestion, assimilation, energization, and excretion. It must be good for us all day. Some diet changes are deceptive in that they initially make us feel good, but after a few months they turn out to be toxic to us. For example, many people do well initially on the traditionally recommended high-protein, hypoglycemia, or weight-loss diet, but they often call the Tree of Life two months later asking for help in finding some other diet because they feel so toxic. A meat diet, although detrimental in the long run, can also sometimes make us feel good initially because the excess protein reverses the uncomfortable detoxification process that we may be experiencing, and the uric acid in meat, which is close to caffeine in its structure, can act as a temporary stimulant. It is said that Gandhi, in order to observe the long-term effects of each change in diet, would only change his diet every four months.

The sensory effects that give us immediate feedback about whether we are eating the wrong food or amount are such basics as a full stomach, gas and bloating from putrefaction and fermentation, increased mucus production, sluggish mind, and a feeling of enervation (decrease in nerve energy leading to toxicity). The data on this level are not subtle if we are willing to pay attention.

At the level of the more refined sensitivity of our spiritual unfolding, some additional criteria are of value. It is useful to eat what increases our experience of our Love Communion with God. If the energy in our body is unimpeded by our diet pattern so that we can focus on the Communion, then we are on the right track. If we are eating too much or eating the wrong foods, too much energy is involved in digesting and assimilating the foods. This draws energy away from our focus on the Communion. If our Love Communion is blocked before, during, or after the meal, this is feedback that we are not on the right track. If our ability to sustain meditation is enhanced, then the diet is appropriate for us. If, while preparing and eating our food, we experience a greater harmony with the forces of Nature, this is a sign of right diet. If we experience ourselves as becoming better and better superconductors of the cosmic energy, this is positive feedback. If our experience of the movement of Kundalini in the body is blocked, this is feedback that we need to reconsider our program. In general, if our diet obstructs the pranic flow of energy in the body, whether or not the Kundalini is awakened, so that our mind and body feel sluggish and unclear in a way that we are not able to focus our attention on the Divine, the diet is not appropriate.

Self-Awareness and the Individualized Diet

As our awareness expands, the physical needs of our body change. It is important to be able to sense when to make a dietary shift to maintain harmony with our spiritual evolution. Intuition, guided by subtle changes in taste, response to textures, quantities, and appetite for different types of foods is key for this. It requires that we be free enough to distinguish between immediate needs and responses secondary to habitual eating patterns, ego needs, and peer pressure. These decisions to eat less or differently are not meant to deprive us but to teach us to eat in harmony with our evolutionary unfolding. This is the art of Spiritual Nutrition.

The art of Spiritual Nutrition is the process of self-study applied in the exploration of the basic guidelines discussed in this book and in the context of a full spiritual life. The creation of right diet is the letting go of nonfunctional patterns of relating to food. For many of us, food is associated with psychological cues. For example, as a kid, the author used to love his mother's cherry pie. Over the years, this food transference, psychological attachment to a particular food based on a previous psychologically associated experience, has led the author to order several organic, baked cherry pies that, according to his empirical post-eating response, were not appropriate for him to be eating. Because of the negative feedback of the post-eating experiences and his awareness of the transference, the author has overcome his desire for cherry pie. In loftier terms, he has transcended his desire for (or, in a different case, aversion to) a psychologically associated food and is no longer controlled by it. Through self-study, we are able to sort out the signals that have a nonnutritional basis. In this process we become more aware of our subtle inputs, food transferences, and post-eating results. This constant attunement to our overall food and energy needs allows us to shift our diet to be in harmony with our evolving process. It allows us to be free to reorganize it at each stage of spiritual evolution to enhance greater states of health and awareness.

Some of this shifting of diet seems to happen spontaneously as our consciousness evolves. This was suggested by a 1986 survey the author made in conjunction with MSH Associates, who have developed a program called Synchronicity, the Recognitions Experience that helps the expansion of consciousness by the use of holographically programmed audiotapes. The survey was filled out by 110 people who had been in the program for three to eighteen months. The main finding was that 63 percent were conscious of making some degree of shift toward a healthier diet. The majority of these shifts seemed to be away from junk foods and other foods of the bioacidic category, toward healthier foods within their established diet pattern. Eight percent of the group described a major shift toward eating less food and 7 percent became vegetarians. Before they started on the Recognitions Experience, 47 percent were using alcohol, coffee, or tobacco. In this survey, 35 percent had decreased their use of these toxins. In the Recognitions Experience, there was no formal teaching about diet. These people were not told in advance that a study would be done. It is the author's feeling that the higher evolutionary forces naturally draw us in the direction of health. The art of Spiritual Nutrition is the conscious act of cooperating with this natural transition.

An approach to right diet that involves self-study and cultivation of an artful self-awareness becomes a spiritual practice on its own. It is part of the skill of self-awareness required to develop a right life in harmony with all our worldly functions such as work, play, family, and world social responsibility.

Transitional Detoxification Phenomena

As we shift to healthier diets, the stored toxins in the system begin to be excreted. This is called detoxification. As part of our nutritional and environmental background, it can be safely said that all of us have some degree of toxicity. In a simplistic but accurate way, detoxification can be understood via the analogy of diffusion. In the process of diffusion, elements move from areas of higher concentration to areas of lower concentration. Nutrients and toxins flow into the blood and lymph systems from the intestinal tract. If they are in higher concentrations than the toxins in the cells, they "diffuse" their way into the cells and even precipitate as crystals or bind to intracellular protein complexes, which is how the cell tries to keep them out of circulation. When we decrease our toxicity level by a cleansing diet or fasting, the diffusion concentrations shift and there are fewer toxins in the bloodstream than inside the cells. The result is that toxins are drawn out of the cells into the bloodstream and lymph systems. This essentially corresponds to the process described by the Wendt Doctrine, in which the protein-clogged basement membranes begin to clear when the protein in the diet is decreased. The toxins that come out of the cells are excreted from the body via the eliminative organs (kidneys, lungs, skin, and bowels).

In the process of this toxin elimination, so much toxic substance is in the blood and lymph that we may not feel or smell good. Many people, if they detoxify too quickly, have a healing crisis in which they appear to get sick. Disease, as defined by J. H. Tilden, M.D., is simply a toxemia crisis.[1] The crisis usually occurs when the vitality of the body reaches a point where there is enough energy to throw off the toxins. The crisis may last for a three-day cycle or it may go on for weeks. The author's clinical experience is that, if a person slowly detoxifies over the years rather than trying to do it in a few months, the discomfort of a major healing crisis is minimized. The recovery from the healing crisis is accelerated by daily enemas, plenty of rest, alkalinizing fluids such as vegetable juices, and maintaining a positive attitude. After the healing crisis passes, we level off at a feeling of well-being correlated to the diet level at which we are eating. At each new stage of purity we experience more flow of energy, Love, and Light in our system, and more energy is available for the focus on the transcendental awareness that is so important for our spiritual evolvement.

Although we are focusing on diet, the key to toxemia is more than diet. Dr. Tilden points out that any habit of body or mind that decreases our nerve energy (enervation) results in the build-up of toxins. This is because enervation slows or stops the natural body process of detoxifying, and therefore results in the accumulation of toxins in the system.[2] Poor diet is one of the major stresses on the system, but to really detoxify and create harmonious health, we need to develop a right life that keeps us totally in Communion with the Divine. A good detoxification program involves a change of lifestyle that gives us time for meditation, exercise, rest, sunshine, fresh air, and joy in our lives. All these factors, plus an appropriate diet, increase the SOEFs of the body. This increases the nerve energy that Dr. Tilden mentions, and therefore the body becomes better organized so it can function appropriately and detoxify itself naturally. Following this protocol at the Tree of Life, we have created one unique, individual detoxification program. It combines aspects of our group Spiritual Fasting program with multiple non-invasive detoxification treatments. When this is followed by the four-day Zero Point Process Intensive for spiritual, mental, and emotional detoxification, we have an optimal holisitic detox program. In this context the author has seen a minimalization of healing crises and a 400 percent increase in the rate of detoxification, compared to fasting alone. (This research was done with electrodiagnostic technologies.)

It is important to understand that toxin production is also a normal part of metabolism. For example, exercise produces lactic acid and protein metabolism produces sulfuric and phosphoric acid. As long as the body and mind have full vitality, these normal poisons are readily eliminated without a build-up in toxins. The idea is not to compulsively spend our time avoiding toxins, but to reach an appropriate body balance in which they are eliminated as they come into the system. Sometimes we get ahead of our system and become too pure. For example, if the basement membranes become porous like those of a baby, and all foreign proteins such as those in polluted air pass into our system readily and cause sensitization reactions, our diet is not correct, no matter how pure it is. If we are not able to function adequately in our worldly roles, or are too reactive to the pollution, to experience the Love Communion with the Divine, then it is important to let go of our purity concepts and make the necessary dietary adjustments. The key guideline is to find the diet that best supports the flow of spiritual energy in our system, the Love energy of Communion, and at the same time supports our function in the world. In the art of Spiritual Nutrition, our concern is not with the ideal of the purest diet, but with the most appropriate diet for our living situation.

Transition Diets

Learning to eat the right amount to energize the system, to maintain whatever flow of cosmic energy we have into our system, and to maintain our present level of Love Communion with the Divine is a basic principle that applies to any level of diet. The place to start our diet transition is with our immediate diet pattern. Unless we have hypoglycemia, it is an aid to the digestive system to cut down to three meals a day with only juices or an occasional piece of fruit or vegetable between meals. Chewing our food well and creating a peaceful, joyful atmosphere in which to eat and to digest our food for ten to fifteen minutes after the meal immediately improves digestion.

There are several major stages of transition diets. Each stage may take as little as one season in the yearly cycle, or it may take years. It is the responsibility of each of us to choose our own rate of transition. The author uses the word *transition* because we are all in transition on every level of our body-mind-spirit function. The word transition creates the possibility of continual and conscious change in our life. It keeps the doors open to evolution.

Stage I Diet

This transition is from all bioacidic foods. It means letting go of processed, irradiated, genetically engineered, adulterated, fast foods, and junk foods such as white sugar, white bread, candy, frozen dinners, pastries, soft drinks, coffee, any non-organic meats treated with nitrites and nitrates, pasteurized milk and cheeses, baked goods containing refined oils, foods containing additives, and alcohol. The stage I diet includes organically raised red meats, fowl, fish, vegetables, fruits, grains, legumes, nuts, seeds, eggs, and unpasteurized (raw) dairy products. It is a basic shift away from a tamasic diet to whole, natural, organically grown foods. It is a time to begin our awareness of food combining.

This stage takes time. It requires discovering and thinking about what has been put in the foods. It requires learning where to shop to get healthy foods. In this stage we may want to fast from all flesh foods for one week two times per year.

Stage II Diet

In this stage we eliminate all red meats and begin to add more fruits and vegetables into our diet. These are important because their alkalinizing minerals help the system begin to rebalance and detoxify from the acid production of red meats. In this stage we may want to fast on fruits and vegetables and their juices for a seven-day spring and fall cleansing. This stage could be part of a one-season transition after stage I, or it could take years to make the transition.

In considering this transition, it is important to remember that flesh foods slow down the spiritualizing action of the Kundalini in the body.

Stage III Diet

This is the first stage of vegetarianism. We completely stop eating all red meat, fowl, fish, and any other sort of seafood, animal life, or eggs. Although eggs are a lighter protein than flesh foods, they still have an animal vibration. They are part of the transition step between stage II and III. In stage III we become lactovegetarian or vegetarian. Our diet includes raw dairy products, fruits, grains, legumes, nuts, seeds, seaweeds, and vegetables. The two best-known diets that approximate the early part of this stage are the macrobiotic diet and Paavo Airola's lactovegetarian diet, which is the basic diet eaten by cultures around the world that are known for their health and longevity. Airola's diet recommends eating lots of grains, nuts and seeds, vegetables, and fruits. Although today he would be against the use of dairy because of the possibility of mad cow disease, previously he allowed minimal use of cultured raw dairy products from healthy, organic cows. He suggests one to two tablespoons of cold pressed oils, plus some supplemental foods such as kelp, yeast, a little uncooked honey, and low-potency organic minerals and supplements.[3]

The standard macrobiotic diet recommended by Michio Kushi suggests that every meal consist of cooked grains, as 50 percent of the volume of the meal; soup, preferably miso, as 5 percent; vegetables, with two-thirds cooked and one-third raw, 20–30 percent; and cooked beans and seaweed, 10–15 percent.[4] The macrobiotic diet emphasizes the 50/50 balancing of the yin/yang energies of food. This diet is complex and requires some training in order to master the system and to cook the foods properly. The major difference between standard macrobiotics and the diet that Airola recommends is that Airola advises 80 percent live foods and more raw nuts and seeds. He also suggests only one grain meal per day and some raw dairy, although in the U.S. the quality of dairy is so poor, he recommended being a vegan in the U.S.[5]

In stage III the awareness of and knowledge about food combining, high- or low-protein diet according to constitution, how to prepare vegan foods, and the proper timing and amounts of foods become more refined. It is the beginning stage of learning about sprouting skills and the meaning of rejuvenating foods. The refined stage III is primarily a shift to 60–80 percent bioactive (raw) and biogenic (life-generating) foods and 20–40 percent biostatic (cooked) foods. The cooked foods are usually beans, grains, and hard vegetables such as broccoli and cauliflower. The biogenic foods – soaked and sprouted nuts, seeds, and legumes – make up 20–30 percent of the diet. It is a stage of much exploration about what works and what does not work. At this level one could begin to fast on juices for seven days twice a year. For many people this stage lasts a long time or is the diet chosen as the maintenance diet. Practiced in its purest and most refined form of 80 percent live and biogenic food and 20 percent biostatic food, it will provide a gradual detoxification over the years, so that our bodies will slowly increase their ability to act as superconductors for the cosmic energy and will support and nurture the purifying action of the Kundalini. It is a diet that is fully adequate for and supportive of spiritual life.

Stage IV Diet

This stage marks the difference between a diet that nurtures and aids spiritual development and a diet that accelerates our readiness for the Kundalini to awaken, increases the spiritualizing power of the Kundalini when it is awakened, and is an intense form of spiritual practice on its own. The difference between stages III and IV is like the difference between hiking, jogging, and other forms of aerobic exercises, which quite adequately tone and maintain the cardiovascular system, and training intensively for intercollegiate athletics. The latter part of stage IV is more like training for the Olympics versus intercollegiate athletics. We are spiritual athletes training for and participating in the event of the planetary transformation of consciousness.

Stage IV begins with a complete vegan diet of grains and bioactive foods such as raw seeds, nuts, vegetables, and fruits. Added to the diet is an increasing amount of life-generating foods such as all forms of soaked or sprouted grains including sprouted wheat, seeds, nuts, legumes, and grasses such as wheatgrass. As we detoxify and the yin expansion of consciousness continues, there is a progressive decrease in yang acid-forming cooked grains until there are none in the diet. There is a progressive increase in the percentage of bioactive and biogenic foods. Because the nutrients are able to move more easily into the cells, the total amount of food we eat will spontaneously decrease. The diet progresses to approximately 40–45 percent biogenic, 55–60 percent raw, and 5 percent undercooked hard vegetables. These are averages. There may be times when it is 100 percent raw. This is the diet we serve at the Tree of Life Café. Each of us must find our own optimal percentages. The author is not able to detect a significant difference between a 100 percent live-food diet and one that is 95 percent, in terms of day-to-day energy and Love Communion in his clients. There may be a difference in terms of ultimate physical longevity, but this is not our primary focus. The 5 percent gives us a certain amount of social flexibility and helps us to feel less constricted by the conceptual purity of 100 percent. If

99–100 percent live food is natural, easy, and peaceful as it is for the author, then such a diet is optimal!

Within this dietary progression there is an increasing amount of green vegetables and some low-glycemic fruit. They increase to about 35–40 percent of the diet. These have a high percentage, 70–90 percent, of structured water, which helps to dissolve toxins and increase the transport of nutrients into the cells. The biogenic foods are the most oxygenated foods, and thus improve health. The juicier the diet is with vegetables and fruits, the less liquid we have to drink. The increase in biogenic greens such as wheatgrass, buckwheat, and sunflower greens is important because they may contain the most rejuvenating energy on the planet. This is the "intercollegiate" diet. It is highly energizing and restorative to our SOEFs. It will create steady and excellent health, increase vitality, and allow experience of the Divine Love Communion to be maintained easily. It enhances the total body-mind-spirit experience of the bliss of Light and Love. By increasing the flow of the prana into and through the system, this diet significantly increases the potential for the critical energy level to be reached for awakening the Kundalini. This diet also accelerates the purifying and spiritualizing action of the Kundalini once it is awakened.

Contrary to other diets, it is very simple to follow. The author has arrived at this diet over thirty years of experimentation. The live foods are a constant reminder of our connection to the living planet and the cycles of Nature. Having been on the Spiritual Nutrition/Rainbow Green Live-Food Cuisine diet since 1983, the author's body has transformed into enough of a superconductor that there is minimal blockage to the full flow of the cosmic prana entering and moving through the system. This seems to also be the case for other people on this diet. Although less than his football playing days, the author's weight has stabilized within the norm established by the life insurance height and weight averages and is the same as his high school graduation weight. Part of the reason for this is that this diet supplies more than sufficient nutrients, compared to the RDA values established by the U.S. Department of Agriculture. The late Ann Wigmore's Hippocrates Diet, with emphasis on green and other fresh juices and fermented food preparations, compared the nutrients in her diet to the RDA values. She found that her almost 100 percent live-food diet had six times the vitamin C, two times the B-complex vitamins, ten times more vitamin A, seven times more iron, two times the calcium, and an amount of B_{12} equal to that of the

RDA.[6] Taken to its heavier side, she found that it could supply almost twice the protein but with half the fat. It is important to remember that in the process of our transmutation, less and less physical food is needed to maintain the physical body adequately, so too much focus on RDA values misses the point of the art of Spiritual Nutrition. Her data leaves no doubt about the adequacy of this type of diet for those still thinking in terms of the materialistic-mechanistic concept of nutrition.

Ann Wigmore's book, *The Hippocrates Diet,* and Viktoras Kulvinskas's book, *Survival into the Twenty First Century,*[7] both give a detailed and clear discussion of how to prepare and grow many of the biogenic foods referred to here. The author supports the use of green and fresh juices, but in many of our lives it is one step beyond what most of us are regularly willing to do. Although good for health, it is not clear that daily green juices are necessary for our primary spiritual focus. Carefully monitored and pre-seeded with healthy culture, the fermented seed preparations are an additional way to have a source of easily assimilated and tasty protein. By increasing the protein and fat with biogenic seed cheeses, soaked nuts and seeds, avocados, and ground flax, we can even increase our weight. Learning to adjust these nutrients to maintain optimal physical function and strength for our worldly work is part of the art of Spiritual Nutrition.

The "Olympic" part of stage IV includes Spiritual Fasting during three to four seven-day fasts per year. It may also include at least one forty-day fast at some point in our evolution. As discussed in Chapter 23, these are times of increased meditation and fasting from worldly activities. This is a powerful spiritual practice that enhances the transformational process. Spiritual Fasting, with increased meditation, most effectively turns our system into a superconductor for the Kundalini. After we reach a certain point of purification, the fasting program is no longer done for purification. By following the 40–percent-biogenic, 95–100-percent live-food diet, our body is able to purify at a rate equal to the internal metabolic toxin production and the environmental pollution exposure. One then begins to use the fasting to further enhance the superconductive Kundalini flow and transcendent transformation.

Supplementation

Supplements can be used to help correct deficiencies, to prevent deficiencies, and to act as an antioxidant protection against pollution. In high potencies, they can act as a drug to stimulate healing of the system, as well as compensate for stress in our daily lives. In stages I and II, people often use high-potency multivitamins to compensate for their enervating diets and lifestyles. We may use some supplements in stage III, but in this stage we start to tune into the subtleties of organic versus synthetic vitamins and our own internal harmony. Almost all vitamins are synthetics. One way to recognize the few natural vitamins and minerals on the market is by their low potencies. For example, natural B vitamins usually do not exceed 10 milligrams of B_1, B_2, and B_6. From the theoretical viewpoint of the SOEFs, synthetic vitamins have crystalline structures as do the natural vitamins, but they have weak SOEFs and bond less well to the appropriate sites in the body. To bond and act effectively in the body, they take energy from our own SOEFs. Initially, because of their higher concentrations, we get a stimulating effect. For some, this stimulating effect may last a few months or even several years. If the high synthetic potencies are taken for a long time, our SOEFs may become depleted and the system thrown into imbalance. As we get healthier, we also need fewer and fewer supplements. For these reasons, at stage III, it is recommended to minimize intake of high potency synthetic supplements, and focus on the use of concentrated food supplements and foods that have high amounts of nutrients, such as kelp and dulse, for minerals. Dulse, because it is much higher than kelp in potassium and lower in sodium and is purple, makes a good addition to the evening meal. It is generally good to soak the dulse to get rid of excess sea salt. If one chooses to take yeast, which the author does not recommend, it is useful to take 250 milligrams of calcium to counterbalance the high phosphorus. Lecithin and vitamin E are well supplied by germinated nuts, seeds, beans, and bee pollen so they are not necessarily needed as supplements. As we move into stage IV, the increased ability of our body to absorb nutrients from food and the higher quality of the foods allows us to even decrease the concentrated food supplements. There may be some vitamin or mineral, however, that our body, because of its own individualized biochemistry, is not adequately absorbing from food. For example, the author seems to consistently need magnesium. We need to observe closely if any mineral or vitamin deficiencies occur in the dietary shifts and with fasting. If you need help, your holistic physician or nutritionist can determine deficiencies. Until further research proves otherwise, the author recommends all vegans take B_{12} supplementation.

The key to stage III and IV supplements is that they contain the living vibration of the nutrient so that they have optimal resonance with our living cells.

A supplement the author has found to be expansive for consciousness is a blue-green algae, technically known as Aphanae-Klamathomenon flos-aquae (AFA). It is grown in pure and highly structured water in Upper Klamath Lake, which comes from underground streams. It has an extremely high SOEF field that regenerates mind, body, and immune forces. In about 70–80 percent of the people who use it, it seems to particularly activate mind-brain function. Currently the author is using E3 Live and phycomin, an extract of E3 Live. It has been a boon to some people who do much mental work and want renewed energy for meditation. The author has published a preliminary paper in the *Journal of the Orthomolecular Medical Society,* reporting that AFA partially reversed one case of Alzheimer's disease and halted the progression of another.[8] This is probably because of its specific enhancement of brain-mind SOEFs. These classes of supplements can be of use in the adjustment phases of stage IV. AFA is the only vegan source to rebuild and activate the hypothalamus. It also contains and stimulates production of DHA and EPA, which are essential long-chain Omega-3 fatty acids necessary for optimal health.

Final Perspectives

> For the Kingdom of God is not food and drink, but righteousness, and peace, and joy in the holy spirit.
>
> (Romans 15:17)

No diet without the full context of the Six Foundations will bear full spiritual fruit. We cannot eat our way to God. Although our understanding is esoteric, we are dealing with a most basic and practical life process – eating. Diet is not religion or searching for the Truth; it is simply a part of the Six Foundations. It is important for developing right diet as a support for spiritual life. Once this is achieved, just as with any foundation, we no longer have to focus on it. It becomes an expression of our awareness and way of Being. On this level the art of Spiritual Nutrition in developing a right diet is simply appropriate and supportive. It is one in a context of life practices that opens the door to our focus on harmony and Love Communion with God. Optimal health is not the goal but a by-product of this goal. For some of us, Spiritual Nutrition is also a practice of self-awareness that deepens our understanding of right life. For others, it is also a powerful spiritual practice of diet, fasting, and meditation that accelerates our spiritual unfolding by increasing the cosmic prana entering all the subtle bodies and the physical body. As this universal prana increases within us, the awareness of our own Enlightenment is increased. Spiritual Nutrition is a Whole Person Enlightenment approach that includes the spiritualization of the body as well as the mind and spirit.

Right diet is an expression of our natural attunement with the laws of Nature as manifested by the Oneness of God. When we are attuned with these laws, our health and spiritual life are supported. A spiritually appropriate diet is both the cause and the result of our state of Being. Because proper diet is the expression of our Being and state of harmony, it manifests less appropriately if it is subjected to external formulas for diet or even recipes. The only formula that we need to follow is the thoughtful and intelligent application of the art of Spiritual Nutrition. The main guideline to developing our diet is our inner experience of the Kundalini, or simply that while eating or after eating, our body-mind complex should feel energized and good throughout the day. Diet approached in this way is a common-sense personal harmony. This is why the author maintained some vagueness about the details of the diet and focused on the principles in this book.

The direct transcendental awareness of our True Nature as that who is Light, Love, and the non-dualistic Truth of God supersedes any dietary practice, purity consciousness, or dietary awareness. Throughout the Torah and New Testament, food was an offering to God. It was an ancient symbol of God Communion: "Whatever, therefore, ye eat or drink, do all things for God's glory" (Corinthians 10:32). Therefore, in the aware state we live as a Love offering to God, and we live on that Love as the primary food in our lives. In this way we become that Love and that consciousness of dual/non-dual awareness. Without this awareness, there is never enough food to feed a hungry soul.

Summary, Chapter 31

1. Six purposes for developing an individualized diet for spiritual life are reviewed.
2. Ten beneficial aspects of the Spiritual Nutrition approach are listed.
3. There are so many factors important to our process of developing an individualized diet that the only computer able to correlate them is that of our inner sensitivity. To use it effectively, we need to become our own laboratory.
4. By stabilizing the patterns of the time we eat, the physical and emotional environment in which we eat, how much we eat, and what we eat, we can consciously begin the process of self-awareness and diet.
5. Our "feedback" system on the gross physical level is feeling good all day after eating or experiencing the ill effects of gas, bloating, and nausea from a diet that is inappropriate for us.
6. On a more subtle level, if the Love Communion with the Divine is blocked before, during, or after the meal, this is "feedback" that we are not on the right diet.
7. Diet is not static. It needs to evolve in a way that supports and maintains harmony with our spiritual evolution.
8. The art of Spiritual Nutrition is the process of self-study applied to the basic guidelines of Spiritual Nutrition in the context of a full spiritual life of the Six Foundations. The creation of right diet involves letting go of nonfunctional patterns of relating to food such as food transferences.
9. Some of this shifting of diet happens spontaneously as our spiritual life evolves.
10. An approach to right diet that involves self-study and cultivation of an artful self-awareness becomes a spiritual practice on its own.
11. In the process of dietary purification we may go through a detoxification process, which may be mild or severe depending on how rapidly we proceed.
12. Learning to eat the right amount of food to be in harmony with all levels of our nutritional and spiritual needs applies to any stage of diet.
13. There are four main stages of transition diet.

14. Stage I is the removal of all bioacidic foods from the diet. It incorporates flesh foods that are organically grown.
15. Stage II is the removal of all red meats from the diet.
16. Stage III is a vegetarian diet with no fish, fowl, seafood, or eggs. It may be lactovegetarian or macrobiotic initially. By the end of stage III, we have evolved to a diet equal to 80 percent raw and 20 percent cooked foods, with 20–30 percent of the diet made of biogenic foods. This diet is fully supportive of and adequate for spiritual life.
17. Stage IV is a diet level that both accelerates spiritual development and is a spiritual practice on its own. It is a 95–100 percent live-food diet that is approximately 40–45 percent biogenic, 55–60 percent fruits and vegetables, and up to 5 percent cooked vegetables. It involves fasting one day per week or three days per month, and four seven- to ten-day seasonal fasts per year.
18. No diet without the full context of right life, right fellowship, Love, and meditation will bear spiritual fruit.
19. Diet is an expression of our natural attunement with the laws of Nature, as manifested from the Oneness of God. By attuning to these laws, we support health and spiritual life.
20. Diet is both the cause and result of our state of Being.
21. One cannot eat their way to God.

Epilogue

In the process of writing this book, the author realized that he was not writing about Spiritual Nutrition or the awakening and evolution of Kundalini. He realized that this book is emerging as part of the rising spiral of planetary consciousness preparing itself to take a quantum leap into mass world Enlightenment. We are transforming from a dysfunctional, self-centered awareness to a new global awareness centered in Divine Love Communion with God and in the Unity awareness that everyone on this planet is of one body in the Self of All. We are almost ready to give up our individual and planetary dysfunctional patterns of wasting food and of world hunger, of hoarding resources and world poverty, of individual violence and world terrorism, and of individual alienation and nations fighting nations. The historical phase that emphasized personal salvation and planetary Enlightenment is merging into a new historical period of mass salvation and Enlightenment, in which we have the potential to realize as a unified planetary group our individual and collective God nature (which we have been all along).

Spiritual Nutrition is a blueprint of some of the conscious technology and evolutionary processes that we may use or experience in our individualized yet collective way. The transforming process of the Six Foundations for Spiritual Life in the joy of God Communion is a way of deliberately and consciously choosing to cooperate with the patterns of individual and collective evolution. It is a way of choosing to be synchronous with the Will of God in the process of evolution. These patterns are not new. They have always been available to the masses, but few have taken advantage of them. God's Grace has always been on this planet. These patterns, or teachings, are universal in their application and ageless in their wisdom. They were practiced by the Essenes several centuries before the time of the Essene-trained one known as Jesus and by the ancient Egyptians. They are practiced in the Zend Avesta of Zarathustra, in the teachings of Buddha, Mohammed, Lao Tzu, Yoga, Hinduism, Torah and Kabbalah, the Pythagoreans, and the Tibetan Wheel of Life. God's universal laws and patterns of evolution remain unchanged and are as applicable now as before. These teachings were given to accelerate the opening of the doors to the higher states of God Consciousness. The only difference between now and then is that these teachings and the transformational processes are now beginning to be used by the public on a mass basis. This book is a small sharing of some of that eternal and simple wisdom. The author chose to share some of his transformational experiences as part of a more personal and detailed expression of the teachings, to make them more real. These teachings help us develop ourselves as small holographic units of God awareness, capable of resonating with Cosmic Consciousness on a mass scale to uplift the planet.

At each stage of evolution there is a more progressive synergy. Initially, atom was attracted to atom, then cell to cell. Then human Kundalini merged into the Oneness of the crown chakra with the synchronization of right and left brain and male and female awareness. This creates a dualistic/non-dualistic world experience in which there is no separation between humans. It is an awareness that allows human to be attracted to human and social system synchronized to social system, as members of the same Divine Body of God. We are about to make a quantum leap via a social synergy centered in the Love of Unity Awareness. This is our destiny. This book is an invitation for all to enjoy the celebration.

Glossary

To assist the reader in understanding the terminology presented in this glossary, most terms have been marked with an (S) for Sanskrit or an (H) for Hebrew.

agni (S) – inner subtle fire
Ah Cah Tah triangle (S) – vision from within the soma chakra (part of the crown chakra)
Ahaparinirvana Sutra (S) – an ancient Vedic scripture
ahimsa (S) – proactive process of creating and sustaining peace on every level
Ajna chakra (S) – sixth chakra; brow or third-eye chakra
Akasha (S) – space, or ether
ama (S) – physical toxin, in Ayurvedic medicine
amrita (S) – Divine nectar; literally, of the moon or nectar of immortality; also called soma
amrita chakra (S) – another name for soma chakra; source of Divine nectar
anandakanda (S) – space of bliss in the etheric heart
anandamaya kosha (S) – bliss layer of the mind; sixth kosha
anna (S) – food
annamaya kosha (S) – food layer of the mind; first kosha
Anuhata chakra (S) – heart chakra
anupaya (S) – the practice of direct knowing
apana (S) – downward flow of prana
artha (S) – wealth
asana (S) – Yoga posture

Asee'Yah (H) – physical world in Kabbalistic tradition
ashram (S) – a physical location for spiritual study and evolution
Atik Yoman (H) – the grandmother; also "Face of God," Grace of God, the Unknowable
atimanasa kosha (S) – layer of the mind associated with intuitive inspiration; fourth kosha
Atman (S) – The Divine Self beyond the body-mind-I AM complex
Atz'ilut (H) – fourth world in Kabbalah; associated with direct apperception of God
aura – energetic field composed of the subtle bodies
avadut (S) – a Liberated Being who lives wild, free, often alone in the forest
avadut moksha (S) – A completely God-merged Being
avatar (S) – a Liberated Being who comes to the planet to raise consciousness on a mass level
Ayurveda (S) – 5,000-year-old healing tradition from India; considered the complete knowledge of how to live daily life in harmony with cosmic life
azamara (H) – the practice of finding a point of Light in all situations; seeing the Divine in all things
B'lee mah (H) – the Nothing
B'riYah (H) – second world in Kabbalah; associated with a plane of angels and demons; the astral plane
Baal Shem Tov (H) – founder of the Hasidic movement in Europe who lived 1700–1760; a great shamanic saint
Bala Krishna (S) – child expression of the Divine
Bhagavad-Gita (S) – great Indian epic spiritual story
bhajan (S) –devotional Yogic chant
bhakti Yoga (S) – Yoga of Love and devotion
bhikshu (S) – spiritual seeker
bija (S) – seed sounds
binah (H) – one of the three higher sephirot energies; Divine understanding
bioacidic – life-destroying, processed foods full of additives and preservatives
bioactive – raw, life-sustaining foods
biogenic – raw, high-energy, life-giving foods; especially sprouted greens, nuts, legumes, and immature greens
biostatic – cooked or non-fresh raw foods that are life-slowing

body-mind-I AM complex – ego structure linked to time, space, and Being
brahma nadi (S) – the central nadi in the sushumna
brahma rhandhra (S) – space of the void between the right and left side of the brain
Brahma (S) – Absolute Reality
breatharianism – sustaining human life without the intake of food or water
bruhu – lower level shaman
chaitanya mantra (S) – an energized and awakened mantra
chakra (S) – a vortex energetic field that connects endocrine and nervous system plexus, as well as to other subtle systems
Chandogya Upanishad (S) – a section of one of the Vedas
chandra (S) – moon
chashmal (H) – small, silent voice often heard in meditation or prayer
chavurah (H) – group to support spiritual life
Chaya Yehida (H) – oscillation of dual/non-dual consciousness; Self-realization; Liberation
chesed consciousness (H) – the consciousness of Love and open-heartedness
chi – prana; energy
ching – deep stored sexual energy in the Chinese system
chit Kundalini (S) – the second of the three granthis associated with the etheric heart
chitti (S) – consciousness at the level of the mind
chitrini nadi (S) – moon nadi, located within the vajrini nadi, which is within the sushumna nadi
chitta (S) – activities of the conscious and unconscious mind
chittavahini (S) – nadis that are connected to the flow of consciousness and Self
chitta vritti nirodha (S) – stilling the activity of the mind
chochma (H) – one of the ten sephirot, associated with direct knowledge of God; knowing
colloid – suspension of equal-sized particles in solution; maximal size is 0.001 micron
darshan (S) – audience with the spiritual teacher
Deveikut (H) – merging with God; cleaving to God
dharana (S) – concentration
dharma (S) – right living, including right livelihood and spiritual practice
dhatus (S) – seven tissues in the Ayurvedic system

dhyana (S) – meditation
dosha (S) – psycho-physiological energies that go out of balance as kapha, pitta, and vata
Ein Sof (H) – highest level of the Absolute beyond comprehension
ekadashi (S) – dry fast on the eleventh day after the new and full moon
Essenes (H) – esoteric, Kabbalistically oriented Jewish sect
etheric – beyond physical form
eyn-zu-lo-to (H) – Nothing but God
Ganeshpuri Ashram – Swami Muktananda's original ashram sixty-two miles outside of Bombay, India
granthi (S) – subtle energetic knot associated with regulating the flow of Kundalini
guna (S) – qualities of consciousness
guru (S) – spiritual teacher
guru tattva (S) – the guru principle; the world is the guru
hagiya (H) – mantra repetition
Haniha (H) – Shaktipat
hara (S) – an energy center below the navel; a focus for martial arts and some Chinese and Japanese religions
Hasidic (H) – mystical form of Judaism started by the Baal Shem Tov
hatha Yoga (S) – the practice of Yoga asanas
hiranyamaya kosha (S) – bliss layer of the mind; sixth kosha
hishtavut (H) – equanimity, non-attachment, vairagya, Being in witness consciousness while fully immersing oneself in the play of the world; seeing the Divine in all things
hitbodedut (H) – seclusion from the world; meditation
hrit pundarik (S) – heart lotus; the etheric heart
I AM consciousness – witness consciousness connected to the sixth chakra; prior to the mind; just prior to Self-realization; where time and space dissolve
I AM THAT awareness – the Absolute Eternal Nothing; non-Being awareness; where time, space, and Being dissolve; state of Liberation
ida (S) – one of three major nadis; associated with lunar or yin energies
Indra (S) – Hindu God, head of the Devis
Inner Guru – the Divine Self within
inedia – breatharianism
involution – the contraction of cosmic Kundalini energy into Shakti Kundalini stored at the base of the spine waiting to be awakened
Jainism (S) – ancient Indian religion with focus on ahimsa or non-violence

jivanmukti (S) – Liberated while in the body
jnana Yoga (S) – Yoga of the mind
ka – Egyptian word for the Light body
Kabbalah (H) – esoteric spiritual path in the Jewish tradition of God-merging; receiving the Divine to share the Divine; Kabbalah is not a book, but a tradition of awakening
Kadosh (H) – a holy person in the Jewish tradition; more evolved than a tzadik
kama (S) – pleasure
kamamaya kosha (S) – pleasure layer of the mind; second kosha
kanda (S) – fibrous area below the base chakra from which the Kundalini emanates
kapha (S) – water-mud-mucus dosha
karma (S) – law of cause and effect
Kavanah (H) – spiritual intention
kaya kalpa (S) – An Ayurvedic procedure that reverses aging
kedusha (H) – holiness
kehila (H) – spiritual community
Keter (H) – one of the ten sephirot of the Tree of Life; associated with the Divine Will
khor-lo – Tibetan word for chakra
kippah (H) – skullcap
klipot (H) – shell of negativity
Kmeshdara (S) – Lord Shiva as Lord of the desire principle
Kmeshdari (S) – form of Kundalini as Goddess of desire
kosha (S) – layers of the body-mind complex
kriya (S) – spontaneous movement of body, emotions, mind, or spirit when Kundalini is awakened
Kundalini (S) – spiritualizing force within each person
Kundalini Shakti (S) – Kundalini potential residing at the base of the spine, which becomes activated as awakened Kundalini
Kundalini Shaktipat initiation (S) – the descent of Grace through an awake Kundalini spiritual master
latifa – a work for chakra in the Sufi tradition
lepton – a subatomic particle
Liberation – Self-realization; when the prana and I AM consciousness become one in meditation; merging of Shiva and Shakti
Mah (H) – with; the What (in juxtaposition to the Nothing, or without What – B'lee mah)

Mahabharata (S) – an epic Indian poem story
Malchut (H) – One of the seven lower sephirot in the Tree of Life; Kingdom of God
manas (S) – emotional, sensory, and cognitive mind
Manipura chakra (S) – solar plexus chakra
manna (H) – mystical food for elevating consciousness; activates pituitary and pineal glands
mannahuna – keepers of the manna in the Hawaiian tradition
manomaya kosha (S) – layer of mind associated with emotional, sensory, and cognitive function; third kosha
manovahini nadis (S) – subtle channels associated with the flow of mind energies
mantra (S) – sacred word or name of God repeated by the spiritual aspirant
Manusmriti (S) – ancient Yogic scripture
maya (S) – the illusion of the three-dimensional world; Illuminated Maya is the expansion of the world as the Divine in every form
meridian – energy circuits or lines used in acupuncture
merkaba (H) – aligned with Divine Will
messianic era – pertaining to a messiah's coming; thousand years of world peace
mfkzt – Egyptian term for manna
microzyma – protids
mikvah (H) – Jewish spiritual purification pool
Mishna sage (H) – expert in the oral tradition of Judaism
mitzvah (H) – good and holy deed as described in the Torah
mitzvot (H) – plural of mitzvah
mizmor (H) – chanting in a God-focused way
moksha (S) – fullest level of God-merging and Liberation, 100 percent permanent, unbroken merging
mukti (S) – Liberation; Self-realization
Muladhara chakra (S) – base chakra
mundane Kundalini (S) – vital life force
muon – subatomic particle
nada (S) – the Divine sounds
nadi (S) – hollow, subtle channel through which the Kundalini energy moves; 72,000 nadis exist in the human body
neshama (H) – third level of soul; the individual soul
Netzah (H) – sephirotic energy associated with spiritual perseverance

nirvakalpa samadhi (S) – samadhi beyond time, space, and Being; Nothing exists; God-merging
Nityananda (S) – the guru of Swami Muktananda
niyama (S) – physical and mental activity to avoid in spiritual life; the "don'ts" of proper conduct
Nukba (H) – Feminine energy or Shekhinah associated with the sephirot of Malchut
ojas (S) – vital life force energy and reserve of vital energy
"Om Na`mah Shivaya" (S) – a mantra; a name of God
ophanim (H) – physical embodiment (postures) of energies of the Hebrew letters; also a class of angels related to body, shapes, and cycles
Pancha Karma (S) – Ayurvedic system of detoxification and rejuvenation
par'gawd (H) – thin veil that separates us from the Truth; metaphorically called the glass ceiling of consciousness
para Kundalini (S) – the third knot of Kundalini regulation between the third eye and crown chakra
Paramatman (S) – Absolute Reality; I AM THAT
Parinirvana – Enlightenment
pingala (S) – major nadi associated with the sun
pion – a subatomic particle
pitta (S) – fire dosha
prajna pratihara (S) – crimes against wisdom
prana (S) – vital life force
prana Kundalini (S) – the first knot in the Kundalini system; associated with the first chakra
pranayama (S) – Yogic breathing practice to increase prana
pratyahara (S) – withdrawal from the senses
prion – smallest level of protein that are living
prophesy – the experience of God-merging and the delighting in that experience
protid – Smallest living units in the body
purusha (S) – non-dual spirit
rahu (S) – one of the nodes of the moon
raja Yoga (S) – Yoga of the mind
rajasic (S) – one of the three gunas; associated with an outgoing, active energy
Rama (S) – avatar associated with the energy of Vishnu the Sustainer
Rama Krishna Paramahamsa (S) – great spiritual master and Enlightened Being who lived in the late 1800s

Ramana Maharshi (S) – great spiritual master and Enlightened Being who lived in the twentieth century
rasa (S) – life force or "juices"; plasma
reiki – Japanese healing system developed by Dr. Usui
Rigveda (S) – one of the ancient scriptures of India
rishi (S) – an ancient Indian sage
S'micha l'shefa (H) – initiation of Grace in the Jewish-Kabbalistic system; synonymous with Shaktipat,
sadhana (S) – spiritual practice
sahaja samadhi (S) – experience of Oneness while in the waking state
Sahasrara chakra (S) – crown chakra
Sai Baba of Shirdi (S) – a fully God-merged Enlightened Being who left his body in 1918
samadhi (S) – state of Bliss beyond the mind
samahita chitta (S) – a calm, centered mind
samana (S) – one of five pranas; associated with digestive energies
samskara (S) – impression of the mind
sanatana dharma (S) – the natural way of life that leads to Enlightenment
Sanhedrin (H) – the equivalent of a spiritual supreme court; the seeds started with Moses and manifested primarily in Jerusalem
sangha (S) – spiritual group; right fellowship
sankalpa samadhi (S) – state of Oneness while experiencing the Light; subtle awareness of the I AM beyond time and space
Sanskrit (S) – ancient fire (spiritually activating) language of India
satsang (S) – the experience of the Truth in the presence of an awake spiritual teacher
sattvic (S) – one of the three gunas or states; a state of holiness that points one inward to the Divine
Self-realization – knowing I AM THAT; experiencing the Truth of who you are beyond time, space, and Being
sephirot (H) – The ten consciousness centers of the Kabbalistic Tree of Life
seva (S) – service
Shabbat (H) – holiest day of year one time per week; a time of complete rest from worldly activity; starts Friday night at sunset and ends Saturday night at sunset
Shakti (S) – energy of the One expressed as Divine Mother of all creation
Shaktipat initiation (S) – awakening of the Kundalini energy through a Liberated, spiritual master who has become a vehicle of Grace
shaman – a medicine and spiritual healer/teacher in an indigenous culture

shechitah (H) – proper and holy kosher rituals for animal slaughter and food in general
shefa (H) – the down pouring of cosmic spiritual energy
sheirut (H) – service
Shekhinah (H) – Hebrew name for the energy associated with the sacred feminine; equivalent to the Shakti
shem-an-na – the term for manna during the ancient historical times of Lemuria
Shiva (S) – Hindu name for Cosmic Consciousness; also associated with the God of transformation
Shiva samhita (S) – scriptures on Shiva Consciousness
Shochet (H) – a kosher butcher; plural is shochtim
Shrii Shrii Ananda Murti (S) – a God-merged saint who left his body in 1991; founder of Ananda Marga
Shulhan Arukh (H) – the set table; the coded do's and don'ts in the Jewish tradition
shukra (S) – deep sexual energy; reproductive fluid and tissue
Shurangama Sutra (S) – a Buddhist text
siddhis (S) – miraculous powers
soma (S) – the Divine nectar dripping from the soma chakra; also an herb giving longevity
soma chakra (S) – a sub-chakra in the lower part of the Sahasrara; it is associated with Divine nectar
spiritual Kundalini (S) – the cosmic form of Kundalini
Sri Ganapati Satchidananda Swamiji – a living God-realized Being and expression of nada Yoga (Divine music), whose base is in Mysore, India
structured water – water that is alive and has a high degree of energetic organization
subtle bodies – energetic bodies that surround the physical body
surya nadi (S) – sun nadi
sushumna (S) – central nadi through which the Kundalini moves, located along the inside of the spine in the etheric body
svadharma (S) – the way of life that leads you to know I AM THAT, or the Truth;
Svadhishthana chakra (S) – throat chakra
svarupa (S) – to know one's True state
Swami Jnanananda (S) – a disciple of Swami Nityananda who became God-merged in his nineties, and who attained moksha

Swami Muktananda (S) – Gabriel's first guru; the Enlightened Being who gave him Shaktipat

Swami Prakashananda Saraswati (S) – the first person, in 1969, to be acknowledged by Swami Muktananda to be Enlightened; Gabriel's guru "uncle" and second guru

tachyon – energy moving faster than speed of light, just before it slows to speed of light

t'ai chi – Chinese practices that sustain and balance the chi or prana

tamasic (S) – one of three gunas or states; the state associated with inertia; a veil of ignorance; sloth; junk food

tantra (S) – the Yogic practice of celebrating the Divine in all things

Tao Te Ching – classical text in the Taoist tradition

Tefirot (H) – the sephirot of perfect balance; located at the level of the etheric heart

tefila (H) – prayer

teheru (H) – the void in the Jewish-Kabbalistic system

tejas (S) – one of the three vital essences in Ayurveda associated with subtle fire and electricity; the subtle aspect of pitta

Ten Speakings – the correct translation of what is thought of as the "Ten Commandments"

Tikkun Olam (H) – healing of the world

Torah (H) – the five books of Moses

Tree of Life – The ten sephirotic energies

tridoshic (S) – a state when either all three doshas are perfectly balanced or when they all go out of balance very easily

T'shukat Deveikut (H) – a form of God-merging

tzadik (H) – a saintly, righteous being in the Jewish tradition

Tzava'at Harivash (H) – a book containing English translation of some of the Baal Shem Tov's basic teachings as he personally wrote them

tzedaka (H) – charity

udana (S) – upward moving prana

Universal prana (S) – the cosmic life force

urdhdareta (S) – rising upward of the semen in the sushumna

vairagya (S) – non-attachment

vajrini nadi (S) – inner nadi of the sushumna associated with the sun; thunderbolt nadi

vasana (S) – deep thought form groove made from repetitive vrittis; imbalanced, repeated mental impression

vata (S) – one of the psychophysiological states or doshas in the

Ayurvedic system; associated with anxiety, fear, and imbalanced energies

"Vav Mem Bet" (H) – Kabbalistic prayer for blessing water

Vedas (S) – ancient Hindu scriptures

vijnanamaya kosha (S) – the layer of the mind associated with viveka and vairagya; causal mind; fifth kosha

virtual energy state – place of zero point energy

Vishuddha chakra (S) – throat chakra

viveka (S) – wisdom to tell the difference between the Real and unreal

void – beyond time and space

vritti (S) – a specific activity of the mind

vyana (S) – associated with circulation

vyutthita chitta (S) – an unstable, or "provoked," mind

witness consciousness – the ability to step back and see the ego at play and feel separate from it; I AM consciousness

Yah (H) – the name of God connecting the spirit of God as breath

Yajur Veda (S) – one of the ancient Vedic scriptures

yamas (S) – the "do's" of proper conduct in Yoga

yang – the outward flowing energy in the Chinese system of duality

yantra (S) – a symbolic, energized, spiritual drawing

yechidut (H) – satsang or sangha

Yetzirah (H) – second level of four worlds (astral plane); associated with angels and demons

YHWH (H) – "Yod Hey Wah Hey"; the most sacred name of God in the Jewish tradition; the mantra of Liberation in the West

yin – inward, quiet energies in the Chinese system of duality

Yoga (S) – the path of Union/Liberation in the Hindu traditions

Yoga asanas (S) – Yogic postures

Yoga chitta vritti nirodha (S) – "Yoga is the stilling of the activity of the mind"

yukta triveni (S) – three streams; the place below the base chakra where the sushumna, ida, and pingala begin; coming together of the three main nadi

Zeir Anpin (H) – the partzufim (Face of God) associated with the six lower sephirot energies above Malchut

Zero Point Process – a form of Western jnana Yoga taught by Gabriel

Zohar (H) – considered the most powerful and holy Kabbalistic text

Notes

PART I: ENERGETICS, EVOLUTION, AND SPIRITUAL ANATOMY

Chapter 1: The Mystical Kundalini and the Six Foundations for Spiritual Life

1. Jung, Carl. *Psychological Commentary on Kundalini*. New York: Spring Publications, 1975 (Part I) and 1976 (Part II).

2. Krishna, G. *Kundalini: The Evolutionary Energy in Man*. Berkeley, CA: Shambhala, 1971.

3. Muktananda. *Kundalini: The Secret of Life*. New York: SYDA Foundation, 1979.

4. Ibid.

5. Katz, R. "Education for Transcendence: Lessons from the !Kung Zhu/Twasi," *Journal of Transpersonal Psychology*. Volume 2, 1973, pp. 136–155.

6. Luk, C. *The Secrets of Chinese Meditation*. New York: Samuel Weiser, 1972.

7. Rohrbach, P. *The Search for St. Thérèse*. New York: Dell, 1963.

8. Sannella, Lee. *Kundalini: Psychosis or Transcendence?* San Francisco: Sannella, 1976.

9. Ibid.

10. Ibid.

11. Ibid.

12. Muktananda. *Kundalini: The Secret of Life*. New York: SYDA Foundation, 1979.

13. Ibid.

14. Murphy, Michael and White, Rhea A. *The Psychic Side of Sports*. Menlo Park, CA: Addison-Wesley, 1978.

Chapter 2: Evolution and Fruition of Kundalini into Liberation

1. Tirtha, Vishnu, Swami. *Devatma Shakti*. Darya Ganj, Delhi: Swami Shivom Tirth, 1974.

2. Muktananda. *Kundalini: The Secrets of Life.* New York: SYDA Foundation, 1979.

3. Tsu, Lao. *Tao Te Ching.* Translation by Gia-Fu Feng and Jane English, New York: Vintage Books, 1972.

4. Murthy, T. S. *Anantha Maharaj.* San Rafael, CA: The Dawn Horse Press, 1972.

5. Tirtha, Vishnu, Swami. Op. cit.

6. Singh, Renu Lal. *Right Life: Teachings of the Shivapuri Baba.* North Yorkshire, England: Coombe Springs Press, 1984.

7. Nisargadatta, Maharaj. *I AM THAT.* Bombay: Sudhakar S. Dikshit, 1976.

8. Winkler, Gershon. *Magic of the Ordinary.* Berkeley, CA: North Atlantic Books, 2003.

9. Kaplan, Aryeh. *Gems of Rabbi Nachman.* Jerusalem: Chaim Kramer, 1980.

10. Kapleau, Roshi. *The Three Pillars of Zen.* Garden City, NY: Anchor Books, 1980.

Chapter 3: The Chakra System

1. Motoyama, Hiroshi. *Theories of the Chakras: Bridge to Higher Consciousness.* Madras, India/London, England: The Theosophical Publishing House, 1985.

2. Joy, W. Brugh. *Joy's Way.* Los Angeles: J.P. Tarcher, Inc., 1979.

3. Bagley, L. "New Method for Locating Acupuncture Points and Body Field Distortions," *American Journal of Acupuncture.* Vol. 12, no. 3, July-September 1984, pp. 219–228.

4. Motoyama, Hiroshi. Op. cit.

5. Joy, W. Brugh. Op. cit.

6. Leadbeater, C.W. *The Chakras.* Wheation. IL: Theosopical Publishing House, 1980.

7. Motoyama, Hiroshi. Op. cit.

8. Joy, W. Brugh. *Joy's Way.* Los Angeles: J. P. Tarcher, Inc., 1979.

9. Colton, Ann Ree. *Kundalini West.* Glendale, CA: Arc Publishing, 1978.

10. Anandamurti, Shrii Shrii. *Discourses on Tantra, Vol. 1.* Calcutta, India: A'nanda Marga Publications, 1993

11. Anandamurti, Shrii Shrii. *Ananda Margon Caryacarya,* 4th edition. Calcutta, India: Krsnatmananda Avaduta, 1992.

12. Ranade, Dr. Subhash. *Natural Healing through Ayurveda.* Salt Lake City, UT: Passage Press, 1993.

13. Bahadur, Rai and Vasu, Shrisha Chandra. *Shiva Samhita.* Varanasi, India: Pilgrims Publishing, 2002.

Chapter 4: Healing Unbalanced Kundalini Energy

1. Cousens, Gabriel, M.D. *Rainbow Green Live-Food Cuisine.* Berkeley, CA: North Atlantic Books, 2003.

Chapter 6: Subtle Organizing Energy Fields, a New Concept

1. Tompkins, Peter. *The Secret Life of Plants.* New York: Harper Perennial Publishing, 1989.

2. Vogel, Marcel. Personal communication, 1986.

3. Beardon, T. E. *The New Tesla Electromagnetics and the Secrets of Electrical Free Energy.* Millbrae, CA: Tesla Book Co., 1982.

4. Trombley, Adam. Personal communication, 1986.

5. Department of Defense Program Solicitation for FIY, 1986 AF 86–77.

6. Callahan, Philip. *Tuning into Nature.* Old Greenich, CT: Devin-Adair Press, 1975.

7. Wagner, David and Gabriel Cousens, M.D. *Tachyon Energy: A New Paradigm in Holistic Healing.* Berkeley, CA: North Atlantic Books, 1999.

8. Wall, Ernst. *The Physics of Tachyon.* Palm Harbor, FL: Hadronic Press, 1995.

9. Toben, Robert. *Space, Time, and Beyond.* New York: E.P. Dutton and Co., Inc., 1975.

10. Cousens, Gabriel, M.D. *Rainbow Green Live-Food Cuisine.* Berkeley, CA: North Atlantic Books, 2003.

11. Bearden, T. E. *Toward a New Electromagnetics, Part Ill: Clarifying the Vector Concept.* Millbrae, CA: Tesla Book Co., 1983.

12. Sheldrake, Rupert. *A New Science of Life.* Los Angeles: J. P. Tarcher, Inc., 1981.

13. Friedman, H. L., Krishman, C. Y., and Jolicoeur, C. "Ionic Interactions in Water." *Ann. N. Y. Academy of Science,* 1972, no. 204, pp. 77–99.

14. Clegg, James. "Metabolism and the Intracellular Environment: The Vicinal Water Network Model," in *Cell Associated Water* (Drost-Hansen, W. and James Clegg, Eds.). New York: Academic Press, 1979, pp. 363–413.

15. Cope, Freeman. "Structured Water and Complexed Na+ and K+ in Biological Systems Water Structure at the Water-Polymer Interface." *Proceedings of American Chemical Society Symposium,* edited by H. H. Jellinek. New York: Plenum Press, 1972, pp. 14–17.

16. Ling, Gilbert. "Water Structure at the Water-Polymer Interface." *Proceedings of American Chemical Society Symposium,* ed. by H. H. Jellinek. New York: Plenum Press, 1972, pp. 4–13.

17. Hansen, J. Yellin. "W. NMRand Infra Spectroscopic Studies of Stratum Corneum Hydration." *Proceedings of American Chemical Society Symposium,* ed. by H. H. Jellinek. New York: Plenum Press, 1972, pp. 19–28.

18. Clegg, James. "Metabolism and the Intracellular Environment: The Vicinal Water Network Model," in *Cell Associated Water* (Drost-Hansen, W. and James Clegg, Eds.). New York: Academic Press, 1979, pp. 363--413.

19. Ibid.

20. Ibid.

21. Hazelwood, Carlton. "A View of the Significance and Understanding of the Physical Properties of Cell Associated Water," in *Cell Associated Water* (Drost-

Hansen, W. and James Clegg, Eds.). New York: Academic Press, 1979, p. 165.

22. Mikesell, Norm. "Cellular Regeneration." *Psychic Research Newsletter,* 1985, pp. 1–10.

23. Ibid.

24. Bachechi, Orie. *When Light Touches Many Changes Take Place.* Albuquerque, NM: Kiva, Inc., 1984.

25. Ibid.

Chapter 7: Subtle Anatomies

1. Master Charles, MSH Associates. Personal communication, 1986.

Chapter 8: Aberrant Biological Phenomena

1. Nisargadatta, Maharaj. *I Am That.* Bombay: Sudhakar S. Dikshit, 1976.

2. Hotema, Hilton. *Higher Consciousness.* Mokelumne Hill, CA: Health Research, 1962.

3. Yogananda, Paramahansa. *Autobiography of a Yogi.* Los Angeles: Self-Realization Fellowship, 1972.

4. Chia, Mantak and Winn, Michael. *Taoist Secrets of Love.* New York: Aurora Press, 1984.

5. Ibid.

6. Airola, Paavo. *Worldwide Secrets for Staying Young.* Phoenix, AZ: Health Plus, 1982.

7. Ibid.

8. Hotema, Hilton. *Higher Consciousness.* Mokelumne Hill, CA: Health Research, 1962.

9. Murthy, T. S. Anantha. *Maharaj.* San Rafael, CA: Dawn Horse Press, 1972

10. Zevin, Rabbi S. Y. *A Treasury of Chassidic Tales.* New York: Mesorah, 1981.

11. Ibid.

12. Yogananda, Paramahansa. *Autobiography of a Yogi.* Los Angeles: Self-Realization Fellowship, 1972.

13. Ibid.

14. Ibid.

15. Ibid.

16. Ibid.

17. Ibid.

18. Burkus, J. *Terese Neumanaite.* Chicago: Suduvos Press, 1953.

19. Chia, Mantak and Winn, Michael. *Taoist Secrets of Love.* New York: Aurora Press, 1984.

20. Yogananda, Paramahansa. *Autobiography of a Yogi.* Los Angeles: Self-Realization Fellowship, 1972.

21. Manek, Hiran Ratan. From his website.

22. Lo'ez, MeAm. *The Torah Anthology.* New York /Jerusalem: Maznaim, 1977.

23. Ibid.

24. Ibid.

25. Szekely, Edmond Bordeaux. *The Essenes by Josephus and His Contemporaries.* San Diego, CA: International Biogenic Society, 1981.

26. Murthy, T. S. Anantha. *Maharaj.* San Rafael, CA: Dawn Horse Press, 1972.

27. Ibid.

28. Airola, Paavo. *Worldwide Secrets for Staying Young.* Phoenix, AZ: Health Plus, 1982.

29. Ibid.

30. Wallace, R. K. "Effects of the TM and TM Sidhi Program on the Aging Process," *International Journal of Neuroscience,* 16(1), 1982, pp. 53–58.

31. Little, W. A. "Superconductivity at Room Temperature," *Scientific American,* 212(21), 1965.

32. Barr, Frank, M.D. "Melanin as Key Organizing Molecule," *Brain Mind Bulletin,* Aug. 1983, pp. 1–8.

33. McClare, C. W. F. "Resonance in Bioenergetics," *Annals of the New York Academy of Sciences,* 227, 1974, pp. 74–91.

34. Kervan, C.L. and Abehsera, M. *Biological Transmutations.* New York: Swan Publishing Co., 1972

35. Yogananda, Paramahansa. *Autobiography of a Yogi.* Los Angeles: Self-Realization Fellowship, 1972.

36. Ibid.

37. *The Lost Books of the Bible and the Forgotten Books of Eden.* New York: World, 1972.

Chapter 9: The Human Crystal

1. Vogel, Marcel. Personal communication, 1986.

2. Rein, Glen. "Biological Crystals," presented at the First International Crystal Congress, San Francisco, CA, June 1986.

3. Ibid.

4. Vogel, Marcel. Personal communication, 1986.

5. Basset, Andrew C. "Biophysical Principles Affecting Bone Structure," in *The Biochemistry and Physiology of Bone.* New York: Academic Press, 1971, pp. 1–76.

6. Basset, Andrew C. "Biological Significance of Piezoelectricity," *Calc. Tiss. Res.,* vol. 1, 1968, pp. 252–272.

7. Basset, Andrew C. "Biophysical Principles Affecting Bone Structure," in *The Biochemistry and Physiology of Bone.* New York: Academic Press, 1971, pp.1–76.

8. Basset, Andrew C. "Biological Significance of Piezoelectricity," *Calc. Tiss. Res.,* vol. 1, 1968, pp. 252–272.

9. Ibid.

10. Bassett, L. S., Tzitzikalakis, G., Pawluk, R. J., and Bassett, C. A. L. "Prevention of Disuse Osteoporosis in the Rat by Means of Pulsing Electromagnetic Fields," in *Electrical Properties of Bone and Cartilage: Experimental Effects and Clinical Applications.* C. T. Brighton, J. Black, and S. R. Pollack, eds. New York: Grune and Stratton, 1979, pp. 605–630.

11. Bassett, C. A. L., et al. "Modification of Fracture Repair with Selected Puls-

ing Electromagnetic Fields," *The Journal of Bone and Joint Surgery,* vol. 64-A, no.6, July 1982, pp. 888–895.

12. Basset, Andrew C. "Biophysical Principles Affecting Bone Structure," in *The Biochemistry and Physiology of Bone.* New York: Academic Press, 1971, pp. 1–76.

13. Bassett, C. A. L. "Pulsing Electromagnetic Fields: A New Approach for Surgical Problems," in *Metabolic Surgery.* Henry Buchward, M.D. and Richard L. Varcho, M.D., eds. New York: Grune and Stratton, 1978, pp. 255–306.

14. McClare, C. W. E. "Resonance in Bioenergetics," *Annals of the NY Academy of Sciences,* 227, 1974, pp. 74–91.

15. Johnson, J. E. and Porter, R. S., eds. *Liquid Crystals and Ordered Fluids.* New York: Plenum Press, 1970.

16. Miksell, Norman. "Structured Water: Its Healing Effects on the Diseased State," San Jose, CA: PRI, 1985, pp. 1–10.

17. Rapp, P. R. "An Atlas of Cellular Oscillators," *Journal Exp. Biol,* vol. 81, 1979, pp. 281–306.

18. Gurudas. *Gem Elixirs and Vibrational Healing,* vol. 1. Boulder, CO: Cassandra Press, 1985.

Chapter 10: Bioenergetic Assimilation

1. Steiner, Rudolf. *Agriculture: A Course of Eight Lectures.* London: Biodynamic Agricultural Association, 1977.

2. Vogel, Marcel. Personal communication, 1986.

3. Schmidt, Gerhard. *The Dynamics of Nutrition.* Providence, RI: Bio-Dynamic Literature, 1980.

4. Ibid.

5. Nisargadatta, Maharaj. *I Am That.* Bombay: Sudhakar S. Dikshit, 1976.

6. Rein, Glen. "Biological Crystals," presented at First International Crystal Conference, San Francisco, CA, 1986.

7. Gurudas. *Gem Elixirs and Vibrational Healing,* vol. 1. Boulder, CO: Cassandra Press, 1985.

8. Basset, Andrew C. "Biophysical Principles Affecting Bone Structure," in *The Biochemistry and Physiology of Bone.* New York: Academic Press, 1971, pp. 1–76.

9. Basset, Andrew. "Biological Significance of Piezoelectricity," *Calc. Tiss. Res.,* vol. l, 1968, pp. 252–272.

10. Basset, Andrew C. "Biophysical Principles Affecting Bone Structure," in *The Biochemistry and Physiology of Bone.* New York: Academic Press, 1971, pp. 1–76.

11. Lipton, Bruce. "Liquid Crystal Consciousness: The Cellular Basis of Life," presented at First International Crystal Conference, San Francisco, CA, 1986.

12. Marshal, Robert, PhD. Personal communication. 2004.

Chapter 11: The Chemistry of Stress and the Alchemy of Meditation

1. Hawkins, David and Pauling, Linus. *Orthomolecular Psychiatry—Treatment*

of Schizophrenia. San Francisco: W. H. Freeman and Company, 1973.

2. Levine, Steve and Kidd, Paris. *Antioxidant Adaption: Its Role in Free Radical Pathology.* San Francisco: Biocurrents Press, 1985.

3. Ibid.

4. Ibid.

5. Ibid.

6. Ibid.

7. Ibid.

8. "Science, Consciousness and Aging," *Proceedings of the International Conference,* West Germany: MERU, 1980, pp. 6–80.

9. Ibid.

10. Ibid.

11. Murthy, T. S. Anantha. *Maharaj.* San Rafael, CA: Dawn Horse Press, 1972.

12. Tsu, Lao. *Tao Te Ching.* Translation by Gia-Fu Feng and Jane English, New York: Vintage Books, 1972.

13. Hubbard, Barbara Marx. *Manual for Co-Creators of the Quantum Leap.* Gainesville, FL: New Visions, 1984.

14. Szekely, Edmond Bordeaux. *The Essenes by Josephus and His Contemporaries.* San Diego, CA: International Biogenic Society, 1981

15. Hertz, O. R., and Joseph, H. *Pirke Aboth.* New York: Benjamin House, Inc.

16. Kirschner, H. E. *Nature's Seven Doctors.* Riverside, CA: H. C. White Publications, 1972.

17. Ibid.

18. Ibid.

19. Ibid.

20. Singh, Renu La!. *Right Life: Teachings of the Shivapuri Baba.* England: Coombe Springs Press, 1984.

Chapter 12: Nutrition, Kundalini, and Transcendence

1. Newbrough, John Ballou. *Oahspe.* Montrose, CO: Essenes of Kosmon, 1935.

2. Ibid.

3. Ibid.

4. Da Free, John. *The Dawn Horse Testament.* San Rafael, CA: Dawn Horse Press, 1985.

PART II: THE SPIRITUAL NUTRITION PARADIGM

Chapter 13: The Need for a New Nutritional Paradigm

1. Kervan, C. L. and Abehsera, M. *Biological Transmutations.* New York: Swan House Publishing Co., 1972.

2. Ibid.

3. Ott, Tru. Personal communication. 2004

4. Kervan, C. L. and Abehsera, M. *Biological Transmutations.* New York: Swan House Publishing Co., 1972.

5. Ibid.

6. Ibid.

7. Szent-Gyorgyi, Albert *Introduction to Submolecular Biology.* London: Academic Press, 1960.

8. Kervan C. L. and Abehsera, M. *Biological Transmutations.* New York: Swan House Publishing Co.,1972.

9. Williams, Roger. *Biochemical Individuality.* New York: McGraw-Hill, 1998.

10. Kervan, C. L. and Abehsera, M. *Biological Transmutations.* New York: Swan House Publishing Co.,1972.

11. Brewer, Richard and Hahn, Erwin. *Scientific American,* vol. 251, Dec. 1984, pp. 50–57.

12. Kervan, C. L. and Abehsera, M. *Biological Transmutations.* New York: Swan House Publishing Co., 1972.

Chapter 15: Nutrients: The Many and the One

1. *The Lost Books of the Bible and the Forgotten Books of Eden.* New York: World, 1972.

2. Wurtman, Richard J. "The Effects of Light on the Human Body," *Scientific American,* vol. 233, no.1, July 1975, pp. 68–77.

3. Brody, Jane E. "Surprising Health Impact Discovered for Light," in *Science Times. The New York Times,* Nov. 13, 1984.

4. Ibid.

5. Ibid.

6. National Institute of Mental Health. *Biological Rhythms in Psychiatry and Medicine.*

7. Ibid.

8. Downing, John. Personal communication, 1986.

9. Wurtman, Richard J. "The Effects of Light on the Human Body," *Scientific American,* vol. 233, no.1, July 1975, pp. 68–77.

10. National Institute of Mental Health. *Biological Rhythms in Psychiatry and Medicine,* pp. 120–132.

11. "Melanin as Key Organizing Molecule," *Brain Mind Bulletin,* vol. 8, no.12/13, July 11/Aug. 1, 1983, pp. 1–8.

12. Ibid.

13. Levine, Steven. "Oxygen, Bioelectricity and Life," *American Chiropractor,* July 1986, pp. 1–8.

14. Levine, Steven. "Oxygen Immunity, Cancer, and Candida," presented at Society of Environmental Medicine. Clearwater, FL: Oct. 1986, pp. 1–10.

15. Babior, B. M. "The Role of Active Oxygen in Microbial Killing by Phagocytes" in *Pathology of Oxygen,* A. P. Antoe, ed. New York: Academic Press, 1982.

16. Levine, Steve and Kidd, Paris. *Antioxidant Adaption; Its Role in Free Radical Pathology.* San Francisco: Biocurrents Press, 1985.

17. Ibid.

18. Heritage, Ford. *Composition and Facts About Food.* Mokelumne Hill, CA: Health Research, 1968.

19. Kamen, Betty, "Vitamin O: The Oxygen Nutrient," *Let's Live,* vol. 54, no.7, July 1986, pp. 1–8.

20. Kazuhiko, Asai. *Miracle Cure, Organic Germanium.* Japan: Japan Publications, Inc., 1980.

21. Ibid.

22. Chia, Mantak and Winn, Michael. *Taoist Secrets of Love.* New York: Aurora Press, 1984.

23. Kornfield, Jack. "The Sex Lives of Gurus," *The Yoga Journal,* vol. 63, July/Aug. 1985, pp. 26, 27, 28, and 66.

24. *The Teachings of Bhagavan Sri Ramana Maharshi in His Own Words.* Arthur Osborne, ed. Madras, India: T. N. Venkataraman, 4th ed., 1977.

25. Dubrov, A. P. *The Geomagnetic Field and Life.* New York: Plenum Press, 1978.

Chapter 16: Food for a Quiet Mind

1. Maharshi, Ramana. *Be As You Are.* New York: Penguin Books, 1985.

2. Ibid.

3. Schochet, Jacob Immanuel. *Tzava'at Harivash.* Brooklyn, NY: Kehot Publication Society, 1998.

4. Maimonides, Moses. *Hilchos De'os* 3.3

5. Ibid.

6. *Health, United States.* Hayattsville, MD: U.S. Dept. of Health and Human Services, 2003.

7. Hawkins, David and Pauling, Linus. *Orthmolecular Psychiatry.* San Francisco: W. H. Freeman and Company, 1973.

8. Ibid.

9. Pfeiffer, Carl C. *Mental and Elemental Nutrients.* New Canaan, CT: Keats Publishing, Inc., 1975.

10. Ibid.

11. *Diet Related to Killer Diseases, V.* Hearing Before the Select Committee on Nutrition and Human Needs of the United States Senate, U.S.: June 22, 1977.

12. Mandell, Marshall and Scanlon, Lynne Waller. *5-Day Allergy Relief System.* New York: Pocket Books, 1979.

13. Ibid.

14. Airola, Paavo. *Hypoglycemia: A Better Approach.* Phoenix, AZ: Health Plus, 1977.

15. Schmidt, Gerhard. *The Dynamics of Nutrition.* Providence, RI: Bio-Dynamic Literature, 1980.

16. Ibid.

17. Health Implications of Obesity, NIH Consens Statement Online. 1985 Feb 11–13; 5(9):1–7

Chapter 17: Veganism Is the Key

1. Hua, Hsuan, Translator. *Shurangama Sutra.* Burlingame, CA: Buddhist Text Translation Society, 1st ed edition, 2003.

2. Cousens, Gabriel, M.D. *Conscious Eating.* Berkeley, CA: North Atlantic Books, 2000.

3. Yukteswar, Sri. *Holy Science.* Los Angeles: Self Realization Fellowship Publishers, 7th edition, 1990.

4. Altman, Nathaniel. *Ahimsa.* Wheaton, IL: Theosophical Publishing House, 1981.

5. Mykoff, Moshe (translator) and Chaim, Kramer (annotator). *Likutei Moharan.* Breslov Research Institute, Jerusalem, 1997, volume 5.

6. Cousens, Gabriel, M.D. *Conscious Eating.* Berkeley, CA: North Atlantic Books, 2000.

7. Ibid.

8. Ibid.

9. Ibid.

10. Ibid.

11. Ibid.

12. Ibid.

13. Ibid.

14. Ibid.

15. Kulvinskas, Viktoras. *Survival into the 21st Century.* Woodstock Valley, CT/Fairfield, IA: 21st Century Publications, 1975.

16. Cott, Allan. *Fasting: The Ultimate Diet.* Toronto, New York, London, Sydney: Bantam Books, 1981.

17. Scharffenberg, John A. *Problems with Meat.* Santa Barbara, CA: Woodbridge Press, 1979.

18. Ibid.

19. Ibid.

20. Airola, Paavo. *Are You Confused?* Phoenix, AZ: Health Plus, Publishers, 1974.

21. Ibid.

22. Cousens, Gabriel, M.D. *Conscious Eating.* Berkeley, CA: North Atlantic Books, 2000.

23. Weissberg, Steven M., M.D., and Christiano, Joseph, A.P.P.T. *The Answer Is in Your Blood Type.* Lake Mary, FL: Personal Nutrition USA, Inc., 1999.

24. Powers, Laura, Ph.D. Personal communication, 2000.

25. Quoted in Barnard, Neal. *The Power of Your Plate.* Summertown, TN: Book Publishing Company, 1990.

26. "Eating According to Your Blood Type: A Bloody Bad Idea," *Tufts University Health and Nutrition Letter,* August 1997..

27. Schmidt, Gerhard. *The Dynamics of Nutrition.* Providence, RI: Bio-Dynamic Literature, 1980.

28. Swank, Roy, and Pullen, Mary-Helen. *The Multiple Sclerosis Diet Book.* New York: Doubleday and Company, Inc., 1977.

29. Schmidt, Gerhard. *The Dynamics of Nutrition.* Providence, RI: Bio-Dynamic Literature, 1980.

30. Ibid.

Chapter 18: High- Versus Low-Protein Diet

1. Airola, Paavo. *Are You Confused?* Phoenix, AZ: Health Plus, Publishers, 1974.

2. Ibid.

3. Ibid.

4. Ibid.

5. Kulvinskas, Viktoras. *Survival into the 21st Century.* Woodstock Valley, CT/Fairfield, IA: 21st Century Publications, 1975.

6. Airola, Paavo. *How to Get Well.* Phoenix, AZ: Health Plus, Publishers, 1974.

7. Ibid.

8. Ibid.

9. Wendt, L., Wendt, T., and Wendt, A. "Protein Transport and Protein Storage in Etiology and Pathogenesis of Arteriosclerosis," *Ernahrungswiss.* Dietrich Steinkopff Verlag, 1975, pp. 1–38.

10. Levine, Steve and Kidd, Paris. *Antioxidant Adaption: Its Role in Free Radical Pathology.* San Francisco: Biocurrents Press, 1985.

11. Airola, Paavo. *Are You Confused?* Phoenix, AZ: Health Plus, Publishers, 1974.

12. Airola, Paavo. *How to Get Well.* Phoenix, AZ: Health Plus, Publishers, 1974.

13. Kulvinskas, Viktoras. *Survival into the 21st Century.* Woodstock Valley, CT/Fairfield, IA: 21st Century Publications, 1975.

14. Airola, Paavo. *Are You Confused?* Phoenix, AZ: Health Plus, Publishers, 1974.

Chapter 19: B_{12}

1. Messina, M. and Messina, V. *The Dietician's Guide to Vegetarian Diets.* Gaithersburg, MD: Aspen Publishers, Inc., 1996.

2. Donaldson, M. S. "Metabolic Vitamin B-12 Status on a Mostly Raw Vegan Diet with Follow-Up Using Tablets, Nutritional Yeast, or Probiotic Supplements," *Ann. Nutr. Metab.*, vol. 44, no. 5–6, 2000, pp. 229–34. And personal communication with author, Jan. 31, 2002.

3. Kuhne, T., Bubl, R., and Baumgartner, R. "Maternal Vegan Diet Causing a Serious Infantile Neurological Disorder Due to Vitamin B_{12} Deficiency," *Eur. J. Pediatr.*, vol. 150, no. 3, Jan. 1991, pp. 205–208.

4. Nelen, W. L., Blom, H. J., Steegers, E. A., denHeijer, M., and Eskes, T. K. "Hyperhomocysteinemia and Recurrent Early Pregnancy Loss: A Meta-Analysis," *Fertil. Steril.*, vol. 74, no. 6, Dec. 2000, pp. 1196–1199.

5. Guyton, A. C. and Hall, J. E. *Textbook of Medical Physiology*, 9th ed. Philadelphia: W. B. Saunders, Co., 1996, pp. 845–847.

6. Grattan-Smith, P. J., Wilcken, B., Procopis, P. G., and Wise, G. A. "The Neurological Syndrome of Infantile Cobalamin Deficiency: Developmental Regression and Involuntary Movements" *Mov. Disord.*, vol. 12, no. 1, Jan. 1997, pp. 39–46.

7. von Schenck, U., Bender-Gotze, C., and Koletzko, B. "Persistence of Neurological Damage Induced by Dietary Vitamin B-12 Deficiency in Infancy," *Arch. Dis. Child.*, vol. 77, no. 2, Aug. 1997, pp. 137–139.

8. Ashkenazi, S., Weitz, R., Varsano, I., and Mimouni, M. "Vitamin B-12 Deficiency Due to a Strictly Vegetarian Diet in Adolescence," *Clinical Pediatrics*, vol. 26, Dec. 1987, pp. 662–663.

9. Sanders, T. A. and Purves, R. "An Anthropometric and Dietary Assessment of the Nutritional Status of Vegan Preschool Children," *J. Hum. Nutr.*, vol. 35, no. 5, Oct. 1981, pp. 349–357.

10. Hokin, B. D. and Butler, T. "Cyanocobalamin (Vitamin B-12) Status in Seventh-Day Adventist Ministers in Australia," *Am. J. Clin. Nutr.*, vol. 70, no. 3 Suppl, Sept. 1999, pp. 576S–578S.

11. Areekul, S., Pattanamatum, S., Cheeramakara, C., Churdchue, K., Nitayapabskoon, S., and Chongsanguan, M. "The Source and Content of Vitamin B-12 in the Tempehs," *J. Med. Assoc. Thai*, vol. 73, no. 3, March 1990, pp. 152–156.

12. Bar-Sella, P., Rakover, Y., and Ratner, D. "Vitamin B_{12} and Folate Levels in Long-Term Vegans. *Isr. J. Med. Sci.*, vol. 26, 1990, pp. 309–312.

13. Tungtrongchitr, R., Pongpaew, P., Prayurahong, B., Changbumrung, S., Vudhivai, N., Migasena, P., and Schelp, F. P. "Vitamin B_{12}, Folic Acid and Haematological Status of 132 Thai Vegetarians," *Int. J. Vitam. Nutr. Res.*, vol. 63, no. 3, 1993, pp. 201–207.

14. Campbell, M., Lofters, W. S., and Gibbs, W. N. "Rastafarianism and the Vegans Syndrome," *BMJ (Clin. Res. Ed.*), vol. 285, no. 6355, Dec. 4, 1982, pp. 1617–1618.

15. Crane, M. G., Sample, C., Pathcett, S., and Register, U.D. "Vitamin B_{12} Studies in Total Vegetarians (Vegans)," *Journal of Nutritional Medicine*, vol. 4, 1994, pp. 419–430.

16. Crane, M. G., Register, U. D., Lukens, R. H., and Gregory, R. "Cobalamin (CBL) Studies on Two Total Vegetarian (Vegan) Families," *Vegetarian Nutrition*, vol. 2, no. 3, 1998, pp. 87–92.

17. Haddad, E. H., Berk, L. S., Kettering, J. D., Hubbard, R. W., and Peters, W. R. "Dietary Intake and Biochemical, Hematologic, and Immune Status of Vegans Compared with Nonvegetarians," *Am. J. Clin. Nutr.*, vol. 70(suppl), 1999, pp. 586S–593S.

18. Woo, J., Kwok, T., Ho, S. C., Sham, A., and Lau, E. "Nutritional Status of Elderly Chinese Vegetarians," *Age Ageing*, vol. 27, no. 4, July 1998, pp. 455–461.

19. Dong, A. and Scott, S. C. "Serum Vitamin B_{12} and Blood Cell Values in Vegetarians," *Ann. Nutr. Metab.*, vol. 26, no. 4, 1982, pp. 209–216.

20. Rauma, A. L., Torronen, R., Henninen, O., and Mykkanaen, H. "Vitamin B-12 Status of Long-Term Adherents of a Strict Uncooked Vegan Diet ("Living

Food Diet") Is Compromised," *J. Nutr.,* vol. 125, no. 10, Oct. 1995, pp. 2511–2515.

21. Donaldson, M. S. Op. cit.

22. Bernstein, L. "Dementia Without a Cause," *Discover,* February 2003, p. 31.

23. Lovblad, K., Ramelli, G., Remonda, L., Nirkko, A. C., Ozdoba, C., and Schroth, G. "Retardation of Myelination Due to Dietary B_{12} Deficiency: Cranial MRI Findings," *Pediatr. Radiol.*, vol. 27, no. 2, Feb. 1997, pp. 155–158.

24. Von Schenck,U., Bender-Gotze,C., and Koletzko, B. "Persistance of Neurological Damage Induced by Dietary Vitamin B-12 Deficiency in Infancy." *Arch.Dis.Child,* vol.77, no.2:Aug. 1997, pp. 137–139.

25. Goraya, J. "Letter About Persistence of Neurological Damage Induced by Dietary Vitamin B_{12} Deficiency," *Arch. Dis. Child.*, vol. 78, no. 4, 1998, pp. 398–399.

26. Specker, B. L., Miller, D., Norman, E. J., Greene, H., and Hayes, K. C. "Increased Urinary Methylmalonic Acid Excretion in Breast-Fed Infants of Vegetarian Mothers and Identification of An Acceptable Dietary Source of Vitamin B-12," *Am. J. Clin. Nutr.,* vol. 47, no. 1, Jan. 1988, pp. 89–92.

27. Kuhne, et al. Op cit.

28. Drogari, E., Liakopoulou-Tsitsipi, T., Xypolyta-Zachariadi, A., Papadellis, F., and Kattamis, C. "Transient Methylmalonic Aciduria in Four Breast Fed Neonates of Strict Vegetarian Mothers in Greece," *Journal of Inherited Metabolic Disease,* vol. 19S, 1996, Abstract, p. A84.

29. Lovblad, et al. Op cit.

30. Davis, J. R., Goldenring, J., and Lubin, B. "Nutritional Vitamin B_{12} Deficiency in Infants," *Am. J. Dis. Child.*, vol. 135, June 1981, pp. 566–567.

31. Lovblad, et. al. Op. cit.

32. Sanders, T. A. "Vegetarian Diets and Children," *Pediatr. Clin. North Am.*, vol. 42, no. 4, Aug. 1995, pp. 955–965.

33. Sanders and Purves. Op. cit.

34. Fulton, J. R., Hutton, C. W., and Stitt, K. R. "Preschool Vegetarian Children. Dietary and Anthropometric Data," *J. Am. Diet. Assoc.*, vol. 76, no. 4, April 1980, pp. 360–365.

35. Crane, et al., 1994. Op. cit.

36. Ibid.

37. Dong and Scott. Op. cit.

38. Rauma, et al. Op. cit. Also Donaldson, M. S. Op. cit.

39. Hokin and Butler. Op. cit.

40. Areekul, S., Churdchu, K., and Pungpapong, V. "Serum Folate, Vitamin B_{12} and Vitamin B_{12} Binding Protein in Vegetarians," *J. Med. Assoc. Thai.*, vol. 71, no. 5, May 1988, pp. 253–257.

41. Bar-Sella, et al. Op. cit.

42. Tungtrongchitr, et al. Op. cit.

43. Crane, et al., 1994. Op. cit.

44. Woo, et al. Op. cit.

45. Harman, S. K. and Parnell, W. R. "The Nutritional Health of New Zealand

Vegetarian and Non-Vegetarian Seventh-Day Adventists: Selected Vitamin, Mineral and Lipid Levels," *NZ Med. J.*, vol. 111, no. 1062, Mar. 27, 1998, pp. 91–94.

46. Alexander, D., Ball, M. J., and Mann, J. "Nutrient Intake and Haematological Status of Vegetarians and Age-Sex Matched Omnivores," *European Journal of Clinical Nutrition,* vol. 48, 1994, pp. 538–546.

47. Brants, H. A., Lowik, M. R., Westenbrink, S., Hulshof, K. F., and Kistemaker, C. "Adequacy of a Vegetarian Diet At Old Age (Dutch Nutrition Survellance System)," *J. Am. Coll. Nutr.*, vol. 9, no. 4, Aug. 1990, pp. 292–302.

48. Campbell, et al. Op. cit.

49. Herbert, V. "Vitamin B-12: Plant Sources, Requirements, and Assay," *Am. J. Clin. Nutr.,* vol. 48, 1988, pp. 852–858.

50. Areekul, et al., 1990. Op. cit.

51. van den Berg, H., Dagnelie, P. C., and van Stveren, W. A. "Vitamin B-12 and Seaweed," *Lancet,* Jan. 30, 1988.

52. Specker, et al. Op. cit.

53. van den Berg, et al. Op. cit.

54. Areekul, et al., 1990. Op. cit.

55. Herbert, V. " Vitamin B_{12}: plant sources requirements in assay." *Am. J. Clin. Nutr.* 1988; 48: 852–8.

56. Mozafar, A. "Enrichment of Some B Vitamins in Plants with Application of Organic Fertilizers," *Plant & Soil,* vol. 167, 1994, pp. 305–311.

57. Areekul, et al., 1988. Op. cit.

58. Hathcock, J,N. and Troendle, G.J. "Oral Colbalamin for Treatment of Pernicious Anemia?" *JAMA* 1991 Jan 2, vol.; 265, no. 1, pp. 96–97.

59. Shinwell, E.D. and Gorodischer, R. "Totally Vegitarian Diets and Infant Nutrition," *Pediatrics,* vol. 70, no. 4, Oct. 1982, pp. 582–586.

Chapter 20: The Light of Live Foods

1. Howell, Edward. *Food Enzymes for Health and Longevity.* Woodstock Valley, CT: Omangod Press, 1946.

2. Wigmore, Ann. *The Hippocrates Diet.* Wayne, NJ: Avery Publishing Group Inc., 1984.

3. Howell, Edward. Op. cit.

4. Ibid.

5. Ibid.

6. Schroeder, Henry A. *The Trace Elements and Man: Some Positive and Negative Aspects.* Boulder, CO: Shambala Publications,1974.

7. Howell, Edward. Op. cit.

8. Ibid.

9. Ibid.

10. *Journal of Medical Hypothesis,* vol. 51, 1998, pp. 179–221.

11. Pottenger, E. M. "The Effect of Heat Processed Foods and Metabolized Vitamin D Milk on the Dento-Facial Structure of Experimental Animals," *American J. Orthodontics and Oral Surgery,* Aug. 1946, pp. 467–485.

12. Cousens, Gabriel. *Rainbow Green Live-Food Cuisine.* Berkeley, CA: North Atlantic Books, 2003, p. 117.

13. Popp, F.A. "Biophoton Emission: New Evidence for Coherence in DNA." *Cell Biophysics,* March 1984, vol. 6: 32–52.

14. Kulvinskas, Viktoras. *Survival into the 21st Century.* Woodstock Valley, CT/Fairfield, IA: 21st Century Publications, 1975.

15. Ibid.

16. Airola, Paavo. *Are You Confused?* Phoenix, AZ: Health Plus, Publishers, 1974.

17. Szekely, Edmond Bordeaux. *The Essene Gospel of Peace, Book One.* San Diego, CA: International Biogenic Society, 1981.

18. Howell, Edward. Op. cit.

19. Kouchakoff, Paul. "The Influence of Cooking Food on the Blood Formula of Man," *Proceedings: First International Congress of Micro Biology,* Paris: 1930.

20. Kulvinskas, Viktoras. Op. cit.

21. McCluskey, C. "The Little-Finger Test," *The Lancet,* Dec. 29, 1973, p. 1503.

22. Szekely, Edmond Bordeaux. *The Chemistry of Youth.* San Diego, CA: International Biogenic Society, 1977.

23. Szekely, Edmond Bordeaux. *The Essenes by Josephus and His Contemporaries.* San Diego, CA: International Biogenic Society, 1981.

24. Szekely, Edmond Bordeaux. 1977. Op. cit.

25. Szekely, Edmond Bordeaux. *The Essene Way Biogenic Living.* San Diego, CA: International Biogenic Society, 1978.

26. Howell, Edward. Op. cit.

27. Ibid.

28. Wigmore, Ann. Op. cit.

29. Szekely, Edmond Bordeaux. 1977. Op. cit.

30. Ibid.

31. Szekely, Edmond Bordeaux. *The Chemistry of Youth.* San Diego, CA: International Biogenic Society, 1977.

32. Cousens, Gabriel. *Rainbow Green Live-Food Cuisine.* Berkeley, CA: North Atlantic Books, 2003, p. 117.

33. Ibid.

34. Airola, Paavo. *How to Get Well.* Phoenix, AZ: Health Plus, Publishers, 1974.

35. Kulvinskas, Viktoras. Op. cit.

Chapter 21: Feeding Our Genes: A Key to Understanding Live Foods

1. Lindquist, S. The Heat-Shock response. *Ann Rev Biochem* 55: 1151–1191, 1986.

2. Lindquist, S., Craig, E.A. The heat shock protines. *Annu Rev Genet* 22: 631–677, 1988.

3. Morimoto, R.I., Jurivich, D.A., Kroeger, P.E., Matheur, S.K., Murphy, S.P., Nakai, A., Sarge, K., Abravaya, K., Sistonen, L. The regulation of heat shock gene expression by a family of heat shock factors. In: *The Biology of Heat Shock Proteins*

and Molecular Chaperones. Morimoto, A.I., Tissieres, A., Georgopoulos, C. eds. Cold Spring Harbor, NY: Cold Spring Harbor Laboratory Press, 1994.

4. Lindquist (1986), Lindquist and Craig (1998), and Morimoto (1994). Op. cit.

5. Green, S., Wahli, W. Peroxisome proliferators activated receptors:finding the orphan a home. *Mol Cell Endocrinol* 100: 149–153, 1994.

6. Keller, H., and Wahli, W. Peroxisome proliferators-activated receptors: A link between endocrinology and nutrition? *Trends Endocrinol Metab* 4: 291–296, 1993.

7. Green (1994) and Keller (1993). Op. cit.

8. Cotton, V.C., Wilkinson, G. *Advanced Inorganic Chemistry, A Comprehensive Text.* New York: John Wiley and Sons, 1980.

9. Lippard, S.J., Bioinorganic chemistry: a maturing frontier. *Science* 261: 699–700, 1993.

10. Vallee, B.L., Auld, D.S. Zinc coordination, function, and structure of zink enzymes and other protines. *Biochemistry* 29: 5647–5659, 1990.

11. Vallee, B.L., Faluchuk, K.H. The biochemical basis of zink physiology. *Physiol Rev* 73: 79–118, 1993.

12. Searle, P.F., et al. Regulation, linkage and sequence of mouse metallothionein I and II genes. *Mol Cell Biol* 4: 1221–1230 (1984).

13. Baeuerle, P.A., editor. *Inducible Gene Expression,* Volume 1, Boston, MA: Birkhauser Boston, 1995

14.Towle, H.C. and Kaytor, E.N. Regulation of gene expression of lipogenic genes by carbohydrate, *Ann. Rev. Nutr.,* 17, 405, 1997.

15. Ibid.

16. Girard, J., Ferre, P., and Foufelle, F., Mechanisms by which carbohydrates regulate expression of genes for glycolic and lipogenic enzymes, *Ann. Rev. Nutr.,* 19, 63, 1999.

17. Oskouian, B., Rangan, V.S., and Smith, S., Transcriptional regulation of the rat fatty acid synthase gene:identification and functional analysis of positive and negative effectors of basal transcription, *Biochem. J.,* 317, 257, 1996.

18. Ibid. SeeJump, D.B., Clark, S.D., Thelen, A., Liimatta, M., and Ben, B., Dietary poly-unsaturated fatty acid regulation of gene transcription, *Prog. Lipid Res.,* 35, 227, 1996.

19. Mariash, C. N., Kaiser, F. E., and Oppenheimer, J. H., Comparison of the response characteristics of four lipogenic enzymes to 3,5,3'-triiodothyronine administration: evidence for variable degrees of amplification of the nuclear 3.5.3'-triiodothyroine signal, *Endocrinology,* 106, 22, 1980.

20. Diamant, S., Gorin, E., and Shafrir, E., Enzyme activities related to fatty acid synthesis in liver and adipose tissue of rats treated with triiodothyronine, *Eur. J. Biochem.,* 26, 553, 1972.

21. Iritani, N., Sugimoto, T., and Fukuda, H., Gene expressions of leptin, insulin receptors and lipogenic enzymes are coordinately regulated by insulin and dietary fats, *J. Nutr.,* 130, 1183, 2000.

22. Yin, D., Clark, S.D., Peters, J. L., and Etherton, T.D., Somatotropin-depen-

dant decrease in fatty acid synthase mRNA abundance in 3T3-F442A adipocytes is the result of a decrease in both gene transcription and mRNA stability, *Biochem. J.*, 331, 815, 1998.

23. Donkin, S.S., McNall, A.D., Swencki, B. S., Peters, J. L., and Etherton, T. D., The growth hormone-dependent decrease in hepatic fatty acid synthase mRNA is the result of a decrease in gene transcription, *J. Mol. Endocrinol.*, 16, 151, 1996.

24. Grobin, A.C., Matthews, D.B., Devaud, L.L. and Morrow, A.L., The role of $GABA_A$ receptors in the acute and chronic effects of ethanol, *Psychopharmacol.* 139, 2, 1998.

25. Aprison, M. H. and Daly, E. C., Biochemical aspects of transmission at inhibitory synapses: the role of glycine, *Adv. Neurochem.*, 3, 203, 1978.

26. Nevo, I. And Hamon, M., Neurotransmitter and neuromodulatory mechanisms involved in alcohol abuse and alcoholism, *Neurochem. Int.*, 26, 305, 1995.

27. Crabbe, J. C., Phillips, T. J., Feller, D. J., Hen, R, Wenger, C. D., Lessov, C. N., and Schafer, G. L., Evevated alcohol consumption in null mutant mice lacking 5 HT1B serotonin receptors, *Nature Genet.*, 14, 98, 1996.

28. Hill, E. M., Stoltenberg, S. F., Burmeister, M., Closser, M., and Zucker, R. A., Potential associations amoung genetic markers in the serotonergic system and the antisocial alcoholism subtype, *Exp. Clinical Psychopharmacol.*, 7, 103, 1999.

29. Lappalainen, J., Long, J. C., Eggert, M., Ozaki, N., Robin, R. W., Brown, G. L., Naukkarinen, H., Virkkunen, M., Linnoila, M., and Goldman, D., Linkage of antisocial alcoholism to the serotonin 5-HT1B receptor gene in 2 populations, *Arch. Gen. Psychiatr.*, 55, 989, 1988.

30. Druse, M. J., Kuo, A., and Tajuddin, N., Effects of in Utero ethanol exposure on the developing serotonergic system, *Alcohol Clin. Exp. Res.*, 15, 678, 1991.

31. Eisenhofer, G., Szabo, G., and Hoffman, P. L., Opposite changes in turnover of noradrenaline and dopamine in the CNS of ethsnol-dependent mice, *Neuropharmacology*, 29, 37, 1990.

32. Campbell, A. D. and Erwin, V. G., Chronic ethanol administration downregulates neurotensin receptors in long- and short-sleep mice, *Pharmacol. Biochem, Behav.*, 45, 95, 1993.

33. Lewohol, J. M., Wang, L. Miles, M. F. Zhang, L. Dood, P. R., and Harris, R. A., Gene expression in human alcoholism: microarry analysis of frontal cortex, *Alcohol Clin. Exp. Res.*, 24, 1873, 2000.

34. Ruiz-Lozano, P., Smith, S. M., Perkins, G., Kubalak, S. W., Boss, G. R., Sucov, H. M., Evans, R. M., and Chien, K. R., Energy deprevation and a deficiency in downstream metabolic target genes during the onset of embryonic heart failure in RXR -/- embryos, *Development*, 125, 533, 1998.

35. Fechner, H., Schlame, M., Guthmann, F., Stevens, P.A., and Rustow, B., Alpha and delta-tocopherol induced expression of hepatic alpha-tocopherol-transfer-protein mRNA, *Biochem. J., 15, 577, 1998.*

36. Wilmut, I., Schnieke, A.E., McWhir, J., Kind, A.J., Campbell, K.H.S. "Viable Offspring Derived from Fetal and Adult Mammalian Cells," *Nature.* Vol. 385, 810–813, 1997.

37. Pauling, L., Itano, H. "Sickle Cell Anemia, a Molecular Disease," *Science*. Vol. 110, 543–647, 1949.

38 Ibid.

39. Bishop, Jerry and Waldholz, Michael. *Genome*. Lincoln, NE: iUniverse, 1999.

40. Bland, Jeffrey. *Genetic Nutritioneering*. Lincolnwood, IL: Keats, 1999.

41. Lin, H.J. "Smokers and Breast Cancer. 'Chemical Individuality' and Cancer Predisposition," *Journal of the American Medical Association*. Vol. 276, 1511–12, 1996.

42. Pyeritz, R.E. "Family History and Genetic Risk Factors. Forward to the Future," *Journal of the American Medical Association*. Vol 278, 1285–86, 1997

43. Williams, R. *Biochemical Individuality*. New York: McGraw-Hill, 1998.

44. Sullivan, J. "Salt-Sensitivity: Definition, Conception, Methodology, and Long-Term Issues." *Hypertension*. Vol 17 (suppl.) 173–74, 1991.

45. Bland, Jeffrey. Op. cit.

46. Ibid.

47. Franz, M.J. "Protein: Metabolism and Effect on Blood Glucose Levels," *Diabetes Education*. Vol. 18, 1–29, 1992.

48. Block, G. "Dietary Guidelines and the Results of Food Consumption Surveys," *American Journal of Clinical Nutrition*. Vol 53, 56–57S, 1991.

49. Milner, J.A. "Garlic: Its Anticarcinogenic and Antitumorigenic Properties," *Nutrition Reviews*. Vol 54, 82–86.

50. Xu, Y.X., Pindolia, K.R., Janakiraman, N, et al. "Circumin, a Compound with Anti-Infalmmatory and Anti-Oxidant Properties, Down-Regulates Chemokine Expression in Bone Marrow Stromal Cells," *Experimantal Hematology*. Vol 25, 413–22, 1997.

51. Chan, N.M., Ho, C.T., Huang, H.I. "Effects of Three Dietary Phytochemicals from Tea, Rosemary and Turmeric on Inflammation-Induced Nitrite Production," *Cancer Letters*. Vol. 96, 23–29, 1995.

52. Sato, M, Miyazaki, T., Kambe, F., et al. "Quercetin, a Bioflavonoid, Inhibits the Induction of Interleukin 8 and Monocyte Chemoattractant Protein-1 Expression by Tumor Necrosis Factor-*a* in Cultured Human Synovial Cells," *Journal of Rheumatology*. Vol 24, 1680–84, 1997.

53. Ibid.

54. Ambrosone, C.B., Freudenheim, J.L. Graham, S., et al. "Cigarette Smoking, N-Acetyltransferase 2 Genetic polymorphisms, and Breast Cancer Risk," *Journal of the American Medical Association*. Vol. 276, no. 18, 1494–1501, 1996.

55. Ryberg, D., Skaug, V, Hewer, A., et al. "Genotypes of Glutathione Transferase M1 and P1 and Their Significance for Lung DNA Adduct Levels and Cancer Risk," *Carcinogenesis*. Voll. 18, no. 7, 1285–89, 1997.

56. Quick, A.J. "The Conjugation of Benzoic Acid in Man," *Journal of Biological Chemistry*. Vol. 92, 65–85, 1931.

57. Nijhoff, W.A., Grubben, J.A., Nagengast, F.M., et al. "Effects of Consumption of Brussels Sprouts on Intestinal and Lymphocytic Glutathione S-transferase in

Humans," *Carcinogenesis*. Vol. 16, no. 9, 2125–28, 1995.

58. Finch, C. "Genetics of Aging," *Science*. Vol. 278, 407, 1997.

59. Mitchell, Terri. "Resveratrol: Cutting-Edge Technology Available Today." *Life Extension Magazine*. Dec 2003.

60. Ibid.

61. Richter, C., Park, J.W., Ames, B. "Normal Oxidative Damage to Mitochondrial and Nuclear DNA is Extensive," *Proceedings of the National Academy of Sciences*. Vol. 85, 6465–67, 1988.

62. Suzuki, Y.J., Forman, H.J., Sevanian, A. "Oxidants as Stimulators of Signal Transduction," *Free Radical Biology and Medicine*. Vol. 22, 269–85, 1997.

63. Palmer, H.J., Paulson, K.E. "Reactive Oxygen Species and Antioxidents in Signal Transduction and Gene Expression," *Nutrition Reviews*. Vol. 55, 353–61, 1997.

64. Beal, M.F. "Aging, Energy, and Oxidative Stress in Neurodegenerative Disease," *Annals of Neurology*. Vol. 38, 357–66, 1995.

65. Kamat J.P., Davasagayam, T.P. "Tocotrienols from Palm Oil as Potent Inhibitors of Lipid Peroxidation and Protein Oxidation in Rat Brain Mitochondria," *Neuroscience Letters*. Vol. 195, 179–82, 1995.

Chapter 22: Undereat!

1. Hoffman, Edward. "The Father of Holistic Healing," *East West Journal*, April 1986, pp. 26–29.

2. Airola, Paavo. *How to Get Well*. Phoenix, AZ: Health Plus, Publishers, 1974.

3. Szekely, Edmond Bordeaux. *The Essene Gospel of Peace, Book One*. San Diego, CA: International Biogenic Society, 1981.

4. Kramer, Penny. "Health and Longevity: What Centenarians Can Teach Us," *Yoga Journal*. Berkeley, CA: Goodfellow Publishers, Sept./Oct. 1983, pp. 26–30.

5. Cornaro, Luigi. *Discourses on the Sober Life*. Mokelumne Hill, CA: Health Research, 1942.

6. Szekely, Edmond Bordeaux. *Essene Science of Fasting and the Art of Sobriety*. San Diego, CA: International Biogenic Society, 1981.

7. Cousens, Gabriel. *Rainbow Green Live-Food Cuisine*. Berkeley, CA: North Atlantic Books, 2003.

8. Kulvinskas, Viktoras. *Survival into the 21st Century*. Woodstock Valley, CT/Fairfield, IA: 21st Century Publications, 1975.

9. Howell, Edward. *Food Enzymes for Health and Longevity*. Woodstock Valley, CT: Omangod Press, 1946.

10. Life Extention Magazine, Nov 1999.

11. Fahy, Gregorym, and Kent, Saul. Reversing Aging Rapidly with Short-Term Calorie restriction. *Life Extention*. May 2001.

12. Berger, Stuart. *Forever Young*. New York: HarperCollins, 1989.

Chapter 23: Spiritual Fasting

1. Cott, Allan. *Fasting: The Ultimate Diet.* Toronto, New York, London, Sydney: Bantam Books, 1981.
2. Ibid.
3. Szekely, Edmond Bordeaux, translator. *The Essenes by Josephus and His Contemporaries.* San Diego, CA: International Biogenic Society, 1981.
4. *Essene Science of Fasting.* Channeled by Kevin Ryerson. Audiotape.
5. Szekely, Edmond Bordeaux. *The Essene Gospel of Peace, Book One.* San Diego, CA: International Biogenic Society, 1981.
6. Kaplan, Arye. *Gems of Rabbi Nachman.* Jerusalem: Chaim Kramer, 1980.
7. *Mathew the Poor—The Communion of Love.* Foreword by Henri J. M. Nouwen, Crestwood, New York: St. Vladimir's Seminary Press, 1984.
8. Airola, Paavo. *How to Keep Slim, Healthy and Young with Juice Fasting.* Phoenix, AZ: Health Plus, 1974.
9. Ibid.
10. Ibid.
11. Ibid.
12. Gurudas. *Gem Elixirs and Vibrational Healing,* Vol. 1. Boulder, CO: Cassandra Press, 1985.
13. Gurudas. *Gem Elixirs and Vibrational Healing,* Vol. II. Boulder, CO: Cassandra Press, 1986.
14. Gurudas. *Flower Essences and Vibrational Healing.* Albuquerque, NM: Brotherhood of Life, 1983.
15. *Essene Science of Fasting.* Op. cit.

Chapter 24: The Ayurvedic Tridosha System

1. Thakkur, Chandrashekhar G. *Introduction to Ayurveda.* San Francisco, CA: Red Wheel/Weiser, 1974.
2. Ibid.
3. Haas, Elson M. *Staying Healthy with the Seasons.* Millbrae, CA: Celestial Arts, 1981.
4. Lad, Vasant. *Ayurveda: The Science of Self-Healing.* Santa Fe, NM: Lotus Press, 1984.
5. Ballentine, Rudolph. *Diet and Nutrition.* Honesdale, PA: The Himalayan Intl. Institute, 1982.

Chapter 25: Ayurvedic Insights into Live Foods

1. Frawley, David. *Yoga and Ayurveda.* Twin Lakes, WI: Lotus Press, 1999.
2. Drapeau, Christian. Personal communication. 2004.
3. Airola, Paavo. *Worldwide Secrets for Staying Young.* Phoenix, AZ: Health Plus Publishers, 1982.
4. Maas, James B. *Power Sleep.* New York, NY: Perennial Currents, 1999.
5. Glenmullen, Joseph. *Prozac Backlash.* New York: Simon & Schuster, 2000.

6. Ibid.

7. Ibid.

8. Primary Pulmonary Hypertension from Fenfluramine and Dexfenfluramine: A Systemic review of Evidence," *Journal of the American Medical Association* 278 (1997): 666–72.

9. Westphalen, R. I. And Dodd, P. R. "The Regeneration of d,l-Fenfluramine-Destroyed Serotonergic Nerve Terminals," *European Journal of Pharmacology* 238 (1993): 399–402.

10. McCann, U. D. Op. cit.

11. Fischer, C., Hatzidimitriou, G., Wlos, J., Katz, J., and Ricaurte, G. "Reorganization of Ascending 5-HT Axon Projections in Animals Previously Exposed to the Recreational Drug (3), 4-Methylenedioxymethamphetamine (MDMA, 'Ecstacy')," *Journal of Neuroscience* 15 (1995): 5476–85.

12. Ibid. Wrona, M. Z., Yang, Z., Zhang, F., and Dryhurst, G. "Potentail New Insights into the Molecular Mechanisms of Methamphetamine-Induced Neurodegeneration," *National Institute on Drug Abuse Research Monograph Series* 173 (1997): 146–74.

13. Grob, Charles and Metzner, Ralph. Personal communication. 2004.

14. Frawley, David. Op. cit.

15. Ibid.

16. Cousens, Gabriel, M.D. *Conscious Eating*. Berkeley, CA: North Atlantic Books, 2000.

17. Ibid.

18. Ibid.

19. Airola, Paavo. *Are You Confused?* Phoenix, AZ: Health Plus Publishers, 1971.

20. Anandamurti, Shrii Shrii. *Beyond the Superconscious Mind.* Calcutta: Ananda Marga, 1987.

21. Ibid.

Chapter 26: The Rainbow Diet

1. Hunt, Roland. *The Seven Keys to Colour Healing*. Rochester, KY: C.W. Daniel Company Ltd., 1971.

2. Babbitt, Edwin. *The Principles of Light and Color.* Whitefish, MT: Kessinger Publishing, 1942.

3. Ott, John. *Health and Light.* Columbus, OH: Ariel Press, 2000.

Chapter 27: Low-Glycemic Eating

1. Airola, Paavo. Personal communication. 1976.

2. Airola, Paavo. *Hypoglycemia: A Better Approach.* Phoenix, AZ: Health Plus, 1977.

3. Williams, Roger. *Biochemical Individuality.* New York: McGraw-Hill, 1998.

4. Buckley, Robert E. "Hypoglycemic Symptoms and the Hypoglycemic Experience," *Psychosomatics,* vol. X, Jan./Feb. 1969, pp. 7–14.

5. Airola, Paavo. Op. cit.

6. Lesser, M. *Proceedings, World Congress of Biological Psychiatry,* Buenos Aires: 1977.

7. Fariss, B. "Prevalence of Post-Glucose Load Glycosuria and Hypoglycemia in a Group of Healthy Young Men," *Diabetes,* vol. 23, 1974, pp. 181–191.

8. Airola, Paavo. Op. cit.

9. Ibid.

10. *Diet Related to Killer Diseases,* Nutrition and Mental Health, Hearing Before the Select Committee on Nutrition and Human Needs of the United States Senate, June 22, 1977.

11. Schauss, Alexander. *Diet, Crime and Delinquency.* Berkeley, CA: Parker House, 1980.

12. Yaryura-Tobias, J.A. and Neziroglu, B. A. "Aggressive Behavior, Glucose, and Brain Dysfunction," *Diet Related to Killer Diseases,* V Nutrition and Mental Health, Hearing before the Select Committee on Nutrition and Human Needs of the U.S. Senate, June 22, 1977, pp. 193–199.

13. Bland, Jeffrey S. *Genetic Nutritioneering.* Lincolnwood, IL: Keats, 1999, Chapter 7, note 9.

14. Considine, R.V., Sinha, M.K., Heiman, M.L., et. Al. "Serum Immunoreactive-Leptin Concentrations in Normal-Weight and Obese Humans," *New England Journal of Medicine.* vol. 334, pp. 292–95, 1996.

15. Brown, I. "Complex Carbohydrates and Resistant Starch," *Nutrition Reviews.* vol. 54, pp.S115–19, 1996.

16.Girard, J., Gerre, P., Foufelle, F., "Mechanisms by Which Carbohydrates Regulate Expression of Genes for Glycolytic and lipogenic Enzymes," *Annual Review of Nutrition.* vol. 17, pp. 405–33, 1997.

17.Spiller, G.A., Jensen, C.D., Pattison, T.S., et al. "Effect of Protine Dose on Serum Glucose and Insulin Response to Sugars," *American Journal of Clinical Nutrition.* vol. 46, pp, 474–80, 1987.

18.Rattan, S.I. "Synthisis, Modifications, and Turnover of Protines During Aging," *Experimental Gerentology.* vol. 31, pp. 33–47, 1996.

19. Wolff, S.P., Bascal, Z.A., Hunt, J.V. " 'Autoxidative Glycosylation': Free Radicals and Glycation Theory," *Progress in Clinical Biology Research.* vol. 304, pp.259–75, 1989.

Chapter 28: Minerals—Frequencies of Light

1. United States Senate document 264, 74th Congress, second session, 1936.

2. Ott, A. Tru. *Wellness Secrets for Life: An Owner's Manual for the Human Body.* Cedar City, UT: Cedar Mountain Publishing, 1999.

3. "Vital Signs." *Southwest Airlines Spirit.* December 2003.

4. Murray, Maynard. *Sea Energy Agriculture.* Austin, TX: Acres U.S.A., 2003.

5. Jensen, Bernard. *The Chemistry of Man.* Escondido, CA: Bernard Jensen International, 1983.

6. Ott, A. Tru. Op. cit., p. 71

7. Fischer, William L. *How to Fight Cancer & Win.* Baltimore, MD: Health Books., 2000, p. 278.

8. Ott, A. Tru. Op. cit.

9. Ibid.

10. Wolfe, David. *Eating for Beauty.* San Diego, CA: Maul Brothers Publishing, 2003.

11. Ibid.

12. Jensen, Bernard. Op. cit.

13. Wolfe, David. Op. cit.

14. Jensen, Bernard. Op. cit.

15. Opitz, Christian. *The Miracle of Krystal Salt.* Mount Shasta, CA: Krystal Web Matrix, Inc., p. 12.

16. Jacob, Stanley, Laurence, Ronald, M., and Zucker, Martin. *The Miracle of MSM.* New York: Berkeley Publishing Group, 1999.

17. Wolfe, David. Op. cit., p. 39.

18. Jensen, Bernard. Op. cit.

19. Baeuerle, P. A., editor. *Inducible Gene Expression,* Volume 1. Boston: Birkhauser Boston, 1995, footnote by Valle & Falchuck 1993, Chapter 7.

20. Baeuerle, P. A., editor. Op. cit., footnote by Valle & Auld 1990, Chapter 7.

21. Baeuerle, P. A., editor. Op. cit., footnote by Cotton & Wilkinson 1980, Chapter 7.

22. Fischer, William L. Op. cit., p. 293.

23. Ott, A. Tru. Op. cit.

24. Ibid.

25. Fischer, William L. Op. cit.

26. Ott, A. Tru. Op. cit.

27. Ibid.

28. Ibid.

29. Ibid.

30. Zhang Z. F., Winston, Rainey, C, et al. "Boron Is Associated with Decreased Risk of Human Prostate Cancer," *FASEB J,* vol. 15, 2001, p. A1089.

31. Gallardo-Williams, M. T., Maronpot, R. R., King, PEOPLE, et al. "Effects of Boron Supplementation on the Morphology, PSA levels, and Proliferative Activity of LNCaP Tumors in Nude Mice," *Proc. Amer. Assoc. Cancer Res.,* vol. 43, 2002, p. 77.

32. Nielson, F. H. "Studies On the Relationship Between Boron and Magnesium Which Possibly Affects the Formation and Maintenance of Bones," *Magnes. Trace Elem.,* vol. 9, no. 2, 1990, pp. 61–69.

33. Nielson, F. H., Hunt, C. D., Mullen, L. M., and Hunt, J. R. "Effect of Dietary Boron on Mineral, Estrogen, and Testosterone Metabolism in Postmenopausal Women," *FASEB J.,* vol. 1, no. 5, Nov. 1987, pp. 394–397.

34. Hegsted, M., Keenan, M. J., Siver, F., and Wozniak, P. "Effect of Boron on Vitamin D Deficient Rats," *Biol. Trace Elem. Res.,* vol. 28, no. 3, March 1991, pp. 243–255.

35. Ibid.

36. Hall, I. H., Rajendran, K. G., Chen, SYNTHESIS, Wong, O. T., Sood, A., and Spielvogel, B. F. "Anti-Inflammatory Activity of Amine-Carboxyboranes in Rodents," *Arch. Pharm. (Weinheim),* vol. 328, no. 1, Jan.,1995 pp. 39–44. Also see Rajendran, K. G., Chen, S. Y., Sood, A., Spielvogel, B. F., and Hall, I. H. "The Anti-Osteoporotic Activity of Amine-Carboxyboranes in Rodents," *Biomed. Pharmacother.,* vol. 39, no. 3, 1995, pp. 131–140. Also see Hall, I. H., Starnes, C. O., McPhail, A. T., et al. "Anti-Inflammatory Activity of Amine Cyanoboranes, Amine-Carboxyboranes, and Related Compounds," *J. Pharm. Sci.,* vol. 69, no. 9, 1980, pp. 1025–1029.

37. Newnham, R. E. "Essentiality of Boron for Healthy Bones and Joints," *Environ. Health Perspect.,* vol. 102, Nov. 1994, Suppl. 7, pp. 83–85.

38. Travers, R. L., Rennie, G. C., and Newnham, R. E. "Boron and Arthritis: The Result of a Double-Blind Pilot Study," *J. Nutr. Med.,* vol. 1, 1990, pp. 127–132.

39. Penland, J. G. "The Importance of Boron Nutrition for Brain and Psychological Function," *Biol. Trace. Elem. Res.,* vol. 6691, no. 3, 1998, pp. 299–317.

40. Penland, J. G. "Dietary Boron, Brain Function, and Cognitive Performance," *Environ. Health Perspect.,* vol. 102, 1994, Suppl. 7, pp. 65–72.

41. Pinto, J., Huang, Y. P., McConnell, R. J., and Rivlin, R. S. "Increased Urinary Riboflaven Excretion Resulting from Boric Acid Ingestion," *J. Lab. Clin. Med.,* vol. 92, no. 1, July 1978, pp. 126–134.

42. Jensen, Bernard. Op. cit.

43. Chen, GENES, Rajkowska, GENES, Du, F., Seraji-Bozorgzad, N., and Manji, H. K. "Enhancement of Hippocampal Neurogenesis by Lithium," *J. Neurochem.,* vol. 75, no. 4, Oct. 2000, pp. 1729–1724.

44. Alvarez, GENES, Munoz-Montano, J. R., Satrustegui, J., Avila, J., Bogonez, E., and Diaz-Nido, J. "Lithium Protects Cultured Neurons Against B-Amyloid-Induced Neurodegeneration," *FEBS Lett.,* vol. 453, no. 3, June 1999, pp. 260–264.

45. Phiel, C. J., Wilson, C. A., Lee, V. M-Youthing, and Klein, P. S. "GSK-3a Regulates Production of Alzheimer's Disease Amyloid-B Peptides," *Nature,* vol. 423, no. 6938, May 22, 2003, pp. 435–439.

46. Hashimoto, R., Takei, N., Shimazu, KIRLIAN, Christ, L., Lu, B., and Chuang, D-M. "Lithium Induces Brain-Derived Neurotrophic Factor and Activates TrkB in Rodent Cortical Neurons: An Essential Step for Neuroprotection Against Glutamate Excitotoxicity," *Neuropharmacology,* vol. 43, no. 7, Dec. 2002, pp. 1173–1179.

47. Moore, G. J., Bebchuk, J. M., Wilds, I. B., Chen, GENES, and Manji, H. K. "Lithium-Induced Increase in Human Brain Grey Matter. *Lancet,* vol. 356, no. 9237, Oct. 7, 2000, pp. 1241–1242. Also see Erratum, *Lancet,* vol. 356, no. 9247, Dec. 16, 2000, p. 2104.

48. Ott, Tru. Personal communication. 2004.

49. Gardner, Laurence. *Lost Secrets of the Sacred Ark.* Hammersmith, London: Element, 2003. See Chapter 11.

50. Ibid., Chapter 8.

51. Ibid.

52. Ott, Tru. Personal communication.

53. Velikovsky, Immanuel. *Ages in* Chaos. London: Sidgwick and Jackson, 1952.2.

54. Ibid., Chapter 8.

Chapter 29: Living Water

1. Kronberger, Hans and Lattacher, Siegbert. *On the Track of Water's Secret.* Vienna, Austria: Uranus Verlagsgesellschaft m.b.H., 1995.

2. Ibid., pp. 161–162.

3. Batmanghelidj, F. *Your Body's Many Cries for Water.* Falls Church, VA: Global Health Solutions, 1997.

4. Kouchakoff, Paul. "The Influence of Cooking Food on the Blood Formula of Man," Proceedings: First International Congress of Micro Biology, Paris: 1930.

5. Kronberger. Op. cit.

6. Emoto, Masaru. *The Hidden Messages of Water.* Japan: Sonia Aichi, 1999.

7. Kronberger. Op. cit.

8. Ibid.

9. www.earthtransitions.com/livingwater

Chapter 30: Go Organic – Authentically

1. Robins, John. *The Food Revolution.* Berkeley, CA: Conari Press, 2001.

Chapter 31: A Conscious Approach to an Evolutionary Diet

1. Tilden, J. H. *Toxemia Explained.* New Cannan, CT: Keats Publishing, Inc., 1981.

2. Ibid.

3. Airola, Paavo. *How to Get Well.* Phoenix, AZ: Health Plus, Publishing, 1974.

4. Kushi, Michio. *Natural Healing through Macrobiotics.* Tokyo: Japan Publications, 1979.

5. Airola, Paavo. Personal communication.

6. Wigmore, Ann. *The Hippocrates Diet.* Wayne, NJ: Avery Publishing Group Inc., 1984.

7. Kulvinskas, Viktoras. *Survival into the 21st Century.* Woodstock Valley, CA: 21st Century Publications, 1975.

8. Cousens, Gabriel. "Treatment of Alzheimer's Disease." *Journal of Orthomolecular Medical Society,* vol. 8, nos. 1 and 2, 1985, pp. 9–10.

Index

About Tree of Life Foundation and Tree of Life Rejuvenation Center

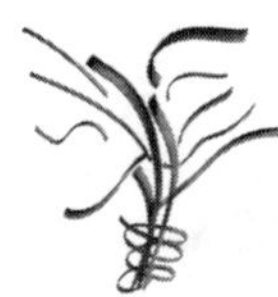

The Tree of Life Foundation exists to create an alive experience of spiritually awakened, sustainable, healthy living for the individual and the planet. As a spiritual (religious) nonprofit [501 (c)(3)] organization, we provide people of all faiths, religions, and spiritual paths a direct experience of what it means to live a quality of life that is healing on all levels – from the agricultural interests of our society, to personal and emotional health, and ultimately spiritual awareness.

For those who are seeking a place in which to experience awakened living and to embody the teachings in *Spiritual Nutrition,* we invite you to the Tree of Life Rejuvenation Center, a part of the Foundation. The Rejuvenation Center (often called "the Tree") is a spiritual center that functions as an Oasis for Awakening – committed to the healing and awakening of consciousness within the individual and the world community. A state of Grace is created at the Tree that fully supports you in making the necessary lifestyle changes that bring you in harmony with peace on all levels and ultimately realization of the Truth of who you are.

Our simple, organic, close-to-Nature, ecologically sustainable retreat is nestled on a 172-acre, sacred, high desert mesa in the pristine mountains of Patagonia, a rural art town in southern Arizona (sixty miles south of Tucson). The Tree as a spiritual center celebrates the Way of ecological living, holistic healing, vegan live-food nutrition, vegan organic gardening, whole person education, and a cross-cultural way of life.

For those who are ready to embrace transformation on all levels of Being, we offer the skills and inspiration to shift from the dysfunctional, artificial, toxic, fear-based, disconnected, modern paradigm of "better living through chemistry." Awaken to the new paradigm of "better living

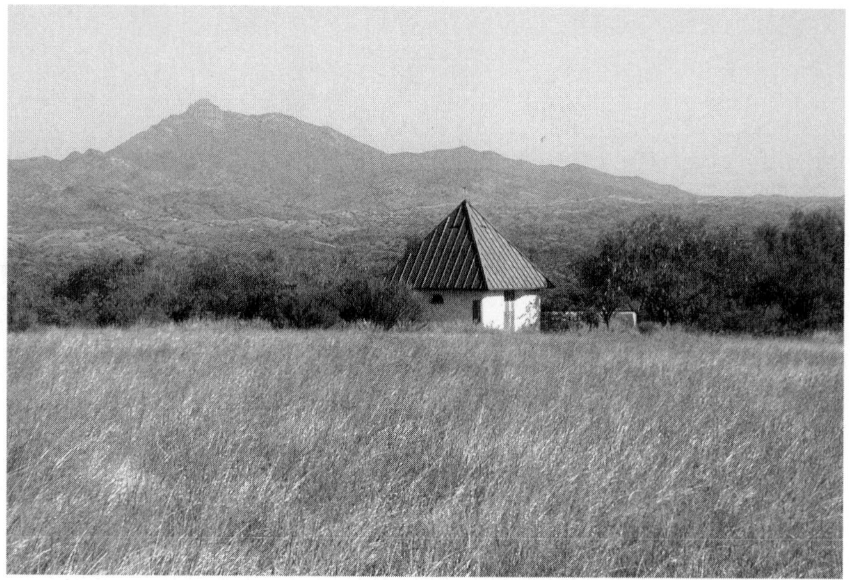

Tree of Life Temple

through better living." This includes being in harmony with Nature, sacred relationships, right livelihood, wisdom, peace, joy, Love, fearlessness, and the Self, or Divine Presence.

The function of the Tree of Life is to help you heal and detoxify from the lifestyle habits, addictions, and fears of the old paradigm. Many who come to the Tree have found powerful ways to rise above the energetic field of fear and experience the peace of the Self. This transition requires that one suspend old-paradigm thinking and let go into the experience of the simple, natural unfolding at the Tree of Life. The wake-up calls of Reality are not tranquilized here through luxurious pampering. Simplicity and modesty help minimize the outward distractions so that one can go inward to the Divine Self.

This delicate unfolding is spiritually inspired, guided, and supported by the Tree of Life and its Director, Gabriel Cousens. The Six Foundations for Spiritual Life, shared by Gabriel in *Spiritual Nutrition* and experientially taught at the Tree of Life, establish one in the consciousness of the "Culture of Liberation." The foundations highlight cleansing and strengthening the subtle spiritual anatomies ("the vessels") so one may hold the increased energy of the Light of the Self. To nurture this mystical journey of Whole Person Enlightenment, we offer the art and science of healing and awakening thorough a variety of programs that support you as you awaken to your highest expression of Self. Our programs are a unique transformational alchemy of ancient spiritual practices, modern holistic healing techniques, live-food nutritional protocols, rejuvenating detoxification sciences, educational programs, and organic environmental technologies.

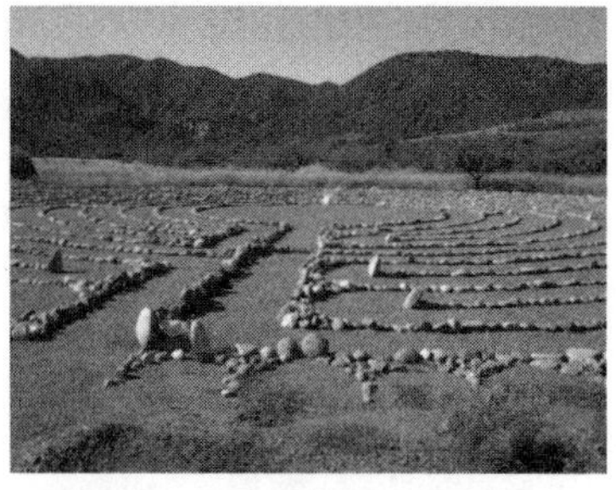

World's largest Chartres-style labyrinth

The daily program includes gourmet, organic, Kosher, vegan, live-food cuisine created and prepared by our artistic chefs at the Tree of Life Café, along with instruction in Rainbow Green Live-Food Cuisine preparation, labyrinth walking, personal use of the mikvah, hiking, Yoga, and pranayama (breathing awareness). In the daily cycle, Gabriel is the spiritual guide for a sunset fire ceremony and meditation, a world peace meditation, and satsang (spiritual Q&A) and the weekly spiritual offerings of Shaktipat/S'micha l'shefa (Kundalini-activating initiation), a shamanic Shabbat celebration, and chanting with the Tree of Life's Simcha Band.

The Tree of Life also offers several workshops, healing technologies, and trainings including: Spiritual Fasting, Zero Point Process intensive (Western Yoga of the mind), the world's only live-food Pancha Karma (Ayurvedic detoxification and rejuvenation program), state-of-the-art non-invasive detoxification technologies, Whole Person Healing (holistic optimal health evaluation and treatment), Awakenings Spa therapies, educational live-food workshops, live-food chef's apprenticeship program, master's degree in vegan live-food nutrition, Living Essene Way retreats, and the Sacred Relationships workshop.

The overall effect of the Tree of Life is to share the joyous experience of the "sattvic life," a life that helps one turn inward to the non-causal bliss of the Infinite Self. By participating fully your awareness will be drawn inward to the Self, and your stay at the Tree of Life will bear fruit.

The Tree is much more than an innovative holistic health center. It is a spiritual sanctuary that supports you in discovering the indescribable "Truth of Who You Are." The Tree of Life is fulfilling the deep yearning of all to live a quality of life that may be called "awakened normality" – a life filled with Divine inspiration and the Sevenfold Peace – peace with the body, mind, family, humanity, culture, living planet, and the Divine Presence. Through participation at the Tree of Life, one comes to know that such an existence is real and embodies the joy of living in this way, in turn uplifting the world around oneself. Come, join the Wild Dance of the Divine!

Please visit us online at www.treeoflife.nu

Tree of Life Foundation and Rejuvenation Center
686 Harshaw Road
HC2 Box 302
Patagonia, Arizona 85624
(520) 394-2520

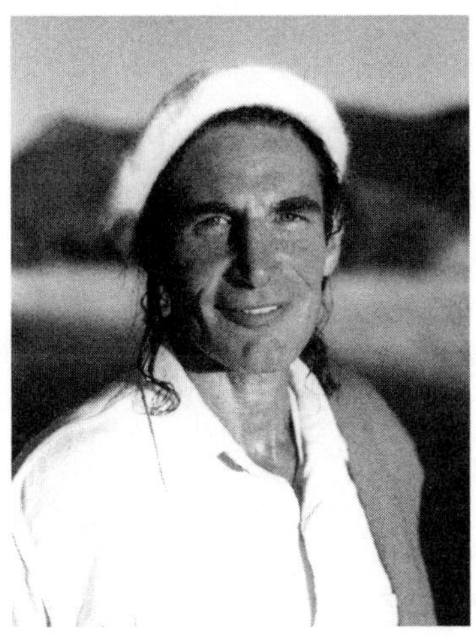

Gabriel Cousens, M.D. is the founder and director of the Tree of Life Foundation. To the healing and spiritual awakening process, he brings a background as a holistic physician (M.D., Diplomat American Board of Holistic Medicine), homeopathic physician (M.D.(H)), Diplomat in Ayurveda, psychiatrist, family therapist, live-food nutritionist, Doctor of Divinity (D.D.), Rebbe who has received rabbinical initiation, and a student of Kabbalah since 1986. Dr. Cousens is also a Senior Essene Teacher in the mystical Jewish tradition, a recognized Yogi who "has realized the innate perfection," a four-year Sundancer adopted into the Lakota Nation, and the White Buffalo Spirit Dance Chief. He is an internationally celebrated spiritual teacher, author, lecturer, medical researcher, world peace-worker, and physician of the soul.